Standard Textbook of Cosmetology

STUDENT SHOULD FILL IN THIS PAGE AT ONCE

If this book should get lost, will the finder please call or notify nearest address at once, and the owner will call for same. I thank you very much for this courtesy.

Collene Greveldinge
____
Student's Name

____
Street Address

Fayetteville
____
City   State

____
Telephone Number

____
Name of School

____
Address of School

____
City   State

____
Telephone Number

____

Standard Textbook of Cosmetology

A practical course on
the scientific fundamentals
of beauty culture
for students and
practicing cosmetologists

Completely Revised 1981

Revised by
Milady Textbook Educational Board

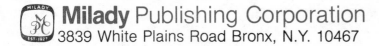

Milady Publishing Corporation
3839 White Plains Road Bronx, N.Y. 10467

EDITOR: Israel Rubinstein

ILLUSTRATOR: Shiz Horii

ART DIRECTORS: Martin Ventura and Gail Drillings

Illustrations based on many Warren Meek drawings

Design Consultant: John P. Fornieri

Cover Illustration: Reina Gillson

ISBN 0-87350-096-2

1981
Completely Revised Edition

© Copyright 1938 - 1954 - 1959 - 1965
            1967 - 1972 - 1981

MILADY PUBLISHING CORPORATION
Bronx, N. Y.

Printed in United States of America

Dedicated to the Advancement of Cosmetology Education

CONTENTS

(continued)

(continued)

(continued)

PREFACE

The material contained in this edition of the Standard Textbook of Cosmetology has been completely revised and modernized with respect to both the science and the art of cosmetology.

The **science of cosmetology** denotes the great fund of knowledge available in this field. The science of cosmetology has been developed into a systematic and coherent body of related cosmetology information.

The **art of cosmetology** refers to the actual performance of the many beauty culture practices. The art of cosmetology varies with the degree of skill developed by the cosmetologist.

The basic theory and information contained in this text have been prepared to allow great flexibility and adaptability to whatever system or routine is followed in either school or salon. The materials presented are not designed nor intended to standardize all cosmetology practice. They are not designed nor intended to in any way stifle initiative in cosmetology education or method. Rather they are presented in such a manner as to encourage teachers to be flexible, modern, and alert to change and improvements.

Certain theory and techniques that are not in common usage in the modern practice of cosmetology have been retained, in modified form, for reference purposes.

This text contains many new features, such as chapter learning objectives and the metric system, to enhance and broaden the scope of the information contained herein.

Cosmetology school graduates who used this text in their studies will find themselves better prepared to cope with the great demands of the modern practice of cosmetology.

We wish to express our sincerest appreciation to the many state board members, cosmetology educators, and stylists who contributed their time, knowledge, and talents to the revision of this textbook.

THE AUTHOR

Printed in the U.S.A.

WELCOME TO THE COSMETOLOGY PROFESSION

Congratulations for making the decision to study cosmetology. By enrolling for a course of study in this school, you have taken the first important step toward a most interesting and satisfying career.

Cosmetology (beauty culture) offers the opportunity for a lifetime career in one of our largest and most respected industries. After completing a comparatively short training period, you will be prepared to embark upon a career that can offer you a good income for your entire working life.

OPPORTUNITIES FOR MEN AND WOMEN

The opportunities available are far greater in the field of cosmetology than in any other field comparable in preparation time and expense. Cosmetology offers a lucrative, exciting, and growth-filled future for the alert and ambitious individual. Furthermore, the practice of cosmetology offers the rare opportunity for a career filled with personal pleasure and satisfaction. It appeals to the artistic and esthetic needs of the cosmetologist. It encourages the free exercise of his or her personal talent and ability. And, most important, it combines job satisfaction with financial stability.

To a young woman, cosmetology presents a vocation that can be tailored to fit into the pattern of her private life. When she is ready to raise a family, she can leave, then return at a later date to continue her career. She can maintain a normal married family life and work at her own convenience.

THE FUTURE OUTLOOK

The future for the cosmetology industry appears to be most promising. New techniques, new products, and new opportunities appear every day. The number of patrons who visit beauty salons and the amount of money they spend for services are constantly increasing.

With reference to your own future, there seems to be no limit to the progress you can make or to the amount of money you can earn. There is no other industry with such a constant demand for qualified, well-trained school graduates, nor is there any other industry that offers comparable opportunities for an individual to start his or her own business.

How fast and how far you go will depend primarily on the effort you make and on the seriousness with which you approach your training. While in school, you should also concentrate on improving your personal habits, grooming, poise, personality, and ability to get along well with people. All these are essential to your achieving success in the "world of work."

WELCOME

We extend a most sincere welcome to you. We are certain that you will be pleased with your decision in selecting this fascinating career. The field and its opportunities are unlimited. You have opened the door to a new, exciting world; now, enter.

CAREER OPPORTUNITIES

Many career opportunities are available to the well-trained cosmetologist. Acquiring a license to practice cosmetology opens doors to a great variety of lucrative careers. The following tables list many of the income areas available to cosmetologists.

I. BEAUTY SALON OPPORTUNITIES

    A. General Cosmetologist

    B. Specialties

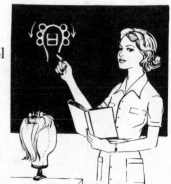

        1) Permanent Wave Technician
        2) Hairstylist
        3) Wig Stylist
        4) Hair Straightening Technician
        5) Hair Colorist
        6) Hair and Scalp Specialist
        7) Skin Care Specialist (Esthetician)
        8) Manicurist
        9) Makeup Artist
       10) Electrologist

Hair Coloring Expert

Hairstylist

    C. Management
        1) Salon Owner
        2) Salon Manager or Supervisor
        3) Concessionaire (Beauty Salon, Department Store, Chain of Salons)

II. EDUCATIONAL OPPORTUNITIES

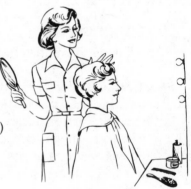

    A. School Management
        1) Owner or Director of Private School
        2) Department Head in Public School
        3) Supervisor or Dean

    B. Teaching-Guidance
        1) Teacher of Cosmetology
        2) Teacher of Related Subjects
        3) Teacher of Specialties
        4) Guidance Counsellor
        5) Trainer of Teachers

Cosmetology Teacher

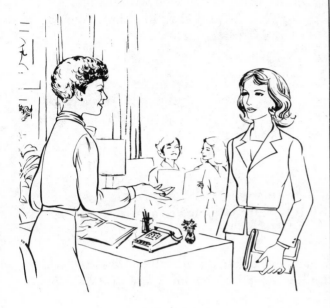

Receptionist

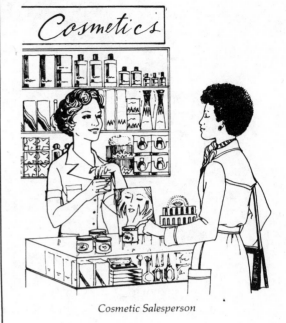

Cosmetic Salesperson

C. Government
    1) State Board Member
    2) State Board Inspector
    3) State Board Examiner

D. Miscellaneous-Educational
    1) Educational Director for Manufacturer
    2) Guest Artist

III. INDUSTRY AND WRITING OPPORTUNITIES

A. Merchandising
    1) Buyer and Assistant Buyer
    2) Salesperson — Direct Seller

B. Scientific and Manufacturing
    1) Demonstrator or Manufacturer's Representative
    2) Researcher — Assistant
    3) Trade Technician

C. Writing
    1) Beauty Editor — Assistant
    2) Promotional Writer
    3) Free-Lance Writer

SUMMARY

Cosmetology is as exciting as it is profitable. It represents to many men and women a profession that will bring much happiness and financial independence.

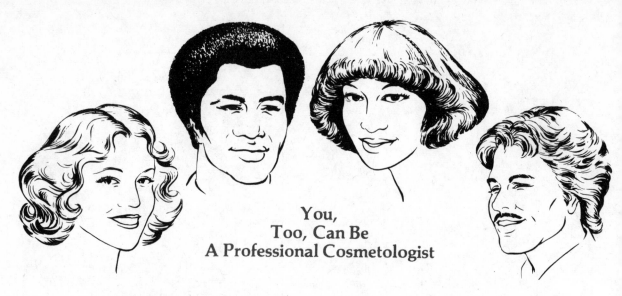

You, Too, Can Be A Professional Cosmetologist

Note: TO BE SUCCESSFUL - you must learn to do the little things that will make patrons like you, in addition to being well-groomed and proficient in your work.

TERMS USED INTERCHANGEABLY

A number of terms are used interchangeably throughout this text. This is done to avoid repetition and to acquaint you with the many terms that are used in the field.

The following terms all refer to the professional performing services in the beauty salon: (1) Cosmetologist (2) Practitioner (3) Artisan (4) Hairstylist (5) Stylist (6) Technician (7) Hairdresser (8) Operator (9) Beautician. The preferred term, cosmetologist, is generally used in this text.

The practice of enhancing the appearance of beauty salon patrons is referred to as (1) Cosmetology (2) Beauty Culture (3) Hairdressing (4) Hairstyling.

The premises where this enhancement takes place is called a (1) Beauty Parlor (2) Beauty Salon (3) Beauty Shop.

(The cosmetology profession enlists the services of both men and women. The pronouns "she" and "he" are used in this text for convenience only and do not indicate the preference of one over the other.)

KEY TO PRONUNCIATION

The accent mark (') following a syllable denotes that this syllable is to receive more emphasis than the other syllables.

(For metric equivalents used in this text and conversions to metric measurements, turn to page 485.)

Chapter 1

HYGIENE AND
GOOD GROOMING

CHAPTER LEARNING OBJECTIVES

The student successfully mastering this chapter will know:
1. *The principles of hygiene and good grooming.*
2. *The rules of cleanliness.*
3. *The details of good grooming.*
4. *The relationship of cleanliness to good health and success as a cosmetologist.*

Good health is required for the successful practice of cosmetology. Without it, one cannot work efficiently nor enjoy the pleasures of life. With it, constructive work and happiness are made possible.

In keeping with the profession, cosmetologists should be living examples of good health, so that they will increase their value to themselves, to their employers, and to the community.

Hygiene is a science that deals with healthful living. It includes both personal and public hygiene.

Personal hygiene concerns the intelligent care taken by the individual to preserve health by following the rules of healthful living, such as:

1. Cleanliness.
2. Oral hygiene.
3. Good posture.
4. Sufficient exercise.
5. Relaxation.
6. Adequate sleep.
7. Balanced diet.
8. Wholesome thoughts.

Public hygiene, or **sanitation,** refers to the steps taken by the government to promote public health. The government takes the responsibility of protecting the health, safety, and welfare of its citizens, by seeing that they are provided with:

1. Pure air.
2. Pure food.
3. Pure water.
4. Adequate sewerage.
5. Control of disease.
6. Adequate medical facilities.

Beauty problems also may become **health problems.** A clear complexion, fine-textured skin, sparkling eyes, and luxuriant hair may project a healthy condition. A dull, sallow complexion may be indicative of:

1. Sluggish circulation.
2. Lack of fresh air.
3. Irregular elimination.
4. Improper diet.
5. Poor health.

HYGIENIC RULES

To improve your health and appearance, you must follow hygienic rules of living.

Eating well-balanced meals at regular intervals and drinking a sufficient amount of water will keep the digestive system functioning properly and produce better elimination. However, one of the basic causes of poor health is a faulty diet. Avoid such poor eating habits as:

1. **Not eating enough** of the **right kinds** of food, which may lead to loss of weight, lower resistance, or nutritional diseases.
2. **Overeating,** which taxes the digestive system and organs of elimination.

Exercise and **recreation,** in the form of running, walking, dancing, sports, and gym activities, develop endurance and keep the body fit. A few of the benefits resulting from regular exercising are:

1. An improvement in the body's absorption of food.
2. An improvement in blood circulation.
3. A larger supply of life-giving oxygen to the body, due to the increased action of the heart and lungs.

Moderate amounts of sunshine add vigor and help to supply the body with essential vitamin D.

Fatigue, caused by work, exercise, mental effort, or worry, should always be followed by a period of rest or relaxation. Overexertion and lack of rest tend to drain the body of its vitality. Therefore, an adequate amount of sleep, not less than seven hours, is necessary. This allows the body to recover from the fatigue of the day's activities and replenish itself with renewed energy.

HEALTHY THOUGHTS

The mind and body operate as a unit. A healthy body and mind contribute to a good life. A healthy body is one in which all organs perform their functions normally. Healthy thoughts can be cultivated by self-control. Worry and fear should be replaced by the health-giving qualities of cheerfulness, courage, and hope. Outside interests and recreation relieve the strain of monotony and hard work.

Thoughts and **emotions** influence bodily activities. A thought may cause the face to turn red and increase the heart action. It may either stimulate or depress the functions of the body. Strong emotions, such as worry and fear, have a harmful effect on the heart, arteries, and glands. Depression weakens the functions of the organs, thereby lowering the resistance of the body to disease.

A WELL-GROOMED FEMALE COSMETOLOGIST

A well-groomed cosmetologist is one of the best advertisements of an effectively run salon.

To keep your appearance at its best, you must give daily attention to all the important details that make for a clean, neat, and charming personality.

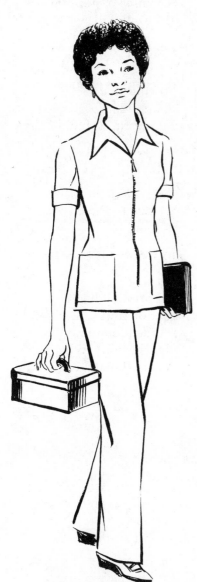

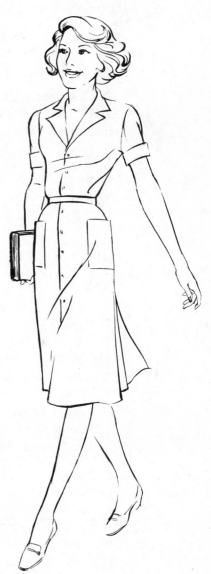

Daily Bath and Deodorant
Keep the body cleansed and odor free by taking a daily shower or bath and by using an underarm deodorant.

Oral Hygiene
Clean and brush the teeth regularly. Use mouth wash to sweeten the breath.

Hairstyle
Keep the hair clean and lustrous. Wear an attractive and practical hairstyle at all times.

Clothes
Wear a uniform that is spotlessly clean, neat, and properly fitted. Wear fresh underclothes.

Facial Makeup
Use the correct cosmetics to match your skin tone. Keep your makeup fresh, eyebrows and lips well-shaped.

Hands and Nails
Keep your hands clean and smooth, and always have your nails well-manicured.

Jewelry
Avoid gaudy jewelry. A wristwatch is permissible.

Shoes and Hosiery
Wear low-heeled shoes that are well-fitted and sensibly styled. Keep the shoes shined and in good condition. Wear clean hose. Watch out for hosiery runs and wrinkles.

Many beauty salon owners consider appearance, visual poise, and personality to be as important as technical knowledge and manual skills.

A WELL-GROOMED MALE COSMETOLOGIST

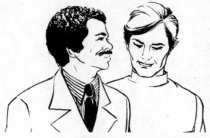

Proper grooming is also important to male cosmetologists. Give careful attention to cleanliness of uniform, skin, hair, hands, and teeth. Keep beard and mustache neatly trimmed. Keep breath sweet with mouth wash. Keep your body free of odor by taking a shower or bath daily, and by using an underarm deodorant.

MAINTAIN GOOD HEALTH

In order to maintain good health, observe the following rules:
1. Get as much clean and fresh air as you can.
2. Drink a sufficient amount of water each day.
3. Follow a balanced diet. Do not overeat.
4. Develop regular elimination habits.
5. Stand, sit, and walk with good posture.
6. Engage in recreation and outdoor exercise, and get adequate sleep.
7. Have regular physical examinations.

SUMMARY

The cosmetologist must observe cleanliness in the following ways:
1. Keep the body clean by taking a daily bath or shower.
2. Avoid body odor by using a deodorant.
3. Keep teeth and gums in good condition. Brush teeth at least twice daily.
4. Have a dental examination every six months.
5. Avoid bad breath by rinsing your mouth with a good mouth wash.
6. Never wear shoes without clean hose or peds.
7. Keep shoes clean and in good condition.
8. Wear clean undergarments and a clean uniform each day.
9. Keep hair well-groomed.
10. Keep hands and fingernails in good condition.
11. Wash hands before and after serving each patron.
12. Avoid the common use of towels, drinking cups, cosmetics, hairbrushes and combs.

REVIEW QUESTIONS

HYGIENE AND GOOD GROOMING

1. Define: a) hygiene; b) personal hygiene; c) public hygiene; d) oral hygiene.
2. List eight basic requirements for good personal hygiene.
3. List six steps taken by the government to assure good public health.
4. Which three mental qualities help to promote good health?
5. Which two emotions can injure health?
6. A daily bath or shower keeps the body . . . .
7. Avoid body odors by using a . . . .
8. Avoid bad breath by rinsing mouth with a good . . . .

Chapter 2

VISUAL
POISE

CHAPTER LEARNING OBJECTIVES

The student successfully mastering this chapter will know:
1. *The benefits of good posture.*
2. *The difference between good and bad posture.*
3. *The influence of good posture on health, appearance, and physical well-being.*

Most of your time as a professional cosmetologist will be spent on your feet. Correct posture, therefore, is very important, as it helps to prevent fatigue, improves your personal appearance, and permits you to move with ease and grace in relation to your everyday work.

Good posture is an important part of personal care. Its continued practice assists in the prevention of many physical problems. In addition, it is a self-disciplinary factor that contributes to the development of other good habits, which are determining elements of a gracious and pleasing personality. When present, they indicate a poised, well-ordered individual.

Many beauty salon owners consider appearance, visual poise, and personality to be of equal importance as technical knowledge and manual skills.

STAND CORRECTLY

Regular exercise keeps the muscles of the body in good condition and assists in forming the habit of good posture. Practice will train the muscles to hold the body correctly. Good posture is a matter of habit. Avoid slouching, humped shoulders, and spinal curvature while working. To walk and stand correctly, distribute the body weight so that you achieve proper body balance that is graceful to the eye.

For the basic standing position:
1. Turn the left foot out at a 45° (0.785 rad.) angle.
2. Point the right foot straight ahead on a straight line.
3. Bend the right knee slightly over line of the left knee.
4. Flex the left knee slightly.

GOOD POSTURE

CENTER LINE

Extends from center of
head, through neck,
shoulder, hip, knee, and
arch of foot

BODY WEIGHT

Is balanced along this
center line and supported
by the weight-bearing
arches of the feet

GOOD POSTURE

Head up
Chin level with floor
Chest up
Shoulders relaxed
Lower abdomen flat

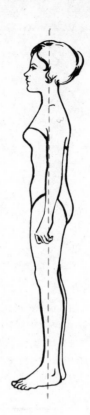

FIVE DEFECTIVE BODY POSTURES

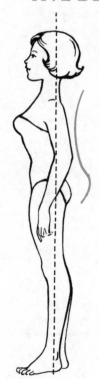
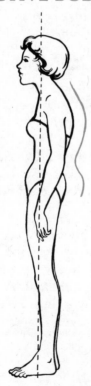
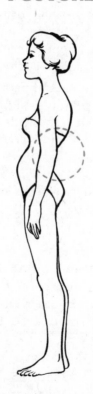
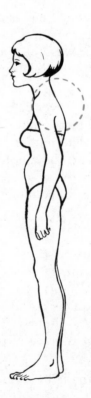
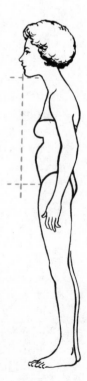

Stiff-rigid—
poor posture.

Slumped-humped—
poor posture.

Sway-back or
lordosis (lor-do'sis).

Drooped shoulders—
kyphosis (ki-fo'sis).

Sway-back and
drooped shoulders—
scoliosis (sko-le-o'sis).

POSTURE WHEN GIVING A SHAMPOO

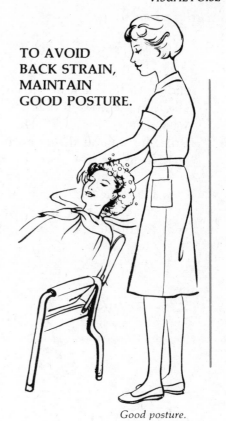

TO AVOID
BACK STRAIN,
MAINTAIN
GOOD POSTURE.

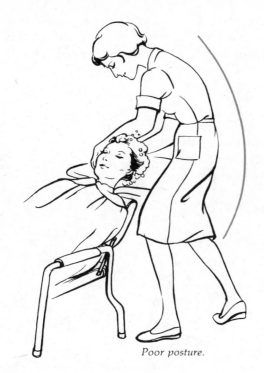

Poor posture.

Good posture.

COMFORT FOR PATRON AND COSMETOLOGIST

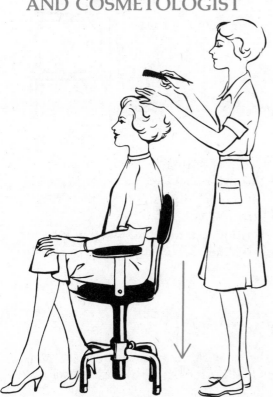

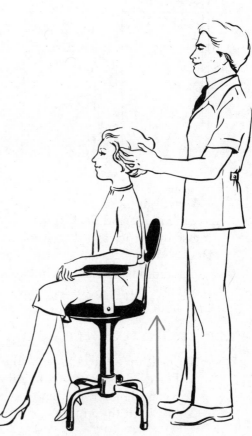

*Short cosmetologist,
tall patron—
lower the chair.*

*Short patron,
tall cosmetologist—
raise the chair.*

CORRECT BODY USE

CORRECT SITTING TECHNIQUE

Never fall into a chair. Glide gracefully into a sitting position. When sliding to the back of the chair, place both hands on the front edge of the chair, at the sides of the hips. Raise the body slightly and slide back. Do not wiggle back.

Rules for a good sitting position:
1. Keep the feet close together.
2. Keep the knees together.
3. Place the feet out slightly farther than the knees.
4. Never push your feet under the chair.
5. Keep the soles of your shoes on the floor.

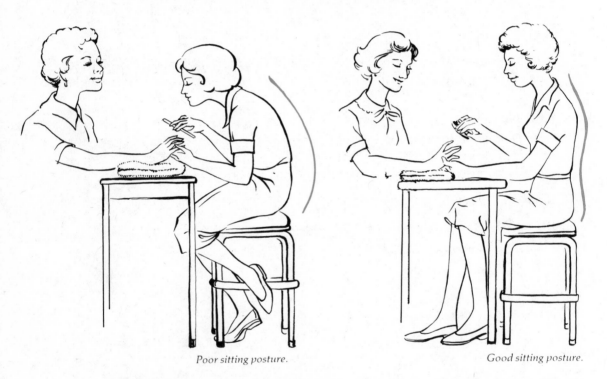

Poor sitting posture.   Good sitting posture.

When giving a manicure, assume a correct sitting position, in order to avoid fatigue and back strain. Sit with the lower back against the chair, leaning slightly forward. If a stool is used, sit on the entire stool. Keep chest up. Rest body weight on the full length of the thighs.

To avoid back strain while reading, writing, or studying, whether it be in school, at business, or at home, sit towards the back of the chair. Do not sit in a slouching position at any time.

CORRECT STOOPING TECHNIQUE

To pick up an article from the floor:
1. Place your feet close together.
2. Keep the back perpendicular to the floor as the knees bend.
3. Lift with the muscles of your legs and buttocks, not with the back.

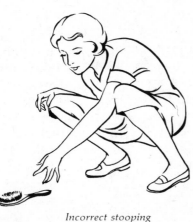

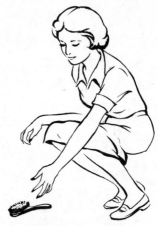

*Incorrect stooping
position.*

*Correct stooping
position.*

CORRECT LIFTING TECHNIQUE

When you lift something heavy, be sure to use the weight-lifter's method, or you may cause a rupture or a slipped disk. Lift with your back straight, pushing with the heavy thigh muscles, never the back muscles.

CAUTION:

Have some idea of the weight of the object you are lifting. You can hurt your back just as severely by lifting a light object your muscles expect to be heavy as you can by lifting a heavy object incorrectly.

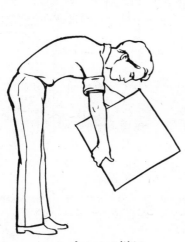

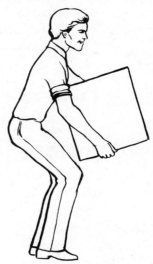

*Incorrect lifting
position.*

*Correct lifting
position.*

CARE OF THE FEET

High heels are often responsible for poor posture, malformed feet, and aching backs. The weight of the body is thrown forward, putting a strain on the feet and back.

Low, broad heels give the body support and balance which help to maintain good posture. Low-heeled shoes are more comfortable and tend to offset fatigue resulting from prolonged standing.

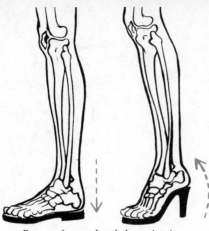

The cosmetologist should give her feet the following daily care:

1. After bathing, apply cream or oil and massage each foot for five minutes.
2. Remove cream and apply an antiseptic foot lotion.
3. Keep the toenails filed smooth.
4. Corns, bunions, or ingrown nails should receive care from a podiatrist.

Wearing well-fitted, low-heeled shoes and giving the feet a few minutes of daily care are also steps to good posture and success.

For comfort and to help maintain good posture, wear well-fitted, low-heeled shoes.

NORMAL AND WEAK ARCHES

Normal arch.

A **normal foot** is narrow in the middle and wide at the heel and toes. Good arches are characteristic of the normal footprint.

Weak arch.

A **weak foot** is caused by a weak arch. Its footprint is wider in the middle than a normal footprint.

Fallen arches, or **flat feet,** is a common foot ailment. The flat foot leaves a footprint that is almost the same throughout its entire length.

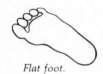

Flat foot.

Weak and flat feet may be strengthened by means of massage and exercise, or may be helped by the wearing of arch supports and proper shoes. These remedial measures should be taken only after consultation with a foot specialist.

REVIEW QUESTIONS

VISUAL POISE

1. What are three benefits of correct posture?
2. How does regular exercise assist in forming the habit of good posture?
3. In a basic stance or standing position, place the left foot at a . . . . degree angle and point the right foot straight ahead.
4. For a good standing posture, keep the head . . . .; chin level with . . . .; chest . . . .; shoulders relaxed and lower abdomen . . . .
5. For a good sitting posture, keep the feet and knees close . . . .
6. For a comfortable sitting posture, keep the soles of the feet on the . . . .
7. When giving a manicure, sit with the lower back against the . . . .
8. Why is a correct sitting position important when giving a manicure?
9. How should one sit to avoid back strain?
10. Why should the cosmetologist wear low, broad-heeled shoes?
11. The cosmetologist who stands for long periods of time should wear well-fitted, ... shoes.
12. Why should the cosmetologist give his/her feet daily care?

Chapter 3

PERSONALITY DEVELOPMENT

CHAPTER LEARNING OBJECTIVES

The student successfully mastering this chapter will know:
1. *The reasons for cultivating a pleasing personality.*
2. *The qualities needed for a pleasing personality.*
3. *The relationship of personality to success as a cosmetologist.*

Your **personality** is the key to a successful career in cosmetology. Personality can be defined as the outward reflection of your inner feelings, habits, attitudes, and values. It is the total effect you have on other people.

Only you can form the pattern of the "ideal individual" you hope to be. Only you can develop a personality that will help open the door to a life filled with pleasant and useful experiences.

A pleasant personality and a good character are as vital to a successful career in cosmetology as are expert technical ability and an attractive appearance.

Without a pleasing personality, a cosmetologist's fine workmanship or attractive appearance will be overlooked. People are not born with personalities; they are acquired according to the way individuals meet their everyday problems. By developing the ability to handle both the good and the bad experiences of life, you will develop a better personality.

DESIRABLE QUALITIES TO CULTIVATE

Attitude has a great deal to do with personality. It influences your likes and dislikes and your response to people, events, and things. People who meet difficult situations with calmness, and who are cheerful, pleasant, and easy to get along with, are said to have a healthy attitude toward life.

Behavior. Control your temper. Once you have spoken, you cannot recall a single word. One person with his controls off balance can throw others into a state of confusion. Everything you say or do (good or bad) starts a chain of reactions that can have a continuing and lasting effect. When you become master of your own behavior, you can cultivate those characteristics that are desirable, and discard those that are unwanted.

Thoughts. How and what you think are parts of your personality, so do everything you can to improve the quality of your thoughts. If you want people to listen when you speak, know what you are talking about and be able to say it well. Increase your word power by reading good newspapers, magazines, and books. Learn new words each day by looking up in the dictionary the unfamiliar ones you encounter in conversation and reading.

A **pleasant voice** is needed; words alone will not suffice. If speech is to be fluent and pleasing, a properly pitched tone of voice must be used. A **monotone** voice is dull and uninteresting.

Emotional stability is something everyone strives for. Those who achieve it realize how much it contributes to their appreciation of life. If you want to be admired, develop the ability to live life to its fullest. Emotional stability will help you in this task. Learn to suppress the signs that betray emotions, such as facial expressions or gestures of anger, impatience, envy, or greed.

Be gracious. Learn to display pleasant emotions. A smile of greeting and a word of welcome, the willingness to assume the responsibilities of friendship, fitting into new environments, and meeting new people with charm and grace, all express the quality of graciousness.

Good manners are a reflection of your thoughtfulness of others. Good manners should be easy to follow for they include all the little things, such as saying "Thank you," "Please," treating other people with respect, exercising care of other people's property, being tolerant and understanding of other people's efforts, and being considerate of those with whom you work. Courtesy is one of the keys to a successful career.

Be well-groomed. The first impression you have of a person is how he or she is groomed. This is true of the impression the other person has of you. To meet good grooming requirements the cosmetologist's hair should be clean and attractively styled. Your grooming goes hand-in-hand with good posture, whether standing, walking, or sitting. Your clothing should be immaculately clean, your hands smooth, and your nails properly cared for.

Have a sense of humor. Cultivate your sense of humor. Take yourself less seriously. When you can laugh at yourself, you will have gained the ability to properly evaluate your position in society.

Remember, your personality is the key to success. Be sure to develop yours to the utmost.

VOICE AND CONVERSATION

A pleasant **voice,** interesting **conversation,** and the use of good **English** contribute to success. The use of good English and interesting conversation will serve you well as a professional cosmetologist because patrons will enjoy being with you and will seek your services.

Success is not attained within the beauty salon alone, but also depends on personal contacts, membership in associations, and active participation in many social and cosmetology functions, such as association meetings, trade shows, conventions, workshops, and social gatherings with the people who create, develop, and direct cosmetology activities.

Your voice should project your most attractive characteristics. These are:
1. **Sincerity** — honesty of mind or intention.
2. **Intelligence** — the act of understanding.
3. **Friendliness** — friendly behavior.
4. **Vitality** — vigor and liveliness.
5. **Flexibility** — pliable, not rigid, in voice tones.
6. **Expressiveness** — the expression of one's individuality.

The **tone of voice** can be used to express the emotions of anger, joy, hate, love, jealousy, friendliness, and envy. Your voice should be used to present you in the most favorable light possible. It should be clear and understandable. If the spoken words cannot be understood, a good voice tone is useless.

To be successful, a pleasing voice is needed:
1. To greet the patrons.
2. For conversation.
3. To sell yourself.
4. To sell services and products.
5. To build business.
6. To talk on the telephone.

Conversation involves the use of voice, words, intelligence, charm, and personality.

The correct use of words is vital to the art of conversation. The most serious violations of good speech are the use of slang, vulgarisms, and poor grammar.

Topics of conversation should be as non-controversial as possible. Friendly relations are easily achieved through pleasant conversations. Such relationships build a better business.

Topics to discuss in conversation:
1. Patron's interest in herself, her personal grooming, and cosmetic needs.
2. Patron's own activities.
3. Fashions.
4. Literature.
5. Art.
6. Music.

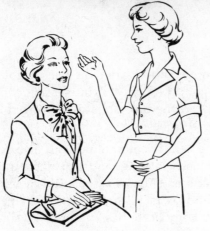

7. Education.
8. Travel.
9. Civic affairs.
10. Vacations.

Try to understand the patron's state of mind and the kind of person she is. Your conversation should be directed toward her interests. Fit your conversation to the patron's mood.

Ability to carry on a pleasant conversation with a patron is an asset to the cosmetologist.

HOW TO ACQUIRE CONVERSATIONAL CHARM

The following steps can help you achieve the charm that contributes so much to success in the beauty culture profession:
1. Guide the conversation.
2. Do not be argumentative.
3. Be a good listener.
4. Do not monopolize the conversation.
5. Do not pry into personal affairs.
6. Talk about ideas rather than people.
7. Use simple language that can be understood.
8. Never gossip. It is small talk used by uninteresting people.
9. Be pleasant.
10. Use good English.

Never discuss the following topics:
1. Your own personal problems.
2. Religion.
3. Other patrons' bad behavior.
4. Your love affairs.
5. Your own financial status.
6. Poor workmanship of fellow workers.
7. Your own health problems.
8. Information given you in confidence.

Unpopular persons annoy or irritate others. To become popular, develop a desirable personality by adhering to the following rules:
1. Do not be bossy.
2. Do not be sarcastic.
3. Do not ridicule people.
4. Do not lose your temper.
5. Do not be rude to others.
6. Do not start an argument.
7. Do not talk continually.
8. Do not spread gossip.
9. Do not use profanity, slang, or poor grammar.
10. Do not monopolize the conversation.

YOUR PERSONALITY CHART

An **attractive personality** is one of your greatest assets in life. It is the charm revealed in your speech, appearance, behavior, and manners. It is the total effect you have on other people. How you behave in school, business, or social life can either add or take away from your personality.

Try to make your answers to the following questions project a true picture of your inner and outer self. First evaluate yourself. If your rating is low, consult your teacher, friends, or doctor to find out what can be done to enrich and improve it. Analyze your personality every three months to find out what progress you are making.

PERSONALITY QUIZ

Check the proper boxes in this Personality Quiz to find out if you have the personality qualities listed below:

1. **Female.** Do you give careful attention to personal grooming, such as your clothes, hair, makeup, hosiery, and shoes?
   ☐ Always   ☐ Sometimes   ☐ Never

   Male. Do you give careful attention to personal grooming, such as your clothes, socks, shoes, hair, shave, mustache, hair in nose?
   ☐ Always   ☐ Sometimes   ☐ Never

2. Do you check your posture when sitting, standing, and walking?
   ☐ Always   ☐ Sometimes   ☐ Never

3. Do you change undergarments daily and avoid halitosis and body odor at all times?
   ☐ Always   ☐ Sometimes   ☐ Never

4. Are you loyal to others?
   ☐ Always   ☐ Sometimes   ☐ Never

5. Are you friendly and courteous to others?
   ☐ Always   ☐ Sometimes   ☐ Never

6. Are you truthful in dealing with others?
   ☐ Always   ☐ Sometimes   ☐ Never

7. Can you get along and work well with others?
   ☐ Always   ☐ Sometimes   ☐ Never

8. Can you accept responsibility?
   ☐ Always   ☐ Sometimes   ☐ Never

9. Do you have confidence in your knowledge and ability?
   ☐ Always   ☐ Sometimes   ☐ Never

10. Do you have a good tone of voice and choice of words?
   ☐ Always   ☐ Sometimes   ☐ Never

Give yourself 10 points for **Always**; 5 points for **Sometimes**; and zero (0) for **Never**. Compare your final rating with the following standards:

Excellent Personality 85-100%
Good Personality 75- 85%
Fair Personality 60- 75%
Poor Personality .... 59% or less

Note: About two-thirds of all job dismissals are due to bad manners, poor personality and inability to get along with people. It would be to your advantage, therefore, to do all you can to improve your personality.

REVIEW QUESTIONS

PERSONALITY DEVELOPMENT

1. Define personality.
2. How is a pleasing personality developed?
3. Why should the student develop a pleasing personality?
4. What are two personality characteristics that reflect graciousness?
5. What is the foundation of good manners?
6. Your personality is the key to ....
7. What are six characteristics a voice should project?
8. How does a pleasant voice, interesting conversation and the use of good English help a cosmetologist succeed?
9. Vitality in a speaking voice means vigor and ....
10. List the five essentials of good conversation.
11. The most serious errors of good English are slang, vulgarisms, and poor ....
12. Which of the following topics can be pleasantly discussed in conversation?

    ☐ Fashions   ☐ Religion
    ☐ Health problems   ☐ Education
    ☐ Personal grooming   ☐ Literature
    ☐ Love affairs

13. Personality is revealed in your speech, appearance, behavior, and
    ....

Chapter 4

PROFESSIONAL ETHICS

CHAPTER LEARNING OBJECTIVES

The student successfully mastering this chapter will know:
1. *The cosmetologist's code of ethical conduct.*
2. *How ethics contribute to success.*
3. *How to maintain a professional attitude toward patrons.*

Cosmetology refers to the scientific study and practice of beauty culture. As a professional career, cosmetology offers many opportunities and rewards to those students who receive a thorough training, develop an attractive appearance and a charming personality, and observe professional ethics.

ETHICS

Ethics deal with the proper conduct and business dealings of cosmetologists in relation to their employers, patrons, and co-workers. Simply stated, a cosmetologist's code of ethical conduct is based on the "Golden Rule," namely, "Do unto others as you would have them do unto you."

Ethical conduct helps to build confidence and increase patronage. The individual cosmetologist should live up to the following rules of ethics:
1. Give courteous and friendly service to all patrons.
2. Treat all patrons honestly and fairly; do not show favoritism.
3. Be fair, courteous, and show respect for the feelings and rights of others.
4. Keep your word and fulfill your obligations.
5. Cherish a good reputation. Set an example of good conduct and behavior.
6. Be loyal to your employer, manager, and associates.

7. Practice only the highest standards of sanitation at all times.
8. Obey all provisions of the state cosmetology laws.
9. Believe in the cosmetology profession. Practice it faithfully and sincerely.
10. As a student:
    a) Be loyal to, and cooperate with, school personnel and fellow students.
    b) Comply with school and clinic rules and regulations.

Questionable practices, extravagant claims, and **unfulfilled promises** violate the rules of ethical conduct. They cast an unfavorable light on cosmetology in general and upon the individual student, cosmetologist, and beauty salon in particular.

A PROFESSIONAL ATTITUDE TOWARD PATRONS

Greet a patron by name, with a pleasing tone of welcome in your voice. See that her personal belongings are cared for. See patron to her seat. Study her mood. Often the patron will prefer quiet and relaxation. Confine your own conversation to her cosmetic needs. If the patron wishes to talk, be a good listener. Never repeat a tidbit of gossip to her as she may lose confidence in you. **Never gossip about anyone.**

Off-color stories are distasteful to most women and have no place in a beauty salon.

Good habits and practices acquired during your school training lay the foundation for a successful career in cosmetology. To become successful, you should:

1. Be ethical by following the rules of proper personal behavior.
2. Make a good impression on others.
3. Cultivate charm, confidence, and a pleasing personality.
4. Pay attention to the minor details that will make patrons like you.
5. Be cordial when greeting patrons in person or over the telephone.
6. Cultivate a pleasing voice.
7. Listen attentively when others speak.
8. Address patrons by their names — Miss or Mrs. Smith. Never use "Honey," "Dearie," etc.
9. Handle all patrons with tact. Develop an even temperament.
10. Set a good example for what you are selling. An attractive personal appearance is your best advertisement.
11. Train yourself to be capable and efficient in your work.
12. Be punctual in arriving at work and keeping appointments.
13. Plan each day's schedule. Avoid long waiting periods.
14. Learn to talk intelligently about your work.
15. Develop business and sales abilities along with common sense. Use tact when suggesting additional services to patrons.
16. Avoid criticizing, condemning, or complaining.
17. Be prompt and judicious in adjusting patrons' complaints.

TO BE SUCCESSFUL . . .

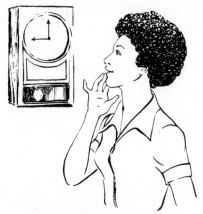

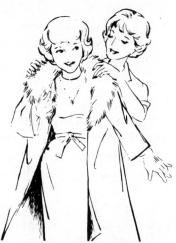

BE PUNCTUAL.
Get to work on time and you won't miss any patrons.

TARDINESS never pays.

BE COURTEOUS.
Treat people with the same kindness you would want to be treated, and everyone will like you.

DISCOURTESY is inexcusable.

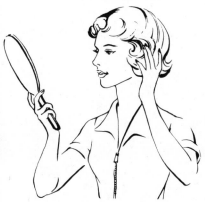

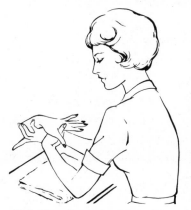

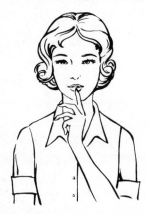

BE NEAT, CLEAN, AND ATTRACTIVE.
Be good to look at, and patrons will admire you.

SLOVENLINESS in dress or hygiene is offensive.

BE GENTLE. You will be remembered for this valued characteristic.

HARSH, rough treatment chases patrons away.

MIND YOUR OWN BUSINESS. Patrons will trust you.

GAB and they won't like you.

TO BE SUCCESSFUL you must learn to do the little things that will make people like you and want to come back to see you again and again.

To be successful the cosmetologist should avoid:
1. Bad breath and body odor.
2. Chewing gum and smoking in the presence of patrons.
3. Speaking in a loud or harsh voice.
4. Criticizing the services of fellow workers.
5. Discussing personal problems with patrons.
6. Lounging on the arms of chairs, table tops, or in the reception room.
7. Poor posture when working; shuffling of feet when walking.
8. Playing the television or radio loudly in the presence of patrons.
9. Spreading gossip, or using profane or sarcastic language.
10. Making statements that are untrue or unduly critical; this lowers the dignity of cosmetology as a profession.
11. Know the rules and regulations that govern the practice of cosmetology in your state.

Nobody likes a person who gossips.

The successful cosmetologist extends **courtesy** to state board members and inspectors. These people are acting in the line of duty and they contribute to the higher standards of cosmetology.

The successful cosmetologist must know the laws, rules, and regulations that govern cosmetology and must comply with them. By such compliance, the cosmetologist is contributing to the health, welfare, and safety of the community.

REVIEW QUESTIONS

PROFESSIONAL ETHICS

1. Define ethics.
2. Check which of the following you consider to be ethical practices.
   - ☐ Courtesy
   - ☐ Honesty
   - ☐ Extravagant claims
   - ☐ Unfulfilled promises
   - ☐ Obeying the cosmetology laws
   - ☐ Keeping your word
3. Why should the cosmetologist never repeat gossip to patrons?
4. Why should a cosmetologist always be neat and clean?
5. Why is it desirable that the cosmetologist always be gentle in the performance of services?
6. Why is it important to avoid statements that are untrue or unduly critical?
7. Why should the cosmetologist extend courtesy to state board members?
8. Why should the cosmetologist comply with cosmetology laws?

Chapter 5

BACTERIOLOGY

CHAPTER LEARNING OBJECTIVES

The student successfully mastering this chapter will know:
1. *Why an understanding of bacteriology is necessary.*
2. *The various types and classifications of bacteria.*
3. *How bacteria grow and reproduce.*
4. *The relationship of bacteria to the spread of disease.*

Bacteriology (bak-te-re-ol'o-je), **sterilization** (ster-i-li-za'shun), and **sanitation** (san-i-ta'shun) are subjects of practical importance to cosmetologists, because they have a direct bearing on their own as well as on their patrons' welfare. To protect individual and public health, cosmetologists should know when, why, and how to use good sterilization and sanitation practices.

In order to understand the importance of sanitation and sterilization, a basic understanding of how **bacteria** (bak-te're-ah) affect our daily lives is most helpful.

BACTERIOLOGY

Bacteriology is the science that deals with the study of **micro-organisms** (mi'kro-or-gan-izms) called **bacteria.**

Cosmetologists should understand how the spread of disease can be prevented, and they must become familiar with the precautions necessary to protect their own and their patrons' health. Knowledge of the relationship between bacteria and disease will help students understand the need for school and salon cleanliness and sanitation.

State boards of cosmetology and health departments require the use of sanitary measures while serving the public. Contagious diseases, skin infections, and blood poisoning are caused either by the conveyance of infectious bacteria from one individual to another, or by unsanitary implements (such as combs, brushes, hairpins, clippies, rollers, etc.) used first on an infected person and then on others. Dirty hands and fingernails are other sources of infectious bacteria.

BACTERIA

Bacteria are minute, one-celled vegetable micro-organisms found nearly everywhere, and are especially numerous in dust, dirt, refuse, and diseased tissues. Bacteria are also known as **germs** (jermz) or **microbes** (mi'krobs).

Bacteria can exist almost anywhere, and are found on the skin of the body, in water, air, decayed matter, secretions of body openings, on clothing, and beneath the nails.

Bacteria can be seen only with the aid of a **microscope** (mi'kro-skop). Fifteen hundred rod-shaped bacteria will barely reach across a pinhead.

TYPES OF BACTERIA

There are hundreds of different kinds of bacteria. However, bacteria are classified into two types, depending on whether they are beneficial or harmful.

1. **Non-pathogenic** (non-path-o-jen'ik) **organisms** (beneficial or harmless types) constitute the majority of all bacteria. They perform many useful functions, such as decomposing refuse and improving the fertility of the soil. To this group belong the **saprophytes** (sap'ro-fyts), which live on dead matter and do not produce disease.

2. **Pathogenic** (path-o-jen'ik) **organisms** (microbes or germs) are harmful, and although in the minority, produce disease when they invade plant or animal tissues. To this group belong the **parasites** (par'ah-syts), which require living matter for their growth.

It is because of pathogenic bacteria that cleanliness and sanitary conditions are necessary in a beauty school or salon.

PRONUNCIATIONS OF TERMS RELATING TO PATHOGENIC BACTERIA

Singular	**Plural**
coccus (kok'us)	cocci (kok'si)
bacillus (bah-sil'us)	bacilli (bah-sil'i)
spirillum (spi-ril'um)	spirilla (spi-ril'ah)
staphylococcus (staf-i-lo-kok'us)	staphylococci (staf-i-lo-kok'si)
streptococcus (strep-to-kok'us)	streptococci (strep-to-kok'si)
diplococcus (dip-lo-kok'us)	diplococci (dip-lo-kok'si)

treponema pallida (trep-o-ne'mah pal'i-dah)

syphilis (sif'i-lis)

CLASSIFICATIONS OF PATHOGENIC BACTERIA

Bacteria have distinct shapes which aid in their identification. Pathogenic bacteria are classified as follows:

Cocci

1. **Cocci** are round-shaped organisms which appear singly or in the following groups:

    a) **Staphylococci** are pus-forming organisms which grow in bunches or clusters. They cause abscesses, pustules, and boils.

THREE GENERAL FORMS OF BACTERIA

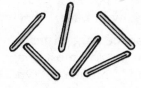
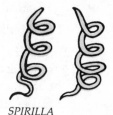

COCCI   BACILLI   SPIRILLA

GROUPINGS OF BACTERIA

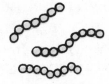

DIPLOCOCCI   STREPTOCOCCI   STAPHYLOCOCCI

SIX DISEASE-PRODUCING BACTERIA

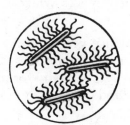
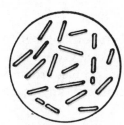
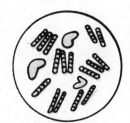

TYPHOID BACILLUS
SHOWING FLAGELLA

TUBERCLE BACILLUS
(Tuberculosis)

DIPHTHERIA
BACILLUS

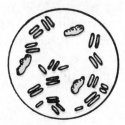
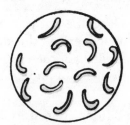
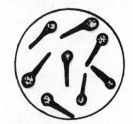

INFLUENZA
BACILLUS

CHOLERA
(Microspira)

TETANUS BACILLUS
WITH SPORES

TO AVOID THE SPREAD OF DISEASE

KEEP YOURSELF CLEAN. KEEP YOUR SURROUNDINGS CLEAN. KEEP EVERYTHING YOU COME IN CONTACT WITH CLEAN. SEE THAT EVERYTHING YOU USE IS CLEAN.

Bacilli

b) **Streptococci** are pus-forming organisms which grow in chains. They cause diseases, such as blood poisoning.

c) **Diplococci** grow in pairs. They cause pneumonia.

2. **Bacilli** are rod-shaped organisms which are either short, thin, or thick in structure. They are the most common and produce diseases, such as tetanus (lockjaw), influenza, typhoid fever, tuberculosis, and diphtheria. Many bacilli are **spore** producers.

Spirilla

3. **Spirilla** are curved or corkscrew-shaped organisms. They are further subdivided into several groups, of chief importance being the **treponema pallida**, which cause **syphilis**.

BACTERIAL GROWTH AND REPRODUCTION

Bacteria generally consist of an outer cell wall and internal protoplasm. They manufacture their own food from the surrounding environment, give off waste products, and grow and reproduce.

Bacteria may exhibit two distinct phases in their life cycle: the **active** or **vegetative** stage, and the **inactive** or **spore-forming** stage.

Active or Vegetative Stage

During the active stage, bacteria grow and reproduce. These micro-organisms multiply best in warm, dark, damp, or dirty places where sufficient food is present.

When conditions are favorable, bacteria reproduce very fast. As food is absorbed, the bacterial cell grows in size. When the limit of growth is reached, the bacterial cell divides crosswise into halves, thereby forming two cells. From one bacterium as many as sixteen million germs may develop in half a day.

When conditions are unfavorable, bacteria die or become inactive.

Inactive or Spore-Forming Stage

Certain bacteria, such as the anthrax and tetanus bacilli, form **spherical spores** with tough outer coverings during their inactive stage, in order to withstand periods of famine, dryness, and unsuitable temperature. In this stage, spores can be blown about and are not harmed by disinfectants, heat, or cold.

When favorable conditions are restored, the spores change into the active or vegetative form, then grow and reproduce.

Movement of Bacteria

The ability to move about is limited to the bacilli and spirilla; the cocci rarely show active motility (self-movement). Motile bacteria use hairlike projections, known as **flagella** (fla-jella') or **cilia** (sil'ya), which extend from the sides, or both sides and end, to move about. A whiplike motion of these hairs propels bacteria about in liquid.

BACTERIAL INFECTIONS

Pathogenic bacteria become a threat to health when they enter the body. An **infection** occurs if the body is unable to cope with the bacteria and their harmful toxins. A **local infection** is indicated by a boil or pimple that contains pus. A **general infection** results when the bloodstream carries the bacteria and their toxins to all parts of the body, as in blood poisoning or syphilis.

The presence of **pus** is a sign of infection. **Staphylococci** are the most common pus-forming bacteria. Found in pus are bacteria, waste matter, decayed tissue, body cells, and blood cells, both living and dead.

A disease becomes **contagious** (kon-ta′jus) or **communicable** (ko-mu′ni-kah-bl) when it spreads from one person to another by contact. Some of the more common contagious disorders which would prevent a cosmetologist from working are tuberculosis, common cold, ringworm, scabies, head lice, and virus infections.

The chief sources of contagion are unclean hands, unclean implements, open sores, pus, mouth and nose discharges, and the common use of drinking cups and towels. Uncovered coughing or sneezing and spitting in public also spread germs.

There can be no infection without the presence of **pathogenic** bacteria.

Pathogenic bacteria may enter the body by way of:
1. A break in the skin, such as a cut, pimple, or scratch.
2. The mouth (breathing or swallowing air, water or food).
3. The nose (air).
4. The eyes or ears (dirt).

The **body fights infection** by means of:
1. Unbroken skin, which is the body's first line of defense.
2. Body secretions, such as perspiration and digestive juices.
3. White blood cells within the blood that destroy bacteria.
4. Antitoxins that counteract the toxins produced by bacteria.

Infections can be prevented and controlled through personal hygiene and public sanitation.

Other Infectious Agents

Filterable viruses (fil′ter-ah-bl vi′ru-sez) are living organisms so small that they can pass through the pores of a porcelain filter. They cause the common cold and other **respiratory** (re-spir′ah-to-re) and **gastro-intestinal** (gas-tro-in-tes′ti-nal) infections.

Parasites are organisms that live on other living organisms without giving anything in return.

Plant parasites or **fungi** (fun′ji), such as molds, mildews, and yeasts, can produce contagious diseases, such as ringworm and **favus** (fa′vus).

Animal parasites are responsible for contagious diseases. For example, the itch mite causes **scabies** (ska′bees) and the louse causes **pediculosis** (pe-dik-u-lo′sis).

Contagious diseases caused by parasites should never be treated in a beauty school or salon. Patrons should be referred to their physicians.

IMMUNITY

Immunity (i-mu'ni-te) is the ability of the body to resist infection by destroying bacteria once they have gained entrance. Immunity against disease may be natural or acquired and is a sign of good health. **Natural immunity** means natural resistance to disease, which is partly inherited and partly developed by hygienic living. **Acquired immunity** is achieved after the body has overcome certain diseases by itself, or when it has received inoculations against these diseases.

Human disease carrier is a person who is personally immune to a disease yet harbors germs that can infect other people. **Typhoid** (ti'foid) **fever** and **diphtheria** (dif-the're-ah) may be transmitted in this manner.

Bacteria may be destroyed by disinfectants, and by intense heat achieved by boiling, steaming, baking, or burning, and ultra-violet rays. (This subject is covered in the chapter on **Sterilization and Sanitation.**)

REVIEW QUESTIONS

BACTERIOLOGY

1. Define bacteriology.
2. Why is a basic understanding of bacteriology important to the cosmetologist?
3. What are bacteria?
4. By what other terms are bacteria known?
5. Why can bacteria only be seen with the aid of a microscope?
6. Name and briefly describe two types of bacteria.
7. What are: a) parasites; b) saprophytes?
8. Name three general forms of bacteria and the shape of each.
9. Which bacteria grow in: a) clusters; b) chains?
10. How do bacteria multiply?
11. Name two common pus-forming bacteria.
12. a) Briefly describe spore-forming bacteria. b) Name two.
13. What causes an infection?
14. What is the difference between local infection and general infection?
15. What is a contagious or communicable disease?
16. Name four common contagious diseases that prevent a cosmetologist from working.
17. Name four principal routes through which bacteria may enter the body.
18. In which four ways does the body resist infection?
19. How can infection be prevented?
20. What is immunity?
21. Differentiate between natural and acquired immunity.
22. What is a human disease carrier? Give two examples.
23. What will destroy bacteria?

Chapter 6

STERILIZATION AND SANITATION

CHAPTER LEARNING OBJECTIVES

The student successfully mastering this chapter will know:
1. *The various methods of sterilization.*
2. *The difference between sterilization and sanitation.*
3. *How the spread of disease can be prevented.*
4. *The methods of sanitation employed in the beauty salon.*
5. *Why good sanitation practices in the beauty salon are necessary.*

STERILIZATION

Sterilization is the process of making an object germfree by the destruction of all kinds of bacteria, whether beneficial or harmful.

Health departments and state boards of cosmetology recognize that it is impossible to completely sterilize all implements and equipment in the beauty school or beauty salon. Therefore, it is generally recognized that implements and equipment are sanitized and not sterilized.

Throughout the entire text the term "sanitize" will be used to indicate all forms of sanitation.

Sterilization and sanitation are of practical importance to the cosmetologist because they deal with methods used either to prevent the growth of germs or to destroy them entirely when possible, particularly those which are responsible for infections and communicable diseases.

DEFINITIONS PERTAINING TO SANITATION

Antiseptic (an-ti-sep'tic)—a chemical agent that may kill or retard the growth of bacteria.

Asepsis (ah-sep'sis)—freedom from disease germs.

Bactericide (bak-te'ri-sid)—a chemical agent having the power to destroy bacteria (germs or microbes).

Disinfect (dis-in-fekt')—to destroy bacteria on any object.

Disinfectant (dis-in-fek'tant)—a chemical agent having the power to destroy bacteria (germs or microbes).

Fumigant (fu'mi-gant)—vapor used to keep clean objects sanitary.

Germicide (jer'mi-sid)—a chemical agent having the power to destroy germs (bacteria or microbes).

Sanitize (san'i-tiz)—to render objects clean and sanitary.

Sepsis (sep'sis)—poisoning due to pathogenic bacteria.

Sterile (ster'il)—free from all germs.

Sterilize (ster'i-liz)—to make free from all bacteria (harmful or beneficial) by the act of sterilizing.

METHODS OF STERILIZATION AND SANITATION

There are five well-known methods of sterilization and sanitation. These may be grouped under two main headings:

1. **Physical agents:**

   a) **Moist heat.**

      1. **Boiling water** at 212° Fahrenheit (100° Celsius) for 20 minutes. (This method is no longer used in beauty salons.)

      2. **Steaming** requires a steam pressure sterilizer. It is used in the medical field to kill bacteria and spores.

   b) **Dry heat** (baking) is used in hospitals to sterilize sheets, towels, gauze, cotton, and similar materials.

   c) **Ultra-violet rays** in an electrical sanitizer are used in beauty salons to keep sanitized implements sanitary.

2. **Chemical agents:**

   a) **Antiseptics** and **disinfectants** are presently used in beauty salons.

   b) **Vapors** (fumigants) in a cabinet sanitizer are used to keep sanitized implements sanitary in beauty salons.

Chemicals are the most effective sanitizing agents used in beauty salons for destroying or checking the growth of bacteria. The chemical agents used for sanitizing purposes are antiseptics and disinfectants.

1. An **antiseptic** is a substance that may kill bacteria or retard their growth without killing them. As a general rule, antiseptics can be used with safety on the skin.

2. A **disinfectant** destroys most bacteria and is used to sanitize implements.

Several chemicals can be classified as both antiseptic and disinfectant. A **strong solution** may be used as a disinfectant and a **weak solution** as an antiseptic. [Examples: **formalin** (for'ma-lin), alcohol, or **quats** (kwats).]

Requirements of a good disinfectant:

1. Convenient to prepare.
2. Quick acting.
3. Practically odorless.
4. Non-corrosive.
5. Economical.
6. Non-irritating to skin.

There are many prepared and ready for use chemical disinfectant agents on the market. If these are used, select the ones that have been approved by your board of health or state board of cosmetology. Chemicals commonly used in the beauty salon are:

1. **Quaternary ammonium compounds** (quats) (kwa-ter'nah-re ah-mo' ne-um kom'pounds—(kwats)—to sanitize implements.
2. **Formaldehyde** (for-mal'de-hid)—to sanitize implements.
3. **Alcohol**—to sanitize sharp cutting instruments and electrodes.
4. **Prepared commercial products** that clean floors, sinks, and toilet bowls.

A **wet sanitizer** is any receptacle large enough to hold a disinfectant solution in which the objects to be sanitized can be completely immersed. A cover is provided to prevent contamination of the solution. Wet sanitizers can be obtained in various sizes and shapes.

Before immersing objects in a wet sanitizer containing a disinfectant solution, be sure to:

1. Remove hair from combs and brushes.
2. Wash them thoroughly with hot water and soap.
3. Rinse them thoroughly.

This procedure prevents contamination of the solution. In addition, soap and hot water remove most of the bacteria.

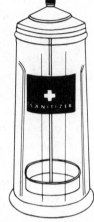

Wet sanitizer.

After the implements are removed from the disinfectant solution, they must be rinsed in clean water, wiped dry with a clean towel, and stored in a dry cabinet sanitizer until needed.

A **dry** or **cabinet sanitizer** is an airtight cabinet containing an active fumigant. The sanitized implements are kept clean by being placed in the cabinet until needed.

How to prepare a fumigant. Place 1 tablespoonful (15 ml) of borax and 1 tablespoonful (15 ml) of formalin on a small tray on the bottom of the cabinet. This will form formaldehyde vapors. Replace chemicals regularly as they lose their strength, which depends on how often the cabinet door is opened and closed.

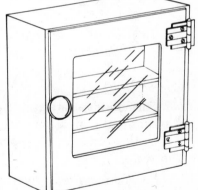

Dry or cabinet sanitizer.

Formalin is also available in tablet form. Follow manufacturer's directions.

Ultra-violet ray electrical sanitizers are effective for keeping combs, brushes, and implements clean until ready for use. Combs, brushes, and implements must be sanitized before they are placed in the ultra-violet sanitizer. Follow manufacturer's directions for proper use.

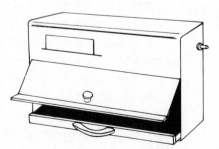

Ultra-violet ray sanitizer.

CHEMICAL SANITIZING AGENTS

QUATERNARY AMMONIUM COMPOUNDS (QUATS)

These compounds are effective as disinfectants. They are available under different trade and chemical names.

The advantages claimed for them are short disinfection time, odorless and colorless, non-toxic, and stable. A 1:1000 solution is commonly used to sanitize implements. Immersion time ranges from 1-5 minutes, depending on the strength of the solution used.

CAUTION

Before using any quat, read and follow the manufacturer's directions on label and accompanying literature. Find out if the product can be used in naturally soft or hard water, or water that has been softened. Inquire whether it contains a rust **inhibitor** (in-hib'i-tor). Should the product lack a rust inhibitor, the addition of ½% of **sodium nitrite** (so'de-um ni'trit) to the solution prevents the rusting of metallic implements.

HOW TO PREPARE A 1:1000 STRENGTH SOLUTION OF A QUATERNARY AMMONIUM COMPOUND

If the product contains:

10% active ingredient, add 1¼ oz (37.5 ml) quat solution to 1 gallon (3.8 l) of water.

12½% active ingredient, add 1 oz. (30 ml) quat solution to 1 gallon (3.8 l) of water.

15% active ingredient, add ¾ oz. (22.5 ml) quat solution to 1 gallon (3.8 l) of water.

FORMALIN

Formalin is a safe and effective sanitizing agent which can be used either as an antiseptic or disinfectant, depending on its percentage strength. As purchased, formalin is approximately 37% to 40% of formaldehyde gas in water.

Formalin is used in various strengths, as follows:

25% solution (equivalent to 10% formaldehyde gas)—used to sanitize implements. Immerse implements in the solution for at least 10 minutes. (Preparation: 2 parts formalin, 5 parts water, 1 part glycerine.)

10% solution (equivalent to 4% formaldehyde gas)—used to sanitize combs and brushes. Immerse them for at least 20 minutes. (Preparation: 1 part formalin, 9 parts water.)

5% solution (equivalent to 2% formaldehyde gas)—used to cleanse the hands after they have been in contact with wounds, skin eruptions, etc. Also used to sanitize shampoo bowls and chairs. (Preparation: 1 part formalin, 19 parts water.)

SANITIZING WITH CHEMICAL DISINFECTANTS

1. Wash implements thoroughly with soap and hot water.
2. Use a plain hot water rinse to remove all traces of soap.
3. Immerse implements in a wet sanitizer (containing approved disinfectant*) for the required time.
4. Remove implements from wet sanitizer, rinse in water, and wipe dry with clean towel.
5. Store sanitized implements in individually wrapped cellophane envelopes in cabinet sanitizer or in ultra-violet ray cabinet until ready to be used.

SANITIZING WITH ALCOHOL

To sanitize **electrodes** and **implements,** use 70% alcohol or 99% isopropyl alcohol.

70% alcohol refers to ethyl or grain alcohol.
99% isopropyl alcohol is the same strength as 70% ethyl alcohol.

Implements having a fine cutting edge are best sanitized by rubbing the surface with a cotton pad dampened with 70% alcohol. This application prevents the cutting edges from becoming dull.

Electrodes (e-lek'trods) may be safely sanitized by gently rubbing the exposed surface with a cotton pad dampened with 70% alcohol. Then place the articles into a dry sanitizer or ultra-violet ray sanitizer until ready for use.

SANITIZING FLOORS, SINKS, AND TOILET BOWLS

To sanitize floors, sinks, and toilet bowls in the beauty salon use a commercial product, such as Lysol or pine needle oil. **Deodorants** also are useful to offset offensive smells and to impart a refreshing odor.

Whichever disinfectant is used, make sure that it is properly diluted, as suggested by manufacturer.

IT IS ALWAYS A PLEASURE FOR PATRONS TO RECEIVE SERVICES IN A BEAUTY SALON THAT IS SPOTLESS. GET INTO THE HABIT NOW. KEEP EVERYTHING CLEAN AND IN ORDER.

PROPORTIONS FOR MAKING PERCENTAGE SOLUTIONS

100% Active Liquid Concentrate	Strength
5 drops of liquid to 1 oz. (30 ml) water or	
1 teaspoon (5 ml) of liquid to 12 oz. (.36 l) water	1%
10 drops of liquid to 1 oz. (30 ml) water or	
2 teaspoonfuls (10 ml) of liquid to 12 oz. (.36 l) water . . . . : .	2%
4 teaspoonfuls (20 ml) of liquid to 12 oz. (.36 l) water	4%
5 teaspoonfuls (25 ml) of liquid to 12 oz. (.36 l) water	5%
10 teaspoonfuls (50 ml) of liquid to 12 oz. (.36 l) water	10%

---

* Consult your state board of cosmetology or health department for list of approved disinfectants to be used in beauty salons.

Table of Equivalents

Ordinary Measured Glass	8 oz. (.237 l)
1 Pint	16 oz. (.475 l)
1 Quart	32 oz. (.95 l)
½ Gallon	64 oz. (1.9 l)

SAFETY PRECAUTIONS

The use of chemical sanitizing agents involves certain dangers, unless safety measures are taken to prevent mistakes and accidents. Follow these safety rules:

1. Purchase chemicals in small quantities and store them in a cool, dry place; otherwise, they could deteriorate when exposed to air, light, and heat.
2. Carefully weigh and measure chemicals.
3. Keep all containers labeled, covered, and under lock and key.
4. Do not smell chemicals or solutions because some of them have pungent odors and may irritate the membranes of your nose.
5. Avoid spilling when diluting chemicals.
6. Prevent burns by using forceps to insert or remove objects from the source of heat.
7. Keep a complete first aid kit on hand.

SANITIZING RULES

Chemical solutions in sanitizers should be changed regularly.

Manicuring implements must be kept in a disinfectant solution (70% alcohol) during a manicure.

All articles must be clean and free from hair before being sanitized.

Combs and **brushes** must be sanitized after each patron has been serviced.

Shampoo bowls must be sanitized before and after each use.

All manicuring implements must be sanitized after use on a patron.

Sanitize electrical appliances by rubbing surface with a cotton pad dampened with 70% alcohol.

All cups, finger bowls, or **similar objects** must be sanitized prior to being used for another patron.

IMPORTANT

The immersing of implements in a chemical solution should conform to state board of cosmetology regulations issued by your state.

DISINFECTANTS COMMONLY USED IN BEAUTY SALONS

NAME	FORM	STRENGTH	HOW TO USE
Quaternary Ammonium Compounds (Quats)	Liquid or tablet	1:1000 solution	Immerse implements in solution for 1-5 minutes.
Formalin	Liquid	25% solution	Immerse implements in solution for 10 minutes.
Formalin	Liquid	10% solution	Immerse implements in solution for 20 minutes.
Ethyl or Grain Alcohol	Liquid	70% solution	Sanitize sharp cutting implements and electrodes.
Cresol (Lysol)	Liquid	10% soap solution	Cleanse floors, sinks, and toilets.

ANTISEPTICS COMMONLY USED IN BEAUTY SALONS

NAME	FORM	STRENGTH	USE
Boric Acid	White crystals	2-5% solution	Cleanse the eyes.
Tincture of Iodine	Liquid	2% solution	Cleanse cuts and wounds.
Hydrogen Peroxide	Liquid	3-5% solution	Cleanse skin and minor cuts.
Ethyl or Grain Alcohol	Liquid	60% solution	Cleanse hands, skin, and minute cuts. Not to be used if irritation is present.
Formalin	Liquid	5% solution	Cleanse hands, shampoo bowl, cabinet, etc.
Chloramine-T (Chlorazene; Chlorozol)	White crystals	½% solution	Cleanse skin and hands, and for general use.
Sodium Hypochlorite (Javelle water; Zonite)	White crystals	½% solution	Rinse the hands.

Other approved disinfectants and antiseptics are being used in beauty salons. Consult your state board of cosmetology or your health department.

PUBLIC SANITATION

Public sanitation is the application of measures to promote public health and to prevent the spread of infectious diseases.

The importance of sanitation cannot be overemphasized. Professional services bring the cosmetologist in direct contact with the patron's skin, scalp, hair, and nails. By using the best sanitary practices you can insure the protection of the patron's health.

Various governmental agencies protect community health by providing for a wholesome food and water supply and the quick disposal of refuse. These steps are only a few of the ways in which the public health is safeguarded.

Water for drinking purposes should be odorless, colorless, and free from any foreign matter. Crystal clear water still may be unsanitary because of the presence of pathogenic bacteria, which cannot be seen with the naked eye.

The **air within a beauty salon** should not be dry or stagnant, nor have a stale, musty odor. Room temperature should be about 70° Fahrenheit (21° Celsius).

The beauty salon can be ventilated with the aid of an exhaust fan or an air conditioning unit. Air conditioning has the advantage of permitting changes in the quality and quantity of air brought into the salon. The temperature and moisture content of the air can be regulated by means of air conditioning.

A **person with an infectious disease** is a source of contagion to others. Hence, cosmetologists with colds or other communicable diseases must not be permitted to serve patrons. Likewise, patrons obviously suffering from an infectious disease must not be accommodated in a beauty salon. In this way, the best interests of other patrons are served.

The **public** has learned the importance of sanitation and is now demanding that every possible sanitary measure be used in the beauty salon for the promotion of public health.

The **state board of cosmetology** and **board of health** in each state or locality have formulated sanitary regulations governing beauty salons. Every cosmetologist must be familiar with these regulations and obey them.

SUMMARY

Adherence to the following sanitary rules will result in cleaner and better service to the public:

1. Every beauty salon must be well-lighted, heated, and ventilated, and must be kept in a clean and sanitary condition.
2. The walls, curtains, and floor coverings in a beauty salon must be washed and kept clean.
3. All beauty salons must be supplied with hot and cold running water. Drinking facilities (individual paper cups and/or fountain) should be provided.
4. All plumbing fixtures must be properly installed and work effectively.
5. The premises must be kept free from rodents, vermin, flies, or similar insects.
6. The beauty salon is not to be used for eating, sleeping, or living quarters.
7. All hair, cotton, or other waste material must be removed from the floor without delay and deposited in a closed container, then removed from the premises at frequent intervals.
8. The rest rooms must be kept in a sanitary condition and be provided with soap dispenser and with individual paper towels.
9. Each cosmetologist must wear a clean unform while working on patrons.
10. The cosmetologist **must cleanse** his or her hands thoroughly **before** and **after** serving a patron and **after** leaving the **rest room.**
11. A freshly laundered towel must be used for each patron. Clean towels must be stored in a sanitized, closed cabinet. Soiled towels and linens must be placed immediately after use in containers provided for this purpose. Keep dirty towels away from clean towels.
12. Headrest coverings and neck strips **must be changed** for each patron.

13. **Do not permit** the shampoo cape to come in contact with the patron's skin.
14. The common use of powder puffs, lip color, cheek color, solid soap, sponges, combs, brushes, or styptic pencils is **prohibited.**
15. Keep lotions, ointments, creams, and powders in clean, closed containers. Use clean spatula to remove creams or ointments from jars. Use sterile cotton pledgets to apply lotions and powders. Re-cover cosmetic containers after each use.
16. For manicuring, provide a sanitary container or finger bowl with an individual paper cup for each patron.
17. Discard emery boards after use on a patron.
18. Soiled combs, brushes, towels, or other used material must be removed from tops of work stations immediately after use.
19. Clippies, hairpins, or bobby pins must not be placed in the mouth.
20. Combs or implements must not be carried in pockets of the uniform.
21. Hairnets must not be carried in pockets or cuffs of the uniform.
22. Hairnets must be washed after each use.
23. Clippies, curlers, bobby pins, or hairpins must be sanitized after each use.
24. All implements and articles used must first be sanitized and then placed in a dustproof or airtight container, or in a cabinet sanitizer.
25. Objects dropped on the floor are not to be used until they are sanitized.
26. Dogs, cats, birds, or other pets should not be permitted in a beauty school or salon.

REMINDERS

1. The **responsibility for sanitation** rests with **each student** in the beauty school and **each cosmetologist** in the beauty salon. The manager must provide the necessities for school and salon sanitation.
2. You **must** obey the rules issued by the health department and the state board of cosmetology regarding acceptable methods of sanitation.

REVIEW QUESTIONS

STERILIZATION AND SANITATION

1. What is sterilization?
2. What term is used by health departments and state boards to indicate cleanliness of implements and equipment?
3. What type of bacteria makes necessary the practice of sanitation in the beauty salon?
4. Effective sanitation prevents the spread of . . . . and . . . . in the beauty salon.
5. Distinguish between asepsis, sterile, and sepsis.
6. What is an antiseptic?
7. Is there a difference in the action of a disinfectant, germicide, or bactericide? Give reasons for your answer.
8. What is a disinfectant?

9. What is a fumigant?
10. Physical and .... agents are used in sanitation.
11. Name two methods of keeping objects clean after they have been sanitized.
12. List six requirements of a good disinfectant.
13. What is the chemical sanitizing agent quaternary ammonium compound commonly called?
14. What is a wet sanitizer?
15. What should be done to combs, brushes, and implements before they are immersed in a wet sanitizer?
16. Why should a wet sanitizer be kept covered at all times?
17. What should be done with implements after they are sanitized in a disinfectant solution?
18. What is a dry or cabinet sanitizer?
19. What is the proper way to produce formaldehyde vapors in a cabinet sanitizer?
20. What are four advantages of using quats as a disinfectant?
21. In what strength are quats commonly used?
22. About how long does it take to sanitize implements when using: a) quats; b) 25% formalin; c) 10% formalin?
23. Formaldehyde is the active gas found in ....
24. What is the composition of formalin?
25. What strength formalin solution is recommended to sanitize implements?
26. What is the best way to sanitize sharp implements and prevent their dulling?
27. What is a safe way to sanitize electrodes?
28. List six safety precautions when using chemical agents.

PUBLIC SANITATION

1. Define public sanitation.
2. Why is it important that the cosmetologist conform with the best sanitary practices?
3. Why is it important to have a pure water supply?
4. Why is it important that a cosmetologist refuse to serve a patron with an infectious diaease?
5. Which two governmental agencies formulate sanitary regulations for beauty schools and salons?
6. How should cotton, hair and other waste material be disposed of?
7. How often should the cosmetologist cleanse her hands?
8. How should clean towels be stored?
9. How often should a headrest cover be changed?
10. What is a sanitary way to remove cosmetic creams from their containers?
11. How are face powders kept, and how are they applied?
12. On whom does the responsibility for sanitation rest within the beauty school?
13. If a towel or an implement is accidentally dropped on the floor, how should it be treated?

Chapter 7

DRAPING

CHAPTER LEARNING OBJECTIVES

The student successfully mastering this chapter will know:
1. *How to protect the patron and her clothing.*
2. *How the protection of the patron affects the cosmetology services being offered.*
3. *How patron satisfaction is affected by the cosmetologist's efforts to protect her.*
4. *The various methods of draping for wet and dry hair work.*

The protection of the patron must be the first consideration at all times. Whenever cosmetology services are being performed, the cosmetologist's primary responsibilities are:

1. To provide for the patron's comfort.
2. To protect the patron's clothing from damage by any of the chemicals or cosmetic solutions being used.
3. To protect the patron from injury.
4. To provide competent, professional services to the patron.

Correctly draping the patron for the various services being given is an important part of the cosmetologist's service to that patron. Properly draping the patron is the "first line of defense" for the protection of the patron's skin and clothing from stains or damage. In addition, the patron feels more confident, relaxed, and comfortable when she knows that the cosmetologist serving her has taken care of her personal safety.

Note: There are many ways to drape a patron for the various salon services. Discussed and illustrated here are only some of the methods. Your instructor may use different techniques which are equally acceptable. Basically, however, every method of draping is designed to accomplish the same objective, which is the protection of the patron and her clothing.

PREPARATION FOR DRAPING

Before draping a patron for any kind of hair service, the following steps should be followed:

1. Seat patron comfortably.
2. Select and arrange the required materials and supplies.
3. Wash and sanitize hands.
4. Ask patron to remove all neck and hair jewelry, earrings and glasses, and place in her purse for safekeeping.
5. Turn dress or blouse collar to the inside, making sure that it is straight and will not wrinkle. (Fig. 1)
6. Place neck strip or towel around the patron's neck.
7. Adjust cape over neck strip or towel.
8. Fold neck strip or towel over cape neck band.
9. Remove all hairpins and combs from the hair.

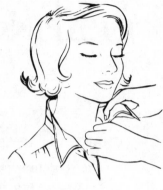

Fig. 1

If towel is short it may be folded on the bias which will not only add length to the towel, but also will give a higher collar and more protection.

Note: The neck strip or neck towel is used for sanitary as well as protective reasons. Regardless of whether a neck strip or towel is used, special care must be exercised to make certain that the cape does not come into direct contact with the patron's skin, because the cape is used on many patrons and it could be a carrier of disease or infection.

DRAPING FOR WET HAIR SERVICES

DRAPING FOR SHAMPOOING, SCALP AND HAIR CARE, AND WET HAIR SHAPING

The method used for draping the patron for a shampoo, a wet hair shaping, or scalp and hair care must be completely effective against any accidental wetting of the patron.

Procedure

1. Place a small towel lenghtwise across the patron's shoulders. Adjust the towel so that about one-third of its width is resting on the neck while the rest is draped over the shoulders. Bring the ends of the towel together under the chin and overlap them in front, similar to a collar on a blouse.
2. Position the shampoo cape in front and in the center of the draped towel. Bring the

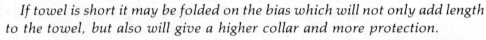

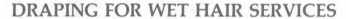

Fig. 2

neck band of the cape around the patron's neck and tie, pin, or clip the ends of the neck band in the back.

3. Fold the part of the towel resting on the patron's neck down over the cape neck band. At no time should the cape touch the patron's skin.

4. Drape a second towel over the shoulders and fasten it in front with a large clip or clamp. (Fig. 2)

The patron is now thoroughly protected.

Alternate Method: Open small towel to its full length. Take opposite ends of towel and fold them over. Place towel across patron's shoulders and criss-cross ends under her chin. Adjust the towel so that about one-third of its width is resting on the neck, while the rest is draped over the shoulders. Ask patron to hold the towel snugly, until the cape is placed over the towel, holding it in place.

DRAPING FOR PERMS, HAIR RELAXING, AND HAIR COLORING

There are several ways in which a patron may be draped for a permanent wave, hair relaxing treatment, hair coloring, and all other wet hair services. It is essential that no chemical lotion be permitted to drip down the patron's neck. The lotion could cause irritation to the skin and might even ruin the patron's clothing. The comfort of the patron and adequate protection of her person and clothing are important during the entire procedure.

The method of draping presented here is only one of many techniques that may be followed.

Procedure

1. Place the cape loosely across the front of the patron. (Fig. 3)

2. Drape towel across the crown area of the patron's head. (Fig. 3)

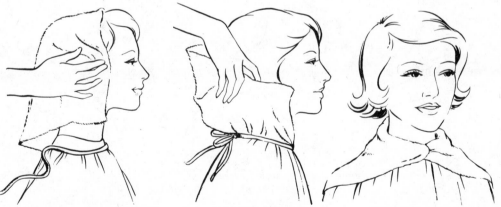

Fig. 3. Placing cape loosely in front of patron. Sliding towel down around patron's neck.

Fig. 4. Adjusting and tieing cape over towel.

Fig. 5. Folding towel over in cape effect.

3. Slide the towel down around the patron's neck, leaving one-third of the

width of the towel draped over the shoulders and two-thirds of the width upright around the neck. (Fig. 4)

4. Adjust the cape over the towel, and tie or fasten the cape neck band at the back of the neck. (Fig. 4)

5. Fold the upright portion of the towel down and over in a cape effect. (Fig. 5)

The patron and her clothing are now completely protected against any dripping liquid.

DRAPING FOR DRY HAIR SERVICES

Draping for dry hair services differs somewhat from the techniques previously outlined. The cape is used in much the same manner, and great care must be exercised to be certain that the cape does not touch the patron's skin. However, in draping for dry hair services, less emphasis is placed on the use of towels, with neck strips more commonly used. The neck strip, of course, is used for sanitary as well as protective purposes.

Procedure

1. Place the neck strip around the neck of the patron. (Fig. 6)

2. Fold the ends of the neck strip and tuck them in. (Fig. 6)

3. Adjust the cape carefully around the patron's neck with the ends of the neck band overlapping at the nape of the neck.

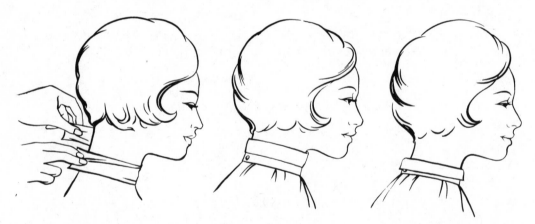

Fig. 6. Placing neck strip around neck; folding ends over and tucking in.

Fig. 7. Tieing, pinning, or attaching cape over neck strip.

Fig. 8. Folding neck strip down over cape neck band. Cape should not touch the patron's skin.

4. Care must be exercised to be certain that the neck band of the cape rests in the center of the neck strip around the entire neck. (Fig. 7)

5. Tie, pin, or fasten the ends of neck band at the back so that the cape fits snugly around the neck. (Fig. 7)

6. Fold the uncovered portion of the neck strip down over the cape neck band, making certain that the cape does not touch the patron's skin. (Fig. 8)

The patron and her clothing are now protected against hair clippings and water drippings.

FIRE HAZARD

When draping for thermal curling or waving, a plastic cape will create a fire hazard. It is advisable to use a cotton or linen cape for these services.

DRAPING FOR A COMB-OUT

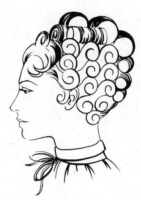

Draping for a comb-out is the same as draping for dry hair shaping. The only differences are that the cape used for a comb-out is usually shorter and is fastened in front to avoid interference with the back and nape comb-out. (Fig. 9)

Comb-out capes do not have to be waterproof and can be made of softer and more colorful material. This type of cape is more attractive and more glamorous to the patron. However, this cape should be laundered more frequently to maintain its freshness and cleanliness.

Fig. 9

DRAPING FOR FACIALS

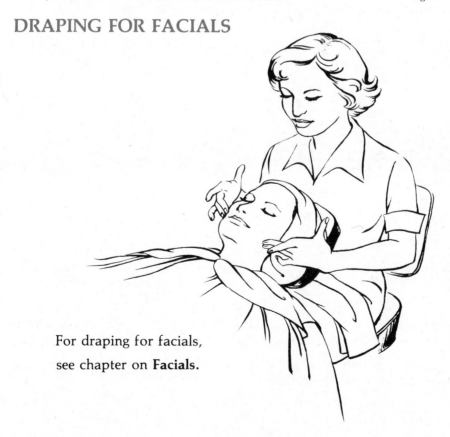

For draping for facials,
see chapter on **Facials.**

REVIEW QUESTIONS

DRAPING

1. What should be the cosmetologist's first consideration at all times?
2. List the four primary responsibilities of the cosmetologist.
3. What is the "first line of defense" for the protection of the patron?
4. List the nine steps followed in preliminary draping for any service.
5. What sanitary purpose is served by a neck strip or neck towel?
6. Why is it important that the cape does not touch patron's skin?
7. How are patrons protected from dripping lotions?
8. What is the major difference between draping for dry hair services and draping for wet hair services?
9. What two purposes are served by the neck strip?
10. How does draping for a comb-out differ from draping for dry shaping?

Chapter 8

SHAMPOOING
AND RINSING

CHAPTER LEARNING OBJECTIVES

The student successfully mastering this chapter will know:
1. *The reasons for good hygienic care of the hair and scalp.*
2. *Why a cosmetologist should have a sound background and knowledge of professional methods of shampooing.*
3. *How to identify the various types of shampoos.*
4. *The procedure for shampoo manipulations.*
5. *The accepted methods of cleansing the hair and scalp with and without water.*
6. *When and how to use the various types of shampoos.*
7. *The effect of hair rinses on the hair.*
8. *How to identify the various types of rinses.*
9. *When and how to use the various types of rinses.*

Shampooing the hair is not only an important preliminary step for various hair services, but it is also the first impression a patron has of the ability of the cosmetologist. In this respect, a shampoo can be considered to be a valuable selling aid, because a patron who is pleased with the way her hair has been shampooed is more likely to look favorably upon a recommendation of additional services made by the cosmetologist. Therefore, the cosmetologist who gives a professional quality shampoo becomes a valuable asset to a salon.

While shampoos are primarily given to clean the hair and scalp, they perform another important function: they initiate the relaxing experience to which the patron has been looking forward with pleasant anticipation. If the cosmetologist can make this expected pleasurable experience a reality, the patron is likely to make her visits to this salon a regular habit.

To be effective, a shampoo must remove all dirt, oils, cosmetics, and skin debris from the scalp and hair shaft, without adversely affecting either the scalp or hair. Shampoos that are strongly alkaline should not be used because they may make the hair dry and brittle.

Unless the scalp and hair are cleansed regularly, the accumulation of oil and perspiration, which mixes with natural scales and dirt, offers a breeding place for disease-producing bacteria. This condition can lead to scalp disorders.

Hair should be shampooed as often as necessary, depending on how quickly the scalp and hair become soiled. As a general rule, oily hair should be shampooed more often than normal or dry hair.

WATER

Chemically, water is composed of hydrogen and oxygen. Depending on the kinds and quantities of other minerals present, it can be classified as either **hard** or **soft** water. The cosmetologist must know the kind of water that is available, whether it is hard or soft, in order to select the right cosmetic products for the services being performed.

Soft water. Rain water, or water that has been chemically softened, contains very small amounts of minerals, and, therefore, lathers freely. For this reason, it is preferred for shampooing.

Hard water contains certain minerals, and, as a result, does not lather very freely. However, it can be softened by a chemical process and made suitable for shampooing.

SELECTING THE CORRECT SHAMPOO

There are many different kinds of shampoos available to the cosmetologist. To make an intelligent choice of shampoo, the cosmetologist should know the composition and action of the shampoo and whether it will do an effective job. To obtain this information, carefully read the label and accompanying literature.

Select the shampoo according to the hair's condition. Hair is not considered normal if it has been:

Lightened	Sun bleached
Toned or tinted	Abused by the use of harsh shampoos
Permanently waved	Damaged by improper care
Chemically relaxed	Damaged by exposure to the elements

REQUIRED MATERIALS AND IMPLEMENTS

Before giving a shampoo, gather all necessary materials and implements. There is nothing more annoying to the patron than to have the cosmetologist wet her hair and leave her stranded while she dashes out to get shampoo or other necessities. Required materials and implements are:

Neck strip	Comb and hairbrush
Towels	Shampoo
Shampoo cape	Hair rinse

DRAPING THE PATRON FOR A SHAMPOO

It is important that the patron be properly draped for the shampoo so that both her person and clothing are properly protected. (For the proper method of draping, consult chapter on **Draping**.)

HAIR BRUSHING

Brushes. Hairbrushes made of natural bristles are recommended for hair brushing. Natural bristles have many tiny imbrications which clean and add luster to the hair, while nylon bristles are shiny and smooth and recommended only for hairstyling.

Thorough brushing of the hair always should be a part of every shampoo and scalp treatment, with the following exceptions:

1. Do not brush before giving a lightening treatment.
2. Do not brush before the application of a tint or toner
3. Do not brush before giving a permanent wave.
4. Do not brush before applying a chemical hair relaxer.
5. Do not brush if the scalp is irritated.

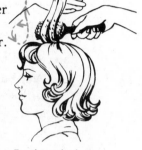

Brushing stimulates the blood circulation to the scalp, helps remove dust and dirt from the hair, and gives hair added sheen. Therefore, the hair should receive a thorough brushing whether the scalp and hair are in a dry or oily condition. **Do not use the comb to loosen scales from the scalp.**

Brushing the hair.

To brush the hair, first part it through the center from front to nape. Then part a section about ½" (1.25 cm) off the center parting to the crown of the head. Holding this strand of hair in the left hand between the thumb and fingers, lay the brush (held in the right hand) with the bristles well down on the hair close to the scalp; sweep the bristles the full length of the hair, turning the wrist slightly in doing so. Repeat three times. Then, part the hair again ½" (1.25 cm) from the first parting, and continue until the entire head has been brushed.

PLAIN SHAMPOO

PREPARATION

1. Seat the patron comfortably.
2. Select and arrange required materials.
3. Wash and sanitize hands.
4. Place neck strip, or towel, and shampoo cape around the patron's neck.
   (Be sure that the dress or blouse collar lays smoothly under the garment before the neck strip is adjusted.)
5. Remove all hairpins and combs from the hair.
6. Ask the patron to remove necklace, ear jewelry, and glasses, and put them into her purse.
7. Examine condition of the patron's hair and scalp.
8. Brush the hair thoroughly.
9. Cover the neck of the shampoo bowl with a folded towel and seat the patron comfortably.
10. Adjust the shampoo cape over the back of the shampoo chair.
11. Adjust the volume and temperature of the water spray.

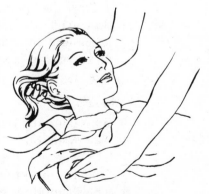

Support patron's head with your right hand and place the cape over the back of the chair.

PROCEDURE

You should be able to use both of your hands with equal ease and work from either side of the patron.

The water you use should be as warm as the patron can comfortably stand. Her preference always should be considered.

Turn on cold water first, and gradually add warm water until you obtain the proper water temperature for your patron's comfort.

Test the temperature of water by spraying it on the inner side of your wrist.

When the spray is turned on , your fingers should be curled over the edge of the nozzle, so that any sudden change in the water temperature can be detected. Proceed as follows:

1. **Wet hair thoroughly** with warm water spray. Lift the hair and work it with the free hand to be sure it is saturated right to the scalp. Shift hand to protect patron's face, ears, and neck from the spray when working around the hairline, as in Figs. 1, 2, and 3.

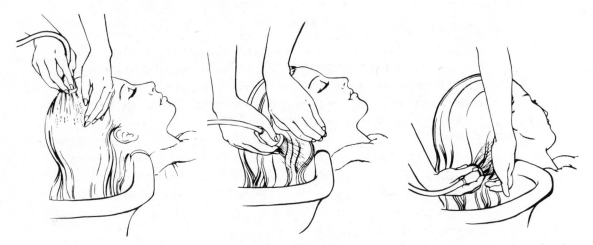

Fig. 1. Protecting the face.   *Fig. 2. Protecting the ears.*   *Fig. 3. Protecting the neck.*

2. **Apply small quantities of shampoo to the hair.** Work each application into a lather until the entire head is lathered.

   Start the application of the shampoo at the front hairline and work down. Lift the patron's head with the left hand, and apply shampoo across the nape area. Using the cushions of the fingers of both hands, and working from front to back, massage the shampoo into a lather over the entire head.

Reminders

In massaging the scalp, **do not use firm pressure if:**
1. The shampoo is to be followed by a lightening treatment.
2. The shampoo is to be followed by a tint treatment.
3. The shampoo precedes a permanent wave.
4. The shampoo precedes a chemical hair relaxing treatment.
5. The scalp is tender or sensitive.
6. The patron requests less pressure.

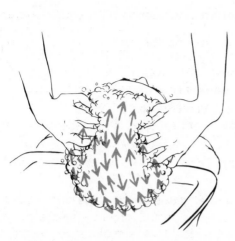

Fig. 4. Manipulating from hairline
to top of head.

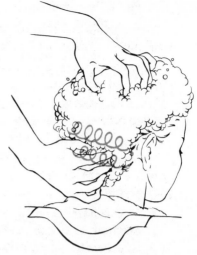

Fig. 5. Lifting patron's head.

3. **Manipulate scalp.**
   a) Starting at the hairline in front of ears (using the cushions of the fingertips of both hands), work in a back-and-forth movement until the top of the head is reached. (Fig. 4)
   b) Continue in this manner to the back of the head, shifting the fingers back 1" (2.5 cm) at a time.
   c) Lift the patron's head, as in Fig. 5, with the left hand controlling movement of her head. With the right hand, start at top of the right ear and, using same movement, work to back of the head.
   d) Drop the fingers down 1" (2.5 cm) and repeat the process until the right side of the head is covered.
   e) Starting at the left ear, repeat steps (c) and (d).
   f) Allow the patron's head to relax, and work around the hairline with your thumbs in a rotary movement.
   g) Repeat these movements until the scalp has been thoroughly massaged.
   h) Remove excess shampoo and foam by squeezing the hair.

4. **Rinse hair thoroughly** with a strong spray, as in Figs. 1, 2, and 3.
   a) Lift the hair at the crown and back with the fingers of the left hand, to permit the spray to rinse the hair thoroughly.
   b) Cup the left hand along the napeline and pat the hair, forcing the spray of water against the base scalp area.

5. **If required, apply shampoo again.**
   a) Apply shampoo again as outlined in Step 2. Loosen the hair before applying the second shampoo application. You will need less shampoo because the shampoo will lather more easily. Follow the same procedure as you did for the first shampoo.

6. **Rinse hair thoroughly** with a strong spray.

7. **Partially towel dry.**
   a) Remove excess moisture from the hair at the shampoo bowl.
   b) Wipe excess moisture from around the face and ears with the ends of the towel.
   c) Lift the towel over the back of the patron's head and drape her head with the towel.
   d) Massage the scalp over the towel with the palms and fingers of both hands, using a circular motion until the hair is partially dry. (Fig. 6)

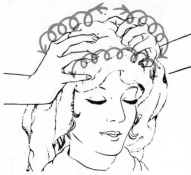

Fig. 6. Towel drying the hair.

COMPLETION

1. Comb hair, starting with the hair ends at the nape of the neck.
2. Set hair in the desired style.
3. Remove the shampoo cape, towel, or neck strip.
4. Dry hair under dryer, and comb out hair in appropriate style.

CLEANUP

1. Discard used materials, and place unused supplies in their proper place.
2. Remove hair from combs and brushes, wash with hot, soapy water, rinse, and place in wet sanitizer for required time.
3. Place used towels in towel hamper.
4. Clean and sanitize shampoo bowl.
5. Wash and sanitize hands.

SHAMPOOING LIGHTENED HAIR

Since lightened hair is likely to mat and tangle when wet, it must be handled with great care. The shampoo used should be mild or low in alkalinity.

Wet the hair with lukewarm water, pour shampoo on hair very slowly, and then lather the hair. Always work with the hands underneath the hair to avoid matting the hair. Rinse hair thoroughly with clear water. Apply a special cream rinse for lightened hair for easier combing. Towel dry hair carefully. Comb the hair gently. Do not force the comb through any tangles.

Note: Hair that has been tinted or damaged should be shampooed with the same care as lightened hair.

SAFETY PRECAUTIONS

1. Do not permit shampoo to get into patron's eyes.
2. Protect patron's ears with pledgets of clean cotton if she is sensitive to water in the ears.
3. Test the water temperature before applying to patron's head.
4. Do not permit the fingernails to scratch the patron's scalp.
5. Always towel blot excess moisture from patron's hair before she leaves the shampoo bowl.
6. Do not permit the shampoo cape to come in contact with patron's skin.
7. Use sanitized combs, brushes, towels, and other implements for each patron.
8. Do not turn the dryer to "hot" if the patron has high blood pressure.
9. Do not permit water to remain on the floor around the shampoo bowl.
10. Clean shampoo bowl, and sanitize the neck of the bowl after each use.

TYPES OF SHAMPOOS

PLAIN SHAMPOO

There are many types of shampoos available to the professional cosmetologist. Only through experience can she learn which type gives the best results. The student should follow the instructor's recommendations at all times.

Plain shampoos are usually clear and transparent, and may have a natural amber shade or colored a greenish yellow. They may contain a plain liquid soap or a detergent-based product. These shampoos seldom contain lanolin or other special agents that may be used to leave a gloss on the hair. If a liquid soap is used, it should be followed by an **acid rinse** to counteract its alkaline reaction on the hair.

A plain shampoo may be used on virgin hair that is in good condition. A plain shampoo should never be used on lightened, toned, tinted, or damaged hair. **It will strip or fade the color, and may further damage the hair.**

Shampoos for **oily** and **normal** hair can be of either the soap or soapless type of plain shampoo. Shampoos for oily hair usually contain a higher concentrate of soap or detergent.

SOAPLESS OIL SHAMPOOS

Soapless oil shampoos are made from synthetic detergents in which the oils have been treated with sulfuric acid. One of the main advantages of soapless shampoos is their effectiveness in both soft and hard water. They also rinse out easily and do not leave soap scum on the hair.

LIQUID CREAM SHAMPOOS

Liquid cream shampoos are usually semi-heavy white liquids and are used primarily on dry hair. As a rule, they are detergent-based products in which soap, or sometimes soap jelly, is used as the thickening agent. **Magnesium stearate** also is used as a whitening agent. Cream shampoos are mostly emulsions. They often contain oily compounds that make the hair feel silky and soft. Use this type of shampoo as directed by your instructor or manufacturer.

CREAM OR PASTE SHAMPOOS

Cream or paste shampoos are essentially the same as the liquid creams, except that more detergent material or more soap is used with less water. Some contain oily compounds to make the hair feel softer. Be guided by your instructor or manufacturer in their use.

ACID-BALANCED (NON-STRIP) SHAMPOOS

Hair and skin are considered to be slightly acid in nature, with a pH of about 5.5. Shampoos with the same pH (5.5) are considered to be acid balanced, and their use will not disturb or have any effect on the pH of the hair or skin.

Acid-balanced (non-strip) shampoos are formulated to prevent the stripping of tints or toners from the hair. They are mild in action, contain conditioners, and are low in alkaline content.

Acid-balanced shampoos also are recommended for brittle, dry, or damaged hair. Follow manufacturer's or instructor's instructions concerning their use.

ANTI-DANDRUFF SHAMPOOS

Anti-dandruff shampoos are used to control a dandruff condition of the scalp. They are made by adding a germicide to a plain shampoo. The appropriate anti-dandruff shampoo should be selected for either a dry or oily scalp condition. It is important that manufacturer's or instructor's directions be followed when using this type of shampoo.

HENNA SHAMPOO

The basic color produced by henna is reddish or auburn. The shade achieved depends on the original color of the hair, the strength of the henna mixture, and the length of time the mixture is left in the hair. Henna shampoo adds brightness to darker shades of hair rather than changes the color.

Note: *Do not use a henna shampoo on blonde, white, or grey hair, as it will give the hair an orange color.*

Materials

In addition to the required materials, you will need a measuring cup, henna powder, bowl, and spoon for mixing.

Procedure

Mix one cup of henna powder with very hot water to form a creamy paste.
1. Give hair a plain shampoo and rinse.
2. Make sure mixture is not too hot.
3. Pour mixture slowly through hair.
4. Work mixture well into hair.
5. Leave mixture on hair 5-15 minutes or longer, depending on desired shade.
6. Rinse with clear, warm water.
7. Shampoo and rinse.
If commercial product is used, follow manufacturer's directions.

LIQUID DRY SHAMPOOS

Liquid dry shampoos are cosmetic products used for cleansing the scalp and hair when the patron is prevented by illness from having a regular wet shampoo. These shampoos are made from benzene or gasoline.

CAUTION

Be sure that the room is well ventilated when using a liquid dry shampoo.

Procedure

1. Brush hair thoroughly and comb lightly.
2. Part hair in 1" (2.5 cm) sections from forehead to crown and crown to nape.
3. Saturate a piece of cotton with the cleaning liquid, squeeze out lightly, then rub briskly along each part. Follow this by swiftly rubbing with a towel along the part. Repeat this procedure all over the head. Next, apply cleaning liquid with cotton pledget down length of hair strands.
4. Rub the hair strands with the towel to remove soil.
5. Remoisten hair lightly with cleaning liquid; then set hair.

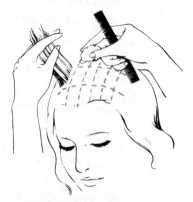

Liquid dry shampoo.

A dry shampoo will freshen the hair and tone the scalp without endangering the patron. (When using any type of shampoo, carefully read and follow manufacturer's directions.)

POWDER DRY SHAMPOO

A powder dry shampoo is usually given when the patron's health will not permit the giving of a wet shampoo.

A commercial powder dry shampoo containing orris root powder is freely sprinkled into the hair and worked in, one section at a time. This powder,

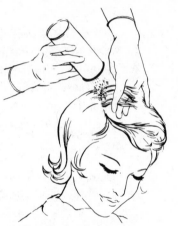

Powder dry shampoo.

which takes up the oil in the hair, is then brushed out of the hair with a long-bristled brush.

Brush the hair, strand by strand, until every trace of powder has been removed. Between strokes, the brush should be wiped on a clean towel to remove the dust and dirt.

If the patron desires and her health permits, a tonic rub may be applied to the scalp after the brushing. Do not give a powder dry shampoo before permanent waving or hair tinting.

SHAMPOOS FOR HAIRPIECES AND WIGS

Prepared wig cleaning solutions are now available. (See chapter on **The Care and Styling of Wigs.**)

OTHER TYPES OF SHAMPOOS

An **egg shampoo** is recommended for dry, brittle, over-lightened, or tinted hair. Commercial egg shampoos, containing small amounts of egg, are available. Apply as directed by manufacturer.

Highlighting shampoos. (See chapter on **Hair Coloring.**)

Castile and **oil shampoos** contain a coconut oil soap solution, dissolved flakes of castile soap, and a small amount of olive oil to prevent the excessive drying produced by the high alkali content of the soap.

They are neutral and mild in action when they contain a high grade castile soap. Be guided by your instructor.

Medicated shampoos contain special chemicals or drugs which are very effective in reducing excessive dandruff. They must be used only with a **physician's prescription** and **instruction**. They must not be used on tinted hair.

HAIR RINSES

A hair rinse consists of water alone or a mixture of water with a mild acid, coloring agent, or special ingredients.

ACID RINSES

Causes of soap scum. Minerals are present in all kinds of water; the more minerals, the harder the water. In soaps, there are fatty acids. The minerals and fatty acids combine to form a soap scum which dulls the hair and makes it difficult to comb.

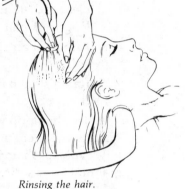

Rinsing the hair.

It is impossible to remove all the soap curds from the hair with ordinary water.

Special acid rinses now on the market actually remove soap curds from the hair, thus making combing easier, and at the same time, adding brilliance to the hair. Follow manufacturer's directions.

The main ingredients of prepared acid hair rinses are:

Citric acid—from the juice of the lime, orange, or lemon.

Tartaric acid—obtained from residues in wine making.

Acetic acid—present in vinegar.

Lactic acid—lactose, or sugar of milk.

Acid rinses are used to dissolve soap curds, separate the hair, and make it soft, pliable, and bright.

An acid rinse also may be used to counteract the alkilinity of hair after a tint, lightener, or cold wave application.

Most acid rinses, whether solid or liquid, are dissolved in water before they are used.

CAUTION

Do not use an acid rinse without diluting it with water, as pure acid can seriously burn the scalp.

Procedure

1. Mix 1 cup (236 ml) of acid rinse with 1 pint (.473 l) of warm water, and apply as the last rinse after a shampoo.
2. Rinse the hair with the mixture several times.
3. Finally, rinse the hair with clear warm water to remove all traces of the acid rinse.

CREAM RINSES

A cream rinse is a commercial product with a creamy appearance, and it is used as a last rinse. It tends to soften the hair, add luster, and make tangled hair easier to comb.

To be effective, cream rinses depend on one or more chemicals having one property in common—they stick to the hair. Some substances adhere to the hair shaft and are not washed off by ordinary rinsing. The result is that the hair has a nice soft feel, and is much easier to comb and handle.

A cream rinse does not have the same function as an acid rinse. Cream rinses are slightly acid in reaction as a result of the nature of the ingredients used. However, the acidity is so low that, in the dilutions used, it would have no effect as a soap (curd) remover.

ACID-BALANCED (NON-STRIP) RINSES

Acid-balanced (non-strip) rinses are formulated to prevent the stripping of color after a tint or toner application. They help close and harden the cuticle imbrications that were swollen and opened by the alkaline tint or toner. Most manufacturers formulate this type of rinse in connection with their own particular tint or toner products.

RECONDITIONING RINSE

A reconditioning rinse is used after a tint application. Follow manufacturer's directions.

MEDICATED RINSES

Medicated rinses are formulated with some medicinal properties to control minor conditions of dandruff. Follow manufacturer's instructions.

COLOR RINSES

Color rinses are used to highlight or add temporary color to the hair. These rinses remain on the hair until the next shampoo. (For additional information see chapter on **Hair Coloring.**)

HENNA RINSE

A henna rinse is used as a final rinse to give an auburn tinge to the hair. It can be used over darker shades, but not over blonde, grey, or white hair.

Procedure

1. Dissolve 1 ounce (28.4 g) of henna powder in 1 quart (.946 l) of very hot tap water.
2. Shampoo the patron's hair and pour solution over her head 3-4 times.
3. Allow the liquid to remain on the hair for about 10 minutes.
4. Rinse it off with warm water.

This will furnish warm subtle highlights to brunette hair, and make it slightly redder in tone.

REVIEW QUESTIONS

SHAMPOOING

1. Why is a cosmetologist who can give a professional shampoo a valuable asset to a salon?
2. In order to be effective, what must the shampoo be capable of doing?
3. Which type of shampoo will have a damaging effect on the hair?
4. Why is it necessary to cleanse the scalp and hair regularly?
5. How often should the hair be shampooed?
6. What two classifications of water are there?
7. What determines the classification of water?
8. Which important steps precede the shampoo?
9. When brushing the hair, why are brushes with natural bristles preferable to brushes with nylon bristles?
10. How does brushing the hair benefit the hair and scalp?
11. List five conditions under which hair brushing is omitted before a shampoo.
12. What are the main steps in shampooing the hair?
13. What is done with leftover supplies after the shampoo?
14. When does the cosmetologist wash and sanitize her hands?
15. List seven types of shampoos.
16. When is a non-strip shampoo recommended?
17. When is a liquid dry shampoo recommended?

RINSES

1. What are hair rinses?
2. What type of rinses remove soap curds from the hair?
3. Name four types of acids used in rinses.
4. What benefits do acid rinses have on the hair?
5. Under what circumstances do acid rinses counteract the alkilinity of hair?
6. How does a cream rinse affect the hair?
7. What is a non-strip rinse?
8. How long do color rinses last?
9. When is a henna rinse used?
10. For what type of hair should a henna rinse not be used?

Chapter 9

SCALP AND HAIR CARE

CHAPTER LEARNING OBJECTIVES

The student successfully mastering this chapter will know:
1. *The purpose of scalp and hair care.*
2. *The normal and abnormal conditions of the scalp and hair.*
3. *The various scalp and hair disorders encountered in the beauty salon.*
4. *The scalp manipulations used, and the techniques required, for corrective scalp and hair treatments.*
5. *The purpose of the cosmetics used in scalp and hair care.*

The purpose of scalp treatments is to preserve the health and beauty of the hair and scalp. They also assist in overcoming disorders of the scalp, such as dandruff and excessive loss of hair.

A basic requisite for a healthy scalp is cleanliness. The scalp and hair should be kept clean by frequent treatment and shampooing. A clean scalp will resist a wide variety of disorders.

Scalp manipulations stimulate the circulation of the blood to the scalp, relax and soothe the nerves, stimulate the muscles and the activity of scalp glands, render a tight scalp more flexible, and help maintain the growth and health of the hair.

While shampooing will keep the hair clean, it will not prevent the hair from becoming dry and brittle. The cosmetologist, therefore, should always recommend the proper cosmetic applications to counteract the danger of either a dry and scaly scalp or an excessively oily condition of the scalp and hair.

Because the scalp and hair are vitally related, many scalp disorders need correction in order to keep the hair healthy. A healthy scalp contributes to the growth of healthy hair. The cosmetologist treats only common and minor conditions.

Do not suggest a scalp treatment:
1. If there are scalp abrasions, or if there is a scalp disorder.
2. Immediately prior to the application of a lightener, tint, toner, permanent wave, or a chemical hair relaxing treatment.

Advise patron to consult a physician for serious or contagious scalp ailments. However, conditions caused by neglect, such as tight scalp, over-active or inactive oil glands, and tense nerves, can be corrected or alleviated by proper scalp treatments.

PREPARATION OF PATRON FOR SCALP TREATMENT

As in any other salon service, first gather all the necessary equipment according to the kind of scalp treatment you are about to give.

Prepare the patron by proper draping, removing all hairpins from the hair, and combing out tangles.

Brush hair. Brushing always should be an essential part of every scalp treatment. Not only will proper brushing, with a good natural bristle brush, help to stimulate circulation to the scalp, it also will help to remove dust and dirt from the hair, and give it added luster and sheen. (For instructions on hair brushing, see chapter on **Shampooing and Rinsing.**)

SCALP MANIPULATIONS

Since the same manipulations are given with all scalp treatments, the cosmetologist should learn to give them with a continuous, even motion, **which will stimulate the scalp and/or soothe the patron's tension.** Scalp massage is most effectively applied as a series of treatments, once a week for normal scalp, and more frequently for scalp disorders, under the direction of a dermatologist.

ANATOMY

Knowing the muscles, the location of blood vessels, and the nerve points of the scalp and neck will help guide the cosmetologist to those areas in which massage movements are to be directed for the most beneficial results.

SCALP MANIPULATION TECHNIQUE

There are several ways in which scalp manipulations may be given. The following routine may be changed to meet your instructor's requirements.

With each massage movement, place the hands under the hair so the length of the fingers, balls of the fingertips and cushions of the palms can stimulate the muscles, nerves, and blood vessels of the scalp area.

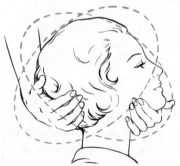

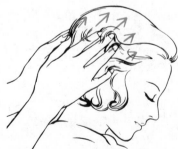

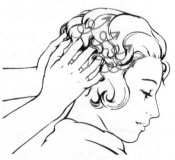

1. RELAXING MOVEMENT. Cup the patron's chin in your left hand; place your right hand at the base of her skull, and rotate head gently. Reverse positions of your hands and repeat.

2. SLIDING MOVEMENT. Place your fingertips on each side of the patron's head; slide your hands firmly upward, spreading the fingertips until they meet at the top of the head. Repeat four times.

3. SLIDING AND ROTATING MOVEMENT. Same as movement No. 2, except that after sliding the fingertips 1", you rotate and move the patron's scalp. Repeat four times.

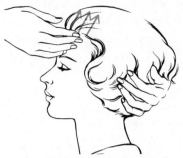

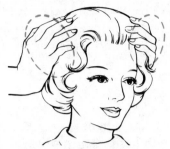

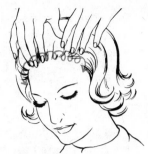

4. FOREHEAD MOVEMENT.
Hold the back of the patron's head with your left hand. Place stretched thumb and fingers of your right hand on the patron's forehead. Move your hand slowly and firmly upward to 1" past the hairline. Repeat four times.

5. SCALP MOVEMENT. *Place the palms of your hands firmly against the patron's scalp. Lift the scalp in a rotary movement, first with your hands placed above her ears, and second with your hands placed at the front and back of her head.*

6. HAIRLINE MOVEMENT. *Place the fingers of both hands at the patron's forehead. Massage around her hairline by lifting and rotating.*

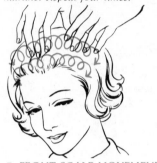

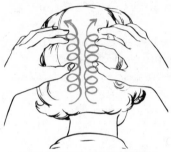

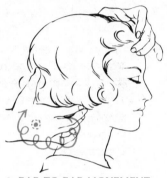

7. FRONT SCALP MOVEMENT.
Dropping back 1", repeat preceding movement over entire front and top of the scalp.

8. BACK SCALP MOVEMENT.
Place the fingers of each hand on the sides of the patron's head. Starting below her ears, manipulate the scalp with your thumbs, working upward to the crown. Repeat four times, Repeat thumb manipulations, working towards the center back of the head.

9. EAR-TO-EAR MOVEMENT.
Place your left hand on the patron's forehead. Massage from the right ear to the left ear along the base of her skull with the heel of your hand, using a rotary movement.

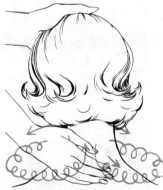

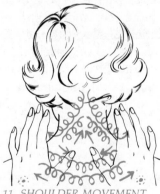

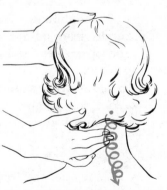

10. BACK MOVEMENT. *Place your left hand on the patron's forehead and stand to the left of her. Using your right hand, rotate from the base of the patron's neck, along the shoulder, and back across the shoulder blade to the spine. Slide your hand up the patron's spine to the base of her neck. Repeat on the opposite side.*

11. SHOULDER MOVEMENT.
Place both your palms together at the base of the patron's neck. With rotary movement, catch muscles in the palms and massage along the shoulder blades to the point of her shoulders, and then back again. Then massage from the shoulders to the spine and back again.

12. SPINE MOVEMENT. *Massage from the base of the patron's skull down the spine with a rotary movement. Using a firm finger pressure, bring your hand slowly to the base of the patron's skull.*

TREATMENT FOR NORMAL HAIR AND SCALP

The purpose of a general scalp treatment is to keep the scalp and hair in a clean and healthy condition. Regular scalp treatments also are beneficial in preventing baldness.

PREPARATION

1. Assemble materials and supplies.
2. Help the patron with her dress or blouse.
3. Prepare patron. (Drape properly.)

PROCEDURE

1. Brush hair for about 5 minutes.
2. Apply scalp pomade or cream.
3. Apply infra-red lamp for about 5 minutes.
4. Give scalp manipulations for 10-20 minutes.
5. Shampoo the hair.
6. Towel dry the hair to remove excess moisture.
7. Apply suitable scalp lotion or tonic.
8. Set, dry, and style hair.
9. Clean up your work station.

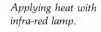

Applying heat with infra-red lamp.

DANDRUFF TREATMENT

The principal signs of dandruff are the appearance of white scales on the hair and scalp which may be accompanied by itching of the scalp. Dandruff may be associated with either a dry or oily scalp condition. The more common causes of dandruff are poor circulation of blood to the scalp, improper diet, uncleanliness, and infection. To prevent the spread of dandruff in the beauty salon, the cosmetologist must sanitize all implements and avoid the common use of combs, brushes, and scalp applicators.

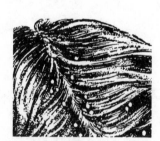

Simple dandruff.

PROCEDURE

1. Prepare the patron as for a normal scalp treatment.
2. Brush the patron's hair for 5 minutes.
3. Apply a scalp preparation according to the scalp's condition (dry or oily).
4. Apply infra-red lamp for about 5 minutes.
5. Give scalp manipulations, using indirect high-frequency current.
6. Shampoo with corrective anti-dandruff lotion.

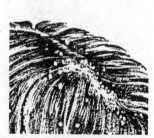

Excessive dandruff.

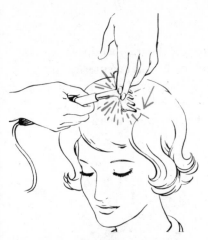

Applying high-frequency with glass rake electrode.

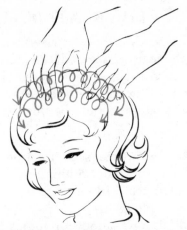

Applying indirect high-frequency current, cosmetologist manipulates the scalp . . .

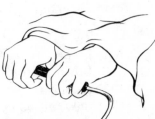

. . . while the patron holds metal electrode.

7. Thoroughly towel dry the hair.
8. Use direct high-frequency current for 3-5 minutes.
9. Apply scalp preparation suitable for the condition.
10. Set, dry, and style the hair.
11. Clean up your work station.

DRY HAIR AND SCALP TREATMENT

This treatment should be used when there is a deficiency of natural oil on the scalp and hair. Select scalp preparations containing moisturizing and emollient materials. Avoid the use of strong soaps, preparations containing a mineral oil or sulfonated oil base, greasy preparations, and lotions with a high alcoholic content.

PROCEDURE

1. Prepare patron as for a normal scalp treatment.
2. Brush patron's hair for about 5 minutes.
3. Apply the scalp preparation for this condition, as directed by manufacturer or your instructor.
4. Apply the scalp steamer for 7-10 minutes, or wrap the head in warm steam towels for 7-10 minutes. Be guided by your instructor.
5. Give a mild shampoo.
6. Towel dry the hair and scalp thoroughly.
7. Apply moisturizing scalp cream sparingly with a rotary, frictional motion.
8. Stimulate the scalp with direct high-frequency current, using the glass rake electrode, for about 5 minutes.
9. Set, dry, and style the hair.
10. Clean up your work station.

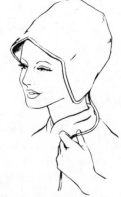

Scalp steamer.

OILY HAIR AND SCALP TREATMENT

Excessive oiliness is caused by the over-activity of the sebaceous (oil) glands. Manipulate the scalp and knead it to increase the blood circulation to the scalp. Any hardened sebum in the pores of the scalp will be removed with the correct degree of pressing and squeezing. To normalize the function of these glands, excess sebum should be flushed out with each treatment.

PROCEDURE

1. Prepare patron as for normal scalp treatment.
2. Brush patron's hair for about 5 minutes.
3. Apply a medicated scalp lotion to the scalp only with a cotton pledget.
4. Apply infra-red lamp for about 5 minutes.
5. Give scalp manipulations. (Optional: Faradic or sinusoidal current may be used.)
6. Shampoo with a corrective shampoo for oily scalp.
7. Towel dry the hair.
8. Apply direct high-frequency current for 3-5 minutes.
9. Apply a scalp tonic containing an astringent base.
10. Set, dry, and style the hair.
11. Clean up your work station.

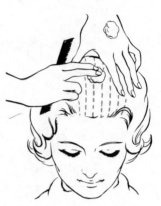

Applying scalp lotion with cotton pledget.

CAUTION

Creams or ointments may be applied **before** using high-frequency current. Hair tonics or lotions with alcoholic content may be applied only **after** the application of high-frequency current.

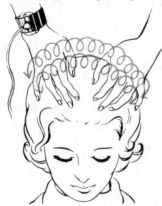

Applying faradic current. Manipulate the scalp while the patron holds the electrode.

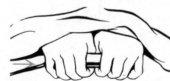

CORRECTIVE HAIR TREATMENT

A corrective hair treatment deals with the **hair shaft,** not the scalp. Dry and damaged hair can be greatly improved by conditioners. Hair treatments are especially beneficial and extremely important when given approximately a week or 10 days before, and a week or 10 days after, a permanent wave, tint, lightener, toner, or chemical hair straightening treatment.

Dry hair may be softened quickly with a conditioning preparation applied directly on the hair shaft. The product used for this purpose is usually an emulsion containing cholesterol and related compounds.

Some conditioners function more effectively when heat is applied to induce penetration into the cortex. The heat applied to the hair opens the cuticle's imbrications, and permits significantly more corrective agents to enter the hair shaft. This provides more conditioning and more lasting benefits.

PROCEDURE

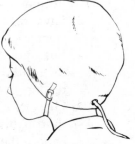

1. Prepare patron as for a normal scalp treatment.
2. Brush the patron's hair for about 5 minutes.
3. Apply a mild shampoo.
4. Towel dry the hair.
5. Apply a conditioner according to manufacturer's directions.
6. Set, dry, and style hair.
7. Clean up your work station.

Applying heat.

TREATMENT FOR ALOPECIA

Alopecia refers to a condition of premature baldness or excessive hair loss. The chief causes of alopecia are poor circulation, lack of proper stimulation, improper nourishment, certain infectious skin diseases, such as ringworm, or constitutional disorders. The treatment for alopecia is directed to stimulating the blood supply to the scalp and reviving the hair papillae involved in hair growth.

PROCEDURE

1. Prepare patron as for a normal scalp treatment.
2. Brush the patron's hair for about 5 minutes.
3. Apply a medicated scalp ointment as directed by a physician.
4. Apply infra-red light for about 5 minutes.
5. Give scalp manipulations. You may use the faradic or indirect high-frequency current.
6. Use a mild shampoo.
7. Towel dry the hair.
8. Apply direct high-frequency current for about 5 minutes.
9. Apply medicated scalp lotion.
10. Repeat scalp manipulations; include neck, shoulders, and upper back.
11. Set hair; dry with warm or cool air, and style hair.
12. Clean up your work station.

REMINDERS AND HINTS ON SCALP AND HAIR CARE

1. An abnormal scalp and hair condition requires very careful analysis in order to give the appropriate scalp and hair treatment.
2. Some scalp conditions may be infectious. Therefore, use only sanitized implements on patrons.

TREATMENT FOR ALOPECIA AREATA

Alopecia areata is a disorder causing baldness in spots. This condition may be treated under the direction of a physician.

PROCEDURE

1. Prepare the patron as for a normal scalp treatment.
2. Give regular scalp manipulations.
3. Shampoo the hair according to its condition; if scalp is very tender, use a mild shampoo.
4. Dry the hair and scalp thoroughly.
5. Expose the scalp to ultra-violet rays for 5-10 minutes, especially the bald spots.

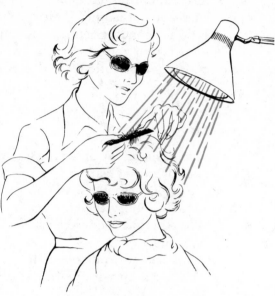

Applying ultra-violet rays.

6. Apply ointment or lotion with light manipulations on the bald spots.
7. Apply high-frequency current for about 5 minutes. If an ointment is used, apply direct current; if a lotion is used, apply indirect current.
8. Style the hair, using a comb only.
9. Clean up your work station.

REVIEW QUESTIONS
SCALP AND HAIR CARE

1. What is the purpose of giving scalp treatments?
2. What benefits are obtained from effective scalp manipulations?
3. Why is a healthy scalp necessary for the growth of healthy hair?
4. Which scalp disorders are commonly treated in the beauty salon?
5. When should a scalp treatment not be given?
6. What benefits are obtained from regular hair brushing?
7. How often should scalp massage be given?
8. Why do normal hair and scalp require scalp treatments?
9. What are the common causes of dandruff?
10. What causes excessive oiliness in hair?
11. What precautions are required when using high-frequency current with hair tonics or lotions?
12. How can dry and damaged hair be improved?
13. What is alopecia?
14. What is alopecia areata?

Chapter 10

HAIR SHAPING

CHAPTER LEARNING OBJECTIVES

The student successfully mastering this chapter will know:

1. *Why professional hair shaping is a foundation for hairstyling or permanent waving.*
2. *The correct use of the basic hair shaping implements.*
3. *Proper hair sectioning, and its relationship to professional hair shaping.*
4. *How to cut and use a guideline in hair shaping.*
5. *The various techniques used in hair thinning.*
6. *The basic techniques for shaping with scissors or with a razor.*
7. *Definitions pertaining to hair shaping.*

The art and technique of hair shaping must be mastered by the student of cosmetology before she can be qualified to work in the better salons. Thorough instruction is required in the proper way to shape the hair, using either regular scissors, thinning shears, or razor. Instruction must be followed by practice under the guidance of the instructor. A good hair shaping serves as a foundation for beautiful coiffures. The cosmetologist's education is not complete until she has acquired the artistic skill and judgment necessary for successful hair shaping.

Modern hairstyles are designed to accentuate the patron's good points while minimizing her poor features. The cosmetologist must be guided by the patron's wishes, as well as by what is best for her personality. In selecting the proper hairstyle, the cosmetologist should take into consideration the patron's head shape, facial contour, neckline, and hair texture.

IMPLEMENTS USED IN HAIR SHAPING

A cosmetologist will find that the quality of the implements she selects and uses in hair shaping is important. To do her best work, the cosmetologist should buy and use only superior implements from a reliable manufacturer.

Improper use quickly will destroy the efficiency of any implement, however perfectly it might be made at the factory.

The following are the implements used in hair shaping:

Regular hair shaping scissors
Thinning shears (single- or double-notched blades)
Straight razors
Razors with safety guards
Combs
Hair clippers

HAIR SHAPING IMPLEMENTS

HAIRCUTTING SCISSORS

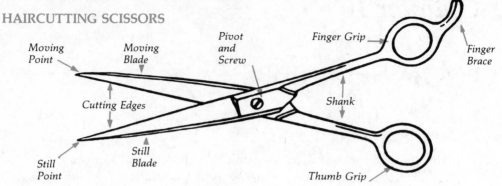

Moving Point · Moving Blade · Pivot and Screw · Finger Grip · Finger Brace · Cutting Edges · Shank · Still Point · Still Blade · Thumb Grip

THINNING SHEARS

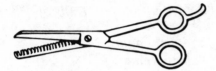

Thinning Shears—One Blade Notched

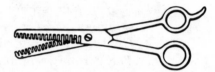

Thinning Shears—Both Blades Notched

STRAIGHT RAZOR

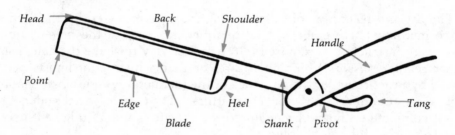

Head · Back · Shoulder · Handle · Point · Edge · Blade · Heel · Shank · Pivot · Tang

RAZORS WITH SAFETY GUARDS

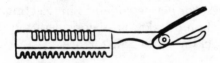

Single Edge Razor with Safety Guard

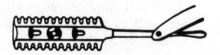

Double Edge Razor with Safety Guard

POPULAR COMBS

Large-Tooth Comb

Tail (Rat-Tail) Comb

All-Purpose Comb

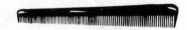

Hair Shaping Comb

SECTIONING FOR HAIR SHAPING

By following a step-by-step practical procedure, the student will soon learn how to give a professional hair shaping. The first step is to section the hair properly. The following illustrations cover the practical and accepted methods for dividing the hair into either four or five sections. In any case, follow your instructor's methods for dry or wet hair shaping.

FOUR SECTION PARTING

Part hair down the center from forehead to nape, and also across the top of the head from ear to ear. Pin up the four sections and leave nape hair to use as a guide.

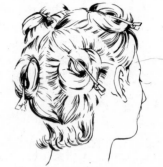

FIVE SECTION PARTING

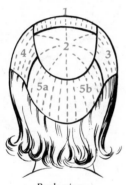

Back view.

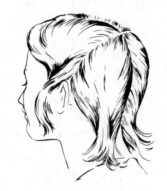

Top section No. 1 may be sub-parted either in a horizontal or vertical direction.

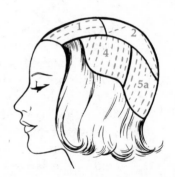

Side view.

Five section parting, with sub-parting panels. Section and pin up hair in the order shown in the illustrations.

The back section (No. 5) may be divided into sections No. 5a and No. 5b for easier handling.

ALTERNATE FIVE SECTION METHOD

Another way to divide the hair into five sections is to part the hair across the crown from ear to ear; then to sub-divide the hair in the same order as shown in the illustration.

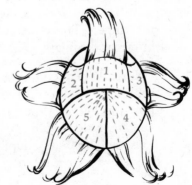

Hair divided into five sections with center back parting.

HOLDING HAIR SHAPING IMPLEMENTS

SCISSORS (SHEARS)

Hair shaping scissors are correctly handled by inserting the third (ring) finger into the ring of the still blade, and placing the little finger on the finger brace. The thumb is inserted into the ring of the movable blade. The tip of the index finger is braced near the pivot of the scissors in order to have better control. (Fig. 1)

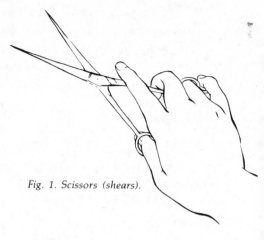

Fig. 1. Scissors (shears).

THINNING SHEARS

Excess bulk is removed from the hair by the use of thinning shears. As can be seen in the accompanying illustration (Fig. 2), they are quite similar to hair shaping scissors, except they have one or both blades notched or serrated. The single notched edge cuts more hair. Which one is used depends on the preference of the cosmetologist. The notches help the cosmetologist control the amount of hair that is removed. Both thinning shears and shaping scissors are held in the same way.

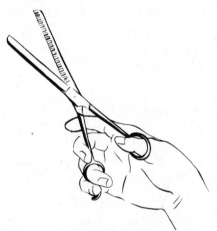

Fig. 2. Thinning shears with one blade notched.

COMB AND SCISSORS

Whenever it is necessary to use the comb during hair shaping, close the blades of the scissors, remove thumb from the ring, and rest scissors in the palm. Hold the scissors securely with the ring finger. The comb is held with the thumb and fingers. (Fig. 3)

Note: When combing the hair, hold comb and scissors in the right hand, as shown in Fig. 3. When shaping (cutting) the hair, hold the comb in the left hand. To speed up hair shaping, do not lay down comb or scissors.

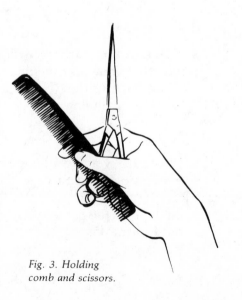

Fig. 3. Holding comb and scissors.

HAIR THINNING

The purpose of thinning the hair is to remove the excess bulk without shortening its length. For best results, use the following suggestions:

1. When using a razor for thinning or shaping, first dampen the hair.
2. When using thinning shears or regular scissors, the hair may be either dry or damp.

The **hair texture** determines the point where thinning should start on the hair strand. As a rule, **fine hair** may be thinned closer to the scalp than coarse hair. Why? Because if coarse hair is thinned too close to the scalp, the short, stubby ends will protrude through the top layer. On the other hand, fine hair is softer and more pliable, and when cut very short will lay flatter on the head.

How much to thin depends on the particular hairstyle to be created. As a guide, start thinning different textures of hair as follows:

1. Fine hair—½-1″ (1.25-2.5 cm) from the scalp.
2. Medium hair—1-1½″ (2.5-3.75 cm) from the scalp.
3. Coarse hair—1½-2″ (3.75-5 cm) from the scalp.

HAIR THINNING AREAS

There are several areas where it is not advisable to thin the hair:

1. At the nape of the neck (ear to ear).
2. At the side of the head, above ears.
3. Around facial hairline. Usually hair is not heavy at hairline.
4. In the hair part. The cut ends would be seen in the finished hairstyle.

Note: Never thin the hair near the ends of a strand; to do so will render the hair shapeless.

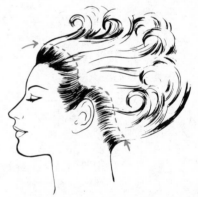

Hair in shaded areas does not require thinning.

REMINDER

Great care must be exercised to avoid removing too much hair in the thinning process. Once the hair has been cut, it is impossible to replace it and it is probable that it might become impossible to develop the desired hairstyle.

THINNING WITH THINNING SHEARS

When using the thinning shears, grip the hair firmly by overlapping the middle finger a trifle over the index finger.

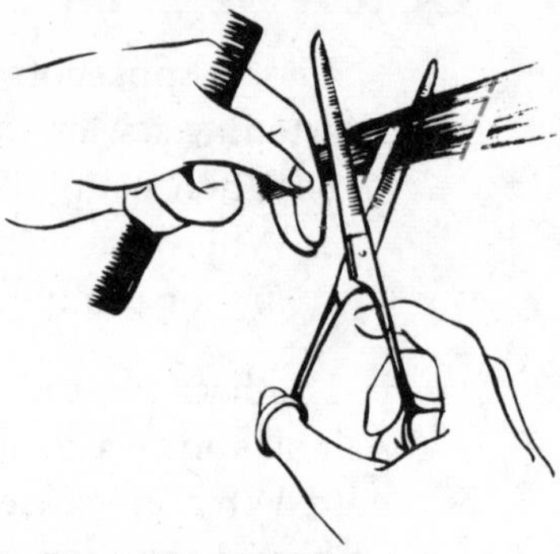

Procedure

1. Pick up a strand of hair from ½-1″ (1.25-2.5 cm) wide by 2-3″ (5-7.5 cm) long, depending on its texture.
2. Hold the strand straight out from the scalp between the middle and index fingers.
3. Place thinning shears 1-2″ (2.5-5 cm) from the scalp.
4. Cut the strand by partly closing the thinning shears 3/4 through the strand. (Fig. 1)
5. Move out another 1½″ (3.75 cm) and cut again.
6. Repeat again if the hair is long enough.

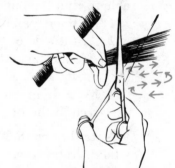

Fig. 1. Thinning with thinning shears.

Note: It is advisable to avoid thinning the top part of the strand.

THINNING WITH HAIRCUTTING SCISSORS (SHEARS)

When using regular haircutting scissors to thin the hair, pick up smaller sections of hair than when using the thinning shears. The technique also is changed. This process of thinning with scissors is known as **slithering.**

Procedure

1. Hold a strand of hair straight out between the middle and index fingers.
2. Place the hair in the scissors so that only the underneath hair will be cut.
3. Slide the scissors about 1-1½″ (2.5-3.75 cm) down the strand, closing them slightly each time the scissors are moved toward the scalp. (Fig. 2)
4. Repeat this procedure twice on each strand.

Fig. 2. Thinning with haircutting scissors (shears).

Note: Alternate method of holding the hair is with the thumb and index finger. (Fig. 3)

Back-combing. The short hair may be back-combed and then slithered, as shown in Fig. 4.

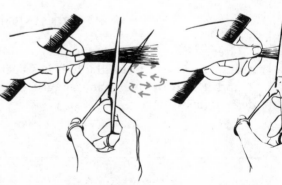

Fig. 3. Holding the hair with thumb and index finger.

Fig. 4. Slithering the hair after back-combing.

HAIR SHAPING WITH SCISSORS

Scissor hair shaping may be done either on dry or wet hair.

Dry shaping. If the hair is shaped while dry, it usually is shampooed after the shaping is completed.

Wet shaping. The hair may be shaped immediately after it has been shampooed.

PREPARATION

1. Seat patron; adjust neck strip and plastic cape.
2. Examine head shape, facial features, and hair texture.
3. Comb and brush hair free of tangles.
4. Shaping may be done on dry or damp hair.

PROCEDURE

1. Divide hair into five sections.
2. Determine the length of the nape guideline hair.
3. Blunt cut guideline strand of nape hair. (Fig. 1)
    a) Blunt cut strand on left side, using the earlobe as guide. (Fig. 2)
    b) Blunt cut strand on right side to match left side. (Fig. 2)

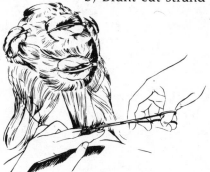

Fig. 1. Blunt cutting strand at center nape to desired length.

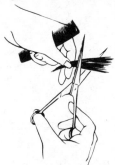

Blunt cutting.

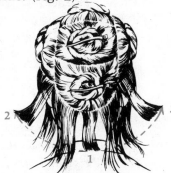

Fig. 2. Following up by cutting all remaining guideline hair.

c) Blunt cut from back center to left front.
d) Blunt cut from back center to right front. For completed guideline, see Fig. 3.

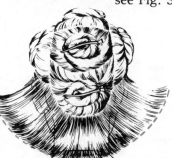

Fig. 3. Properly cut guideline hair.

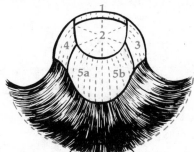

Fig. 4. Divide section No. 5 into two equal parts.

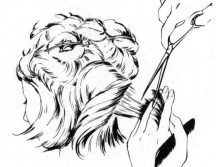

Fig. 5. Blunt cutting section No. 5b.

Let down section No. 5 and divide into two equal parts (No. 5a and No. 5b). Match length with guideline hair. Either left side or right side may be done first (Fig. 4). Hold hair panels out from the head while blunt cutting (Fig. 5). Continue cutting sections No. 3 and No. 4 in the same manner.

CROWN SECTION

Crown section No. 2. Hold pie-shaped strands out from the head; match length by picking up strands from section already cut. Continue around the head, matching length with sides and back hair. (Figs. 6 and 7)

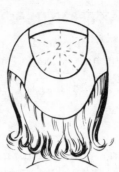

Fig. 6. Crown section.

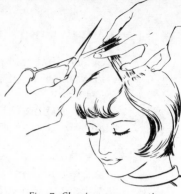

Fig. 7. Shaping crown section.

TOP SECTION

Divide section No. 1 into two parts. Pick up hair from the middle of the section, using previously cut hair as a guide. Maintain the hand movement in a 45° (.785 rad.) arc. Proceed to cut both parts of section No. 1 in the prescribed manner. (Figs. 8 and 9)

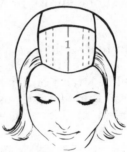

Fig. 8. Top view. Section No. 1 with vertical partings.

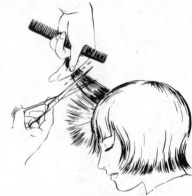

Fig. 9. Shaping top section.

If **bangs** are to be cut, move from side to directly in front of the patron for even cutting. Test hair for bounce (elasticity); then determine desired length. If bangs are to be short, use the bridge of the nose as a guide. If style is to be long, shape strands to blend into the length of the sides.

Reducing bulk. To complete shaping the hair, remove excess bulk by thinning with a razor, thinning shears, or scissors. It is recommended that all hair be checked for proper length.

COMPLETION

Remove neck strip and plastic cape. Thoroughly clean all hair clippings

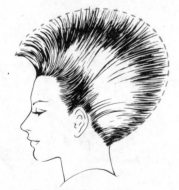

Correct uniform shaping.

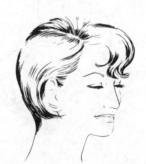

Completed shaping with bang effect and/or off-face style.

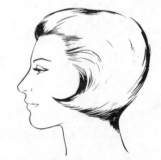

Hair shaping for straight back style.

from cape, patron's clothing, and from work area. You may then proceed with the next professional service desired by the patron.

SHINGLING

Shingling is cutting the hair close to the nape and gradually longer toward the crown, without showing a definite line.

Regardless of the prevailing hair fashion, there always will be a number of patrons who want their hair cut short. To satisfy these patrons, you must know how to shingle the hair. The accompanying illustrations show how shingling is accomplished with the use of shears and comb.

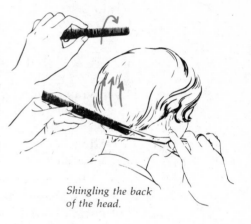

Outlining neckline.

PROCEDURE

Shingling should be done at eye level. Starting at the napeline, cut the hair upward in a graduated effect. After reaching the top of the section being shingled, turn the comb downward and comb the hair. Proceed, section by section, until the entire back of the head is shingled in a smooth, uniform manner.

Note: In shingling, the blades of the scissors are held parallel with the comb; only the top blade moves and does the cutting.

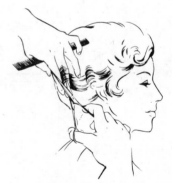

Shingling the back of the head.

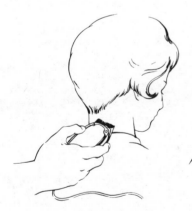

Cleaning neck with clippers.

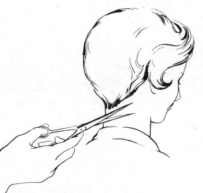

Cleaning neck with points of scissors.

Removing hair ends.

USE OF CLIPPERS

There is a mistaken notion that the use of clippers to clean the neckline has a tendency to make the hair grow thicker on the neck. This is not true, as the amount of human hair can only be as great as the number of follicles in the area, and these do not increase in number with the use of clippers or any other implement.

USING THE RAZOR

The successful cosmetologist must be able to handle all the implements efficiently, including the straight razor.

HOW TO HOLD THE RAZOR

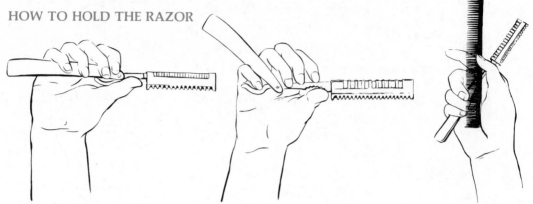

Fig. 1. Finger wrap hold.   Fig. 2. Three finger hold.   Fig. 3. Holding razor and comb.

Finger wrap hold. Place the thumb in the groove part of the shank and fold the fingers over the handle of the razor. The guard faces the cosmetologist while working. (Fig. 1)

Three finger hold. Place three fingers over the shank, the thumb in the groove of the shank, and the little finger in the hollow part of the tang. (Fig. 2)

Note: When combing the hair, hold the razor and comb in the right hand. (Fig. 3) When shaping the hair with a razor, hold the comb in the left hand. Do not put down the comb or razor.

When using the razor, keep the hair damp, in order to avoid pulling the hair, and to prevent dulling the razor.

CHANGING BLADES

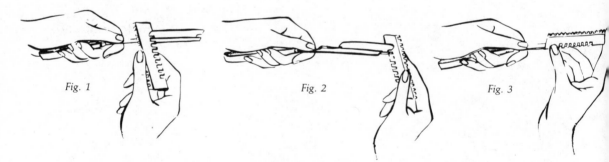

Fig. 1   Fig. 2   Fig. 3

Removing old blade. Remove guard. With left hand, hold shaper firmly above joint. Catch the blade in the teeth of the upper part of guard and push out blade. (Fig. 1)

Inserting new blade. Slide blade into groove, pushing the end with your fingers. Place the tooth end of guard into the blade notch and slide the blade in until it clicks into position. (Fig. 2)

Slide the guard over blade, making sure free or open end is over cutting edge of blade. (Fig. 3)

THINNING WITH RAZOR

Hold a strand of wet hair straight out between the middle and index fingers. Place the razor flat, **not erect,** about 1-2″ (2.5-5 cm) from the scalp (depending on the hair texture), and use short, steady strokes toward the hair ends.

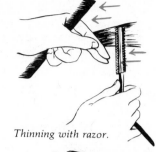

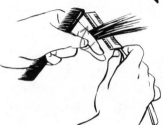

Thinning with razor.

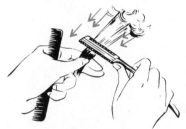

Tapering hair ends after back-combing.

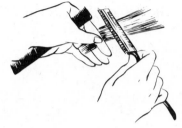

Blunt razor cutting.

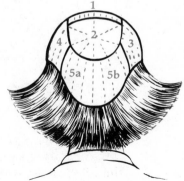

Razor under-cutting with upward stroke.

HAIR SHAPING WITH RAZOR

PREPARATION

1. Seat the patron; adjust neck strip and plastic cape.
2. Examine head shape, facial features and hair texture.
3. Comb and brush the hair free of tangles.
4. Shampoo or wet the hair.

PROCEDURE

1. Divide the hair into five sections.
2. Determine the length of the nape guideline hair.
3. Blunt cut guideline strand of nape hair. (Fig. 1)
   a) Blunt cut strand on the left side; use the earlobe as guide. (Fig. 2)
   b) Blunt cut strand on the right side to match the left side. (Fig. 2)
   c) Use guideline hair to cut from the back center to the left front and back center to the right front. (Fig. 2)
   d) Completed guideline. (Fig. 3)

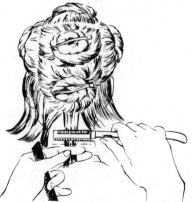

Fig. 1. Blunt cutting a strand at center nape for desired hair length.

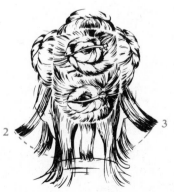

Fig. 2. Following up by cutting all remaining guideline hair.

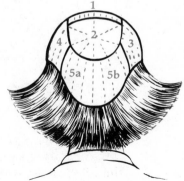

Fig. 3. Completed guideline.

Shaping back section (5a, 5b). Divide section No. 5 into two parts (sections No. 5a and No. 5b). From center of section No. 5a, pick horizontal strands. Pick up a guideline strand for length. When guideline hair falls away, cut hair—moving hands out and upward into a 45° (.785 rad.) arc.

Shaping section 4. Proceed to cut to the left into section No. 4 in the same manner.

Shaping section 3. Return to section No. 5b and cut this section, moving to the right into section No. 3, always lifting hands in an upward 45° (.785 rad.) arc as the hair is cut. **Measure carefully with guideline hair.**

Shaping section 2. Next, proceed to cut section No. 2 (crown), using previously cut hair as a guide.

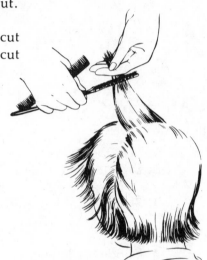

Shaping section No. 5a.

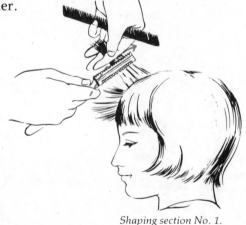

Section No. 2.

Shaping section No. 2.

Shaping section 1. Divide section No. 1 into two parts. Pick up hair from the middle of the section, using previously cut hair as a guide. Maintain the hand movement in a 45° (.785 rad.) arc. Proceed to cut both parts of section No. 1 in the prescribed manner.

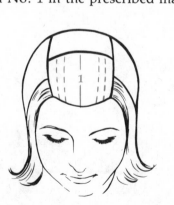

Section No. 1 shown with vertical parting.

Shaping section No. 1.

Bangs. To cut bangs evenly, move your position from the side to directly in front of the patron. Test hair for bounce (elasticity), then determine desired length. If bangs are to be short, use the bridge of nose as a guide. If style is to be long, shape strands to blend into the length of the sides.

Reducing bulk. To complete shaping the hair, remove excess bulk by thinning with a razor, thinning shears, or scissors. It is recommended that all hair be checked for proper length.

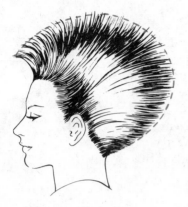
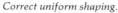

Correct uniform shaping.

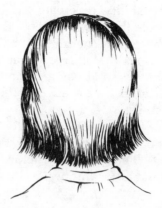

Back view—uniform shaping.

Completion. Remove neck strip and plastic cape. Thoroughly clean all hair clippings from cape, patron's clothing, and work area. You may then proceed with the next professional service desired by the patron.

Note: Cutting the hair properly serves as a foundation for a variety of beautiful hairstyles.

LEARN HOW TO HANDLE CHILDREN

Special consideration should be given to children and teenagers. Hair-stylists who know how to handle children usually will attract the mothers to their salons for their own hairstyling.

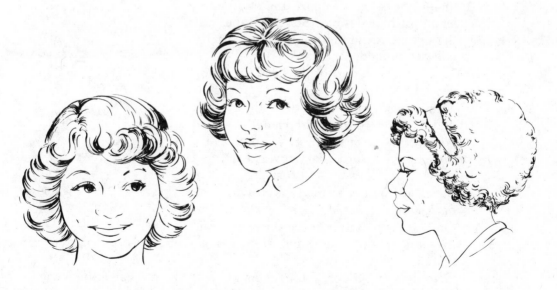

Popular hairstyles for youngsters.

SHAPING OVER-CURLY HAIR

Over-curly hair has its own particular characteristics, as have the other types of hair, which require special techniques for styling. Of prime importance to the hairstylist is the ability to create a hairstyle that will enhance the appearance of the patron and to visualize how the finished hairstyle will look. Knowing the correct shaping and styling techniques, and using common sense in their application, are basic to the success of the hairstylist.

The steps outlined below represent one method of shaping and styling over-curly hair. Where your instructor's methods differ, follow her techniques.

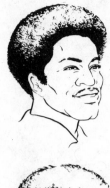

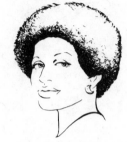

PROCEDURE

1. Drape the patron for hair shaping.
2. Shampoo and dry the hair thoroughly.
3. Apply an emollient product lightly to the scalp and hair to replace lost oil.
4. Using a wide-tooth comb or a hair lifter, comb the hair upward and slightly forward, making the hair as long as possible. Start at the crown, and continue until all hair has been combed out from the scalp and distributed evenly around the head. Combing in a circular pattern will usually help avoid splits.
5. Shape the hair. Visualize the style and length of hair desired. Start by tapering the sides, and cut in the direction the hair will be combed.
6. Taper the back part of the head to blend with the sides.
7. Trim the extreme hair ends of the crown and top areas to the desired length.
8. For an off-the-face hairstyle, comb hair up and backward. For forward movement, comb hair up and forward.
9. Blend side hair with the top, crown, and back hair.
10. Outline the hairstyle at the sides, around the ears, and in the nape area, using either scissors or a trimmer (clipper).
11. Give finishing touch. Fluff the hair slightly with a hair lifter, wherever needed. Spray the hair lightly to give it a natural, lustrous sheen.

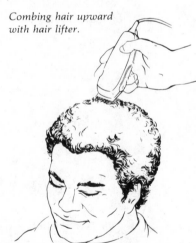

Combing hair upward with hair lifter.

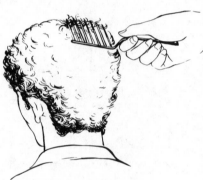

Shaping hair to desired length.

POPULAR HAIRSTYLES

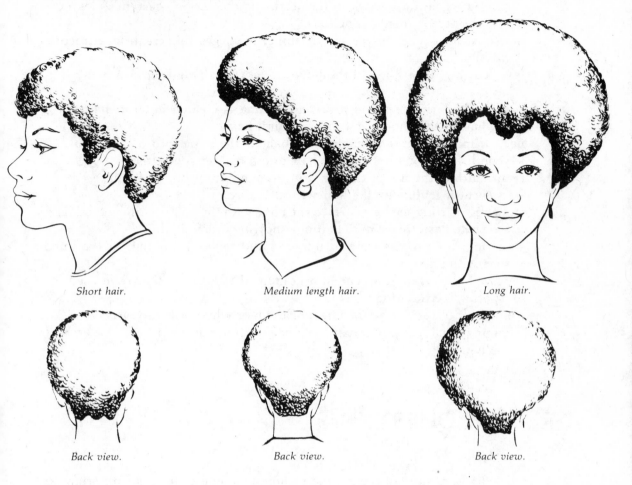

Short hair.   *Medium length hair.*   *Long hair.*

Back view.   *Back view.*   *Back view.*

DEFINITIONS PERTAINING TO HAIR SHAPING

back-combing: combing the short hairs of a strand towards the scalp. Other terms used for back-combing are **teasing, ratting, matting,** and **French lacing.**

basic hair shaping: shaping the hair to a length that is not too long nor too short, in order that it properly fits many different hairstyles.

blunt cutting: cutting the hair straight off, without tapering.

dry cutting: shaping the hair with scissors while it is in a dry condition.

effilating: a French term for **slithering.**

feather edge: when the hair at the nape is shingled in a graceful upward effect and the neck is cleaned with scissors, razor, or clippers.

guideline: a strand of hair at the nape or sides of the head that is cut to a precise length. This cut strand establishes a guide or line to be followed in shaping the balance of the head, and helps to establish the general shaping pattern.

hair shaping: the process of thinning, tapering, and shortening the hair using comb, scissors, thinning shears, or razor in order to mold the hair into a becoming shape. Hair shaping is the commonly used term for **haircutting.**

hairstyling: arranging the hair in various attractive shapes or styles. The contour of the face, shape of the head, and the season's current styles must be considered when styling hair.

hairstylist: one who has the artistic ability to suggest and create an attractive new hair fashion.

layer cutting: tapering and thinning the hair by dividing it into many thin layers.

natural hairline: where no artificial hairline is created in short hairstyles, the hair at the nape is left in its natural hairline.

neck trim: cutting and shaping the hair at the nape into a "V," oval, or round shape, or shingling the hair into a feather edge effect.

razor cutting: the use of the razor in thinning or cutting wet hair.

scissor cutting: shaping the hair with the scissors.

shingling: cutting the hair close to the nape with the hair becoming gradually longer toward the crown, without showing a definite line.

slithering: the process used in thinning and tapering the hair at the same time with scissors.

tapering: shortening the hair in a graduated effect. Another term used for tapering is **feathering.**

thinning: decreasing the thickness of the hair where it is too heavy.

trimming or **clipping:** removing split hair ends or cutting the extreme ends of the hair with the scissors.

REVIEW QUESTIONS

HAIR SHAPING

1. Why is mastery of the art and technique of hair shaping so important to the student?
2. Name the main implements used in hair shaping.
3. What purpose is served by thinning the hair?
4. Why may thin hair be cut closer to the scalp than coarse hair?
5. About how close to the scalp should: a) fine hair; b) medium hair; c) coarse hair be thinned?
6. In which areas is it advisable not to thin the hair?
7. Why is it not advisable to thin hair in the hair part?
8. Why should you avoid removing too much hair during the thinning process?
9. What is shingling?
10. For what purpose is the clipper used?
11. Why should the hair be damp for razor shaping?
12. What does the hairstylist use as a guide when she wants to create short bangs?
13. What is meant by back-combing?
14. What is meant by slithering the hair?
15. What is meant by the term "tapering?"

Chapter 11

FINGER WAVING

CHAPTER LEARNING OBJECTIVES

The student successfully mastering this chapter will know:
1. *The reasons for studying finger waving.*
2. *How to use finger wave lotion, and the purpose for which it is used.*
3. *The techniques employed in correct finger waving.*
4. *The purpose of shadow waving and how it is used.*
5. *How to use finger waves properly in styling hair.*
6. *The precautions, suggestions, and hints for better finger waving.*

Finger waving is the art of shaping and directing the hair into waves and designs using the fingers, comb, waving lotion, and hairpins or clippies.

Training in finger waving is important to students because it teaches them the technique of moving and directing hair. It also helps them develop the dexterity, coordination, and finger strength required for professional hairstyling. In addition, it provides valuable training in creating hairstyles and in molding hair to the curved surface of the head.

PREPARATION

Always wash your hands before giving your patron any salon service. Make sure all necessary implements have been sanitized and towels and other supplies are clean and fresh. Prepare the patron in the same manner as you would for a shampoo.

Shampoo the patron's hair at the shampoo bowl, towel blot the hair, and seat the patron comfortably before a dresserette.

Better soft natural waves are obtained with hair that has a natural wave or has been permanently waved than with straight hair. A finger wave correctly done complements the patron's head as well as her individual features.

FINGER WAVING LOTION

Waving lotion makes the hair pliable and keeps it in place during the finger waving procedure. The proper choice of waving lotion is governed by the texture and condition of the patron's hair. A good waving lotion is harmless to the hair and does not flake on drying.

Part the hair down to the scalp, comb smooth, and arrange it to conform to the planned style. The hair will move much easier if you use the coarse teeth of the comb. Follow the natural growth pattern when combing and parting the hair. You will find the hair easier to mold, and it will not buckle or separate in the crown area.

Waving lotion is applied to the hair while it is damp. This permits the lotion to be distributed smoothly and evenly.

Use an applicator to apply the waving lotion and a comb to distribute it through the hair. Avoid the use of an excessive amount of waving lotion.

Note—Apply lotion to one side of the head at a time; this prevents it from drying and requiring an additional application.

To locate the natural hair growth, comb the hair away from the face, and push hair forward with the palm of your hand. (See **Hairstyling Chapter.**)

The finger wave may be started on either side of the head. However, in this presentation, the hair is parted on the left side of the head and the wave is started on the right (heavy) side of the head.

HORIZONTAL FINGER WAVING

SHAPING THE TOP AREA

Using the index finger of your left hand as a guide, shape the top hair with a comb, using a circular movement. Starting at the hairline, work towards the crown in 1½-2″ (3.7-5 cm) sections at a time until the crown has been reached. (Fig. 1)

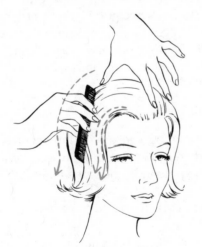

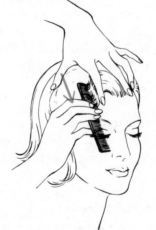

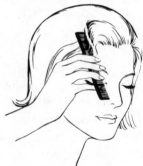

(The left hand is not shown so that you may see the ridge and position of the comb.)

Fig. 1. Shaping top area.

Fig. 2. Drawing hair about 1″ toward fingertip.

Fig. 3. Flattening comb against head.

Forming the first ridge. Place the index finger of the left hand directly above the position for the first ridge. With the teeth of the comb pointing slightly upward, insert the comb directly under the index finger. Draw the comb forward about 1″ (2.5 cm) along the fingertip. (Fig. 2)

With the teeth still inserted in the ridge, flatten the comb against the head in order to hold the ridge in place (Fig. 3).

Remove the left hand from the head and place the middle finger above the ridge and the index finger on the teeth of the comb. Emphasize the ridge by closing the two fingers and applying pressure to the head. (Fig. 4)

CAUTION

Do not try to increase the height of the ridge by pushing or lifting it up with the fingers. Such movement will distort and move the ridge formation off its base.

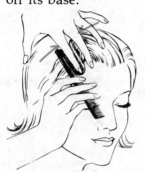

Fig. 4. Emphasizing ridge.

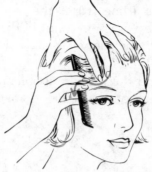

Fig. 5. Combing hair in semi-circular direction.

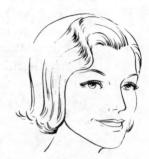

Fig. 6. Completed first ridge at the crown.

Without removing the comb, turn the teeth downward, and comb the hair in a right semi-circular direction to form a dip in the hollow part of the wave. (Fig. 5)

Follow this procedure, section by section, until the crown has been reached, where the ridge phases out. (Fig. 6)

The ridge and wave of each section should match evenly, without showing separations in the ridge and hollow part of the wave.

Forming the second ridge. Begin at the crown area. (Fig. 7) The movements are the reverse of those followed in forming the first ridge. The comb is drawn from the tip of the index finger towards the base of the index finger, thus directing formation of the second ridge. All movements are followed in a reverse pattern until the hairline is reached, thus completing the second ridge. (Fig. 8)

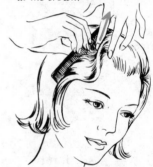

Fig. 7. Starting the second ridge.

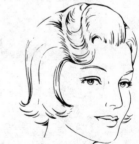

Fig. 8. Completing second ridge.

Forming the third ridge. Movements for the third ridge closely follow those used in creating the first ridge. However, the third ridge is started at the hairline and extended back towards the back of the head. (Fig. 9)

Continue alternating directions until the side of the head has been completed. (Fig. 10)

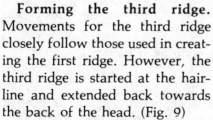

Fig. 9. Starting the third ridge.

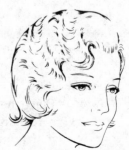

Fig. 10. Completed right side.

LEFT SIDE OF THE HEAD

Use the same procedure for the left (light) side of the head as you used for finger waving the right (heavy) side of the head.

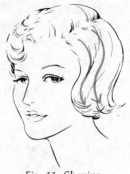

Fig. 11. Shaping for left side.

PROCEDURE

1. First shape the hair as in Fig. 11.
2. Starting at the hairline, form the first ridge, section by section, until the second ridge of the opposite side is reached. (Fig. 12)
3. Both the ridge and the wave must blend without splits or breaks with the ridge and wave on the right side of the head. (Fig. 13)

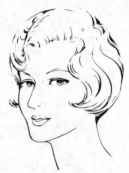

Fig. 12. First ridge starts at hairline.

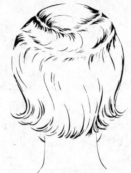

Fig. 13. Ridge and wave matched in the crown area.

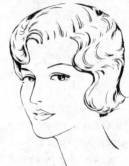

Fig. 14. Left side completed.

4. Start with the ridge and wave in the back of the head and proceed, section by section, towards the left side of the face.
5. Continue working back and forth until entire side completed. (Fig. 14)

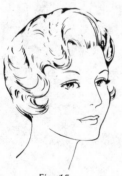

Fig. 15

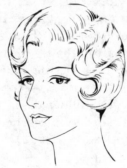

Fig. 16

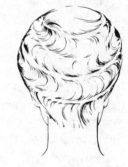

Fig. 17

Figures 15, 16, and 17 illustrate the completed hairstyle.

COMPLETION

1. Place net over hair, secure with hairpins or clippies if needed, and safeguard patron's forehead and ears while under the dryer with cotton, gauze, or paper protectors.
2. Adjust the dryer to medium heat and allow hair to dry thoroughly.

3. Remove patron from under dryer.
4. Remove clippies or pins and hairnet from hair.
5. Comb out and reset waves into a soft coiffure.
6. Clean up booth.
7. Sanitize combs, hairpins, clippies, and hairnet after each use.

ALTERNATE METHOD OF FINGER WAVING

Hair parted on left side. The following is an alternate method in performing finger waving:

1. Shape the top right (heavy) side.
2. Phase out the first ridge starting at the front **right** side, and working around to the crown.
3. Start a ridge on the **left** front side and go all around the head, finishing on the front right hairline.
4. Start another ridge on the front right hairline and finish on the left front side. Continue, left to right and right to left, until the entire head is completed.

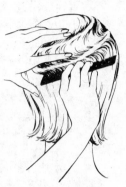

Fig. 1. Finger waving around the head.

This method eliminates the matching of ridges and waves at the back part of the head. (Completion is the same as it is for previous method of finger waving.)

VERTICAL FINGER WAVING

Vertical finger waving differs from horizontal waving in that the ridges and waves run up and down the head, while in horizontal finger waving they go parallel around the head.

Procedure for making vertical ridges and waves is the same as for horizontal finger waving.

1. Make side part, extending from forehead to crown.
2. Form shaping in a semi-circular effect (Figs. 1 and 2).
3. Make first section of ridge and wave (Fig. 3).
4. Continue with additional sections until the part is reached.

Fig. 1

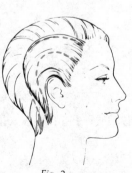

Fig. 2

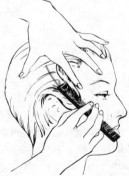

Fig. 3

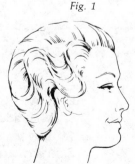

Fig. 4

Start the second ridge at the hair part. Start the third ridge at the hairline. Completed side is shown in Fig. 4. (Completion is the same as it is for horizontal finger waving.)

Since finger waving is the art of directing and molding hair into waves and patterns with the fingers and comb, it is an excellent introduction to hairstyling

SHADOW WAVE

A shadow wave is a shallow wave with low ridges that are not very sharp. The waves are formed in the regular manner, but the comb does not penetrate to the scalp. The hair layers underneath are not waved.

This type of wave is sometimes desirable for a patron who wishes to dress her hair very close to the head.

REMINDERS AND HINTS ON FINGER WAVING

1. Wash hands and have available sanitized implements and supplies.
2. Avoid the use of an excessive amount of waving lotion.
3. Use hard rubber combs with both fine and coarse teeth.
4. Before finger waving, locate the natural or permanent wave in the hair.
5. To emphasize the ridges of a finger wave, press the ridge between the fingers, holding the fingers against the head.
6. To wave the underneath hair, insert the comb through the hair to the scalp.
7. For a longer-lasting finger wave, mold the waves in the direction of the natural growth.
8. To safeguard the patron's forehead and ears from intense heat while under dryer, use cotton, gauze, or paper protectors.
9. Place a net over the hair to protect the setting while it is being dried.
10. Thoroughly dry the hair before combing it out.
11. Prolonged drying under heat will dry the natural oils of the hair and scalp.
12. Finger waves will not remain in place if the hair is combed out before it has been completely dried.
13. Lightened or tinted hair that tangles is easier to comb if a cream rinse is used.
14. Lightly spraying the hair with lacquer will hold the finger wave longer and give the hair a sheen.

REVIEW QUESTIONS
FINGER WAVING

1. What is finger waving?
2. Why is training in finger waving important to the students?
3. What additional valuable training is provided by learning finger waving?
4. How do you protect the patron's clothing?
5. What types of hair will give better soft natural waves?
6. To what advantage is waving lotion used in giving a finger wave?
7. How should the hair be protected while being dried?
8. Why are cotton, gauze, or paper protectors placed over the patron's ears and forehead?

Chapter 12

HAIRSTYLING

CHAPTER LEARNING OBJECTIVES

The student successfully mastering this chapter will know:
1. *Why it is important to have a basic knowledge of hairstyling.*
2. *The technique of hair parting.*
3. *The technique of removing tangles from hair.*
4. *The formation of shapings.*
5. *The styling results of curl placement.*
6. *The basic qualities of good pin curls.*
7. *The various curl bases, and how they are used.*
8. *The styling results of combed out pin curl formations.*
9. *The various types of curls, and the styling effects they create.*
10. *The use of rollers, and the effects that can be created with them.*
11. *The reasons for back-combing and back-brushing.*
12. *How to combine basic hairstyling techniques to produce a hairstyle pattern.*
13. *The various facial types, and the styling patterns that are most becoming.*

The cosmetologist of today must have a basic knowledge of hairstyling in order to keep up with the ever-changing fashions. The successful cosmetologist is capable of giving a personal touch to each coiffure so that it is suitable to the individual.

It is always advisable to examine the patron's hair before starting the shampoo. This gives the cosmetologist the opportunity to do a rough combing and to decide how the hair should be worn in order to produce the most becoming results. It also affords the chance to visualize the desired hairstyle and to plan the proper hair shaping.

The cosmetologist who hopes to become a proficient hairstylist must understand hair structure and the overall importance of hair shaping, permanent waving, hair straightening, thermal waving and curling, hair coloring, hair chemistry, and the action of hair conditioners.

Better styling results can be obtained when the hair is in good condition.

IMPLEMENTS AND MATERIALS USED IN HAIRSTYLING

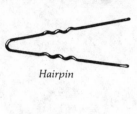

Hairpin

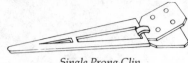

Single Prong Clip

Bobby Pin

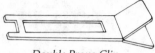

Double Prong Clip

Roller Pin

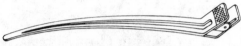

Duckbill Clamp

CYLINDER-SHAPED ROLLERS
One-Half Size

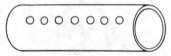

Long

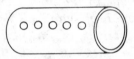

Medium

Short

POPULAR COMBS

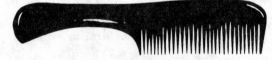

Large-Tooth Comb

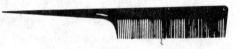

Tail (Rat-Tail) Comb

All-Purpose Comb

Haircutting Comb

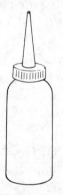

Spout
Plastic Bottle
Dispenser

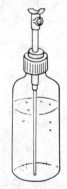

Press-Spray
Plastic Dispenser
Bottle

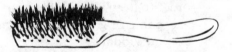

HAIRBRUSHES—NATURAL BRISTLES.
Brushes made from natural boar bristles are
used for brushing out a setting, removing
tangles, or giving a scalp treatment.

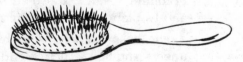

HAIRBRUSHES—SYNTHETIC BRISTLES.
Small, narrow brushes made from synthetic
bristles are used to cushion or lace hair,
smooth out a style, or lock hair in place.

REMOVING TANGLES FROM HAIR

Removing tangles from the hair is very important for successful hairstyling. To prevent damage, tangles must be removed in a systematic manner.

Always begin in the nape area. With the coarse teeth of a comb, section off a small part of hair and comb across and down each strand. (Fig. 1) Work across the back sections in steps, going up to the crown. Size of sections picked up depends on hair elasticity; for fine or lightened hair, pick up smaller sections.

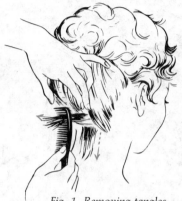
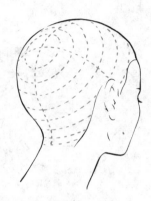
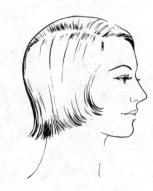

Fig. 1. Removing tangles in nape area.

Fig. 2. Combing pattern for removing tangles.

Fig. 3. Tangles removed.

Fig. 2 shows combing pattern for removing tangles from hair. After tangles are removed, the hair is ready for setting or other service. (Fig. 3)

MAKING A PART

Clean partings are essential to good hairstyling. Comb hair straight back. Hold the comb slightly angled and place it a trifle in front of the hairline. Draw the comb in an even line toward the back until the length of the part is reached. (Fig. 1)

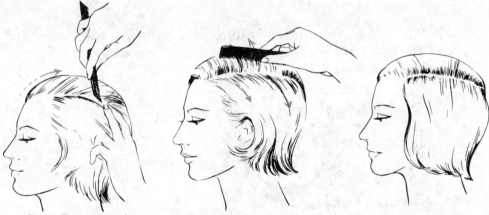

Fig. 1. Drawing comb back full length.

Fig. 2. Combing hair above and below part.

Fig. 3. Hair combed with straight part.

Hold the lower side of the part with the left hand, while combing the hair towards the right, then comb the hair down below part. (Fig. 2) A clean, straight part is illustrated in Fig. 3.

FINDING THE NATURAL PART

If a natural hair part is desired in a hairstyle, it may be made in the following manner:

After shampooing and towel drying the hair, comb it straight back. Place the palm of the left hand on the head and push the hair forward. The hair will separate at the natural part. (Fig. 1) Separate and comb the hair over to the right. (Fig. 2) Then comb the hair below the part. Fig. 3 illustrates a clean, straight part.

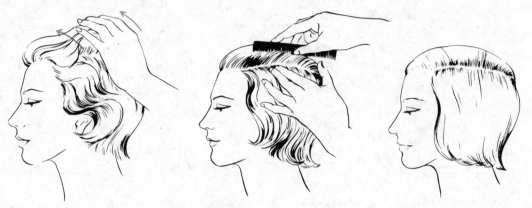

Fig. 1. Finding natural part.

Fig. 2. Combing hair above and below part.

Fig. 3. Hair combed with straight part.

PIN CURLS

Pin curls (also called sculpture curls), when carefully planned in exact patterns, will result in good lines, waves, ringlets, curls, or rolls. Pin curls are suitable for naturally or permanently waved hair. The hair should be properly tapered, and pin curls wound smoothly, to make them springy and longer lasting.

PARTS OF A CURL

Pin curls are constructed of three principal parts: **base**, **stem**, and **circle**. The **base** is the stationary, or immovable, foundation of the curl, which is attached to the scalp.

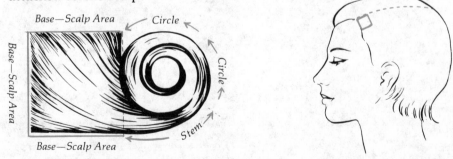

The **stem** is the part of the pin curl, between the base and the first arc (turn) of the circle, which gives the circle its direction, action, and mobility.

The **circle** is the part of the pin curl that forms a complete circle. The size of the curl governs the width of the wave and its strength.

MOBILITY OF A CURL

The mobility of a curl is determined by the **stem,** depending on the amount of movement that takes place in the stem and circle. Curl mobility is classified as no-stem, half-stem, and full-stem.

1. The **no-stem curl** gives the base of the curl a firm immovable position, permitting only the curl to move. It produces a strong, long-lasting curl. The curl is placed in the center of the base.

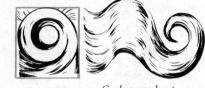

Curl opened out.

2. The **half-stem curl** permits freedom of movement, since the half stem allows the circle to move away from its base. It gives good control of the hair and produces softness in the finished wave pattern. The curl is placed one-half off its base.

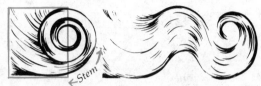

Curl opened out.

3. The **full-stem curl** permits the greatest mobility to the curl. It gives the lines and

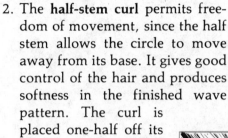

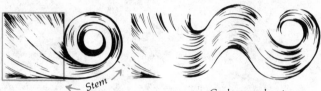

Curl opened out.

direction as much freedom as the length of the stem will permit. It is used when a strong direction of the hair and a weaker wave pattern is desired. The base may be parted in a square, triangular, half-moon, or rectangular section, depending on the area of the head in which the full-stem curls are used. The circle is placed completely off its base.

The type of curl used will determine whether the design is to be close to or away from the head.

PIN CURL COMB-OUT

The size of the curl determines the size of the wave.

Note the difference in the size between the combed out wave of a pin curl set with a closed center and that with an open center.

To obtain an even, smooth wave and a uniform end curl, the **open center curl** is recommended.

A **closed center** is recommended for fine hair if a fluffy comb-out is desired.

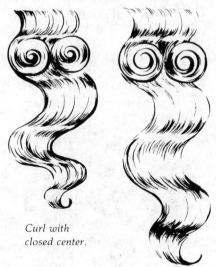

Curl with closed center.

Curl with open center.

CURL AND STEM DIRECTION

The stem direction may be toward the face, away from the face, upward, downward, or diagonal. However, the stem direction is determined by the finished hairstyle desired.

Curl and stem direction in relation to the face is referred to as:

1. **Forward movement**—toward the face.
2. **Reverse (backward) movement**—away from the face.

Up-stem reverse curl

Back-stem reverse curl

Down-stem reverse curl

Down-stem forward curl

Up-stem forward curl

Back-stem forward curl

Comb-out.

Up-stem reverse curl

Back-stem reverse curl

Up-stem forward curl

Down-stem reverse curl

Back-stem forward curl

Down-stem forward curl

Comb-out.

These illustrations are only intended to show stem directions and curl placements, and are not intended to be illustrations of pin curl patterns.

CLOCKWISE AND COUNTER-CLOCKWISE CURLS

Some hairstylists prefer to use the terms "clockwise curls" and "counter-clockwise curls."

Curls formed in the same direction as the movement of the hands of a clock are known as clockwise (C) curls.

Curls formed in the opposite direction to the movement of the hands of a clock are known as counter-clockwise (CC) curls.

Clockwise curls.

Counter-clockwise curls.

SHAPING FOR PIN CURL PLACEMENTS

A shaping is a section of hair that has been molded into a design to serve as a base for a curl or wave pattern. The exact point from which the hair is directed in forming a shaping is the **pivot**.

Shapings may be classified as **forward** and **reverse**.

FORWARD SHAPINGS

A forward shaping is one in which the hair is directed toward the face. This type of shaping is oval in form and is larger in size at its **closed end** than at its **open end**.

Side Forward Vertical Shaping

The hair is directed in a circular motion, following the side hair part, downward and towards the face, as shown in the illustration. The size of the shaping depends on the setting for the hairstyle being created.

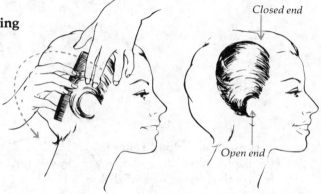

Closed end

Open end

Shaping for right side.

Top Forward Shaping

The hair is comb-directed in a circular motion, **away from the forehead,** in a circular effect towards the face.

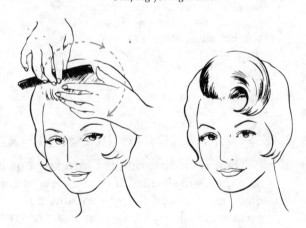

Oval shaping for top forward movement.

DIAGONAL SHAPING

This is similar to the side forward shaping, with the exception that the shaping is formed in a diagonal manner to the side of the head.

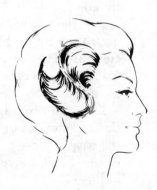

VERTICAL SHAPING

Vertical side shaping is one in which the hair is comb-directed in a down-upward circular motion, away from the face.

LEFT SIDE REVERSE VERTICAL SHAPING

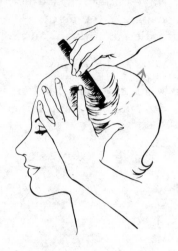

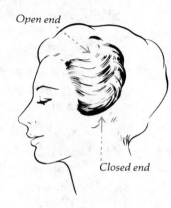

Open end

Closed end

HORIZONTAL SHAPING

Horizontal oblong shaping is one in which the hair is comb-directed parallel with the parting. It is recommended for pin curl parallel construction, and may be used for the first movement in finger waving design.

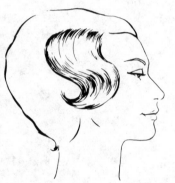

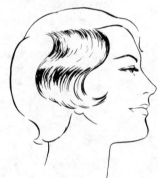

PIN CURL FOUNDATIONS OR BASES

The hair is first divided into sections or panels, and then sub-divided into the type of foundations or bases required for the various curls. The most commonly shaped bases in use are: rectangular, triangular, arc (half-moon or "C" shape), and square.

In order to avoid splits in the hair, the hairstylist must use care in the selection and formation of the curl base. Furthermore, uniformity of curl development only can be achieved if the sections of hair are as equal as possible.

It is important to make certain that each curl lies flat and smooth on its base. If extended too far off the base, a loose curl near the scalp will result. The finished curl, however, is not affected by the shape of the base.

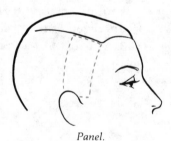

Panel.

Panel with rectangular bases.

RECTANGULAR BASE

Rectangular base pin curls are usually recommended at the side front hairline for a smooth, upsweep effect.

To avoid splits in the comb-out, the pin curls must overlap.

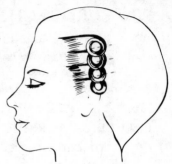

Rectangular base.

TRIANGULAR BASE

Triangular base pin curls are recommended along the front or facial hairline to prevent breaks or splits in the finished hairstyle. The triangular base allows a portion of hair from each curl to overlap the next and comb into a uniform wave without splits.

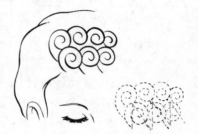

Triangular base.

ARC BASE

Sides. Arc base, also known as half-moon or "C" shape base, pin curls may be carved out of a shaping at the sides of the head.

Back of head. Arc base pin curls also may be used for an upsweep effect or French twist at the lower back of the head.

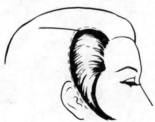

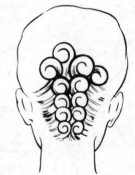

Arc base—side.   *Arc base—back of head.*

SQUARE BASE

Square base pin curls are used for even construction suitable for combing and brushing into curls or waves. They can be used on any part of the head, and will comb out with lasting results.

To avoid splits, stagger the sectioning as shown in the illustration.

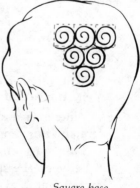

Square base.

PIN CURL TECHNIQUES

Pin curls can be made in several ways. The following drawings illustrate several methods of forming them. Your instructor may demonstrate other methods which are equally correct.

PIN CURLS FOR RIGHT SIDE

Pin curls, carved out of a shaping without disturbing the shaping, are usually referred to as carved curls. To form these curls on the right side of the head, the following procedure is followed:

Procedure

Wet the hair with water or setting lotion; comb smooth and form shaping. Start making curls at the open end of the shaping.

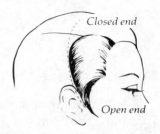

Closed end

Open end

1. Form shaping.

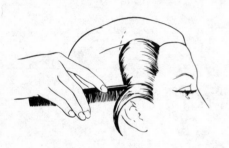

2. Slice strand for first curl.

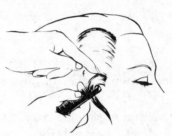

3. Use tip of comb and index finger as buffer.

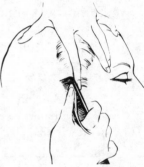

4. Stretch strand by pulling through back of comb.

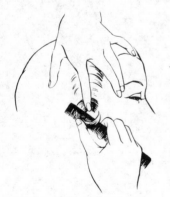

5. Form forward curl.

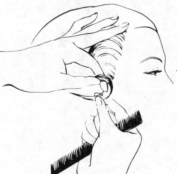

6. Wind curl around index finger.

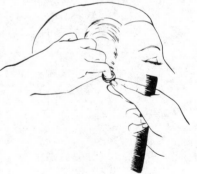

7. Slide curl off finger, keeping the hair ends in center of curl.

Very Important

Whenever a longer-lasting curl movement is desired, the strand should be stretched or tensioned.

This is accomplished by ribboning and stretching the strand. Firmly comb it between the spine of the comb and the thumb in the direction of the curl movement, as in Figs. 4 and 5.

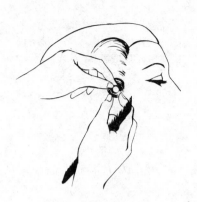

8. *Mold curl into shaping.*

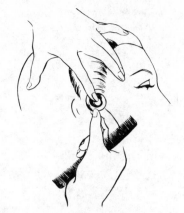

9. *Hold curl in shaping.*

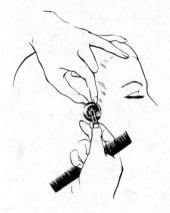

10. *Anchor curl with clippie.*

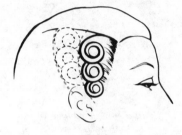

11. *Sculpture curl arrangement backed up with a second row of curls.*

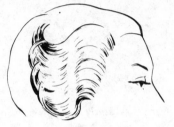

12. *Curls combed into waves with a strong ridge.*

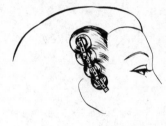

13. *Fine hair usually requires four curls.*

PIN CURLS FOR LEFT SIDE

Making pin curls on the left side of the head requires a different technique than making them on the right side.

Wet the hair with water or setting lotion, comb smooth, and form the shaping. Start at the open end of the shaping.

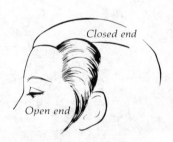

Closed end

Open end

1. *Shaping.*

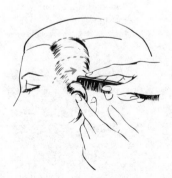

2. *Slice strand out of shaping.*

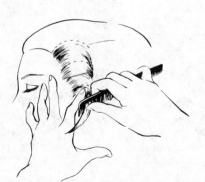

3. *Strand stretched by pulling through backbone of comb.*

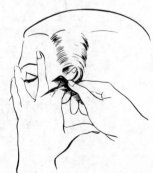

4. *Form forward curl.*

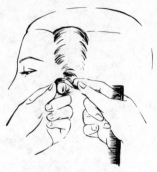 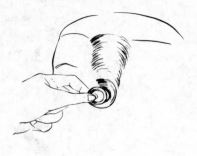 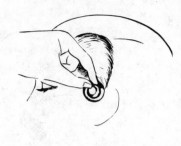

5. Wind strand around index finger.

6. Slide curl off tip of finger and mold into shaping.

7. Hold curl in shaping.

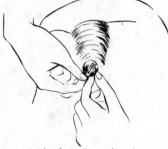 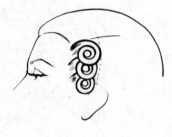 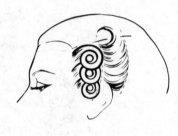

8. Anchor pin curl with clippie.

9. Curls fit within curvature of shaping. Curls overlap. Size of curls graduated.

10. Reverse shaping for back-up curls.

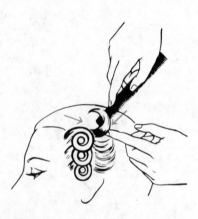 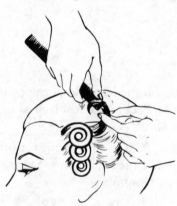 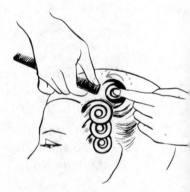

11. To slice strand, tip of comb touches tip of finger half through shaping.

12. Ribbon strand. The use of coarse or fine teeth of comb depends on the texture of the hair.

13. Ribbon tip of strand with fine teeth of comb for neat closing of curl.

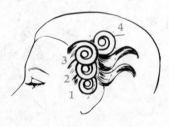 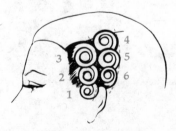 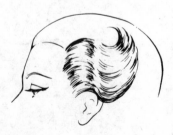

14. Top reverse curl completed and the shaping divided into strands for next two curls.

15. Completed second row of curls within curve of shaping.

16. Comb-out of forward and reverse pin curl setting into a full, wide wave.

ANCHORING PIN CURLS

Anchoring pin curls is an important technique that must be mastered in order to achieve success in hairstyling. It is essential that the curls hold firmly as placed, so that the planned pattern can be followed and developed into the desired coiffure.

Every hairstylist or instructor has his or her own favorite method for inserting clips or clippies. Each one of these professional methods can be considered equally correct. However, it is essential that good common sense be used at all times in the insertion of clips or clippies so that pin curls are anchored securely.

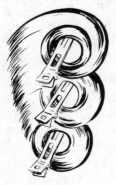

Hairline forward pin curls (clockwise curl).

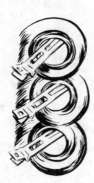

Forward pin curls equal in size. Any place on the head.

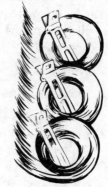

Reverse pin curls (counter-clockwise curls). Equal in size. Any place on the head.

PROCEDURE

To anchor the pin curl correctly, gently slide the clip or clippie through part of the base and/or stem at an angle and across the ends of the curl. This will hold the curl securely without its unfurling, sagging, or flipping over.

1. Clips should be anchored in such a manner so that they do not interfere with the formation or placement of other curls, or with any other step in setting the hair.

2. To avoid indentations or impressions, it is advisable not to pin across the center of the entire curl.

3. The size of clips used should be governed by the size of the curl.

4. To avoid discomfort to the patron during the drying process, do not permit the clips to touch the ears, skin, or scalp. In the event the clips do touch the skin or ears, place cotton under the part of the clips touching these areas.

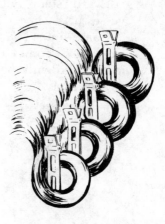

Ridge reverse pin curls (counter-clockwise curls).

EFFECTS OF PIN CURLS

There are a number of pin curl patterns designed to achieve specific effects, several of which are illustrated here.

However, care must be taken that the curls lie evenly and are placed in the direction in which they are intended to be combed; otherwise, a haphazard setting will result, with uneven wave or curl design.

VERTICAL WAVES

To achieve vertical wave effects on the left side of the head, first give a reverse shaping, then follow pin curl pattern as illustrated.

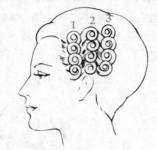 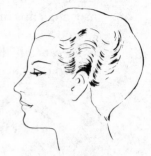

Vertical wave pin curl pattern.   *Vertical wave comb-out.*

HORIZONTAL WAVES

To achieve horizontal waves, the hair is first shaped in a forward semi-circular effect, from the hair part downward. The pin curls are then set as illustrated. This creates a long-lasting wave close to the head.

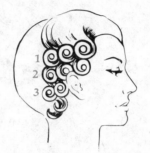 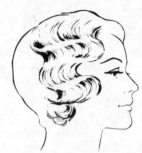

Horizontal wave pin curl pattern.   *Horizontal wave comb-out.*

INTERLOCKING MOVEMENT

1st Row—Back-stem with forward curls.

2nd and 3rd Rows—Forward stem with reverse curls.

Comb-out—The back curls are combed and interlocked with the front row of curls.

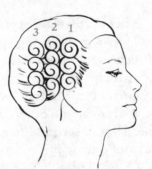 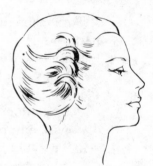

Setting pattern.   *Comb-out.*

WAVED TOP

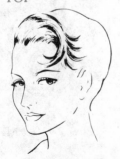 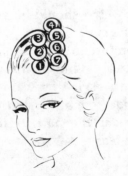 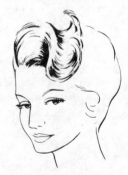

Shaping.   *Setting pattern.*   *Comb-out.*

DIAGONAL WAVES

Shape hair—Oval forward shaping.
Set—Start at open end.
Comb-out—Diagonal waves.

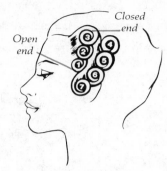

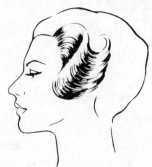

Setting pattern.   *Comb-out.*

WAVED BANGS

Setting for Fine Hair

Shape hair.
Set—1st row.
    2nd row.

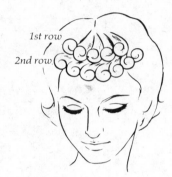

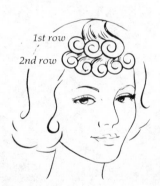

Setting pattern.   *Comb-out.*

Setting for Normal Hair

Shape hair.
Set—1st row.
    2nd row.

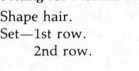

Setting pattern.   *Comb-out.*

FRENCH TWIST

Setting for Normal Hair

Part off back area and make vertical center part. Comb both sections toward center.

Make large **smooth** pin curls, as shown in illustration.

Comb-out. Back-comb each side. Brush or comb one side, fold in ends, and pin.

Brush or comb the other side and fold ends over first section. Pin hair in herringbone fashion, so ends do not show.

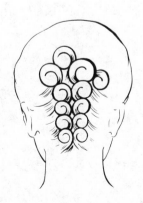

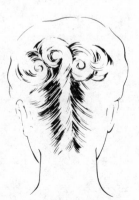

Setting pattern.   *Comb-out and pinning.*

RIDGE CURLS

Ridge curls are pin curls placed behind the ridge of a shaping or finger wave when a loose wave is desired. Care must be taken **not to disturb the ridge** when slicing out the strands for the curls.

Prepare hair. Shape hair and make ridge as for vertical finger wave. Slice strand without disturbing the ridge.

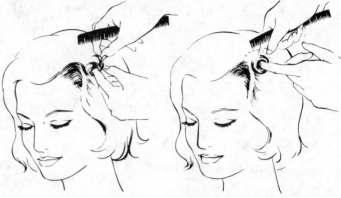

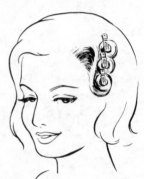

Fig. 1. Wind hair around fingertip.

Fig. 2. Slide strand off finger and roll it to base of ridge.

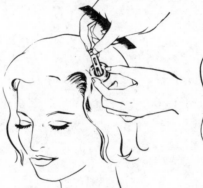

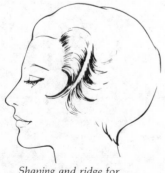

Fig. 3. Anchor curl with clippie.

Fig. 4. Completed ridge curl.

SKIP WAVE

The skip wave is a combination finger wave and pin curl pattern, the pin curls being placed in alternate finger wave formations. This technique is recommended when wide, smooth-flowing vertical waves are desired.

To obtain best results, the hair should be 3-5" in length. It is not recommended for hair that has a tight permanent wave or hair that is fine.

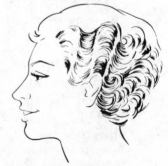

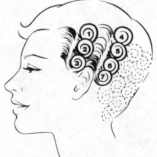

Shaping and ridge for vertical finger wave.

Skip wave pattern for fluff ends.

Comb-out with fluff ends.

CASCADE OR STAND-UP CURL

The cascade curl, sometimes referred to as a **stand-up curl,** is wound from the hair ends to the scalp. The center opening is made large, and the curl is pinned in a standing position.

The stand-up curl provides a great deal of lift to the hair. It can either be used in conjunction with rollers or by itself when volume is desired.

Note: In order to become proficient in hairstyling, the student must learn to make stand-up curls with ease and proficiency.

PROCEDURE

Wet the top section with water or setting lotion.

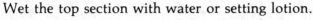

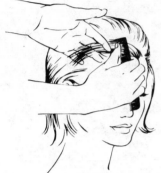

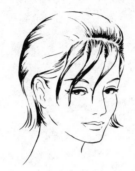

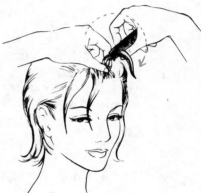

Comb, divide, and smooth strand.

Divide section into strands for easy pickup.

Ribbon strand.

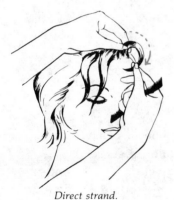

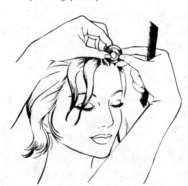

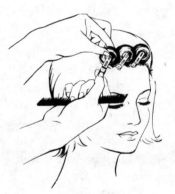

Direct strand.

Wind curl.

Pin curl.

EFFECT OF STAND-UP CURLS

Setting—Stand-up curls for side movement with a side part.

Comb-out—The hair is brushed from the hairline, then sliced off in small sections and flipped over the forehead.

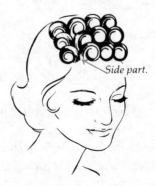

Side part.

Top setting.

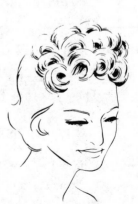

Comb-out.

SEMI-STAND-UP CURLS

Semi-stand-up curls are pin curls that have been carved out of a shaping and pinned into a semi-standing position.

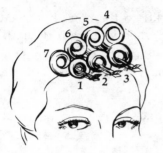

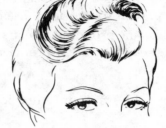

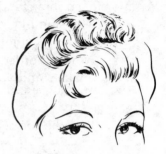

Semi-stand-up curl setting.   *Comb-out.*   *(Alternate) Comb-out.*

Top wave effect may be achieved with stand-up curls by the following procedure:

1. Shape top hair.
2. Make three counter-clockwise curls.
3. Back up with four clockwise curls.
4. Comb-out. The hair may be combed out as shown in the two illustrations.

ROLLER CURLS

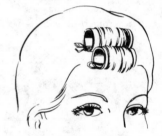

Roller curls are designed to create the same effects as stand-up curls. They are formed over special rollers that come in various sizes to fulfill special needs in a hair design.

The rollers are in effect molds around which curls are formed to create added lift or volume.

Roller curls.

They are especially effective in creating a straight line design with more height and stability than is usually achieved with stand-up curls.

An important difference between roller and stand-up curls is that stand-up curls are formed one at a time, while rollers can accommodate at one time the equivalent of from 2-4 stand-up curls. In addition, the rollers give far more security to the rolled hair while it is in a wet state.

SECTIONING THE HAIR

First, the hair is sectioned into panels, then subdivided into roller bases. The size of the bases should be as near as possible to the length and diameter of the roller.

A good example to follow is if a roller is 3″ (7.5 cm) long and 1″ (2.5 cm) wide in diameter, the base should be 1″ (2.5 cm) wide by 2¾″ (6.875 cm) long, about ¼″ (.625 cm) shorter. If this proportion is followed with the various sizes of rollers, the hair will not be over-crowded, nor will the hair slip off the sides of the rollers.

PREPARATION

The hair is moistened with water or setting lotion in the same manner as for conventional curls. The hair is then sectioned according to the number of rollers that must be used to achieve the hairstyle desired. End papers may be used for easier winding, as in permanent waving.

Roller Setting Technique. Hold strand at 45° (.785 rad.) angle and roll in the manner shown in Figs. 1-4. The roller will sit directly over the base of the rectangle. The curl will be strong and have maximum volume or body.

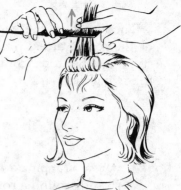

1. Strand preparation.

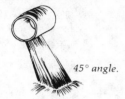

45° angle.

2. Hold strand at 45° angle.

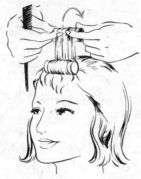

3. Hand position while winding roller.

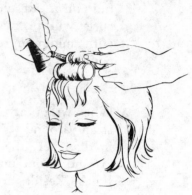

4. Holding roller in position while pinning.

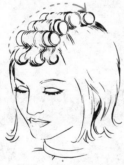

2a. Roll strand on base and anchor with clip.

Complete roller curls from hairline to crown with pin curls for bang effect.

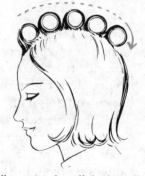

Roller setting for off-the-face effect.

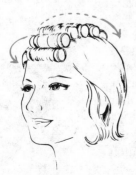

Roller curl pattern for bang effect.

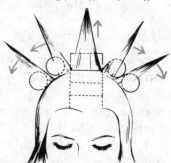

The angle at which the hair is held from the head for roller placement.

103

The length of the hair and the size of the rollers affect the finished hairstyle in the top front area in the following manner:

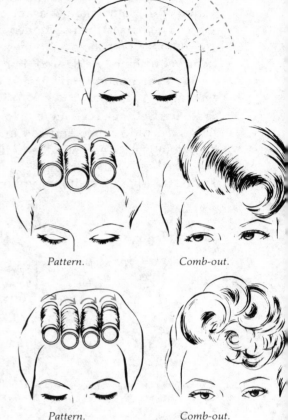

1. When wrapping a 4½" (11.25 cm) strand around a roller 1" (2.5 cm) in diameter, it will go around one full turn. Result: three roller curls will produce a soft puff with minimum curl turned in ends.

Pattern.   *Comb-out.*

2. When wrapping a 4½" (11.25 cm) strand around ¾" (1.85 cm) roller in diameter, the strand will go around about one and one-half times. Result: four rollers will produce a curl fluff with turned in ends.

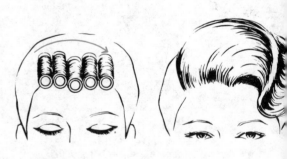

Pattern.   *Comb-out.*

3. Should the size of each roller be small enough to permit the hair strand to be rolled around it twice, five rollers will be needed to adequately curl the area. The use of these rollers will result in a deep, soft wave, because the hair ends are in the opposite direction from the original movement of the hair.

Pattern.   *Comb-out.*

BARREL CURLS

A barrel curl serves as a substitute for a curl formed around a roller. It may be used where there is insufficient room to place a roller. However, it does not provide the tension that is present in roller wrapping.

The barrel curl is made in a similar manner as the stand-up curl, with a flat base and containing much more hair.

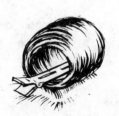

Barrel curl.

VOLUME AND INDENTATION IN ROLLER TECHNIQUE
(With Cylinder Rollers)

CYLINDER SHAPED ROLLERS
(one-half size)

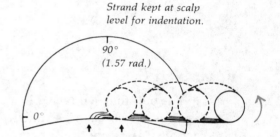

Long   Medium   Short

Modern hairstyling incorporates the use of various devices and methods in order to achieve special designs and effects. One of the most effective devices used in this area is the roller which is available in various sizes and lengths. Rollers are especially important in the creation of volume (lift), and indentation (valleys and hollowness) in the hairstyle.

Note: In order that the rollers be used to their maximum efficiency, the hair length should be over three times their diameter.

VOLUME AND INDENTATION

Volume is created by directing the hair up from the head, rolling the ends under, and then rolling the hair down to the scalp on its base. (Fig. 1)

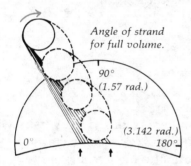

Fig. 1. To create full volume, roller rests on its base.

Fig. 2. To create indentation or hollowness, keep hair close to head and roll to one-half off base.

In order to create indentation, the hair is kept close to the head and rolled over on the rollers. (Fig. 2)

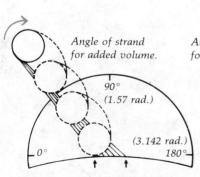

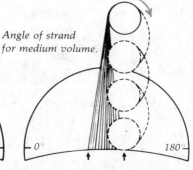

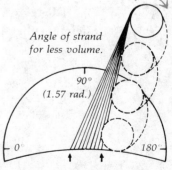

To create maximum volume, roller rests one-half off left side of base.

To create a medium amount of volume, roller rests one-half off the right side of base.

To create a small amount of volume, roller rests off right side of base.

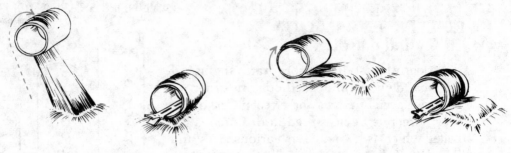

Creates volume.   Creates indentation or hollowness.

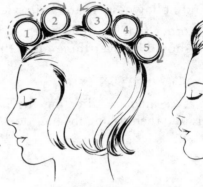

Illustrations

1st two rollers—volume.
3rd roller—indentation.
4th and 5th rollers—volume.

Setting pattern.   Comb-out.

CYLINDER CIRCULAR ROLLER ACTION

The hair that is directed in a circular manner is referred to by hairstylists in various ways, such as radial motion, circular movement, curvature roller action, rotary motion or movement, spotmatic movement, contour movement, and others.

The spot or area from which the hair is directed to form a circular movement also is referred to by any of the following terms: balance point, swing point, terminal point, pivot point, pendulum point, radial point, fulcrum point, radiation point, rotary point, and spotmatic point.

SIDE EFFECTS OF HAIR LENGTHS ON CYLINDER ROLLERS

**Short hair
(slender rollers)**

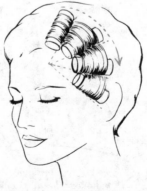

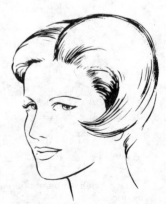

Pattern.   Comb-out.

Medium length hair (medium size rollers)

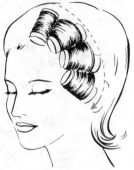

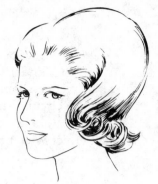

Pattern.

Comb-out.

Long hair (large rollers)

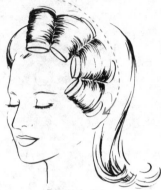

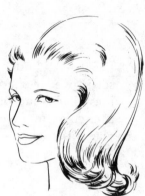

Pattern.

Comb-out.

THE EFFECTS OF SAME SIZE ROLLERS ON DIFFERENT LENGTHS OF HAIR
(Using the same length and diameter roller)

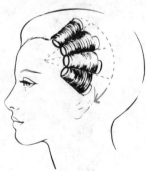

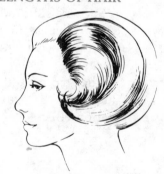

Pattern.

Comb-out— short hair.

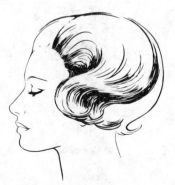

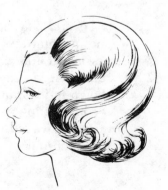

Comb-out— medium length hair.

Comb-out— long hair.

Top—Cylinder rollers set in wedge-shape partings in a circular manner. Comb out in a forward shell effect with bangs.

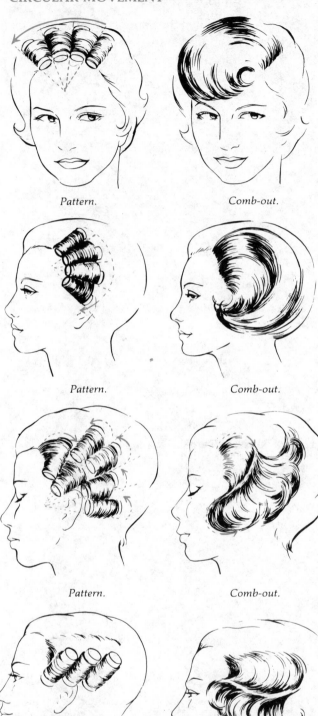

Pattern.　　　　*Comb-out.*

Side—Cylinder rollers set in wedge-shape partings. The comb-out gives a circular movement towards the face.

Pattern.　　　　*Comb-out.*

Special side effects—Side roller setting with sculpture curl in front of ear.

The comb-out produces an "S" wave formation effect.

Pattern.　　　　*Comb-out.*

To create a ridge line and indentation (hollowness), set the hair on rollers at an angle, as shown in illustration.

This setting will produce the waved effect in the comb-out.

Pattern.　　　　*Comb-out.*

TAPERED ROLLERS

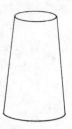

Practically the same styling results may be achieved by using either cylinder or tapered rollers. However, since cylinder rollers must be placed slightly further back from the point of distribution in a pie-shaped parting, the movement of the hair may be weaker. The tapered roller, however, makes it possible to develop a tighter curvature movement.

Size of rollers is governed by the texture of the hair. Example: fine hair takes smaller rollers, while coarse hair takes larger rollers.

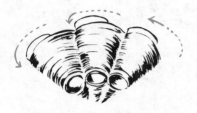 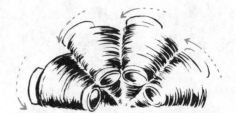

One-quarter circle setting using thinner rollers produces tighter comb-outs.

One-half circle setting using larger (thicker) rollers produces looser comb-outs.

EFFECTS OF TAPERED ROLLERS

Tapered hairline roller setting combs out like a shell shaped front with bangs or curled up ends.

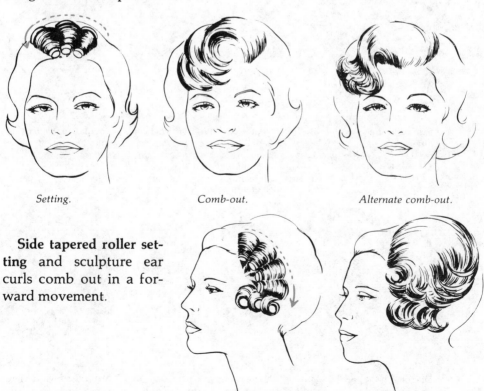

Setting.

Comb-out.

Alternate comb-out.

Side tapered roller setting and sculpture ear curls comb out in a forward movement.

Setting.

Comb-out.

HAIR PARTINGS

The manner of parting the patron's hair should be adjusted to the shape of her head, to her facial type, and to the desired hairstyle. The cosmetologist also must be guided by the natural parting of the patron's hair.

The following are suggested hair partings for various facial types and hairstyles.

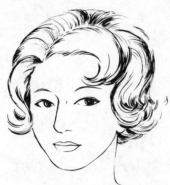

Diagonal part, *used to give height to a round or square face.*

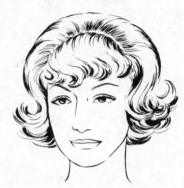

Curved rectangular part, *used for receding hairline or high forehead.*

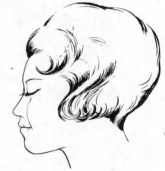

Concealed part, *used for height and a one-sided style effect.*

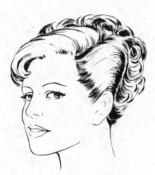

Side part, *used for styles to be directed to one side. Helps to create the illusion of decreasing the width of forehead.*

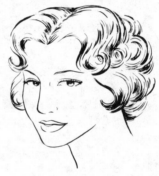

Center part. *No rigid rule can be made for a center part hairstyle. Always try to create a hairstyle that will give an optical illusion of ovalness to the face.*

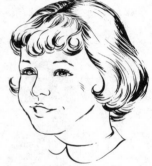

Popular center parting *for children's hairstyles with bangs.*

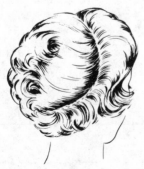

Diagonal back parting, *used to create the illusion of width to crown and back of head.*

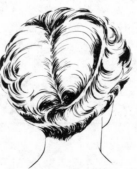

Natural crown parting.

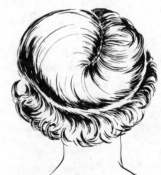

Natural crown parting.
(It would be extremely difficult to create a hairstyle when working against the natural crown parting. Working against the natural parting would cause problems in getting the hair to fall smoothly or to hold the setting.)

BACK-COMBING AND BACK-BRUSHING TECHNIQUES

Back-combing and back-brushing are processes of matting the hair by combing or brushing it toward the scalp so that the shorter hair mats to form a cushion or base for the top or covering hair.

BACK-COMBING

Back-combing also is called **teasing, ratting, matting,** or **French lacing.**

After the basic comb-out is completed, it may need back-combing or back-brushing to achieve the planned hairstyle. When the hair has been brushed and relaxed, analyze the areas that need to be raised.

Procedure

1. Pick up a section of hair about ¾″ (1.875 cm) wide, and hold up firmly from scalp.

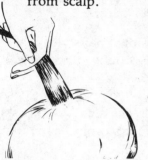 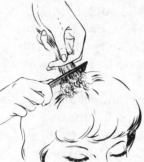 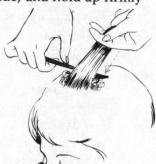

The hair properly held between the index and middle fingers. *Back-combing on top of strand.* *Back-combing in back of strand.*

2. Insert the comb into the strand near its base, press to scalp, and remove.
3. Repeat Step 2 by inserting the comb into the strand a little further away from the scalp, press to scalp, and remove.
4. Repeat Step 3 as many times as necessary, using very small strokes until the desired volume of cushioned hair has been achieved.

BACK-BRUSHING

Back-brushing, also called **ruffing,** is a technique used to build a cushion to a desired volume at the scalp for the top or covering hair.

Procedure

1. Pick up and hold strand straight out from scalp.
2. With a slight amount of slack in the strand, place the brush near the base of the strand. Push and roll the brush with the wrist until it touches the scalp. Then remove the brush from hair with a turn of the wrist.
3. Repeat this procedure by moving the brush about ½″ (1.25 cm) further away from the scalp.
4. Repeat until the desired volume has been achieved.

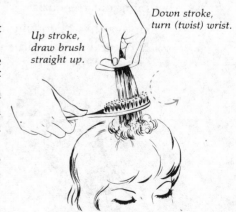

Up stroke, draw brush straight up. *Down stroke, turn (twist) wrist.*

Back-brushing.

Note: *Only the inner edge of the brush is used. The shorter ends of tapered hair are interlocked to form a cushion at the scalp. In order for interlocking to occur, the brush must be rolled.*

COMB-OUT

To achieve success as a hairstylist, the cosmetologist must first master the art and technique of combing and brushing the hair. The creative skills of the stylist can only be realized when the hair has been properly shaped and molded in order to produce an attractive and fashionable coiffure. It should be remembered, however, that most comb-out failures are the result of poorly or improperly set hair.

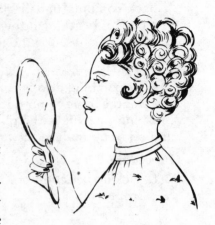

Fast, simple, and effective methods for combing and brushing out hair are very important objectives for the creative hairstylist. The real quality of the truly professional hairstyle, as developed by the capable hairstylist, is most easily and appreciatively recognized by the salon patron.

By applying good combing and brushing skill, the imaginative cosmetologist can artistically create almost any hairstyle desired. It is this skill, this technical ability to handle the comb and brush, that forms the foundation for success as a professional hairstylist.

SUGGESTED PROCEDURE

A definite system or plan, indicating where to start and the procedure to follow, is required for effectiveness in combing out. Such a planned procedure will help to develop the desired finished coiffure.

A suggested procedure is outlined here.

1. Brush out curls.
2. General wave placement.
3. Accentuate and develop lines and style.
4. Finishing steps.

Brushing out the curls

Remove the rollers and clips, and relax the set by brushing out the curls with natural bristle brush. The objective of this technique is to smooth

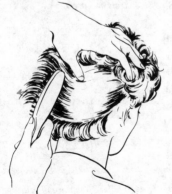

Fig. 1. Brushing back area.

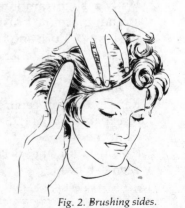

Fig. 2. Brushing sides.

and brush the hair into a semi-flat condition and to remove excess curl. (Figs. 1 and 2) This permits the stylist to position the lines for the planned hairstyle. It is essential that this procedure be correctly executed in order to achieve a smooth, flowing, finished coiffure.

General wave placement

When the brushing is completed, the hair should be combed into the general pattern desired. Lines and direction should be slightly over-emphasized to allow for some expected relaxation during the comb-out process. This may be accomplished by placing the hand on the head and gently pushing the hair forward, in order that the waves fall into the planned design. Any necessary teasing is performed, and volume, indentation, and ridges are created as part of the overall arrangement. (Fig. 3) The entire coiffure is created in exaggerated and over-emphasized lines to provide for the final combing and styling.

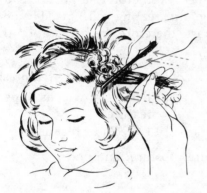

Fig. 3. If desirable, teasing from scalp out to 2" from hair ends.

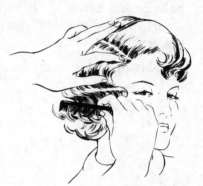

Fig. 4. Molding and combing hair to the desired hairstyle.

Accentuating and developing lines and style

Taking one section at a time, the proper lines, ridges, volume, and indentations are combed and brushed into the finished coiffure. Softness and evenness of flow are created by blending, smoothing, and combing. Exaggerations and over-emphasis are carefully removed. Finished patterns are created, and final evenness and smoothness of line are combed into the final silhouette.

Finishing steps

After the creation of the style has been completed, it is time for the finishing touches. Lightly spray the hair to hold it in place for the final placement. Using the tips of the teeth of the comb, lightly fit any small hairs or loose ends into place. If necessary, lift and blend disarrayed hair with the tips of the fingers, or by carefully lifting with the comb. (Fig. 4) Even movement and touch during the final stage must be very lightly performed. The objective at this point is to smooth out any visible imperfections.

When the finishing touches have been completed, check the entire set for structural balance, and then lightly spray the hair for the desired holding effect.

ARTISTRY IN HAIRSTYLING

The principles of modern hairstyling and makeup are guides to the cosmetologist in selecting what is most appropriate in achieving a beautiful appearance. Best results are obtained when each facial type is analyzed for its own merits and defects.

Each type of face demands a distinctive coiffure that is rightly proportioned, has a balanced line, and correctly

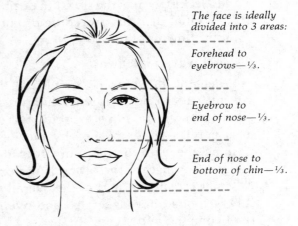

The face is ideally divided into 3 areas:

Forehead to eyebrows—⅓.

Eyebrow to end of nose—⅓.

End of nose to bottom of chin—⅓.

frames the face. Every accomplished cosmetologist possesses a sense of balance and harmony in visualizing and creating coiffures. The essentials of an artistic and suitable hairstyle must, therefore, be based upon the following general characteristics:

1. Shape of the entire head:
   a) Front view.
   b) Profile (side view).
   c) Back view.

2. Characteristics in features:
   a) Perfect as well as imperfect features.
   b) Defects or blemishes.

3. Body structure, posture, and poise.

FACIAL TYPES

The facial type of each patron is determined by the position and prominence of the facial bones. There are seven facial types: oval, round, square, oblong, pear shape, heart shape, and diamond.

To recognize each facial type and be able to give correct advice, the hairstylist should be acquainted with the outstanding characteristics of each.

Oval Facial Type

The oval type is generally accepted as the perfect face. The contour and proportions of the oval face form the basis for modifying all other facial types.

Facial Contour: The oval face is about one and a half times longer than its width across the brow; the forehead is slightly wider than the chin.

Any style can be worn as there are no features to minimize.

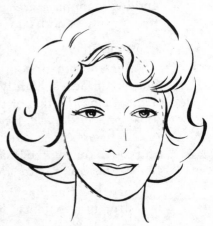

Round Facial Type

Facial Contour: Round hairline and round chinline.

Aim: To create the illusion of length to the face.

Arranging the hair on top of the head and dressed over the ears and part of the cheeks, with bangs to one side, will help to minimize the roundness of the face.

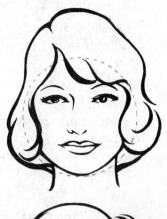

Square Facial Type

Facial Contour: Straight hairline and square jawline.

Aim: To create the illusion of length and offset the squareness of the features.

The problems of the square facial type are similar to those of the round. The style should lift off the forehead and come forward at the sides and jaw, to create the illusion of narrowness and softness in the face.

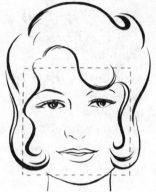

Pear-Shape Facial Type

Facial Contour: Narrow forehead, wide jawline and chinline.

Aim: To create the illusion of width in the forehead.

Keep the hair dressed fairly full and high. Partially cover the forehead with a fringe of waved hair. The hair should be worn with a semi-curl or soft-wave effect over the lower jawline. This arrangement will add apparent width to the forehead.

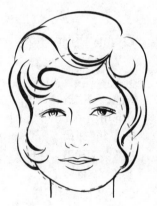

Oblong Facial Type

Facial Contour: Long, narrow face with hollow cheeks.

Aim: To make the face appear shorter and wider.

The hair should be styled fairly close to the top of the head with a fringe of curls or bangs, combined with fullness at the sides. The length of the face will appear to be reduced.

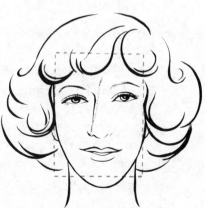

Diamond Facial Type

Facial Contour: Narrow forehead, extreme width through the cheekbones, and narrow chin.

Aim: To reduce the width across the cheekbone line.

Increasing the fullness across the forehead and at the jawline, while keeping the hair close to the head at the cheekbone line will help to create the illusion of ovalness to the face.

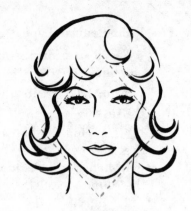

Heart-Shape Facial Type

Facial Contour: Wide forehead and narrow chinline.

Aim: To decrease the width of the forehead and increase the width in the lower part of the face.

To reduce the width of the forehead, a hairstyle with a center part with bangs rolled up or a style slanted to one side is recommended. Add width and softness at the jawline.

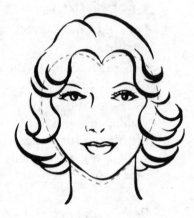

SPECIAL CONSIDERATIONS

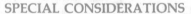

Plump With Short Neck

Aim: To create illusion of length.

Corrective Hairstyle: For the forehead, use forward bangs. Style the crown high to lend the illusion of length. Waved-in sides create a slender effect. A smooth head-hugging napeline emphasizes slenderness from the back and side view.

Avoid hairstyles that give fullness to the nape area.

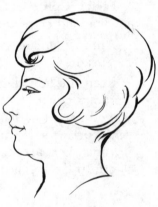

Long, Thin Neck

Aim: To minimize the appearance of a long neck.

Corrective Hairstyle: Cover the neck with soft waves or curls. Avoid styling the hair up from the back of the neck. Keep the nape hair long.

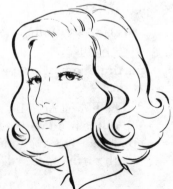

Thin Features

Aim: To minimize thinness of facial features and neck length.

Corrective Hairstyle: A high, soft crown-line, with the sides lifted up and out from the hairline and brushed loosely forward onto the cheeks, will create a softening effect for the face, and develop a soft, fluffy effect at the forehead. Keep the nape hair long and full, to offset the long, thin neck.

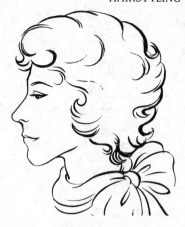

Negroid Features

Follow styling rules that relate to each particular facial type.

Styling the hair. It may be accompanied by one of two different methods of hair straightening or relaxing:

Chemically relaxed. The hair should be wet set with rollers and pin curls. It is then dried and combed out in the usual manner.

Thermal straightened (pressed). Use large barrel curls or curl with thermal (marcel) irons. Then comb the hair into a suitable hairstyle.

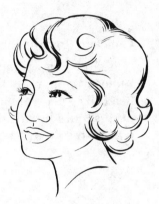

Uneven Features

Aim: To minimize the imperfect features.

Corrective Hairstyle: Uneven features can be minimized by selection of the proper hairstyle. The suggested hairstyle recommended for this model is a soft effect over protruding features, thereby creating evenness on both sides of the face.

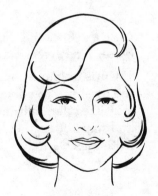

Oriental Features

Follow hairstyling rules that relate to the particular facial shape. The oriental hairstyle is very versatile in that it may be combed into a side-upward movement, or into a loose, fluffy page-boy style. This is achieved by rolling the hair outward or inward.

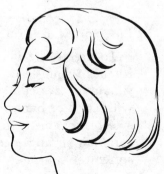

Straight

Usually, all hairstyles are becoming to the straight or normal profile.

A normal profile is neither concave nor convex. It contains neither a prominent protrusion nor a receding feature.

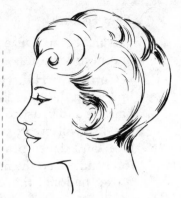

Concave (Prominent Chin)

A close hair arrangement or bangs over the forehead minimizes the bulginess of the forehead. The hair at the sides and nape of the neck should be dressed in small, soft curls or waves to soften the features.

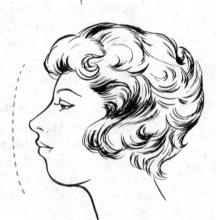

Convex (Receding Forehead, Prominent Nose, And Receding Chin)

Curls or bangs should be placed forward on the forehead to conceal the receding forehead and irregular hairline. The hair at the sides and nape of the neck should be dressed close to the head to give it perfect balance.

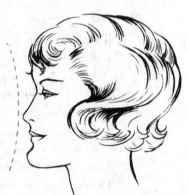

Low Forehead, Protruding Chin

To create the illusion of height to a low forehead and length to the face, the hair should be dressed high on the top of the head with curls or bangs on the forehead. An upsweep movement in the temple area with a soft hair arrangement over the jawline will soften the sharpness of the chin.

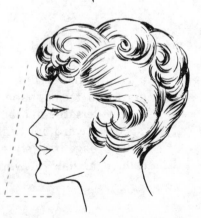

NOSE SHAPES

Closely allied to any profile analysis, in fact a very important part of such study, is the shape of the nose which must be considered both in profile and in full face. (Appropriate makeup for nose shapes will be found in the chapter on **Facial Makeup**.)

TURNED-UP NOSE

This type of nose is usually small and accompanied by a straight profile. To overcome this, the hair should be swept back off the face at the sides, lengthening the line from the nose to the ear.

Top hair is given a forward movement to minimize the appearance of the turned-up nose.

PROMINENT NOSE

A hooked nose, a large nose, or a pointed nose, all come under this classification. The stylist must plan to draw as much attention as possible away from these features.

To minimize the prominence of the nose, bring the hair forward at the forehead with softness around the face.

CROOKED NOSE

To minimize the conspicuous crooked nose, style the hair in an off center manner which will attract the eye away from the nose.

WIDE, FLAT NOSE

A wide, flat nose tends to broaden the face. In order to minimize this effect, the hair should be drawn away from the face.

A hairstyle with a middle part and double curled bangs will draw attention away from the nose.

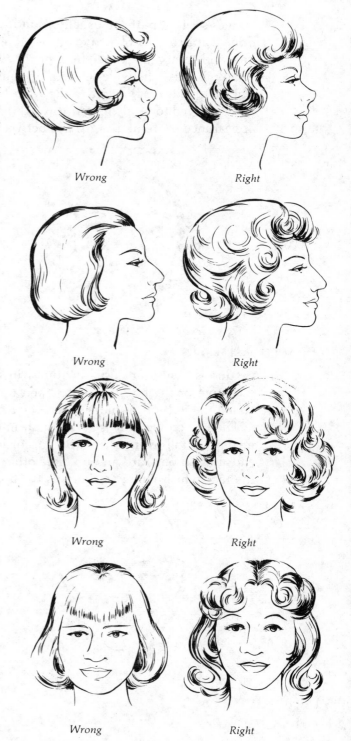

Wrong   *Right*

Wrong   *Right*

Wrong   *Right*

Wrong   *Right*

THE EYES

The eyes are the focal point of all feminine beauty. A professional hairstylist should be qualified to minimize or entirely eliminate any defects in the appearance of the eyes.

WIDE-SET EYES

Eyes set far apart are usually found with round, square, or strong cheekbone features. The objective of the stylist is to effect a better balance for the face and to minimize the effect of the wide space between the eyes.

To minimize the wide-set eyes, lift and fluff the top hair into a side bang. The other side is styled into a dip wave. The rest of the hairstyle is fluff dried and arranged to nestle under, toward the head. The entire hairstyle gives the appearance of minimizing space between the eyes.

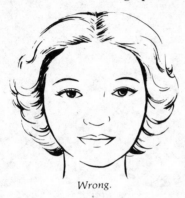
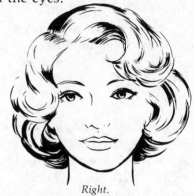

Wrong.　　　　　*Right.*

CLOSE-SET EYES

Close-set eyes are usually found in an oval or long, narrow face. The objective of the hairstyle is to open up the appearance of the face and to create the illusion of more space between the eyes.

The top crown hair is styled high into a pyramid effect. The side movement may fall over either brow, according to the patron's choice, with hair ends turned outward and up. The other side of the hair is styled away from the face which will give the eyes the appearance of being wider apart.

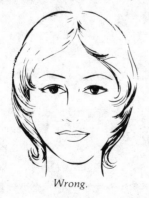
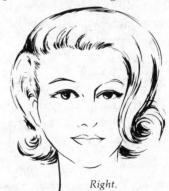

Wrong.　　　　　*Right.*

STYLING FOR WOMEN WHO WEAR GLASSES

Women who wear glasses should be especially careful in their hairstyling and makeup habits. A combination of a becoming hairstyle, the proper makeup, and the correct glasses should be blended together to develop and emphasize the wearer's basic feminine beauty. To the beholder, a face wearing glasses can take on an individualistic, special charm, if all the elements of good grooming are in proper harmony.

The following are a number of basic good grooming rules that should be followed by all women who wear glasses:

1. Glasses should be modern, with large lenses for good vision.
2. Never wear gaudy, over-jewelled, or tricky frames.
3. Do not wear strip false eyelashes. They are too long and function like windshield wipers with every eye movement.
4. Do not use heavy eye makeup. It does not require heavy makeup to bring out the color and the best features of your eyes.
5. Hairstyles that fall naturally around the face, making putting on and taking off glasses easy, are most advantageous.
6. Over-styled hair with many tight curls is impractical for women with glasses.

There are numerous **"do's"** and **"don'ts"** in every area of hair and facial grooming. The following are designed to illustrate some of the **"do's"** for those women who must wear glasses:

THE ROUND, OVAL, OR SQUARE FACE

The natural beauty of the oval, round, or square facial types can be further enhanced with proper glasses and grooming.

Glasses. A woman with big eyes should wear slender frames with large visual lenses to show off eyes and good eye makeup. (Color of frames should be selected carefully to match her hair.)

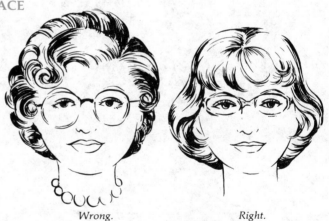

Wrong.   *Right.*

Hairstyle. Wear a bouffant hairstyle in natural balance, a simple, uncluttered style, casual but chic.

Bangs. Wear a slashed bang freely touching the eyebrows.

Jewelry. If earrings are worn, they should be long and dangling.

THE HEART-SHAPE OR DIAMOND-SHAPE FACE

The natural beauty of the heart-shape or diamond-shape face can be emphasized, and the glasses can become an integral part of a very pleasing grooming picture.

Glasses. Wear smart, slender frames that follow or give a lift to the eye-

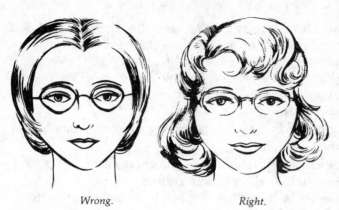

Wrong.   *Right.*

brows. The frames should be of medium thickness to rest gently against the face.

Makup. Wear light makeup shades and delicate eye makeup.

Hairstyle. Wear a full page boy style, or increase the width in the lower part of the face.

Bangs. Wear open, chic bangs which harmonize and balance with the lower part of the face.

THE SMALL, NARROW, OR OVAL FACE

The small, narrow, or oval face has a special, unique charm which should be emphasized by proper grooming.

Glasses. Select large, modern frames that are not too exotic or gaudy.

Makeup. Wear only natural tones of makeup. It is essential that eye makeup be applied very carefully. The eyes are seen and magnified through the glasses. Proper eye makeup emphasizes beautiful, sparkling eyes.

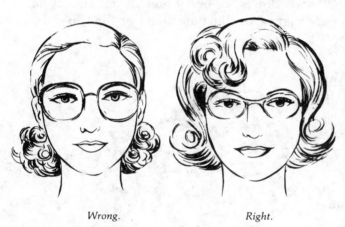

Wrong.   *Right.*

Hairstyle. Since the face is delicate in proportion, it is important that the hairstyle have width and height. The hairstyle should be short, with deep wave shapings on the sides, leaving freedom for control of glasses. Use deep waves and flip curls placed well back of the ears and ending lower at the nape.

Bangs. A side wave bang caressing one eyebrow can compliment the eyes.

THE PEAR-SHAPE FACE

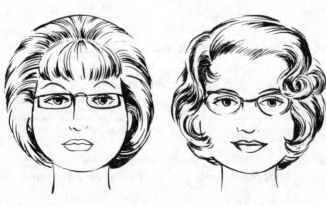

Wrong.   *Right.*

The pear-shape face has attractive features when properly made up and surrounded with an attractive hairstyle.

Glasses. Wear large, oval-shaped frames to let the glasses reveal eyes wearing appropriate makeup.

Hairstyle. This facial contour requires emphasis on length; therefore, wear the hair up and off the face, high in the front and crown. Soft bouffant styling around the face, with softness brushed forward on the cheeks, reduces width and adds beauty.

Bangs. A side wave bang over one eye will add expression and interest.

Proper hairstyling, correct makeup, and the selection of suitable and becoming glasses all contribute to making the woman who wears glasses much more attractive.

SHAPES OF HEADS

The shape of the patron's skull (head) has just as many variations as the rest of her physical features. Again the oval is considered to be the perfect shape. It is the hairstylist's objective to produce this shape by skillfully shaping and arranging the hair. The hairstylist should carefully observe the patron's head shape, and then mentally impose an oval picture over it. Where there is flatness, the volume of the hair should be adjusted to fill the area.

The heavy lines on the diagrams outline the actual shape of the head, and the shaded areas indicate where volume is required. This does not necessarily mean that all heads and all hair designs must be oval. The complete outside shape may be fashioned into many patterns and designs as long as the head shape has been ovalized.

HEAD SHAPES

1. The perfect head shape (oval).
2. The narrow head, flat back.
3. The flat crown.
4. The pointed head shape, hollow nape.
5. The flat top.
6. The small head.

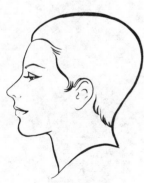
1. Perfect shape.

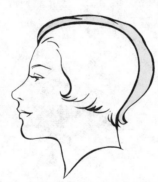
2. Narrow head—flat back.

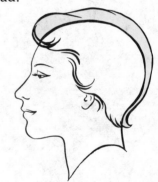
3. Flat crown.

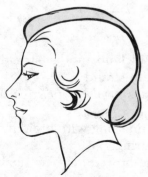
4. Pointed head, hollow nape.

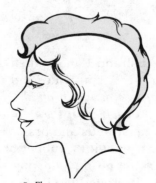
5. Flat top.

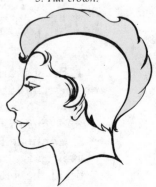
6. Small head.

BRAIDING

Braiding has long been a popular hair grooming technique with both adults and children. The cosmetologist would do well to add the ability to perform this technique to the range of her styling skills. It helps to broaden her professional scope and adds to her versatility as an artist.

There are two different types of braiding:
1. French (invisible) braiding—regular braiding.
2. French (visible) braiding—inverted braiding.

INVISIBLE FRENCH BRAIDING

Invisible French braiding is performed by overlapping the strands on top.

Procedure

1. Part crown section off. Hold out of way with clips or clamps. Back hair: Part hair from center of crown, 1, to nape, 2. (Fig. 1)

2. Divide section evenly into three strands. Start to braid by bringing strand 1 (on the left) over strand 2a (in the center). (Fig. 2) Draw strands tightly.

3. Pick up another strand from the left, about ½" (1.25 cm) wide, as indicated by 2b. (Fig. 3) Join strands 2a and 2b. Tighten strands.

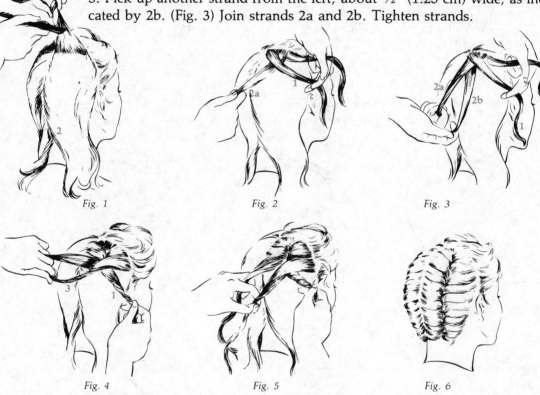

Fig. 1   Fig. 2   Fig. 3

Fig. 4   Fig. 5   Fig. 6

4. Bring strand 3 over strand 1 and tighten. (Fig. 4) Pick up another strand on the right, about ½" (1.25 cm) wide, and place with strand 1.

Note: *To insure a neat braid with all short hair ends in place, twist each strand toward the right or left with the thumb and index finger.*

5. Continue to pick up strands and braid (Fig. 5), finishing with braiding of hair ends at nape. Fasten with a rubber band or string.

Braid the left side of the head, following the same procedure. The final regular French braid is illustrated in Fig. 6.

Alternate method: The regular French braid (invisible) also may be started at the nape and braided toward the top of the head. The ends may be finished into rolls or curls.

Fashion

The braids may be crossed and tucked neatly underneath and held in place with hairpins or bobby pins.

When hair is long enough, braids can be crossed and extended up the back of the head.

Another attractive effect may be obtained by tying the braids with ribbons at the hairline and allowing the ends to fall into clusters of curls.

VISIBLE FRENCH BRAIDING

Inverted French braiding (visible) is done by pleating the strands under, thus making the braid visible.

Procedure

Part and section hair in the same manner as for regular French braid.

1. Divide top right section evenly into three strands. Start to braid the hair strands by placing the right side strand under the center strand, and the left side strand under this one. Draw strands tightly. (Fig. 1)

2. Pick up ½" (1.25 cm) strand on right side and combine with right side strand. Place this combined strand under the center strand. Pick up ½" (1.25 cm) strand on left side and combine with left side strand. Place this combined strand under center strand. (Fig. 2)

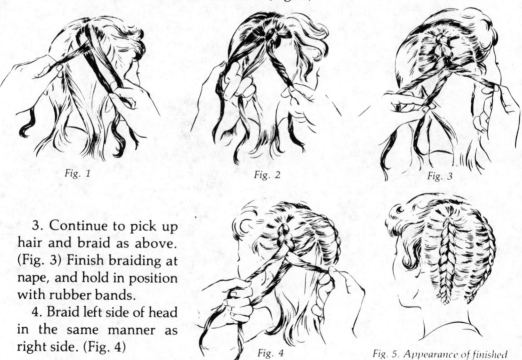

Fig. 1   Fig. 2   Fig. 3

3. Continue to pick up hair and braid as above. (Fig. 3) Finish braiding at nape, and hold in position with rubber bands.

4. Braid left side of head in the same manner as right side. (Fig. 4)

Fig. 4

Fig. 5. Appearance of finished inverted French braid with braids tucked under and held in place with hairpins or bobbi pins.

Fashion

The same suggestions recommended for the regular (visible) French braiding can be utilized for the inverted (invisible) French braiding.

CORN ROWING

Overly-curly hair may be fashioned into visible braids with long, narrow sections, sometimes called corn rows, which are popular with children and adults alike.

The technique is similar to the visible method of French braiding with the following exceptions: ·

1. After a shampoo, apply and distribute conditioner through the hair.
2. Use hand dryer or blow dryer to dry hair. If a hood dryer is used, apply and spread conditioner and then cover hair with a hair net. Have patron sit under dryer.

PROCEDURE

Pre-determine the hairstyle to be achieved.

Part a long, narrow section and braid as outlined for **French visible braids.**

Part another section and braid. Continue until the entire head is completed. (Fig. 1)

Fashion the style to be created so that it will enhance the appearance of the patron.

Corn rowing is a hairstyle for young ladies seeking an individualistic effect. (Fig. 2)

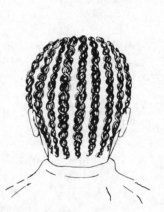

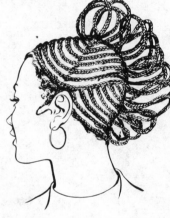

Fig. 1

Fig. 2

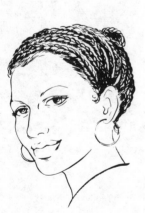

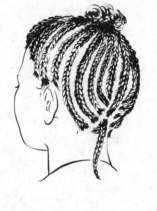

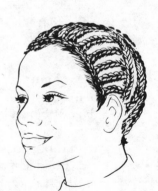

DEFINITIONS PERTAINING TO HAIRSTYLING

back-brushing: the brushing of the hair toward the scalp, so that the shorter hair tangles to form a cushion at the scalp for top covering hair. Other term used for back-brushing is **ruffing.**

back-combing: combing the underside of small sections of hair from the ends toward the scalp, causing the shorter hair to form a cushion at the scalp. Other terms used for back-combing are **teasing, ratting,** or **matting.** (See **French lacing** below.)

barrel curl: a curl that is wound like a roller curl without using a roller.

base: the stationary or immovable foundation of the curl that is attached to the scalp.

bouffant: the degree of height and fullness in a finished hairstyle.

carved curl: a section of hair sliced from a shaping and formed into a curl while holding the strand close to the head.

circle: that part of the pin curl forming a complete circle.

clockwise: the movement of hair, in shapings or curls, in the same direction as the movement of the hands of a clock.

counter-clockwise: the movement of hair, in shapings or curls, in the opposite direction to the movement of the hands of a clock.

curl: a circle or circles within a circle. The size of the curl governs the width of the wave.

direction: the moving of hair in order to form a particular pattern or style.
forward: toward the face.
down-shaping: directing the hair in a downward movement in preparation for a particular pattern or style.
up-shaping: directing the hair in an upward movement in preparation for a particular pattern or style.

extended or **elongated stem:** a space area between two rows of pin curls that permits the first row of curls to unfold without buckling.

finger wave: a wave formed in wet hair with the use of fingers and comb.

flat curl (regular pin curl): gives a flat motion and no lift.

forward curl: a curl that is directed toward the face.

forward shaping: directing the hair towards the face.

French lacing: a term for back-combing the top part of the hair.

hair shaping pivot: the exact point from which the hair is directed in forming a curvature or shaping.

indentation: indicates a curved hollow or valley created in the formation of a hairstyle.

molded (moulded) curl: same as carved curl.

molding (moulding): the forming or directing of the hair in order to create a desired shape or style.

movement: directing and changing the direction of hair.

over-directed: excessive direction of the hair in the formation of finger waves, curls, or shapings.

overlapping curl: a pin curl that is placed to partially cover an adjoining curl.

panel: the area between two partings. Other term used for panel is **section.**

pin curl wave: alternating the direction of rows of pin curls in order to form a wave pattern.

reverse (backward) curl: a curl that is directed away from the face.

reverse (backward) shaping: directing the hair towards the back of the head or away from the face.

ridge curl: a curl placed behind and close to the ridge of a finger wave.

roller curl: a section of wet hair wrapped around a roller.

sculpture curl (pin curl): a strand of hair that is combed smooth and ribbon-like and wound into a circle with the ends on the inside. Sometimes called a **flat** curl.

semi stand-up curl (flair curl): a pin curl carved out of a shaping and pinned into a semi-standing position.

shaping (in haircutting): the process of shortening and thinning the hair into a particular style or to the contour of the head.

shaping (in hairstyling): the formation of uniform arcs or curves in wet hair, thus providing a base for finger waves, pin curls, or various patterns in hairstyling.

skip wave: a pattern formed by a combination of finger wave and pin curl pattern, the pin curls being placed in alternate finger wave formation.

slicing: carefully removing a section of hair from a shaping, in preparation for making a curl. (The remainder of the shaping is not disturbed.)

stand-up curl (cascade curl): a curl with the stem directed straight up or out from the head and pinned in a standing position.

stem: that part of the pin curl between the base and the first arc of the circle.

no stem: the curl is placed in the center of the base.

half stem: the curl is placed one half off its base.

full stem: the curl is placed completely off its base.

stem direction: the direction in which the stem moves from the base to the first arc. (Stem direction may be forward, backward, upward, or downward.)

strand: a section of hair.

under-directed: insufficiently directing the hair in the formation of finger waves, curls, or shapings.

volume: indicates lift or height created in the formation of a hairstyle.

REVIEW QUESTIONS
HAIRSTYLING

1. Why is it important that a cosmetologist know basic hairstyling?
2. What must a cosmetologist understand in order to become a proficient hairstylist?
3. What should be the condition of hair in order to obtain successful results in hairstyling?
4. Why is the correct removal of tangles important for successful hairstyling?
5. By what other names are pin curls known?
6. What prior treatments should the hair receive in order to insure long-lasting and springy curls?
7. What type of hair is best suited for pin curling?
8. List the three principal parts of a pin curl.
9. Define the base of a curl.
10. Where is the stem of a curl located?
11. What is the function of the curl stem?
12. What is the function of the pin curl circle?
13. Which part of the pin curl determines its mobility?
14. Name three lengths of stems that affect the mobility of curls.
15. When is a no-stem curl used?
16. How does a no-stem curl affect its base?
17. When is a half-stem curl formation used?
18. How does a half-stem curl permit movement?
19. When is a full-stem curl used?
20. How can the greatest curl mobility be achieved?
21. What determines the size of the wave?
22. When is an open center curl used?
23. When is a closed center curl recommended?
24. Explain the directions of a forward curl and of a reverse curl in relation to the face.
25. What is a hair shaping?
26. How may shapings be classified?
27. How is the hair directed in a side forward shaping?
28. List the four most commonly shaped bases used in hairstyling.
29. What effect, if any, does the shape of the base have upon the resulting curl?
30. Why are triangular base pin curls used along the front, or facial, hairline?
31. When are square-base pin curls recommended?
32. In what direction are pin curls placed?
33. What are ridge curls?
34. Describe the formation of a skip wave.
35. When and where is the use of skip waves recommended?
36. What hair length is most likely to obtain the best results in skip waving?
37. By what other name is the cascade curl known?
38. Which hairstyle effects may be created with the use of cascade curls?
39. For what purpose are roller curls used?
40. Name one important difference between a roller curl and a stand-up curl.

41. How can a cosmetologist keep hair from slipping off the rollers?
42. What is the function of end papers when used with rollers?
43. When is a barrel curl used?
44. What is meant by volume in a hairstyle?
45. What is meant by indentation in a hairstyle?
46. How is volume created?
47. How is indentation achieved?
48. What governs the size of the roller used?
49. What three factors determine the patron's type of hair parting?
50. What is achieved by back-combing and back-brushing techniques?
51. Give four alternate names for back-combing.
52. What other name is used for back-brushing?
53. Name the four basic steps to follow when combing out the hair.
54. Why is hair spray applied to the hair after a comb-out?
55. List the three general characteristics upon which an artistic and suitable hairstyle may be based.
56. Which is the ideal type of face for any hairstyle to be created?
57. How should the hair be styled for the square and round facial types?
58. In styling a pear-shape facial type, what illusion should be created in the forehead and jawline areas?
59. In styling a heart-shape facial type, what illusion should be created in the jawline and forehead areas?
60. For a short, thick neck, how should the hair at the back of the head be styled?
61. To minimize the long appearance of the neck, how should the hair be styled?

Chapter 13

THE CARE AND STYLING OF WIGS

CHAPTER LEARNING OBJECTIVES

The student successfully mastering this chapter will know:
1. *The difference between handmade and machine-made wigs.*
2. *The procedure in taking wig measurements.*
3. *The technique of blocking a wig.*
4. *The techniques in wig cleaning and conditioning.*
5. *The procedures for adjusting a wig.*
6. *How to shape a wig.*
7. *The procedure for setting and combing out wigs.*
8. *The art of coloring wigs.*
9. *The various types of hairpieces and their uses.*
10. *The safety precautions to be followed in handling wigs.*
11. *The definitions pertaining to wigs.*

Throughout history, wigs have served to enhance women's charm and beauty. The ancient Egyptians first wore wigs in 4000 B.C., primarily to protect their own hair from the sun. From Asia and Europe, wigs spread to America, where they have grown in popularity over the years.

The use of wigs and hairpieces in hairstyling has become an important and exciting part of the beauty industry. The sale, styling, and servicing of all hairpieces can be the source of an important part of the salon's income.

In order to offer the best possible services, the hairstylist must be familiar with the following:
1. How wigs and hairpieces can improve patrons' appearance.
2. How wigs and hairpieces are made and fitted.
3. How to select and style wigs and hairpieces to the patrons' best advantage.
4. How to clean and service wigs and hairpieces.

WHY WIGS ARE WORN

Wigs are worn for three principal reasons:
1. **Necessity**—to cover up baldness and sparse or damaged hair.
2. **Fashion**—for changes in everyday hairstyles, for decorative purposes, and for special occasions.
3. **Practicality**—for quick changes in hair shades and styles to accommodate the busy woman.

TYPES OF WIGS

Wigs can be made from human hair, synthetic or animal hair, or a blend of both.

A simple match test will tell the difference between human hair and synthetic hair. Cut a small piece of hair from the back area of the wig. With a lighted match, burn this hair and observe these characteristics:

1. Human hair burns slowly and gives off a strong odor resembling burnt chicken feathers.
2. Synthetic hair burns quickly and gives off little or no odor. Besides, small, hard beads can be felt in the burnt ash.

Modacrylic is the general term used to describe synthetic wig fibers.

HUMAN HAIR WIGS

The quality of a wig depends to a great extent on whether it is constructed by hand or machine. Expensive, custom-made wigs are hand knotted into a fine mesh foundation. (Figs. 1 and 2) In cheaper weft wigs, hair is sewn by machine into the net cap in circular rows. (Figs. 3, 4, and 5)

The quality of a wig also varies with the kind of hair it contains, the way it is constructed, and how it is fitted to the patron's measurements.

Handmade Wigs (Ventilated Wigs)

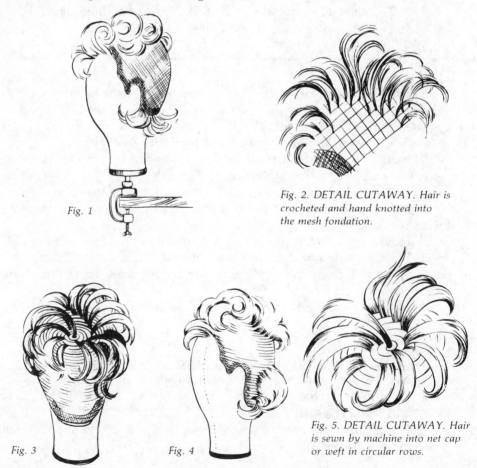

Fig. 1

Fig. 2. DETAIL CUTAWAY. Hair is crocheted and hand knotted into the mesh fondation.

Fig. 3

Fig. 4

Fig. 5. DETAIL CUTAWAY. Hair is sewn by machine into net cap or weft in circular rows.

SYNTHETIC WIGS AND HAIRPIECES

Great improvements have been made in the manufacture of synthetic fibers. Modacrylic fibers, such as dynel, kanekalon, venicelon, and others, have eliminated most of the disadvantages of synthetic hairs. Hair fiber research has developed synthetic hair that closely resembles human hair in texture, resiliency, color acceptance, pliability, durability, sheen, and feel. The fibers have good curl retention, are non-flammable, and do not oxidize and change color in sunlight. In fact, some synthetic fibers so closely resemble human hair that it is difficult to distinguish between them.

Synthetic hairs have a number of advantages that have contributed to their acceptance for the manufacture of wigs and hairpieces. Since the hair is synthetically produced, it is very economical. The supply is unlimited. The wigs and hairpieces are made from long threads that have been rolled on spools, permitting great efficiency in use. They are made with color fasteners in any color or shade desired.

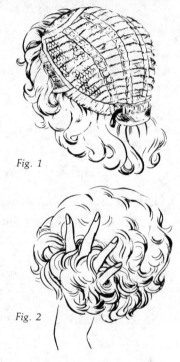

Fig. 1

Synthetic wigs are available as handmade stretch wigs (Fig. 1), as machine-made stretch wigs, and as handmade fitted wigs. Whatever the type of wig, careful selection of quality, proper fit, and good workmanship will give satisfaction in wear, comfort, and style.

Also available is the **no-cap wig** which is composed of rows of wefting sewn to elastic bands. The advantages of no-cap wigs are that they are light and keep the patron's head cooler than other types of wigs. (Fig. 2)

Wig caps and hairpieces are made of cotton, cotton and a synthetic, all synthetic, or reinforced elastic. Hairpieces are generally made with a synthetic base which does not shrink when shampooed. Synthetic hairpieces are available as wiglets, demi-wigs, braids, chignons, cascades, and falls.

Fig. 2

TAKING WIG MEASUREMENTS

To assure a comfortable and secure fit, correct measurements must be taken of the patron's head. First, brush the hair down smoothly and pin it as flat and tight as possible. Keeping close to the head without pressure, take flat measurements with a tape.

PROCEDURE

1. Measure circumference of head. Place tape completely around the head, starting at hairline at middle of forehead; place tape above the ears, around back of head, and return to starting point. (Fig. 1)
2. Measure from hairline at middle of forehead, over top, to nape of neck. Bend head back and measure to point where wig will ride on base of skull at the nape. (Fig. 2)

3. Measure from ear to ear, across forehead. (Fig. 3)

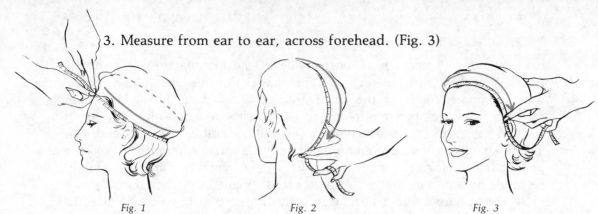

Fig. 1   Fig. 2   Fig. 3

4. Measure from ear to ear, over top of head. (Fig. 4)
5. Place tape across the crown and measure from temple to temple. (Fig. 5)
6. Measure the width of napeline, across nape of neck. (Fig. 6)

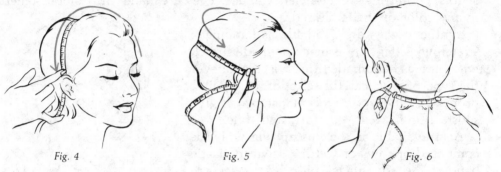

Fig. 4   Fig. 5   Fig. 6

Note: Check to make certain that measurements are accurate.

ORDERING THE WIG

When ordering the wig, keep a written record of the patron's head measurements, and forward a copy to the wig dealer or manufacturer. Also specify what is desired as to:

1. Hair shade. If necessary, submit samples of the patron's hair to the manufacturer. Hair samples should be of hair that has been freshly shampooed, tinted, or rinsed.
2. Quality of hair.
3. Length of hair.
4. Type of hair part and hair pattern.

BLOCKING THE WIG

Good blocking helps obtain professional results when shaping, setting, and combing out a wig. It also reduces the possibility of disturbing the comb-out when T-pins are removed.

Use properly protected canvas blocks for all wig services, because they will stand up under continuous pinning and rough handling. Styrofoam blocks are used for storing the wig. A swivel clamp is used for better block control.

There are six sizes of canvas blocks available: 20, 20½, 21, 21½, 22, and 22½" (50, 51.25, 52.5, 53.75, 55, and 56.25 cm).

The wig should neither be stretched nor hung loosely on a wrong size block, but should fit comfortably. A wig that is stretched and pinned may become larger when the cap is wetted, or if it is hung loosely, it may shrink when the cap is wetted (if made of cotton).

Mount the wig on the correct head size block and pin as follows:

1. At center of the forehead.
2. At each side (temple side). (Fig. 1)
3. At center of the nape.
4. At each corner of the nape. (Fig. 2)

(These illustrations show the proper placement of T-pins.)

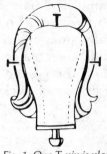

Fig. 1. One T-pin is placed at center of forehead and one at each side.

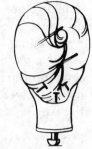

Fig. 2. One T-pin is placed at center of nape and one pin at each corner.

ADJUSTING THE WIG

After the wig has been made according to specific measurements, it may require some adjustments in order to fit the patron's head.

ADJUSTING THE WIG TO A LARGER SIZE

If the wig feels too tight, it may require some stretching. Turn the wig inside out and wet the foundation with hot water. Stretch the wig carefully (without ripping) onto a larger size block and pin securely. Then allow the wig to dry naturally.

ADJUSTING THE WIG TO A SMALLER SIZE

If the wig feels too loose, it must be adjusted to fit properly.

Tucking

Tucks are used to improve the fit of a wig that is too big.

1. **Horizontal tucks** shorten the wig from front to nape. They are made across the back of the wig, in order to remove excess bulk. (Fig. 1)
2. **Vertical tucks** remove width at the back of the wig, from ear to ear. (Fig. 2)

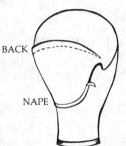

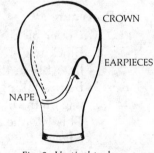

Fig. 1. Horizontal tuck.   *Fig. 2. Vertical tuck.*

Both earpieces must be checked to be certain they are directly across from each other and do not touch the ears. If the wig touches the ear, make a small horizontal tuck over the ear to raise the wig off the ear. If the wig is rubbing or touching the side of the ear, a small vertical tuck behind the ear will pull the wig back and eliminate the problem.

Check the cap fit after each tuck. Excessive tucking will cause the wig to "ride up" and create new fitting problems.

If a wig is too long from forehead to nape, make a tuck approximately ¼" (.625 cm) deep on the weft. Always sew a tuck toward the crown, never down, or hair will stand away from the wig in the comb-out. When tacking a tuck, be certain that as much hair as possible is taken out before the stitching process is completed. The same applies if a wig is too large from crown to ear, where the wig rests on the patron's ear. This can be corrected by stitching horizontally along the wefting.

Note: When adjusting a ventilated or hand-tied wig, the tucks should be sewn on the inside of the foundation. However, when adjusting a machine-made or wefted wig, horizontal tucks can be sewn either inside or outside the wig.

THE ELASTIC BAND

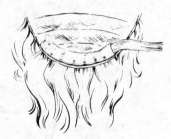
Elastic band.

The final step in the wig adjustment process is adjusting the elastic band at the back of the wig. Pull the elastic band to make the wig fit evenly and snugly at the back of the head and then fasten it.

Some hairstylists favor pinning the ends of the elastic band with a small safety pin, to permit easy adjustments or replacements in the future. The elastic band does require periodic adjustment or replacement, as it stretches or deteriorates because of its exposure to body heat or cleaning fluids over a period of time. Other hairstylists believe that the band should be stitched securely and the stitches broken when additional adjustment or replacement is needed.

CLEANING WIGS

HUMAN HAIR WIGS

A human hair wig should be dry-cleaned every 2-4 weeks, depending on how often it is worn. Also, when a wig is ready for restyling, it should be dry-cleaned.

Procedure
1. Cover block with plastic cover to protect canvas. (Fig. 1)
2. Block wig. Remove back combing, if necessary. Direct hair off the hairline. Brush the hair to loosen dirt and hair spray.
3. Before taking the wig off the block to be cleaned, mark the size of the wig on the block in order to retain the same size after it has been cleaned. This is done by placing a T-pin into the block on an angle next to the edge of the cap and directly in front of the six T-pins securing the wig. (Figs. 2 and 3) Remove the wig, and proceed with the cleaning.

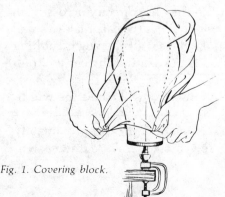
Fig. 1. Covering block.

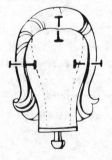
Fig. 2. Front view.

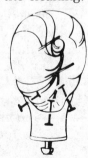
Fig. 3. Back view.

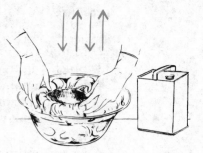

4. Wear rubber gloves to protect your hands. Saturate the wig in a large glass or porcelain bowl containing about 3 ounces (90 ml) of non-flammable liquid cleanser. With the hair side down, dip the wig up and down until it is clean. (Fig. 4)

   Alternate method: *Swirl the wig around in the liquid cleanser. If necessary, clean the edges and inside foundation with a cotton ball or toothbrush.*

Fig. 4

5. Gently shake wig to remove excess fluid. Place the wet wig immediately on the canvas block. Stretch the wig lightly and pin it securely to the block. (Fig. 5)

6. When dry, set and style the wig.

HAND-TIED WIGS

Hand-tied wigs, which are more delicate in structure and far more costly, should be cleaned on the block.

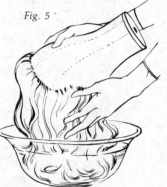

Fig. 5

Procedure

1. Cover canvas block with plastic to protect canvas.

2. Clean edges and inside foundation with a cotton ball or toothbrush.

3. Block the wig.

4. Saturate the wig in a large glass or porcelain bowl containing liquid cleaner. (Fig. 6)

5. Soak the wig for 3-4 minutes.

6. Comb the cleaning solution through length of hair with wide-tooth comb.

7. Work the solution into the entire wig.

8. Carefully towel blot. (Fig. 7)

9. Allow to dry naturally on block for about ½ hour.

10. Give conditioning treatment, if necessary.

11. Set and style the wig.

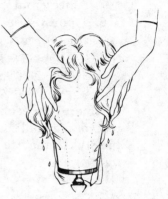

Fig. 6. Saturate wig and work solution through hair.

SYNTHETIC WIGS

Synthetic wigs and hairpieces do not require cleaning as often as human hair wigs. Synthetic fibers are non-absorbent (lack porosity) and do not attract dust and dirt.

Synthetic wigs and hairpieces require cleaning about every three months, depending on the amount of wear and styling. Use tepid or cool water to clean the wig, as hot water will take the curl out of the synthetic wig.

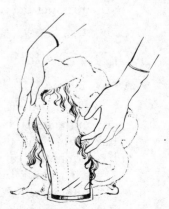

Fig. 7. Towel dry hair.

Procedure

1. Cover appropriate block with plastic to protect canvas.
2. Mount wig on block and outline size.
3. Brush wig free of tangles and wig spray before cleaning.
4. Fill a container with mild shampoo or a specially formulated cleaner (read directions). Use tepid or cool water.
5. Remove the wig from the block. Swish the wig through cleaning solution for a few minutes. Rinse thoroughly in cool water.
6. Use a toothbrush or cotton to clean the foundation.
7. Squeeze out excess water and towel blot. (Do not wring or twist wig.)
8. T-pin wig on proper size block and let dry naturally.
9. Do not brush a synthetic wig when it is wet as the curl may be removed.
10. Do not expose a synthetic wig to heat.
11. When wig is completely dry, brush out hair and spray with conditioner, to add luster.

Note: If it becomes necessary to reduce the drying time, the wig may be placed in a cool dryer with only the fan used. Since most synthetic wigs are pre-styled, they require no further styling.

CONDITIONING THE WIG

A wig differs from hair on the human head because it does not have its own supply of natural oils for self-lubrication. Since wig cleaners usually are very drying to the hair, it is advisable that a conditioning treatment be given after each cleaning, to keep the wig hair from drying and looking dull, and to keep it in good condition. (Fig. 8)

PROCEDURE

1. Cover block with plastic and block wig properly.
2. Apply conditioner. Distribute conditioner evenly to damp, clean hair with a wide-tooth comb. Keep conditioner in hair for the length of time indicated in the instructions accompanying the product being used.
3. Set and style the wig.

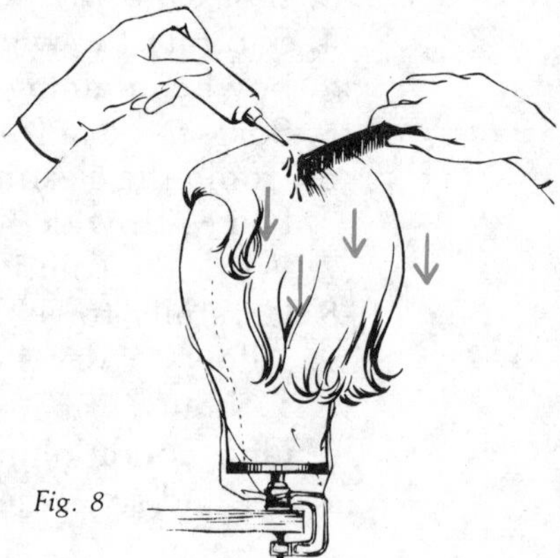

Fig. 8

SHAPING WIGS

SHAPING HUMAN HAIR WIG

Basically, a wig may be shaped (cut) in the same manner as natural hair is cut on the head. However, consideration must be given to the fact that a wig has about twice as much hair as the normal human head. As a result of this large quantity of hair, the failure to thin and taper the wig properly will cause it to look bulky and artificial.

Thinning wig hair may be done with either a razor or thinning shears. Because of the excessive amount of hair in the wig, more bulk must be removed in the top section, in back of the ears, and around the face. These are areas that usually are not thinned on natural hair.

Most of the thinning should be done as close to the wig foundation as possible, without damage to the cap itself. Thin close to the cap to remove more bulk and to be certain that no hair spurs are left to stick out after the hair is styled. Special care must be taken so that all knots on the hand-knotted wig are tight. Equal care must be taken not to cut any of the wefts or sewing threads on the wefted wig.

When cutting the wig, special care must be exercised, because once a wig has been cut the hair will not grow back to cover an error in judgment.

The wig may be cut either on the head, to fit in with the natural hair, or on a canvas block, to facilitate ease and freedom of the hairstylist's movements.

It is a good technique to cut the guideline on the patron's head and then transfer the wig to the block. This assures you that the wig is being cut to the proper length. By moving the wig to the block, you can secure it firmly for the balance of the shaping process.

Cutting on the block also has the advantage of permitting the wig to be pinned securely, thus avoiding possible slippage during the cutting process.

In placing the wig to be cut on the canvas block, it is important that you carefully set it on the block evenly and at the correct hairline distance.

PROCEDURE **(Can be done on a block or on the patron's head.)**

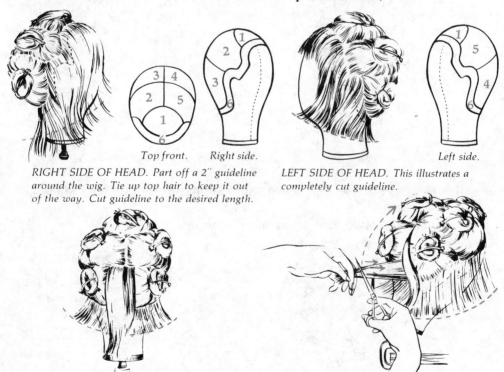

Top front.   *Right side.*   *Left side.*

RIGHT SIDE OF HEAD. *Part off a 2" guideline around the wig. Tie up top hair to keep it out of the way. Cut guideline to the desired length.*

LEFT SIDE OF HEAD. *This illustrates a completely cut guideline.*

BACK OF HEAD. *Let down center back hair. Cut to the same length as guideline.*

BACK OF HEAD. *Pick up a strand of the guideline. With hands arched at a 45° angle, cut into longer hair. Proceed with a sweeping upward motion.*

Continue the shaping process, section by section, until the entire wig has been shaped.

SHAPING SYNTHETIC HAIR WIG

Use only scissors and thinning shears on either synthetic fiber or on a mixture of synthetic and human hair. The durable fiber is extremely dulling to a razor.

Synthetic fiber is solid and does not have the resiliency or flexibility of human hair. As a result, a razor may cause permanent damage to the wig.

Synthetic wigs always should be cut dry, because the fibers may stretch and become mis-shapen if pulled when wet.

SETTING AND STYLING WIGS

SETTING AND STYLING HUMAN HAIR WIGS

Setting wig hair is similar to setting hair on the human head, except for hairline coverage and the need for a tight curl at the nape area.

The added fullness of the patron's hair, plus the hair and foundation of the wig, are factors to be considered when setting and styling the wig.

Note: Remember that pin curls replace rollers on certain parts of the head, in order to keep the style close to the head.

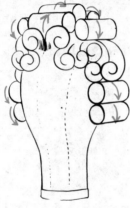

Setting on block.

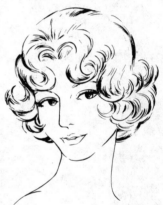

Comb-out.

It is desirable to use T-pins instead of clippies or bobby pins to hold both rollers and curls.

Set, dry, and style hair in the usual manner.

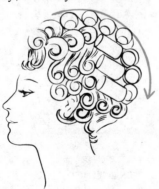

Setting on head.

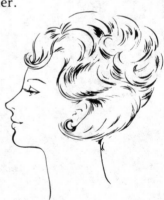

Comb-out.

SETTING AND STYLING SYNTHETIC WIGS

Cutting and styling synthetic wigs differ from human hair wigs in the following ways:

Teasing or back-combing synthetic wigs should be confined solely to the base of the fibers. This is necessary to avoid damage to the fiber, which should be kept perfectly smooth at the wig surface. Damage to the hair shaft (by thinning) will result in a frizzy, fuzzy looking wig.

Synthetic wigs are pre-cut into definite styles when they are manufactured. If the patron desires a change, a good quality synthetic wig may be combed into different styles by a skilled stylist. These comb-out styles are all based on the basic pre-cut factory created style. The synthetic wig never really needs restyling. However, the hairstylist must be guided by the patron's wishes.

PUTTING ON AND TAKING OFF A WIG

A simple, but very important, procedure is the correct way to remove a wig from a block and place it on the patron's head. (It is a good policy to show the patron the proper way to put on and take off her own wig.)

PROCEDURE

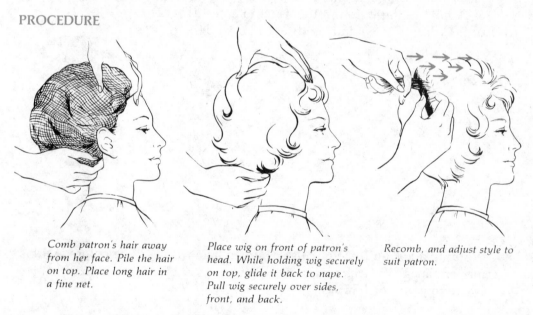

Comb patron's hair away from her face. Pile the hair on top. Place long hair in a fine net.

Place wig on front of patron's head. While holding wig securely on top, glide it back to nape. Pull wig securely over sides, front, and back.

Recomb, and adjust style to suit patron.

To remove a wig from the head, place only the thumb of your right hand under the cap at the nape. **Do not put your fingers into the hair.** Have the patron bend her head down and slide the wig off, catching it in the palm of your left hand.

COMBING PATRON'S HAIR INTO A WIG

Comb patron's hair away from her face. Set a flat row of pin curls at the nape. Anchor pin curls with criss-cross bobby pins. Secure the wig at the nape. Bring it forward and adjust it to the front hairline.

When the wig is comfortably adjusted, draw out approximately 1" (2.5 cm) of the patron's hair from around the front hairline; then comb and blend the hair into the style of the wig.

WIG COLORING

COLOR RINSES

Color rinses are used as temporary coloring on human hair wigs and should be reapplied every time the hair is cleaned. Color rinses can only darken the hair; if a lighter color is desired, a different wig must be worn.

The following method is one way to apply a color rinse. Your instructor's method may be equally correct.

Procedure

1. Pin the wig securely on a plastic covered block.
2. Dampen clean hair, using a spray applicator bottle.
3. Whenever in doubt of which color to use, strand test the color rinse on the back of the wig.

Note: *If a color rinse is applied on dry hair, additional rinse is required for complete coverage.*

4. Spray hair with a color rinse. Distribute it evenly with a downward motion, using a small brush and a wide-tooth comb. (Fig. 1)
5. Apply setting lotion in the usual manner. (Fig. 2)
6. Set, dry, (Fig. 3) and comb out hair to desired style.

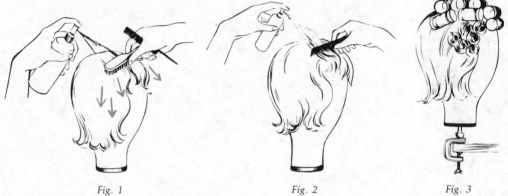

Fig. 1   Fig. 2   Fig. 3

Note: In addition to color rinses, human hair wigs may be colored with a semi-permanent tint. However, it is never advisable to attempt to lighten (bleach) any wig or hairpiece.

SEMI-PERMANENT TINTS

Semi-permanent tints are referred to as six-week tints. They are self-penetrating and require no peroxide. They do not change the basic structure of the hair. The following is one method of application of semi-permanent tints to machine-made wigs.

Procedure

1. Mount wig on appropriate plastic-covered block, and outline size with T-pins.
2. Remove all teasing, tangles, and snarls.
3. Clean wig and comb hair smooth.
4. Remove wig from block.

5. Immerse wig in glass bowl of hot water and semi-permanent tint solution.
6. Leave completely immersed for 10 miinutes.
7. Remove and rinse with cold water.
8. Apply conditioner.
9. Block, set, dry, and comb out in usual manner.

PERMANENT TINTS

Since 100% human hair wigs and hairpieces have been subjected to extensive processing, it is risky to use permanent tints on such hair as the results are unpredictable.

HAIRPIECES

A variety of hairstyles can be created with hairpieces that can be dressed for either daytime or evening wear. These hairpieces come in various forms, such as:

1. **Switches**—long wefts of hair mounted with a loop at the end. They are constructed with 1-3 stems of hair. The better switches are constructed with three stems, to provide greater flexibility in styling and braiding. They may be worked into the hair or braided, to create special styling effects. (Fig. 1)

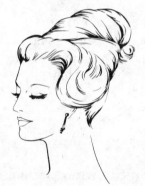 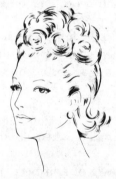 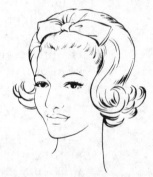

Fig. 1. Switch.　　　　*Fig. 2. Wiglet.*　　　　*Fig. 3. Bandeau type hairpiece.*

2. **Wiglets**—hairpieces with a flat base which are used in special areas of the head. They are used primarily to blend with patron's own hair in order to extend the range of the hair. Wiglets can be worked into the top of the hair in curls or under the hair, to give it height and body. They also are used to create special effects. (Fig. 2)

3. **Bandeau type**—a hairpiece that is sewn to a headband. The headband, which is replaceable and comes in different colors, serves as an excellent disguise for the hairline. The bandeau type hairpiece is usually worn over the hair, and is dressed in a casual, relaxed manner. (Fig. 3)

4. **Fall**—a section of hair, machine wefted on a round base, running across the back of the head and available in various lengths. Falls have a thick, full, and plushy look.

Short falls range from 12-14" (30-35 cm) in length. (Fig. 4)
Demi-falls, 15-20" (37.5-50 cm).
Long falls, 18-24" (45-60 cm).

5. **Demi-fall** or **demi-wig**—a large base hairpiece that is designed to fit to the shape of the head, and generally ranges in length from 15-20" (37.5-50 cm).

6. **Cascade**—a hairpiece on an oblong base which offers an endless variety of styling possibilities. Cascades can be styled in curls, braids or page boy, or can be used as a filler with patron's own hair. (Fig. 5)

7. **Braid**—a switch whose strands are woven, interlaced, or entwined together. Some are prepared with a thin wire inside, in order that they be formed into various shapes. Others, without wire, are permitted to hang loose on the head.

8. **Chignon**—a knot or coil of hair that is created from synthetic hair, and worn at the crown or nape of the head. A chignon is most effective when worn in combination with another hairpiece.

9. **Crown curls**—a group of light curls worn on top of the head.

10. **Frosting curls**—segments of frosted or blended hair pinned into any head of hair to simulate a frosted or streaked head of hair.

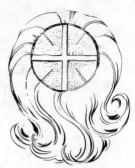

Fig. 4. Short fall.

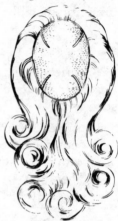

Fig. 5. Cascade.

SAFETY PRECAUTIONS

1. Great care must be taken when combing or brushing wigs to avoid matting.
2. When dry cleaning a wig or hairpiece, never rub or wring cleaning fluid from it.
3. When shaping (cutting) a wig or hairpiece, use great care; once the hair has been cut, it cannot grow back.
4. When combing a freshly set wig, use a wide-tooth comb to avoid abuse to the foundation, and to gain greater control in combing.
5. When cleaning or working with a wet wig, always mount it on a block the same head size as the wig, to avoid stretching.
6. To assure a comfortable and secure fit, correct measurements must be taken of the patron's head.
7. Recondition wigs as often as necessary, to prevent dryness or brittleness of the hair.
8. If required, dry clean wigs before setting and styling.
9. Brush and comb wigs and hairpieces with a downward movement.
10. Never lighten (bleach) a wig or hairpiece.
11. Never give a permanent to a wig or hairpiece.

DEFINITIONS PERTAINING TO WIGS

The following are the technical words commonly used in wig work:

angora: long, silky hair of the Angora goat. It is used primarily in fantasy work.

band wig: a hairpiece that is sewn to a headband which covers the hairline. The foundation of the hairpiece covers about ⅔ of the head, and the overhanging hair covers all the patron's hair. This can be used instead of a full wig.

base: the foundation of a hairpiece.

binding: ribbon used to protect and reinforce the edges of netting.

block (foundation block): a head-shaped block made to hold a wig upon which work is to be done.

cap (wig cap): the combined netting and binding of a wig.

capless wig: wefts of synthetic hair sewn on a cap made of wide straps. Also referred to as **synthetic wig cap.**

carbon tetrachloride (or carbon tet): chemical used for dry cleaning wigs.

caul: open weave netting used in the crown of a wig.

chignon: knot or coil of hair worn at the crown or nape.

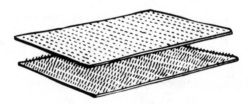

Swivel clamp.

clamp: device that can be attached to a table, and upon which a wig block can be mounted. A **swivel clamp** can be adjusted to hold the block at different angles.

custom-made wig: wig that is fitted to the exact measurements of a patron's head, and styled to her specifications.

dart: tapered seam formed by cutting into a piece of wig net foundation and sewing the cut ends together. A dart is used to reduce the size of a wig cap.

drawing brushes: the brushes used to hold hair for mixing, matching, ventilating, or weaving.

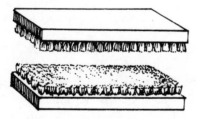

Drawing brushes.

Drawing cards.

drawing cards: two identical rectangles of leather with bent wire protruding throughout the surface area. They are held with the teeth pointed away from the cosmetologist, to create a resistance while the hair is being pulled through. They are used to hold hair and keep it from tangling while a small quantity is being drawn off.

fantasy: hairpiece used for its artiness rather than for its practicality. The stylist uses any design and color combination to achieve an effect.

foundation (base): any supporting material used as a base to attach hair to.

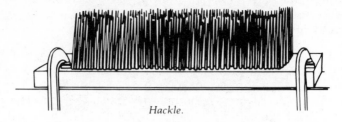

Hackle.

hackle: board with long metal teeth used for combing and mixing hair.

hackling: using a hackle to mix or blend hair.

hairpiece: small wig used to cover the top or crown of the head.

hair roll: a sausage-like shape, in various lengths, used to fill in under the natural hair in order to create special effects.

halo: lengths of layered hair, on a ventilated or wefted foundation band, used either over the top of the head or to encircle the head.

hem: the bent over edge of a piece of material that has been turned under to avoid fraying. In wig work, the netting is so hemmed in order to place the raw edge between the outside netting and the binding.

handmade (or **hand ventilated**) **wig:** wig that is made by hand-knotting hair onto a fine mesh net.

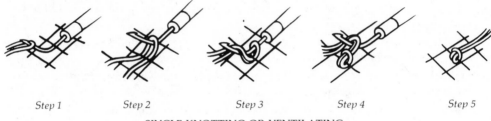

| *Step 1* | *Step 2* | *Step 3* | *Step 4* | *Step 5* |

SINGLE KNOTTING OR VENTILATING

knotting (or **ventilating**): process by which hair is attached to the foundation in the creation of a wig or hairpiece. The actual knotting also is referred to as **ventilating**. Two types of knotting are generally used, single and double. **Single knotting** fastens the hair to the net by a single knot. **Double knotting** uses a double knot.

knotted hair: hair that has been knotted to a wig or hairpiece foundation.

machine-made (or **wefted**) **wig:** hair is sewn onto strips of material by machiine, and then the strips of material are sewn onto a net by machine. The strips of material also are called **wefts**.

mesh: open weave foundation used in wig and hairpiece construction.

mixing: intermingling of hair of different shades or lengths.

modacrylic fibers: synthetic fibers, known as **dynel, kanekalon, venicelon,** etc.

net (or **netting**): see **mesh**.

refined hair: Oriental hair, which is coarse in texture, is often chemically treated to make it more workable and usable.

shield (finger shield): long, pointed metal cap, which is worn to protect the finger from the needle, and used in a manner similar to a thimble. It is used to work in difficult wig areas.

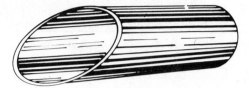

Finger shield.

smocking: length of weft sewn in triangles, diamonds, or loops in order to create the flat, airy base of a hairpiece.

spring (wig spring): spring inserted into a wig or hairpiece foundation to hold the foundation close to the head.

stretch base wig: wig cap (foundation) made of elastic material that stretches to fit various size heads.

styrofoam: lightweight, plastic foam used for a wig block; recommended for storing wigs.

switch: long length of wefted hair mounted with a loop on the end; usually constructed with three stem strands, to provide flexibility in styling.

synthetic hair: artificially produced hair fibers used in the manufacture of wigs and hairpieces.

Syrian hair: mixture of angora and yak hair.

T-pin: pin resembling the letter "T." It is used to secure the hairpiece to the block. It is also called a **block point,** or **wig point.**

topper: hairpiece designed for use on the top of the head, generally made on a round or oval base.

tuck: reduces the size of the wig cap. Netting is folded into a tuck formation, sewn, and folded together.

T-pins.

turning (root): process by which wig hair cuttings or combings are arranged so that all root ends are together and the imbrications face in the same direction.

ventilate: see **knotting.**

ventilating needle: miniature crocheting needle made of spring steel which is used to attach hair to a foundation.

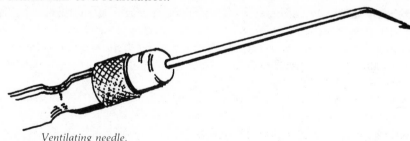

Ventilating needle.

weft: wig fibers sewn to a ribbon of fabric. Wefts are sewn to a base to form the wig.

weft: artificial section of woven (or sewn) hair, used for practice work or as a substitute for natural hair.

wefted wig (machine-made): wig made of wefts of hair sewn into a wig base.

wefting: art of weaving, or sewing, hair strands side by side to form a length of hair.

wig dryers: cabinet dryers used for drying wigs and hairpieces. They provide regulated heat, and can dry many wigs and hairpieces at one time.

wiglet: hairpiece with a flat base which is used to extend the area of hair.

yak: long-haired ox of Tibet and Central Asia. It has long, coarse, silvery hair which is used in the manufacture of wigs.

REVIEW QUESTIONS

THE CARE AND STYLING OF WIGS

1. What four areas of knowledge are required by the cosmetologist in order to give the best possible wig service?
2. Give three reasons that might induce a person to wear a wig or hairpiece.
3. Of what four types of materials are wigs usually made?
4. How can one distinguish between synthetic and human hair?
5. In what three ways does the quality of wigs vary?
6. In what two ways are wigs made?
7. How is the patron's hair prepared before her wig measurements are taken?
8. Why is it important to always work with the proper size block?
9. What type of block is most satisfactory for most wig services?
10. What type of block is used for storing a wig?
11. Why is a swivel clamp used when performing professional services on a wig?
12. Why is it dangerous to hang a wig loosely on a block that is too small?
13. How is the wig adjusted if it feels too tight?
14. What method is usually used to make a wig smaller?
15. Why is it advisable to sew tucks toward the crown and not down?
16. How often should a wig be dry-cleaned?
17. How is the canvas of the wig block protected from damage?
18. What are switches?
19. What are wiglets?
20. What is a bandeau type hairpiece?

Chapter 14

PERMANENT WAVING

CHAPTER LEARNING OBJECTIVES

The student successfully mastering this chapter will know:
1. *The definition of permanent waving.*
2. *The importance of a scalp and hair analysis prior to permanent waving.*
3. *The various chemical products used in permanent waving.*
4. *The reasons for using waving lotions and neutralizers.*
5. *How hair texture, density, and condition affect permanent waving.*
6. *The chemical process involved in permanent waving.*
7. *Why sectioning and blocking are necessary.*
8. *The proper size rods to select.*
9. *The techniques to be used in wrapping the hair.*
10. *The reasons for test curls.*
11. *How to judge processing time.*
12. *The procedure for using cold wave lotions and neutralizers.*
13. *How to handle special problems in permanent waving.*
14. *The procedure for heat permanent waving.*
15. *Safety rules and reminders.*
16. *The importance of maintaining complete records of each patron's services.*

HISTORY OF PERMANENT WAVING

A crude system of permanent waving was practiced by the early Egyptians and Romans. The first real progress in permanent waving was made in 1905 when Charles Nessler invented the heat permanent waving machine. The machine introduced a method of applying heat to pre-formed curls through a series of heaters attached by wires to the machine.

The **spiral permanent wave** was the first method used. It involved winding the hair from the scalp to the ends and was suitable only for long hair.

The **croquignole permanent wave** was introduced in 1926 to meet the needs of short hair. It required that the hair be wound from the hair ends towards the scalp. The hair could be formed into waves finished with end curls.

A **combination** (spiral and croquignole) **permanent wave** soon came into vogue. The crown of the head was given a spiral wave to take care of the longer hair, while the rest of the head received a croquignole wave.

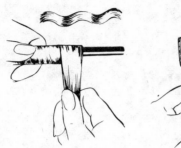
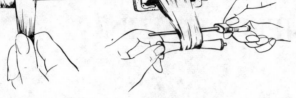
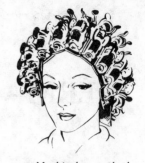

Spiral flat wrap.   *Croquignole wrap.*   *Machineless method (steaming the hair).*

In 1931, the **pre-heat method** of permanent waving was introduced. The procedure was the same as for the croquignole method with the exception of the source of heat. Unlike the machine method, the clamps were first heated by an electrical apparatus, and then clamped over the prepared curls.

Another advance in permanent waving was the **machineless method** which was publicly introduced in 1932. This method required no electrical wires or machines. The source of heat was from the chemical pads which were moistened with water.

COLD WAVING

Cold waving (alkaline type) was first introduce in California during 1938-1939. However, in 1940, a nationwide promotion of cold waving got under way.

Why cold waving is so called. Since cold waving employs no heat and is given at room temperature, the manufacturers had to find a suitable name to distinguish this chemical method of permanent waving from the heat method, and so the name "cold waving" was adopted. As compared to heat permanent waving, cold waving has the following advantages:

1. It is relatively inexpensive since it requires no high priced equipment.
2. The entire procedure is much faster than the heat method.
3. It is more comfortable for the patron.

NEUTRAL AND ACID-BALANCED SOLUTIONS

For many years, manufacturers sought to develop a permanent wave solution that did not require the use of excess ammonia with the salt ammonium thioglycolate. They wanted to minimize the damage caused to hair when permanently waved, and to permit hair that had been damaged by lightening or tinting services to receive a permanent. To achieve these goals, they needed a waving solution that was not highly alkaline.

Neutral and acid-balanced permanent wave solutions were introduced in 1970 which did not contain strong alkalines and, therefore, were less damaging to the hair. These products have a pH of 4.5 to 7.9. Within this range lotions are slow to penetrate hair, and processing time is longer. However, to overcome this problem, **heat** is applied to shorten the processing time.

Note: The word "perm" is now popularly used to indicate permanent waving.

PERMANENT WAVING

All methods of permanent waving involve two major actions on the hair:
1. Physical action—wrapping.
2. Chemical action—processing and neutralizing.

Knowing what takes place as the hair is wrapped around the rods, the chemical action of the waving lotion when applied to the hair, and how the neutralizer re-forms the cross-bonds and rehardens the hair in its new position, is vital to successful permanent waving.

PHYSICAL ACTION

Wrapping. The physical action consists of wrapping the hair around the rods without stretching and with a minimum of tension. When correctly wrapped the hair can expand when completely saturated by the permanent wave solution during processing.

CHEMICAL ACTION

Hair develops and maintains its natural form by means of physical (hydrogen) and chemical (sulfur) cross-bonds in the cortical layer, which hold the hair fibers in position and give the hair its strength and firmness. These physical and chemical bonds must be broken before the shape or contour of the hair can be changed.

Processing. The physical bonds are much the weaker of the two types and are easily broken by the shampooing and rinsing process. However, the chemical action of the permanent waving lotion is required to break the chemical cross-bonds and thus soften the hair. This chemical action permits rearrangement of the inner structure of the hair so that the hair can assume the form of the curlers around which it is wound.

Neutralizing. After the hair has assumed the desired shape, it must be chemically neutralized in order to stop the action of the waving lotion and to re-form the physical and chemical cross-bonds in the cortical layer. This process rehardens the hair and fixes it into its newly curled form. When the neutralizing action is completed, the hair is unwrapped from the rods and permanently assumes its newly curled formation.

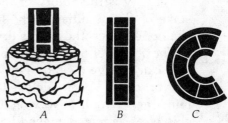

A. Each hair strand is composed of many polypeptide chains. This series of illustrations shows the behavior of one such chain.

B. Hair before processing. Chemical bonds (links) give hair its strength and firmness.

C. Hair wound on rod. The hair bends to the curvature and size of the rod.

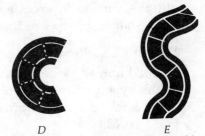

(Permanently waved hair)

D. During processing waving lotion breaks the chemical cross-bonds (links), permitting the hair to adjust to the curvature of the rod while in this softened condition.

E. The neutralizer re-forms the chemical bonds (links) to conform with the wound position of the hair, and rehardens the hair, thus creating the permanent wave.

SCALP AND HAIR ANALYSIS

A very important step before giving a permanent wave is to make a careful analysis of the patron's scalp and hair condition. The professional approach is to learn all the possible facts, such as:

Scalp condition   Hair texture   Hair density
Hair porosity   Hair elasticity   Hair length

SCALP CONDITION

The scalp should be examined very carefully. Abrasions on the scalp can make cold waving dangerous to a patron. An irritated scalp and badly damaged hair are both signs that a permanent wave should be postponed until the condition is corrected.

HAIR POROSITY

Porosity is the ability of the hair to absorb liquids. Since water changes some of the qualities of the hair, this analysis should be made before the shampoo, when the hair is dry.

The ability of hair to absorb is very closely related to the speed with which hair can receive a fluid. This speed of absorption determines the degree of hair porosity. When analyzed properly, porosity can be a measure to determine the strength of waving lotion to use. Unless pre-permanent analysis is closely observed, damaged hair may result.

✗ The **processing time** for any cold wave depends much more on hair porosity than on any other factor. The more porous the hair, the less processing time it takes, and a milder waving solution is required. **The degree at which hair absorbs the cold waving lotion is related to its porosity, regardless of texture.**

Hair porosity is affected by such factors as the patron's health, climate, altitude, humidity, excessive exposure to sun and wind, and the continued use of harsh shampoos, tints, and lighteners.

Porosity Classified

Good porosity—hair with the cuticle layer raised from the hair shaft. Hair of this type can absorb moisture or chemicals in average time.

Moderate porosity (normal hair)—hair that is less porous than hair with good porosity.

Types of Hair and Their Porosity

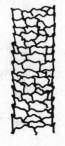 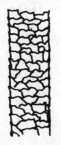 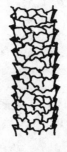 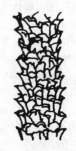

NORMAL
(Moderate porosity)

RESISTANT
(Poor porosity)

TINTED
(Extreme porosity)

DAMAGED
(Over-porous hair)

Poor porosity (resistant hair)—hair with the cuticle layer lying close to the hair shaft. This type of hair absorbs waving lotion more slowly and usually requires a longer processing time.

Extreme porosity (tinted, lightened, or damaged hair)—hair that has been made extremely porous by various hair treatments and abuse. It absorbs the lotion very quickly and requires the shortest processing time. Use either a mild or a very mild lotion for such hair.

Over-porous hair—a result of over-processing. Such hair is extremely damaged, dry, fragile, and brittle. Until the hair has been reconditioned, or removed by cutting, **it should not receive a permanent wave.**

Porosity Test

In order to test accurately for porosity, use three different areas: front hairline, in front of ears, and near the crown.

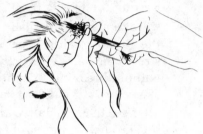

Grasp a small strand of dry hair and comb smooth. Hold the ends firmly with the thumb and index finger of one hand and slide the fingers of the other hand from the ends toward the scalp. If the fingers do not slide easily, or if the hair ruffles up as your fingers slide down the strand, **the hair is porous.** The more ruffles formed, the more porous the hair. The less ruffles formed, the less porous the hair.

Testing for hair porosity.

If the fingers slide easily and no ruffles are formed, the cuticle layer lays close to the hair shaft. This type of hair is least porous, is most resistant, and will require a longer processing time.

Other ways to test for porosity

1. **Cutting dry hair with scissors.** If the scissors cut through dry hair very easily, meeting little resistance, that hair is porous.
2. **Cupping the hair.** If the hair is squeezed and released in the hand and feels completely soft, showing little or no spring, that hair is porous.
3. **Wetting the hair at the shampoo bowl.** If the hair wets easily and thoroughly with the initial spray of water, that hair is porous.
4. **Placing wet hair under dryer.** If hair takes longer than usual to dry, it is porous. The faster the hair dries, the less porosity it has.

HAIR TEXTURE

Hair texture refers to the diameter of the individual hair and its degree of coarseness or fineness. (The texture and porosity are judged together in determining the processing time.) Although porosity is the most important of the two) texture does have an important part in estimating processing time. Fine hair, having a small diameter, will become saturated with waving lotion quicker than hair with a large diameter, if both are equal in porosity. However, when coarse hair is very porous, it will process faster than fine hair that is not porous.

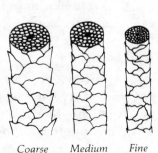

Coarse   Medium   Fine

Hair texture also should be considered in deciding the size of the wave pattern. The texture and density of the patron's hair must be taken into consideration when planning a hairstyle.

Variations in hair texture are due to:

1. **Diameter of the hair shaft:** coarse, medium, fine, or very fine.
2. **Feel of the hair:** harsh, soft, or wiry.

HAIR ELASTICITY

Hair elasticity is a very important factor to consider when giving a permanent wave. Elasticity is the ability of the hair to stretch and contract. All hair is elastic, but its elasticity ranges from very good to poor. Without elasticity, there will be no curl in the hair. The greater the degree of elasticity, the longer the wave will remain in the hair, because less relaxation of the hair occurs.

Testing for Elasticity

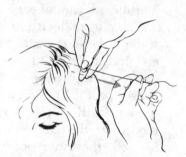

Take a single dry hair and hold it between the thumb and forefinger of each hand. Slowly stretch the hair. The further it can be stretched without breaking, the more elastic it is. If the elasticity is good, the hair slowly contracts after stretching. Hair with poor elasticity will break quickly and easily when stretched.

Testing for elasticity.

Normal hair is capable of being stretched about one-fifth its length, and will spring back when released. However, wet hair can be stretched 40-50% of its length. Porous hair will stretch more than hair with poor porosity.

Poor elasticity. Signs of poor elasticity are limpness, sponginess, and hair that tangles easily.

Limp hair will not develop a firm, strong cold wave. However, there are special waving lotions available for this type of hair. Limp hair requires a smaller diameter rod than hair having good elasticity.

HAIR DENSITY

Hair density is the amount of hair strands per square inch (6.452 sq. cm) on the scalp. Density has nothing to do with the hair's texture. Smaller blockings (sub-sections) and larger rods are often required for thickly growing hair. However, if the hair is thin (fewer hairs per square inch), smaller blockings and smaller (thinner) rods are required in order to form a good wave pattern close to the head.

Avoid blockings that are too large on a thin hair growth, as the strain may cause breakage.

HAIR LENGTH

Hair length is another important factor that must be considered. Waving hair of average length presents no real problem. However, if the patron wears her hair 6″ (15 cm) or longer, follow **Piggyback (Double Rod) Wrap** directions for waving longer hair on page 163.

PRE-PERMANENT SHAPING AND SHAMPOOING

SHAMPOOING FOR A PERMANENT WAVE

Usually, a shampoo is given before a permanent wave. It is advisable to use an acid-balanced or mild shampoo, as suggested by manufacturer. Avoid brushing or massaging, which may cause the scalp to become sensitive to the waving lotion.

Use **extreme care in rinsing,** to make certain that all the shampoo is removed. A residue of shampoo could destroy the effectiveness of the waving lotion. Proper rinsing equalizes the porosity of the hair.

While the hair is still wet, carefully examine for signs of previous permanent. Any hair which indicates that it has recently received a wave could be in a weakened condition and should be treated with extreme caution to avoid hair damage.

SHAPING SUGGESTIONS FOR PERMANENT WAVE

Shaping the hair may be done before or after a shampoo with the use of a razor or scissors.

1. A **razor** may be used to blunt cut damp hair after a shampoo.
2. **Scissors** may be used on dry hair before a shampoo or on damp hair after the shampoo.

SHAPING PRECAUTIONS

The texture of the hair must be considered carefully in planning the shaping procedure.

Coarse or **medium hair.** Taper the hair ends sufficiently to form strong, resilient curls. Excessive tapering may make it difficult to wrap the hair or may cause the hair ends to frizz.

Fine, thin, or **damaged limp hair** should be shaped with the scissors while **in a dry condition.** Use a blunt cut or a short taper. Excessive thinning or tapering will result in frizzy hair ends.

Length of hair. The hair should be long enough to wind around the rods at least two full turns. Otherwise, there will be no wave pattern. If the desired hairstyle requires shorter hair, use smaller diameter rods. If necessary, trim the ends of the hair strands after the permanent is completed.

CAUTION

Slithering the hair prior to the permanent wave may cause some damage to the cuticle, resulting in a poor permanent wave.

In order to avoid distorted wave formation, thinning the hair, if required, should be done after the permanent wave is given.

IMPORTANT REMINDER

The foundation for a professional permanent wave is the careful pre-shaping of the hair.

CURLING RODS

Proper selection of curling rods is essential for successful permanent waving.

The size of the rods controls the shape of the hair during the waving process. Rods are made of a canvas and plastic composition, and vary in diameter, length, and design.

1. Diameter is the distance through the center of the rod.
2. Circumference is the distance around a rod, which is 3.1416 times the diameter of the rod. The circumference is the important factor in determining the size of the wave or curl formation.

Curling rods are available in various lengths: long, medium, and short (3½-1¾" [8.75-4.375 cm] in length).

They also come in varying thicknesses. These range in diameter size from large to very thin (3/4-1/8" [1.875-.3125 cm]).

All rods must have some means of securing the hair on the rod and the rod in the desired position to prevent the curl from unwinding.

TYPES OF RODS

There are two types of rods in general use: concave and straight.

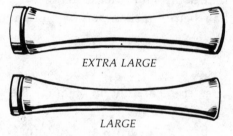

EXTRA LARGE

LARGE

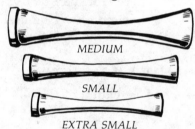

MEDIUM

SMALL

EXTRA SMALL

Concave rods are usually thinner in diameter than the straight rods.

They have a smaller circumference in the center area, which gradually increases to their largest circumference at both ends. Concave rods are used when a close-to-the-head wave pattern is desired.

When hair is wound on a rod, the outside hair of the winding forms a larger curl or wave than the hair next to the rod. This creates a tighter curl or ringlet at the hair ends, which gradually becomes slightly wider as it nears the scalp.

Straight rods are made so that their circumference and diameter are almost the same throughout their entire length. They may, however, taper very slightly toward the center.

This type of rod usually creates the same size curl throughout the entire hair strand.

Large, straight rods are usually used to give a body wave or style wave. They permit the formation of a permanent with a large enough wave to be dressed into any desired hairstyle.

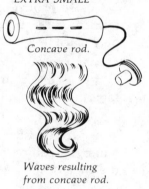

Concave rod.

Waves resulting from concave rod.

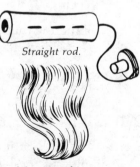

Straight rod.

Waves resulting from straight rod.

CHEMICALS

For successful permanent waving, it is essential that the curling rods and lotion be properly selected. The chemical compounds contained within the waving lotion have an important influence on the procedure to be followed in the waving process.

WAVING LOTIONS

Alkaline waving lotions have as their basic ingredient ammonium thioglycolate, commonly referred to as "thio," which permanently changes the structure of the hair. This compound is prepared by combining ammonia and thioglycolic acid. Other ingredients of the waving lotion may be lanolin and its derivatives, wetting agents, protein, and conditioners. Excess ammonia is added to make the solution alkaline.

Neutral and **acid waving lotions** also contain a thioglycolic acid base. However, their pH range is much lower, 4.5-6.5 for acid lotions, and 7.0-7.9 for neutral lotions. These are not mixed with ammonia and so are not alkaline.

Pre-conditioning. Over-porous or damaged hair may require a pre-conditioning treatment before the application of waving lotion. Special fillers that contain protein are now available which condition the hair and equalize its porosity. Some fillers also contain lanolin and cholesterol, which may help to protect the hair against the harshness of the cold waving lotion.

Conditioners. The alkaline cold waving lotion has a tendency to remove natural oils from the hair, causing it to dry out rapidly through loss of moisture. Mineral oils, lanolin, or lanolin derivatives are added to the waving lotion, or may be used in a separate application, to replace natural oils. By the conditioner remaining in the hair after the lotion has been rinsed out, the moisture content is somewhat preserved, and the feel and appearance of the hair are improved.

The **strength of the waving lotion** can be adjusted by either increasing its pH (alkalinity) or by increasing the amount of active ingredient (ammonium thioglycolate). To adjust the pH of the lotion, the ammonia content is either increased or decreased, not to exceed pH 9.6, which is a strong solution.

Most manufacturers of cold waving products market three or more strengths, such as:

1. **Damaged hair**—weak or mild strength.
2. **Normal hair** (having good porosity)—average strength.
3. **Resistant hair** (less porosity)—stronger strength.
4. **Over-lightened** or **tinted hair** (over-porous)—extra mild strength.

Note: Manufacturers of cold waving products are constantly improving their formulas. It is advisable to follow their directions explicitly.

NEUTRALIZERS

Neutralizers contain either peroxide or sodium bromite, lanolin, and other special ingredients. They come in various forms, such as liquids, powders, and crystals. Depending on the method of application, they may have a thick consistency and may have to be diluted. Conditioners are often incorporated in the prepared liquid neutralizer to give some protection to the hair.

SECTIONING AND BLOCKING

Sectioning is dividing the head into uniform working panels.

Blocking, also known as **sub-sectioning,** is the sub-dividing of panels into uniform individual rectangular rod sections. Uniform wave patterns depend on:

1. Uniformly arranged sections.
2. Equally sub-divided sections (blockings).
3. Clean and uniform partings (length and width).

The size of the blockings is determined by the diameter of the rods.

Depending on the pattern used in hair sectioning, the number of hair blockings may vary with each patron.

The **average blocking** for a standard wave should match the diameter (size) of the rod being used. However, the length of the blocking can be the same as or a little shorter, but not longer, than the length of the rod.

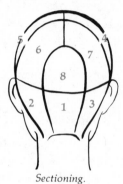

Sectioning.

Blocking (sub-sections).

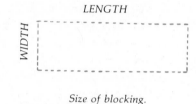

Size of blocking.

LENGTH denotes span of blocking. WIDTH refers to the depth of the blocking. Small or large blockings usually refer to its width.

SUGGESTED HAIR BLOCKINGS AND ROD SIZES

Although the hair elasticity and texture must both be considered in the choice of rods, the texture should be the determining factor.

Coarse hair—good elasticity. Thickly growing hair requires smaller (narrower) blockings and larger rods to permit better arrangements for a definite wave pattern.

Medium hair—average elasticity. Medium or average textured hair requires smaller blockings and medium size rods.

Fine hair—poor elasticity. Thin hair requires smaller blockings and smaller (thinner) rods to prevent strain or breakage and to form a good wave pattern close to the head.

Lightened or **tinted hair**—very poor elasticity. Use smaller hair sub-sections and larger rods. If the lightened or tinted hair is fine in texture, use smaller hair sub-sections and medium rods.

Hair in nape area. Use smaller sub-sections and smaller rods.

Long hair. To permanently wave hair longer than 6″ (15 cm), wrap it smoothly and close to the scalp in smaller blockings. The use of smaller blockings permits the waving lotion and neutralizer to penetrate more easily and thoroughly.

PATTERNS FOR SECTIONING AND BLOCKING

By knowing the texture, elasticity, porosity, and condition of the patron's hair, the cosmetologist is better able to judge how the hair is to be sectioned, blocked, which rods to use, and at what part of the head the application of waving lotion should begin. (**Be guided by your instructor.**)

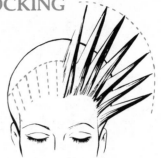

REMINDER

The size of the rods and blockings determines the size of the curl or wave pattern. Processing time has no bearing on the size of the wave pattern.

Four popular blocking (sub-sectioning) patterns:

1. Single Halo
2. Double Halo (Double Horseshoe)
3. Straight Back
4. Dropped Crown

These are known by other names in various areas of the country.

The following patterns are suggested blockings. However, your instructor may suggest different patterns, which are equally correct.

SINGLE HALO

The **single halo** wrap is commonly used for average size heads.

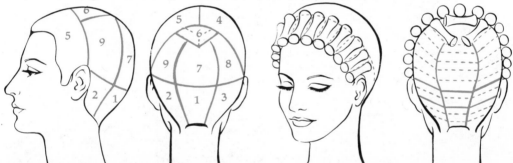

Sectioning diagram.   Blocking (sub-sectioning) pattern.

DOUBLE HALO

The **double halo** wrap is usually used for larger size heads.

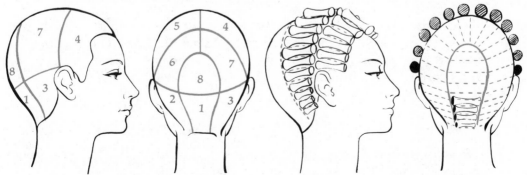

Sectioning diagram.   Blocking (sub-sectioning) pattern.

STRAIGHT BACK

The **straight back** wrap is used to create a rather soft, full, and high style effect, directed off the face.

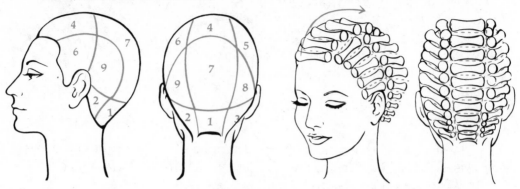

Sectioning diagram.   *Blocking (sub-sectioning) pattern.*

Bangs

To create bangs on the forehead, the first two top front curls are wrapped in a forward direction.

DROPPED CROWN

The **dropped crown** wrap is usually used for longer hair and for a smooth crown effect.

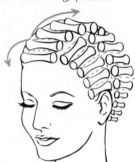

Setting for bangs.

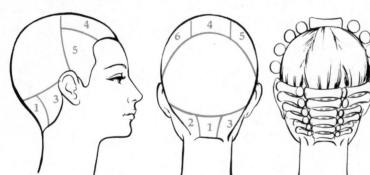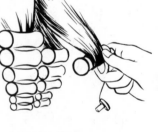

Sectioning diagram.   *Blocking (sub-sectioning) pattern.*   *Wrapping hair ends of crown area.*

The hair is sectioned in the same way as for the straight back pattern. However, in the back area that is not numbered, larger hair sections are made, depending on the amount of hair. Only the hair ends are wrapped on larger curling rods, with the rods resting on the smaller rods in the nape area. (Be guided by your instructor.)

BODY WAVES

A body wave is given with extra large straight rods, solely for the purpose of adding slight body or wave pattern to the hair. For details consult page 172.

WINDING OR WRAPPING THE HAIR

To form a uniform wave with a strong ridge, wrap the hair smoothly and neatly on each rod without stretching. Hair is not stretched because the penetration of waving lotion causes the hair to expand. Tight wrapping or stretching interferes with this expansion and prevents penetration of the waving lotion and neutralizer, which may cause hair breakage.

STRAND RELATION TO THE HEAD

Curl one-half off base. When the strand is held straight out from the head and wound on a curling rod, the curl will rest one-half off base. (Fig. 1)

The hair wound on curling rods in this manner is adaptable to many hairstyles.

Curl off base. When the strand is held in a semi-downward position and wound on a curling rod, the curl will rest off base. (Fig. 2)

The hair wound in this manner will produce a wave that is a little further away from the scalp than hair wound one-half off base. Off base winding produces close-to-the-head hairstyles.

Curl on base. When the strand is held in a semi-upward position and wound on a curling rod, the curl will rest on base. (Fig. 3)

Hair wound in this manner will produce waves close to the head and hairstyles that require fullness, height, and upward movement.

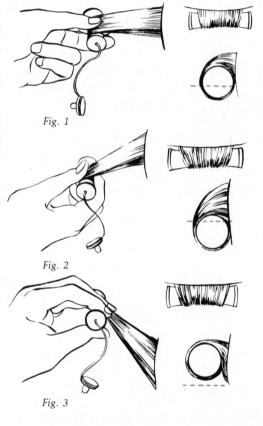

Fig. 1

Fig. 2

Fig. 3

END PAPERS

Porous end papers are very important aids in the proper wrapping or winding of the hair around curling rods. Properly used end papers may help in the formation of smooth and even curls and waves. They help eliminate the possibility of "fishhooks" and minimize the danger of breakage of the hair ends. They are especially important in helping to smooth out the wrapping of uneven hair lengths.

There are three methods of end paper application in general use in the practice of permanent waving. Each method is equally effective, if properly used.

1. The double end paper wrap.
2. The single end paper wrap.
3. The book end paper wrap.

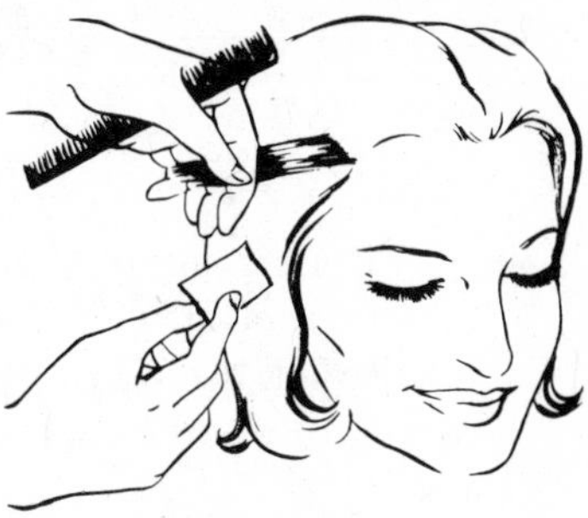

Hair should be moistened (not saturated) with a weak solution of the waving lotion, in the area starting ½" (1.25 cm) from the scalp and up to 1" (2.5 cm) from the hair ends, before being wrapped by any method. However, water should be used instead of waving lotion while practicing, until the student has become proficient in the technique of winding or wrapping the hair.

Procedure

A step-by-step procedure for wrapping and fastening a one-half off base curl is illustrated, using the double end paper wrap method.

Note: *The blocking (sub-section) should not be longer than the length of the rod. If it is, the hair will not wave evenly.*

1. Part and comb sub-section up and out until all hair is evenly directed and distributed. (Fig. 1)
2. Place one end paper beneath the hair strand and the other on top. (Fig. 2)
3. With the right hand, place rod under double end papers, parallel with hair part. Draw both towards hair ends. (Fig. 3)

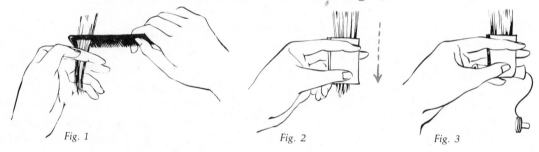

Fig. 1   *Fig. 2*   *Fig. 3*

4. Wind the strand smoothly on the rod to the scalp without tension. (Fig. 4)
5. Fasten band at top of rod. (Fig. 5)

Note: *To prevent breakage, the band should not cut into the hair nor be twisted against the curl.*

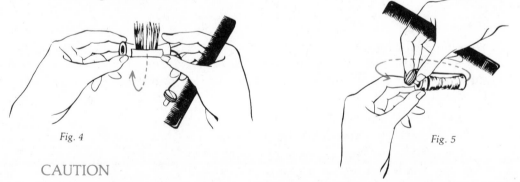

Fig. 4   *Fig. 5*

CAUTION

When wrapping hair, always avoid bulkiness on the rod. Bulkiness prevents the formation of a good curl because the hair cannot conform to the shape of the rod. The end paper goes around the rod on the first turn only. This assures a smooth wave formation and avoids the development of "fishhook" ends.

OTHER END PAPER WRAPS

The preparation and winding of curls for single end paper wrap and the book end paper wrap are the same, with the following exceptions:

Single end paper wrap. Place one end of paper on top and hold it flat between the index and middle fingers to prevent bunching. (Fig. 6) The hair is wound in the same manner as the double end paper wrap. (Figs. 3, 4 and 5)

Book end paper wrap. Hold strand between index and middle fingers; fold and place end paper over strand, forming an envelope. (Fig. 7) The winding of the curl is done as in double end paper wrap. (Figs. 3, 4 and 5)

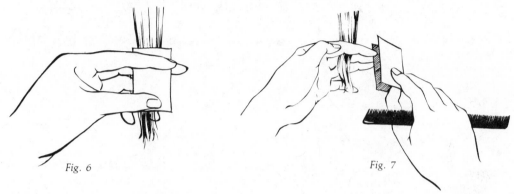

Fig. 6   Fig. 7

THE PIGGYBACK (DOUBLE ROD) WRAP

The piggyback (double rod) method of wrapping is especially suitable for extra long hair. This wrapping technique permits maximum control of the size and tightness of the curl from the scalp to the hair ends. Control of the amount of curl can be exercised by the size of the rods selected. Thus, the use of larger rods will result in a loose, wide wave; while small, or medium rods, will give tighter curls. The following is the procedure for wrapping in the piggyback (double rod) method:

1. Section the head in the usual manner (9 sections).
2. Select rods of the desired size. The rods used in the midpoint to the scalp area should be at least one size larger than those used for the hair ends.

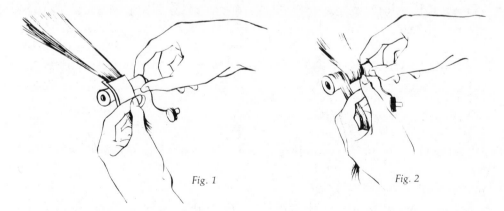

Fig. 1   Fig. 2

3. About halfway up the strand, place porous end papers one on top and one underneath. (Fig. 1)
4. Start at the midpoint part of the strand. Place the larger rod underneath the hair strand and start wrapping. (Fig. 2)

5. Roll the rod toward the scalp and, at the same time, control the hair ends by holding them to the left away from the rod.
6. Secure the wrapped rod at the scalp, leaving the hair ends dangling free from the rod. (Fig. 3)

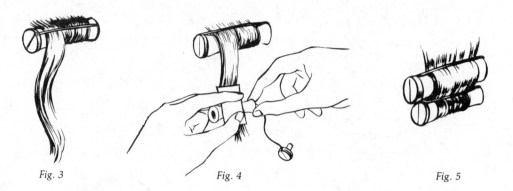

Fig. 3   Fig. 4   Fig. 5

7. Wrap the hair ends. Place an end paper on the hair strand covering the ends. Using the smaller size rod, wrap the hair ends up to the above larger rod. (Fig. 4)
8. Secure the second rod to rest against the first one in piggyback fashion. (Fig. 5)
9. In order to maintain better control over the wrapping and processing, it is advisable to complete the wrapping of each hair strand before proceeding to the next one.
10. Test curls should be taken from the rods closer to the scalp as the hair in this area is more resistant and may require additional processing time.

TEST CURLS

Test curls help to determine in advance how the patron's hair will react to the cold waving process. A test curl gives the cosmetologist information on how to protect the patron's hair and how to obtain the best possible results.

Testing enables the cosmetologist to observe the reaction of hair as to:
1. Speed of wave formation.
2. Overall picture of wave formation.
3. Exact time when peak of wave formation has been reached.
4. Resistant areas.

Test curls may be given before or while waving the entire head.

PRE-PERMANENT TEST CURL METHOD

Pre-permanent test curls should be given if the hair presents any problem, such as damage, poor porosity, or poor elasticity. If the patron has an illness, or if there is any doubt in the mind of the cosmetologist concerning the final results, pre-test curls are important.

Procedure

After the hair has been shampooed and towel dried, wrap two or three curls on the upper back of the head. Each curl is given a complete treatment, with a different strength waving lotion. The action of the lotion is timed and the curl is examined according to manufacturer's directions. After neutralizing and rinsing the curls, judge and record the results.

TEST CURL-WAVE DEVELOPMENT METHOD

This procedure is part of the processing phase of a cold wave. Each head of hair is different. In fact, conditions may vary even on the same head of hair. A patron's hair will not always process in the same length of time for each curl. Neither will one type of curl always process in the same length of time on every head. Curl-wave development should be tested:

1. Immediately after the last rod is secured.
2. Following the re-wet application of lotion.
3. Frequently thereafter, until wave formation has occurred. Frequent testing for wave formation will prevent over-processing. While manufacturer's directions supply a general guide, the cosmetologist should carefully judge individual curl development.

Procedure

1. Thoroughly blot the waving solution from the curl to be tested.
2. Loosen the rod fastener. (Do not let the hair become loose or unravel on the rod. Hold it firmly with thumbs touching on the rod.)
3. Unwind the rod 1½ turns, without pulling on the strand. Since the hair is in a softened condition, pulling or stretching it will spoil the test. Permit the hair to relax into a firm "S"wave pattern.
4. Rewind the test curl.

Continue testing for wave development at regular intervals (every 30 seconds is preferable) until the desired wave pattern has been reached. Test on different areas of the head each time. **Do not use the same curl for retesting.**

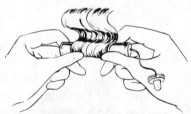

Unwinding hair carefully, without pulling or pushing.

SAFETY PRECAUTIONS

Safety precautions protect the skin and scalp against chemical injury.

1. The cosmetologist must wear protective gloves.
2. For the patron's safety, apply protective cream around the hairline and neck, and cover with a strip of cotton or neutralizing band.
3. Use dry cotton pledgets or neutralizing band between curls to absorb any excess waving lotion.
4. If cotton strips or bands become wet with lotion, remove, blot, and replace with dry material.
5. If the lotion drips on the skin or scalp, absorb with cotton pledgets saturated with cold water or neutralizer.

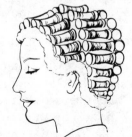

Hairline protected by cotton strips or neutralizing band.

APPLICATION OF WAVING LOTION

APPLICATOR BOTTLE

A **plastic bottle** with a nozzle top makes the most efficient applicator. It dispenses liquid freely, yet permits good control. There is a minimum loss of lotion. A better distribution is achieved throughout the hair.

Note: Bottles should be absolutely clean before being filled with waving lotion. Be certain that there are no traces of leftover chemicals in the bottle, since such leftover chemicals may weaken or spoil the waving lotion.

Protect patron's eyes. If the waving lotion gets into the patron's eyes, rinse immediately with cold water or preparation recommended by your instructor and then take patron to a doctor.

APPLYING THE WAVING LOTION

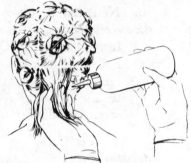

Pre-wrap wetting or moistening. Following shampooing and towel drying, if required by manufacturer, the hair should be moistened with a weak solution of the waving lotion, to facilitate the wrapping procedure. The lotion is applied with a bottle applicator to an entire section at a time. Start about ½" (1.25 cm) from the scalp and extend the lotion to within 1" (2.5 cm) from the hair ends.

Applying lotion ½" from scalp to about 1" from the hair ends.

To assure a complete and even distribution, apply the lotion on the top of the section and comb through from underneath with an upward motion.

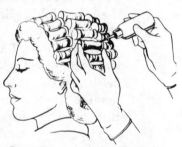

Rewetting or saturation. After subsectioning and winding the curls over the entire head, the hair is ready for rewetting or complete saturation. This procedure is important and essential to assure complete penetration and processing of the entire hair shaft.

Rewetting or second application of waving lotion.

The lotion is thoroughly applied to each curl, following the same order as that used in the pre-wetting step. It is most important to the success of the permanent that each curl be thoroughly and completely saturated.

Note: Be careful not to disturb the wrapping or the placement of curls by dragging the nozzle over the hair. Do not leave the patron alone while the hair is processing. Do not interrupt the rewet or saturation step. Complete it as quickly as possible.

PROCESSING TIME

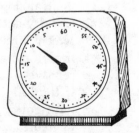

Processing time is the length of time required for the hair strands to absorb the waving lotion and complete the total rearrangement of the chemical bonds in the hair around the rod. The ability of the hair to absorb moisture may vary from time to time on the same individual, even when the same lotions and procedures are used. A record of the previous processing time is desirable, but should be used only as a guide. It is usually safe to anticipate the processing time to be less than that suggested by the manufacturer or a patron's previous record card.

The factors affecting processing time are the strength of the lotion, texture, porosity, length and condition of the hair, atmospheric conditions, patron's body heat, and the working speed of the cosmetologist.

Resaturation step during the processing time. Often, it is necessary to rewet all the rods a second time during the processing time. This may be due to:

1. Evaporation of the lotion or dryness of the hair.
2. Hair poorly saturated by the cosmetologist.
3. No wave development after the maximum time indicated by manufacturer.
4. Improper selection of solution strength for the patron's hair.
5. Failure to follow manufacturer's directions for a specific formula.

A reapplication of the lotion will hasten processing. Watch the wave development closely, since **negligence may result in hair damage.**

WAVE PATTERN FORMATION

The time required to attain the proper depth of the "S" pattern governs the processing time. As the hair is processing, the wave has reached its peak when it forms a well-defined letter "S." The size of the rod used determines the size of the "S" pattern.

The "S" pattern reaches a desirable peak only once. Shortly after the "S" is well formed, unless processing is stopped, the hair could become frizzy. This indicates that the processing time has reached its absolute maximum. Beyond this point the hair becomes **over-processed** and **damaged.**

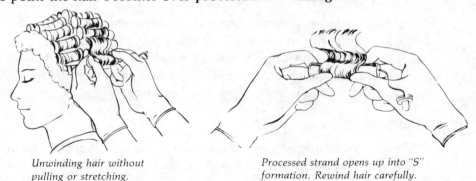

Unwinding hair without pulling or stretching.

Processed strand opens up into "S" formation. Rewind hair carefully.

Different conditions and textures of hair will form different qualities of wave patterns. Hair of good texture will show a firm, strong pattern, whereas hair that is weak or fine will not produce a well defined "S" pattern.

OVER-PROCESSING

Any lotion that can properly process the hair also can over-process it. Lotion left on the hair too long, beyond the best wave formation point, results in over-processing. Another cause of over-processing is when test curls are not made frequently enough or are improperly judged. If neutralizer is used too sparingly, the hair may continue to process, also causing over-processing.

Over-processed hair is easily detected. It is very curly when wet, completely frizzy when dry, and refuses to be combed into a suitable wave pattern. The elasticity of the hair has been excessively damaged and the hair is unable to contract into the wave formation. The hair feels harsh after being dried. Reconditioning treatments should begin immediately.

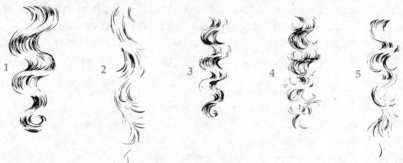

1. *A good permanent wave looks like this.*
2. *Under-processed curl. RESULT:Little or no wave.*
3. *Over-processed curl. RESULT: Narrow waves when wet, no waves when dry.*
4. *Porous ends over-processed. RESULT: Frizzy ends.*
5. *Improper winding; hair ends are wound too tight. RESULT: No wave or curl at hair ends.*

UNDER-PROCESSING

Under-processing results in a limp or weak wave formation. The ridges are not well defined and the hair retains little or no wave formation. Under-processing should be corrected by giving reconditioning treatments. After these treatments, rewrap the hair and apply a milder waving lotion, since the hair has already received some softening. Watch the wave formation closely.

NEUTRALIZATION

The waving lotion produces the curl formation by rearranging the chemical S-bonds in the cortex of the hair shaft into a new alignment. The rods hold the hair in this formation until it is rehardened or fixed by neutralization. The neutralizer stops the action of the waving lotion, re-forms the chemical bonds, and rehardens the hair in its new curled position.

PREPARATION

Most manufacturers require thorough rinsing with warm water in order to remove the waving lotion, followed by careful towel blotting of each curl to remove excess moisture prior to the application of the neutralizer.

To obtain the best results from towel blotting, carefully press the towel with the fingers between each curl. Do not rock or roll the rods while blotting. The hair is in a softened state, so any such movement may cause hair breakage.

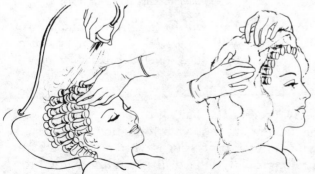

Rinsing waving lotion from the hair.   *Towel blotting.*

METHODS OF NEUTRALIZATION

Neutralizers are packaged in the form of powders, liquid, or crystals and must be prepared and applied as directed by manufacturer immediately before their use.

There are two methods of neutralizer application in general use: the **Direct** or **On-the-Rod Method** and the **Splash-On Method.**

Direct or **On-the-Rod Method** (also referred to as the **Applicator** or **Instant Method**). The neutralizer comes in two forms: ready for use and to be mixed.

1. **Ready for use neutralizer:** cut off tip of applicator bottle and apply.
2. **Neutralizer to be prepared:** mix it according to manufacturer's directions and pour into the applicator bottle and apply.

Direct (On-the-Rod) Method. Apply neutralizer directly to each curl in the same order as that followed in the application of the waving lotion. Start in the top center of the curl and apply in either direction, then apply at the bottom of the curl, making sure that each curl is thoroughly saturated. Repeat if necessary.

Note: A cotton pad saturated with a neutralizer may be placed at the nape of the neck on the rim of the shampoo bowl, to assure that the neckline curls are in constant contact with the neutralizer.

Splash-On Method. Mix neutralizer with water, following manufacturer's directions. Position patron at shampoo bowl in the same manner as for a shampoo.

Use a neutralizing cape with a pocket placed around patron's neck to catch excess neutralizer. With a glass or plastic measuring cup, pour one-half the neutralizer carefully over the curls, thoroughly saturating each curl. The neutralizer is caught in the cape pocket. Using large pads of cotton or sponge, reapply neutralizer, thoroughly saturating each curl. Repeat 2-3 times.

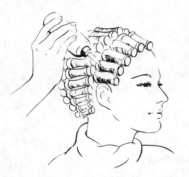

Neutralizing—Direct or On-the-Rod Method.

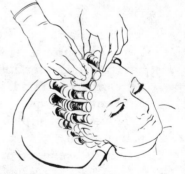

Neutralizing—Splash-On Method.

REMOVING NEUTRALIZER

There are two general methods for removing neutralizers from the hair, whether it be the On-the-Rod or Splash-On Method that was used to apply the neutralizer. (Manufacturer's directions must be followed at all times.)

Method 1. After the neutralizer is thoroughly applied, allow to remain in the hair for 5-8 minutes. Rinse with tepid water followed by a cool water rinse to reharden the hair. Lightly towel blot the hair. Remove the rods carefully, and proceed to set the hair.

Method 2. After the neutralizer is thoroughly applied, allow to set for 5-8 minutes. Carefully remove the rods without stretching the hair and apply the balance of the neutralizer to the hair. Permit an additional minute of neutralizing time and then rinse with cool water. Proceed to set the hair.

Note: Unless the hair is thoroughly and correctly neutralized, the permanent wave will not be successful and all the work done will be wasted. In addition, the hair may be damaged.

COLD WAVING (Alkaline)

A correct analysis for cold waving results should include:

1. Strength of waving lotion.
2. Proper size rods.
3. Blocking and winding the hair.
4. Test curls.
5. Processing time.
6. Neutralization.

There are different methods of giving a cold wave. The suggested outline in this section is one of several ways that may be used. However, it may be changed to meet the requirements of the instructor or cold wave manufacturer.

IMPLEMENTS AND MATERIALS

Applicators	Curling rods	Combs
Porous end papers	Protective cream	Hair clips and pins
Cold waving lotion	Cotton or neutralizing bands	Scissors or razor
Neutralizer	Mild liquid shampoo	Protective gloves
Neutralizing bib	Neutral or cream rinse	Record card
Shampoo cape	Neck strips and towels	Cotton pledgets

If the neutralizer is to be applied by the Splash-On Method, a rinse pan, measuring cup, and quart jar also are needed.

PREPARATION

1. Select and arrange required materials.
2. Wash and sanitize hands.
3. Seat patron comfortably; ask her to remove her earrings and neck jewelry; adjust towel and shampoo cape.
4. Remove all hairpins and combs from patron's hair.
5. Carefully examine condition of scalp and hair. (Check for scalp abrasions.)
6. Seat patron comfortably at the shampoo bowl.

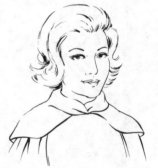

Draping for permanent waving.

DRAPE PATRON

There are several ways in which a patron may be draped for a cold wave. The comfort of the patron, adequate protection of her person and her clothing are important during the entire procedure. One way to drape a patron is to place a small folded towel around her neck, fasten the shampoo cape over it, then place another towel over the cape. Fasten the towel securely. (Your instructor may recommend another method which is equally correct.)

REMINDER

It is important for the student to remember that there are many correct ways to give a permanent wave. The method recommended in this section is merely one suggested way. Always be guided by your instructor or follow manufacturer's directions.

PROCEDURE

1. Shape hair before or after shampoo, as preferred.
2. Shampoo hair lightly (one soaping), rinse thoroughly, and towel dry.
3. If wrapping is to be done after the application of cold waving lotion, apply protective cream and cotton strips around patron's hairline and neck. Wear protective gloves or apply protective cream.

   If wrapping is to be done after conditioner is applied, no protective cream is necessary, nor must you wear protective gloves. **However, you must apply protective cream and wear protective gloves before you apply cold waving lotion to the wound curls.**
4. Section the hair. Sub-divide (block) section and wrap.
5. Apply cold waving lotion as recommended by manufacturer.
6. **Test curl immediately** after saturating hair with cold waving lotion. Take frequent test curls on different areas of the head.
7. Process hair for the required time. If rewetting the curls is necessary, apply the lotion in the same order originally followed. Protect patron with fresh protective cotton strips around hairline and neck.
8. Rinse out waving lotion thoroughly with warm water. Follow manufacturer's directions.
9. Blot excess moisture from hair wound on rods. Do not rock or roll the rods while blotting. Because the hair is in a softened state, any such movement may cause hair breakage.
10. Thoroughly apply neutralizer and retain for required time to re-form cross "S" bonds and reharden the hair.
11. Rinse with tepid water, followed by a cool water rinse. Lightly towel blot.
12. Unwind and remove rods carefully.
13. Apply neutralizer again, if required.
14. Rinse hair again, with cool water, if required.
15. Towel dry, and style the hair.

IMPORTANT REMINDERS

A neutral or acid rinse may be applied to protect the permanent wave and to facilitate the styling of the hair. If manufacturer has included a special rinse with the product, its use will prevent excessive stretching while combing and will counteract any alkaline residue. If used, setting lotion should be of a light consistency. **Avoid excess tension in styling the hair.**

CAUTION

Do not use extreme heat when drying the hair. In handling soft, fine, limp, or damaged hair, it is of utmost importance to use as little tension as possible.

CLEANUP

1. Discard used supplies.
2. Cleanse and sanitize implements.
3. Wash and sanitize hands.
4. Complete perm record card.

BODY (PERMANENT) WAVING

A body (permanent) wave gives the hair softer, wider waves. It is given when a strong curl or wave effect is not desired.

A body wave gives a holding action to the hairstyle, thus permitting the setting to last longer, from one shampoo to another.

Note: Hair texture determines whether or not a body (permanent) wave should be given. If the hair is fine and soft, and the ultimate hairstyle requires curls, a body wave must not be given, as it will not give the hair the desired soft, wide wave effect.

Procedure

Since extra large, straight type rods are used, the wrapping procedure is somewhat different from that followed in using regular size rods. The wrapping should start in the front section. This should be followed by the crown section, leaving the nape section to be wrapped last. Smaller rods should be used in the nape area. (Hair on these rods does not require as much time to curl.)

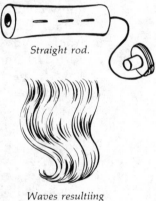

Straight rod.

Waves resultiing from straight rod.

Curling rods. For a body (permanent) wave, use straight rods to give uniform curl formation over the entire strand.

1. For **crown** and **sides**—use large (thick) rods.
2. For **nape area**—use small (thin) rods.
3. For **intermediate areas**—use medium size rods.

PROCESSING AND NEUTRALIZING

Processing and neutralizing closely follow the procedure for a conventional cold wave. However, since the rods are larger in diameter, the lotion and neutralizer used must penetrate thoroughly into the hair shaft.

Each manufacturer has its own formula; therefore, it is important to exactly follow its instructions.

ADVANTAGES

The body (permanent) wave has a number of advantages.

1. The large rods make it almost impossible to kink or frizz the hair ends.
2. The waves created are wide and long lasting.
3. The set or style holds for a longer period of time.
4. It adds body, resilience, and manageability to the hair ends. This permits the hair to work in well and respond to all styling demands.
5. The strong, wide waves relax very slowly and, therefore, the body wave lasts a long time.

HEAT PERMANENT WAVING
(Neutral and Acid-Balanced Lotions)

Neutral permanent waving products have a pH range of 7.0-7.9.

Acid-balanced permanent waving products have a pH range of 4.5-6.5.

ADVANTAGES

1. There is no harsh alkali to damage the hair or skin.
2. There is no swelling of the hair, minimizing damage and breakage.
3. The waving lotion is activated only when heat is applied, thus giving the cosmetologist greater control.
4. No ammonia is used and, therefore, no color is removed from tinted hair.
5. Since no ammonia is used, there is no offensive odor.
6. Since there is greater control, there is less possibility of over-processing.
7. Since no ammonia is used, there is less chance of skin irritation.
8. They produce soft and natural-looking waves.

DISADVANTAGES

1. Curls are not as tight as in the conventional cold thio (alkaline) wave.
2. Curls tend to relax sooner than with the cold thio (alkaline) wave.
3. Within the pH range of these lotions, they are slow to penetrate into the cortex, thus increasing processing time. To overcome this, heat must be applied.

OBJECTIVES OF HEAT APPLICATION

1. To speed up the penetration of the neutral or acid-balanced lotion into the cortex.
2. To increase the processing rate of the lotion within the hair.

METHODS OF APPLYING HEAT

Manufacturers have developed a number of methods of applying the necessary heat to the hair.

1. The pre-heated hair dryer method.
2. The heated clamp method.
3. Thermal cap method.
4. Chemical heat method.
5. Self-heating method.

PRE-HEATED HAIR DRYER METHOD

The pre-heated hair dryer method is very similar to the heated clamp method. The major difference is in the technique used to apply heat.

The hair is saturated with the permanent wave lotion and wound on rods. The hair is then covered with a thin plastic cap to concentrate the heat and to prevent heat loss. The patron is then placed under a pre-heated dryer. Processing begins as soon as the heat is applied.

When the required length of time has elapsed, the plastic cap is removed and the hair rinsed and neutralized in the usual manner.

The pre-heated dryer method has the same three control features as found in the heated clamp method.

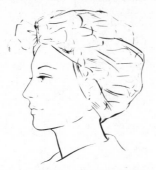

Applying processing cap.

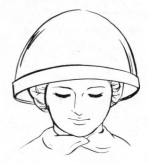

Putting patron under pre-heated dryer.

HEATED CLAMP METHOD

This technique of acid-balanced permanent waving involves the use of heated clamps applied directly to the hair.

The hair is completely wound on rods and thoroughly saturated with the permanent waving solution. During this period, the proper number of rods is being heated for immediate use. After the hair is saturated with lotion and wound on the rods, a pre-heated clamp is placed on each curl. Processing begins as soon as the heat is applied.

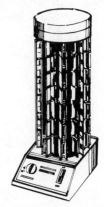

Permanent wave machine.

After the hair has been processed for a pre-determined period of time, the clamps are removed and the hair is rinsed and neutralized in the usual manner.

There are three special control features in the heated clamp method:

1. The temperature of the rods is strictly controlled.
2. The processing does not start until the heat is applied.
3. All curls are processed for exactly the same length of time.

PROCESSING HAIR WITH THERMAL CAP

A thermal cap is frequently used to process a heat-activated formula. It is pre-heated at about the middle of the wrapping step and then placed on the head immediately after the preliminary test curl.

The cap-processing technique can be substituted with the use of a dryer or lamp. The test-curling technique is used by most types of thermal processing unless directions indicate different procedures.

Cover curls first with a plastic covering.

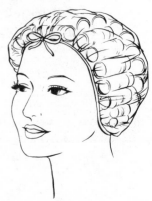

Curls with plastic thermal cap.

CHEMICAL HEAT METHOD

This method uses chemicals that are mixed together to create heat. Heat is generated by a chemical reaction produced by mixing another chemical with the waving solution.

This reaction slightly swells the hair temporarily and causes it to become warm. The moderate heat generated mildly accelerates the waving action.

However, the chemical heat dissipates after it is applied to the hair and is, therefore, not as effective as the heated clamp or pre-heated hair dryer methods.

SELF-HEATING METHOD

This method is used to generate heat by the self-heating technique. The hair is saturated with lotion and wound on rods. A plastic cap is carefully applied to cover the hair and is sealed airtight during processing. Maintaining body heat with no loss during the processing creates enough heat to process the hair.

However, this method has been found to be too slow and uncertain to be effective for professional service.

NEUTRALIZERS

The application of the neutralizer for neutral and acid-balanced permanent waving is very similar to the techniques used for the alkaline permanents. However, manufacturer's directions vary somewhat with different products.

Because each manufacturer has its own formula and special features related to its products, it is essential that manufacturer's instructions be followed carefully.

PERMANENT WAVING FOR MEN

Permanent waving techniques are substantially the same for both men and women.

1. The same chemicals are used.
2. The winding procedures are the same.
3. The placement and fastening of the permanent wave rods are the same.
4. The same processing and neutralizing procedures are followed.

The only differences between permanent waving on female patrons and male patrons are found in the styling patterns. Keep in mind that men do not want end curls. They want waves for control.

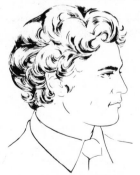 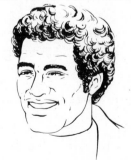 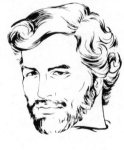

Permanent waving in popular men's hairstyles.

IMPORTANT REMINDER

Permanent waving is one of the most important services a cosmetologist is called upon to give. Proficiency in the techniques outlined in this chapter can only be achieved by constant practice and by taking painstaking care in all details. It is the meticulous worker who becomes the sought-after cosmetologist.

RELEASE STATEMENT

A release statement is used for permanent waving, hair relaxing, or any other type of chemical service. It relieves the salon owner to some extent from responsibility for accidents or damages.

RELEASE FORM

Patron's Name.............................Address...............

Condition of Hair:...

Permanent Wave: Kind.................Given by.......................

I fully understand that the permanent wave treatment that I have requested and am about to receive is ordinarily harmless to normal hair, but may damage my hair because of its present condition.
In view of this, I accept full responsibility for any possible damage that may result, directly or indirectly, to my hair.

Signature of Patron..

Witnessed by...................................Date...............

PERMANENT WAVE RECORD

A record of each permanent wave must be kept for each patron. It is referred to each time the patron is given a permanent. It contains all essential information. It eliminates guesswork. The following is a typical form of permanent wave card.

PERMANENT WAVE RECORD

Name... Tel......................

Address............................... City .... State..................

DESCRIPTION OF HAIR

Form	Length	Texture		Porosity	
☐ straight	☐ short	☐ coarse	☐ soft	☐ very porous	☐ less porous
☐ wavy	☐ medium	☐ medium	☐ silky	☐ moderately porous	☐ least porous
☐ curly	☐ long	☐ fine	☐ wiry	☐ normal	☐ resistant

Condition:

☐ virgin	☐ rewave		☐ dry	☐ oily	☐ bleached

Tinted with...

Previously waved with..system

☐ Original sample of hair enclosed   ☐ not enclosed

TYPE OF PERMANENT WAVE

☐ cold	☐ heat	☐ body wave		☐ other................

No. of curls................. Lotion................ Strength..............

Results:

☐ good	☐ poor	☐ too tight	☐ too loose	☐ sample of finished P.W. enclosed
				☐ sample not enclosed

Date	Operator	Date	Operator
....	....	....	....
....	....	....	....
....	....	....	....

REMINDERS AND HINTS ON PERMANENT WAVING

For the protection of both the patron and the cosmetologist, the following rules should be observed:

1. When giving a permanent wave, always follow manufacturer's directions.
2. Examine scalp for abrasions and lesions.
3. Analyze the hair before every permanent wave.
4. Obtain information concerning patron's permanent wave history.
5. Protect clothing of patron by proper draping.
6. Have the patron remove her glasses, earrings, and neck jewelry.
7. Select a mild shampoo and apply it without irritating the scalp.
8. Eliminate hair brushing or massaging before a permanent wave.
9. Always shape the hair before giving a permanent wave.
10. Use protective cream around patron's hairline and neck.
11. Protect patron's face and neck with cotton strips or neutralizing band during processing.
12. Protect your hands with gloves or protective cream.
13. Use clean applicator bottles for all solutions. Use glass or plastic measuring cups and bowls. Do not use metallic cups or bowls.
14. When in doubt, take pre-permanent test curls.
15. Sub-section hair evenly. Uneven blockings may produce uneven waves.
16. Select proper size rods and correct waving lotion for the hair.
17. Do not stretch the hair when wrapping, or stretch rubber bands over the curls, as hair breakage may result.
18. When applying waving lotion, be sure the curls are thoroughly saturated.
19. Avoid lotion dripping on scalp and skin. Remove lotion drippings by blotting with cotton saturated with cold water, and apply neutralizer.
20. Remove cotton strips or neutralizing bands from face and neck if saturated with waving lotion. If neck towel gets wet with lotion, remove immediately.
21. If waving lotion gets into patron's eyes, wash immediately with cold water, or be guided by your instructor. Take patron to doctor.
22. Do not leave patron alone while the hair is processing.
23. Test wave formation frequently during processing.
24. Neutralize hair thoroughly as directed by manufacturer.
25. Remove drippings from the floor as soon as possible.
26. Do not apply a color rinse, tint, lightener, or any other cosmetic that may cause damage to a new permanent.
27. Do not give a permanent to a patron if she has experienced an allergic reaction during a previous permanent wave.
28. Do not allow patron to sit in draft or near an air conditioner.
29. Complete record carefully and accurately.

SPECIAL PROBLEMS

RECONDITIONING TREATMENTS

Dry, brittle, damaged, or over-porous hair should be given reconditioning treatments. However, avoid any treatment requiring massage or heat just prior to a cold wave. Such treatment could create a sensitive scalp.

SPECIAL PERMANENT WAVE FILLERS

Over-porous or damaged hair must be pre-conditioned before the application of waving lotion. Special fillers that contain protein are available which recondition the hair and equalize its porosity. Some fillers also contain lanolin and cholesterol which help to protect the hair against the harshness of the alkaline cold waving lotion.

AFTERCARE

Reconditioning treatments also have a place in the aftercare of a permanent wave and between permanents.

The aftercare of the permanent wave helps to keep the hair in the best possible condition. It includes regular hair care, as follows:
1. Shampoo hair weekly with mild shampoo and rinse.
2. Use appropriate hair conditioner as directed by manufacturer.
3. Comb and brush the hair daily. Use type of brush best suited to the hair. Avoid excessive brushing or combing in the opposite direction.
4. Suggest patron have hair trimmed and styled at regular intervals, in order to make the hairstyle more serviceable.

WAVING TINTED OR LIGHTENED HAIR

Special precautions are recommended when waving tinted or lightened hair, such as:
1. Shampooing hair with a mild shampoo before waving.
2. Wrapping hair with a special conditioner, as required for damaged hair.
3. Using a special permanent waving lotion according to directions.
4. Giving test curls, using a milder waving solution and a shorter processing time than is used for normal hair.
5. Giving an acid perm which is milder than an alkaline cold wave.

HAIR TINTED WITH METALLIC DYE

Hair tinted with a metallic dye must first be treated with a dye remover to avoid hair discoloration or breakage. Do not wave the hair if the test curls break or discolor. This type of discoloration is very difficult to remove.

CURL REDUCTION

Sometimes a patron is unhappy with her hair after a permanent wave because the hair appears to be too curly. If the hair is fine in texture, do not suggest curl reduction until after two or three shampoos. This type of hair relaxes to a greater extent than normal or coarse hair. Usually, after the second shampoo, the hair has relaxed enough to be satisfactory.

If the hair's texture is normal or coarse, curl reduction may be given either immediately following neutralization or after a few days.

Cold waving lotion may be used to relax the curl, where required. Carefully comb it through the hair to widen and loosen the wave. When sufficiently relaxed, the hair is rinsed, towel blotted, and neutralized.

If curl analysis and proper application is not determined, hair could be damaged and breakage could occur. **Be guided by your instructor.**

CAUTION

Do not attempt curl reduction in hair that has been over-processed. Such a treatment will further damage the hair.

PERMANENT WAVING HAIR WITH PARTIAL PERMANENT

Previously permanently waved hair should be given a reconditioning treatment. Leave the conditioning agent over the old permanent and cover this hair with two or three end papers. Then proceed with the usual permanent wave routine.

This is only one way of waving this type of hair. Your instructor's method is equally correct.

REVIEW QUESTIONS

PERMANENT WAVING

1. List the three advantages of cold permanent waving as compared with heat waving.
2. What are the two major actions on the hair in permanent waving?
3. Name two types of chemical solutions used in permanent waving.
4. What is the main action of a permanent waving solution?
5. The application of which chemical follows the permanent waving lotion?
6. What is the main action of the neutralizer?
7. What is the most important step before giving a permanent wave?
8. List six factors that a scalp and hair analysis should include.
9. Which two hair factors determine the processing time during permanent waving?
10. Why is hair elasticity so important in relation to permanent waving?
11. How does hair density affect the size of hair blockings and the size of rods used?
12. What type of shampoo is advisable for use before giving a permanent wave?
13. Why is it important to use extreme care in rinsing the hair before giving a permanent wave?
14. How does proper rinsing help to assure an even permanent wave?
15. What determines the strength of the waving lotion to be used?
16. Why are special hair conditioners recommended in permanent waving?
17. What strength waving lotion is always recommended for tinted or over-lightened hair?

18. In permanent waving, what determines the size of the blocking (sub-sectioning)?
19. What three factors must be considered in the choice of rods in permanent waving?
20. What determines the size of the curl or wave pattern?
21. Why should hair be wrapped smoothly and without tension on each rod?
22. Why do we avoid stretching the hair in wrapping for a permanent wave?
23. Why is it necessary to give test curls?
24. At what three points should wave development be tested?
25. Why should safety precautions be observed in permanent waving?
26. What must be done if the waving lotion accidentally gets on the skin or scalp?
27. How can you assure a complete and even distribution when applying the permanent wave lotion?
28. When does the complete wave formation reach its peak?
29. What kind of hair texture will not form a firm wave pattern?
30. How is over-processed hair detected?
31. What is the range of the pH value of: a) an acid balanced permanent wave; b) a neutral permanent wave?
32. How do the performance techniques in giving a permanent wave to male patrons differ from those used on female patrons?
33. Why do male patrons want a permanent?
34. Why is it a good practice to obtain a release statement from each patron before giving a permanent wave?
35. Why should a permanent wave record be kept for each patron?
36. How may an over-curly permanent wave be relaxed?

Chapter 15

HAIR COLORING

CHAPTER LEARNING OBJECTIVES

The student successfully mastering this chapter will know:
1. *The reasons for coloring the hair.*
2. *The various hair coloring products and their effect on hair.*
3. *The types of coloring services performed, and the differences among temporary, semi-permanent, and permanent hair coloring.*
4. *The preliminary steps required for tinting.*
5. *The difference between one-step and two-step hair coloring.*
6. *The safety precautions required.*
7. *The theory of hair lightening, the types of lighteners used, and the results obtainable.*
8. *How a lightening retouch is given.*
9. *The purpose of toners, frosting, tipping, and streaking.*
10. *How to apply toners, frosting, tipping, and streaking.*
11. *The problems that are encountered in hair coloring, and the use of fillers and conditioners.*
12. *The procedure involved in eyelash and brow tinting.*
13. *The definitions pertaining to hair coloring.*

Hair coloring (tinting) is both the science and art of changing the color of hair. **Hair coloring** involves the addition of an artificial color to the natural pigment in the hair, or the addition of color to lightened hair. **Hair lightening,** on the other hand, involves a partial or total removal of the natural pigment or artificial color from the hair. (The terms "tinting" and "coloring" are used interchangeably in this text.)

Skill in hair tinting and hair lightening can be accomplished by continuous practice and long hours of study. They can become profitable sources of income in the beauty salon because they represent **repeat business.** The patron who has her hair tinted or lightened usually returns for retouching at regular intervals. Satisfactory service will encourage her to return to the same beauty salon.

Principal reasons for coloring or lightening hair:
1. To restore grey hair to its natural shade.
2. To change the natural shade of hair to a more attractive color.
3. To restore hair to its natural color.
4. To create decorative effects, such as frosting, streaking, or tipping.

The advantages of hair coloring are for:
1. Women and men with prematurely grey hair.

2. Business women and men who may feel that the shade of their hair is a handicap.
3. Women and men who wish to maintain a youthful appearance.

The successful cosmetologist must know:
1. The general structure of the hair and scalp.
2. The proper selection and application of hair tints and lighteners.
3. The chemical reactions to tints and lighteners.

HAIR COLORING

Hair coloring is the application of artificial color to the hair.

Hair coloring falls into three main categories: **temporary, semi-permanent, and permanent.** The professional cosmetologist must know how each group acts on the hair.

CLASSIFICATIONS OF HAIR COLORING

TEMPORARY HAIR COLORING

1. **Color rinses** are prepared rinses used either to highlight the color of or add color to the hair. These rinses contain certified colors, and remain on the hair until the next shampoo.
2. **Highlighting color shampoos** combine the action of a color rinse with that of a shampoo. These shampoos generally contain certified colors, give highlights, and impart color tones to the hair.
3. **Crayons** are sticks of coloring which are available in all shades and compounded with soaps or synthetic waxes. They are used to retouch newly grown hair between tintings.
4. **Hair color creams** are used mostly for theatrical makeup. They rub off easily because of their greasy base.
5. **Hair color sprays** are generally used in gold and silver colors, and are applied from aerosol containers for exotic effects.
6. **Mascara** is used to add color to the eyelashes and eyebrows.

SEMI-PERMANENT HAIR COLORING

Tints that are formulated to last 4-6 weeks are semi-permanent hair coloring agents. They are self-penetrating and are applied without peroxide. They do not change the basic structure of the hair.

Semi-permanent tints are designed to do the following:
1. Cover or blend partially grey hair without affecting its natural color.
2. Enhance the beauty of grey hair without changing its color.
3. Highlight and bring out the natural color of the hair.

PERMANENT HAIR COLORING

1. **Aniline derivative tints** also are called penetrating tints, synthetic organic tints, peroxide tints, oxidation tints, para tints, and amino tints. **Toners** also are classified as penetrating tints.
2. **Pure vegetable tints.** In the past, indigo, camomile, sage, and Egyptian henna were used for hair coloring. They deposited a thin coating on the hair. Today, only henna is still used professionally.

3. **Metallic** or **mineral dyes**, such as lead acetate or silver nitrate, are the **progressive type** known as **color restorers.** They form a metallic coating over the hair shaft and render the hair unsatisfactory for permanent waving, hair lightening, or tinting. Successive applications are made until the proper shade has developed.

4. **Compound dyes,** such as compound henna, are combinations of vegetable dyes with certain metallic salts and other dyestuffs. The metallic salts fix the color. Compound dyes coat the hair shaft and render the hair unfit for permanent waving, lightening, or tinting.

METALLIC DYES

Metallic dyes and compound dyes are never used professionally. However, women do buy and apply such products to their hair. Therefore, the hair colorist must be able to recognize and understand their effects. Such coloring agents must be removed and the hair reconditioned before the application of tints, lighteners, permanent wave, or hair relaxer solutions.

Hair treated with either a metallic dye or compound dye appears to be dull without highlights. It is generally harsh and brittle to the touch. These colorings usually fade into peculiar or unnatural shades. **Silver** dyes have a **greenish** cast; **lead** dyes have a **purple** color, and those containing **copper** dyes turn **red.**

TEST FOR METALLIC SALTS

1. In a glass container, mix one ounce (30 ml) of 20 volume peroxide and 20 drops of 28% ammonia water.
2. Cut a strand of hair from the patron's head. Bind with scotch tape and immerse the hair in the above solution for 30 minutes.
3. Remove from container and observe.

Since most of these products contain lead, silver or copper, look for the following reactions:

Test for lead. Hair will change color immediately. It often turns much lighter very rapidly.

Test for silver. No reaction whatsoever at end of half an hour. A peroxide and ammonia solution cannot lighten the hair because it cannot penetrate the silver coating, while the hair strand with no artificial coloring or penetrating tint will lighten to some degree.

Test for copper. The solution will start to boil within a few minutes. The hair strand feels hot and gives off a very disagreeable odor. After a few minutes, the hair will pull apart easily.

If any of these conditions are present, the metallic coating must be removed before the hair can be successfully colored or given a permanent wave. After the coating has been removed, check the hair strand again in 24 hours by stretching for breakage. If breakage occurs, recondition the hair before any aniline derivative tint, lightener, permanent waving, or relaxer solution is used.

Removing metallic dye. Preparations are available for the removal of metallic dyes and compound dyes. Follow manufacturer's directions.

ANILINE DERIVATIVE TINTS

The aniline derivative tints result in the most successful hair tinting. Most permanent hair coloring is done with aniline derivative tints. These tints remain in the hair until they are removed by chemical means, or until the hair grows out. The coloring penetrates through the cuticle into the cortex of the hair and cannot be washed out.

An aniline derivative tint contains, as its essential ingredient, **para-phenylene-diamine** (par-a-fen'i-len-di-am'in), or a related chemical compound. With this type of preparation, it is possible to duplicate the various shades of human hair without impairing its luster. These tints may be applied successfully over permanently waved and chemically relaxed hair.

Aniline derivative tints are sold in small bottles and in tubes. The stock of these tints should be kept fresh, as they deteriorate when standing.

When the developer (hydrogen peroxide) is mixed with the tint, a chemical reaction, known as **oxidation**, begins. For this reason, the tint mixture must be applied immediately to the hair. After the mixture is applied to the hair, the oxidation continues until the color has developed to the desired shade.

Timing the development of the applied tint requires a **thorough study** of the product being used.

ALLERGY

Allergy to aniline derivative tints is an unpredictable condition. Some patrons may be sensitive to aniline derivative tints. To identify such individuals, a **skin** or **patch test** is required by law for all patrons 24 hours prior to the application of a tint or toner.

A person who has been free of an allergy may suddenly develop one. To be sure, give a patch test to find out if the patron has become sensitive since her last tinting.

The **U.S. Federal Food, Drug and Cosmetic Act** prescribes that a **patch test,** or **predisposition test,** must be given before each application of an aniline derivative tint, whether on a **virgin** head of hair or a **retouch**. This test is required to protect the patron, the hair colorist, and the entire cosmetology profession.

CAUTION

Aniline derivative tints must **never** be used on the eyelashes or eyebrows. **To do so may cause blindness.**

PATCH TEST

The patch test must be given 24 hours before each tinting or toner treatment. The tint used for the skin test must be of the same shade and mixture as the tint intended to be used for the hair tinting service.

Procedure

1. Select test area, either behind the ear extending partly into the hairline, or on the inner fold of the elbow.
2. Wash test area, about the size of a quarter, with mild soap and water.
3. Dry the test area by patting with absorbent cotton or a clean towel.

4. Prepare the test solution by mixing one capful of tint and one capful of 20 volume peroxide, or as directed by the manufacturer.

5. Apply enough test solution with cotton-tipped applicator to cover the area previously cleansed.

6. Allow the test area to dry. Leave it uncovered and undisturbed for 24 hours.

7. Examine the test area for either a negative or positive reaction.

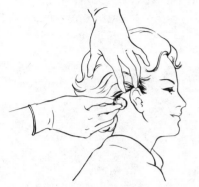 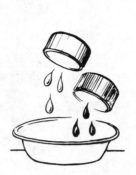 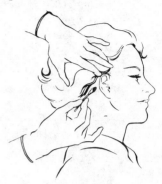

Washing patch test area behind ear.   *Mixing one capful of tint and one capful of peroxide.*   *Applying tint mixture.*

A **negative skin test** will show no sign of inflammation; hence, an aniline derivative tint may be applied.

A **positive skin test** is recognized by the presence of redness, swelling, burning, itching, blisters, or eruptions. A patron showing

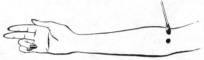

Giving a patch test at the inner fold of elbow.

such symptoms is allergic to an aniline derivative tint, and **under no circumstances should this particular kind of tint be used.**

Symptoms of hair tint poisoning are as follows:

1. Swelling.
2. Itchy red spots spreading all over the body.
3. Tiny blisters from which a liquid oozes.
4. Patron suffering from headaches and vomiting.

Immediate medical attention must be sought by a patron exhibiting the above symptoms.

PREPARATION FOR HAIR TINTING

Color selection. Always consult the patron and consider her color preference before starting to tint the hair. For this purpose, use a well-lighted room, providing either strong natural light or incandescent lighting.

When talking to the patron, find out whether she knows what color suits her age and skin tone. You must consider that skin tones change with age. The natural color of her hair, which harmonized beautifully with her skin coloring at the age of 20 or 30, may be harsh and unbecoming at the age of 40 or 50. For patrons in this age group, keep to the lighter shades of color.

Here are a few general guides to color selection:

1. Women, young in age or appearance, with fair or creamy complexions, can afford to be as daring as they wish when it comes to color selection.

2. Women with florid or pinkish complexions should adhere to the ash tones, either in the pale or darker shades, depending on their skin texture and age.

3. Women with clear olive complexions have a cool-looking skin. The choice of colors ranges from blonde to the warm series of browns, and sometimes to the very dark colors.

4. Women with a yellowish or brownish hue to their skin should avoid the ash colors. Careful study of skin texture is necessary for these skin tones to determine the amount of gold, copper, or red color to be applied.

BASIC RULES FOR COLOR SELECTION

The success or failure of a hair tint depends on the careful selection of the right color. Skill in color selection can best be developed by observing the following basic rules:

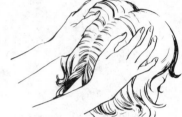

Checking hair color.

1. For color observation, the patron's hair should be clean and dry. If the hair is soiled or wet, the tendency is to select a color that is too dark.

2. Use a color chart to show the product's range of colors, their names and numbers.

3. Compare the patron's hair with the shade that is closest to it on the chart.

4. Determine if her shade, or one more becoming, is to be used.

5. To match the hair color, examine the hair nearest the scalp at the back of the head. This is where the hair is darkest.

6. Always look through, rather than down on, the hair. To see depth as well as highlights, raise the hair by pushing it up with the hands against the scalp.

7. Know the properties and manufacturer's instructions concerning the particular product you are using.

Tint colors are usually divided into four groups, according to the basic tone values:

1. Shades with no red are classified as **drab.**
2. Shades with some red or gold tones are in the **warm** series.
3. Shades with a great deal of red are included in the **very warm** or **red** series.
4. Shades with silver or platinum are classified as the **cool** series.

TESTING FOR COLOR SELECTION

Before applying a tint, give a preliminary strand test, which will indicate:

1. Whether the proper color selection was made.
2. The correct length of time to leave the tint on the hair.
3. Whether the hair is subject to possible breakage or discoloration due to the excessive or faulty use of either a cold waving lotion, relaxer, lightener, tint, metallic dye, or compound dye. If the hair is in a damaged condition, recondition and retest it before applying the tint.
4. Hair in a poor condition, with porous areas, or with streaked or dark ends, should be reconditioned. (For information on reconditioning treatments see section on **Fillers** in this chapter.)

STRAND TEST PROCEDURE

1. Mix a small amount of equal parts of the tint selected and 20 volume peroxide.
2. Apply the mixture to the full length of a dry hair strand. Retain it on the hair until the desired shade is developed.
3. Wash, dry, and examine the hair strand. If the results are satisfactory, proceed with the tinting.

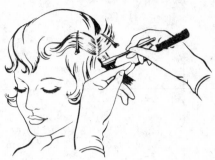

Giving a color strand test.

If the color produced on the test strand is different from the color desired, select another color and strand test again.

If the strand test shows discoloration, which might indicate the presence of a metallic dye, take corrective steps before tint application.

EXAMINING SCALP AND HAIR

Carefully examine the scalp and hair to determine if it is safe to use an aniline derivative tint and whether any special hair tinting problems exist.

The results of such an examination may indicate the need for any of the following:

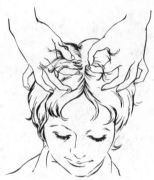

Examining scalp and hair.

1. Reconditioning treatments.
2. Removal of color from the hair.
3. Testing hair for discoloration.
4. Testing hair for breakage.

An aniline derivative tint should not be used if the following conditions are recognized:

1. Signs of a positive skin test.
2. Scalp irritation or eruptions.
3. Contagious scalp or hair disorders.
4. Presence of metallic or compound dyes.

If the scalp and hair are in a healthy condition, observe carefully and record data on a permanent hair tint record card.

Use soft water. When water is used in connection with hair tinting or lightening, be certain that it is **soft** water.

FOLLOW WORKING PLAN IN TINTING

For successful hair tinting with aniline derivative tints, the hair colorist must follow a definite procedure. Such a system makes for the greatest efficiency. Keep a permanent record of each patron's hair tintings. Without a plan, the work takes longer and mistakes may be made. Besides, the patron soon becomes dissatisfied and loses confidence in the hair colorist's ability.

A working plan includes the materials and supplies needed for the tinting service, and a thorough knowledge of the product to be used.

KEEPING HAIR TINT RECORDS

It is of the utmost importance to keep an accurate record so that any difficulties encountered in one treatment may be avoided in subsequent treatments. A complete record should be kept, containing information such as "dries out rapidly," "tint does not develop fast enough," or any other data connected with that particular patron's hair.

HAIR TINT RECORD

Name . . . . Tel. . . . .

Address . . . . City . . . .

Patch Test: Negative ☐   Positive ☐   Date . . . .

DESCRIPTION OF HAIR

Form	Length	Texture	Porosity	
☐ straight	☐ short	☐ coarse	☐ very porous	☐ resistant
☐ wavy	☐ medium	☐ medium	☐ porous	☐ very resistant
☐ curly	☐ long	☐ fine	☐ normal	☐ perm. waved

Condition

☐ normal   ☐ dry   ☐ oily   ☐ faded   ☐ streaked   . . . . . . % grey

Previously lightened with . . . . for . . . . (time)

Previously tinted with . . . . for . . . . (time)

☐ original sample enclosed   ☐ not enclosed

CORRECTIVE TREATMENTS

Color filler used . . . . Corrective treatments with . . . .

HAIR TINTING PROCESS

whole head . . . .   retouch . . . . inches (cm)   shade desired . . . .

Formula: color . . . . lightener . . . .

Results:

☐ good   ☐ poor   ☐ too light   ☐ too dark   ☐ streaked

Date	Operator	Price	Date	Operator	Price
. . . .	. . . .	. . . .	. . . .	. . . .	. . . .
. . . .	. . . .	. . . .	. . . .	. . . .	. . . .
. . . .	. . . .	. . . .	. . . .	. . . .	. . . .

RELEASE STATEMENT

A release statement is used for hair tinting, permanent waving, or any other treatment that may require the cosmetologist's or salon owner's release from responsibility for accidents or damages.

SAMPLE RELEASE

Patron's Name . . . .   Address . . . .

Condition of Hair: . . . .

Hair Coloring: Kind . . . . Given by . . . .

I fully understand that the hair coloring treatment that I have requested and am about to receive is ordinarily harmless to normal hair, but may damage my hair because of its present condition.

In view of this, I accept full responsibility for any possible damage that may result, directly or indirectly, to my hair.

Signature of Patron . . . .

Witnessed by . . . . Date . . . .

TEMPORARY COLOR RINSES

A temporary color rinse is the coating of the hair's cuticle with a thin film of color pigment. Since the color remains on the cuticle and does not penetrate into the cortex, it lasts only a short time, usually from shampoo to shampoo. Temporary color rinses usually contain certified colors.

There are a number of important advantages in the professional use of temporary colorings. They are very useful in helping to:

1. Bring out highlights in the hair.
2. Temporarily restore faded hair to its natural color.
3. Neutralize the yellowish tinge in white or grey hair.
4. Tone down overlightened hair.
5. Temporarily add color to the hair without changing the condition of the hair.

Temporary hair colorings also have several disadvantages:

1. The color is of short duration and must be applied after every shampoo.
2. The coating is very thin and may not cover all the hair evenly.
3. The thin coating of color may rub off on clothing or pillows.

However, for patrons who want to highlight the color of their hair or add beauty to grey hair, a temporary color rinse is very helpful. Color rinses come in various shades: blonde, brown, black, red, silver, and slate. They are applied easily and quickly and are valuable as an introduction to hair coloring.

Methods of Application

There are two methods in general use for the professional application of temporary hair colors. Both methods require that:

1. The patron be properly draped to protect her clothing and skin. (Ask patron to remove her jewelry and glasses.)
2. The hair be shampooed and towel dried.

METHOD A

MATERIALS AND IMPLEMENTS

Neck strip	Towels	Shampoo
Shampoo cape	Comb	Protective gloves
Measuring glass	Color rinse	Plastic applicator bottle

PROCEDURE

After the hair has been shampooed and towel dried:

1. Seat the patron comfortably at the styling station.
2. Apply the color rinse with a plastic applicator bottle. (Fig. 1)
3. Apply the rinse from the roots (scalp area) and comb through to the hair ends.

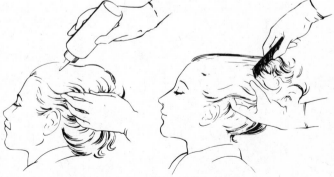

Fig. 1. *Applying temporary rinse with applicator bottle.*

Fig. 2. *Distributing rinse with wide tooth comb.*

4. Using the wide tooth part of the comb, blend the color over every strand to assure complete and even distribution. (Fig. 2)
5. Do not rinse the hair.
6. Set, dry, and style hair in the usual manner.

METHOD B

MATERIALS AND IMPLEMENTS

The same as those used in Method A, with the addition of a rinse brush and cotton applicator.

PROCEDURE

After the hair has been shampooed and towel dried:
1. Prepare the rinse, carefully following manufacturer's directions.
2. At the shampoo bowl, apply the rinse with a brush, cotton swab, plastic applicator, or spray bottle. (Fig. 3)
3. Start the application where hair is lightest or most in need of color.
4. The color rinse application is started nearest the scalp area and completely saturates all hair up to the hair ends.

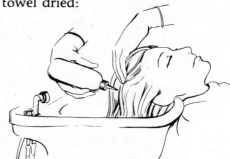

Fig. 3. Applying temporary rinse.

5. If hair ends are porous, dilute mixture before applying to the hair ends.
6. Leave the rinse on the hair from 2-5 minutes, depending on the shade desired.
7. Rinse thoroughly with warm water.
8. Set, dry, and style hair in the usual manner.

Note: For any variations in procedures, follow manufacturer's directions or be guided by your instructor.

CLEANUP

1. Discard all disposable supplies and materials.
2. Close containers, wipe them off, and put them in their proper places.
3. Clean and sanitize implements.
4. Tidy up station.
5. Wash and sanitize hands.

SEMI-PERMANENT TINTS

Semi-permanent tints offer a form of hair coloring suitable for the patron who has previously been reluctant to have her hair color changed.

The semi-permanent tint is a formulated coloring material that fills a gap between a temporary color rinse and a permanent hair color tint, without in any way taking the place of either.

Natural hair that is drab or dull may be improved in color tone by the use of semi-permanent tints, since there is no lightening action on the hair.

A wide range of colors is available and the results obtained will depend mainly on the original color, to a lesser degree on the texture of the patron's hair, and on the length of developing time.

The various shades may be blended to create individual color tones.

There are blue-grey or silver-grey shades specifically designed for hair ranging from 10-100% grey.

Semi-permanent hair colorings are formulated to last from 4-6 weeks. No peroxide is required. The hair fades naturally, provided a **mild non-stripping shampoo** is used. These tints require no retouching.

ADVANTAGES

1. The color is self-penetrating.
2. The color is applied the same way each time.
3. Retouching is eliminated.
4. Color does not rub off because it has penetrated the hair shaft.
5. Hair will return close to its natural color in 4-6 weeks.

Semi-permanent tints require a 24-hour patch test. Some semi-permanent hair colorings require pre-shampooing; others do not. Read manufacturer's directions.

TYPES

1. Semi-permanent tints that cover grey completely, but do not affect the remaining pigmented hair.
2. Semi-permanent tints that make grey hair more beautifully grey without changing the natural pigment.
3. Semi-permanent tints that add color and highlights to hair that is not grey.

MATERIALS AND IMPLEMENTS

Neckstrip	Application bottle	Acid or normalizing rinse
Towels	Cotton	Clips
Tint cape for patron	Mild shampoo	Record card
Protective gloves	Selected color tint	Talcum powder
Comb	Color chart	Plastic cap (if needed)
		Timer

PRELIMINARY STEPS

1. Give preliminary patch test 24 hours before tinting.
2. If the patch test is negative, proceed with the tinting.
3. Assemble all necessary supplies.
4. Prepare patron. Protect her clothing with towel and tint cape. Ask patron to remove her jewelry and glasses.
5. Examine patron's scalp for irritation or abrasions.
6. Select the desired shade of color.

The semi-permanent tint is applied by using the nozzle of an applicator bottle.

Manufacturers' directions vary, so be guided by their directions or by your instructor.

PROCEDURE

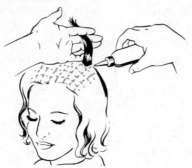

Applying tint to scalp area.

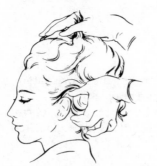

Gently working color through hair.

1. Give a mild shampoo, if required.
2. Towel dry hair (follow manufacturer's directions).
3. Put on protective gloves.
4. Apply tint to the hair throughout the scalp area.
5. Gently work color through the hair with your fingers until the hair is thoroughly saturated. (Do not massage into the scalp.)
6. Pile hair loosely on top of the head.
7. Be guided by the manufacturer whether to use or omit a plastic cap covering.
8. Strand test for color.
9. When color has developed, wet hair with warm water and work up a lather.
10. Rinse with warm water until water runs clear.
11. Give an acid or normalizing rinse.
12. Towel blot hair; set, dry, and style.
13. Fill out record card.

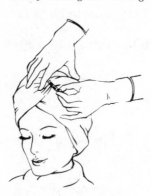

Using plastic covering, if required.

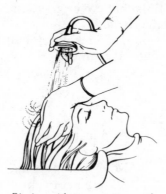

Rinsing with warm water until water runs clear.

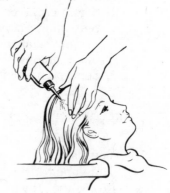

Giving acid or normalizing rinse.

CLEANUP

1. Discard all disposable supplies and materials.
2. Close containers; wipe them off, and put them in their proper places.
3. Clean and sanitize implements.
4. Remove stains from the tint cape.
5. Tidy up station.
6. Wash and sanitize hands.

PERMANENT HAIR COLORINGS

Practically all permanent hair coloring is done with the use of oxidizing-penetrating tints containing an aniline derivative.

These tints penetrate the cuticle of the hair into the cortical layer. Here they are oxidized by the peroxide—which has been added—into color pigments, and are distributed throughout the hair in much the same manner as the natural pigment.

Penetrating tints are also referred to as:

One-step tints, also called one-process or single-application tints.

Two-step tints, also called two-process or double-application tints.

One-step tints (cream or liquid) perform two activities: they lighten and add color to the hair in a single application.

Two-step tints (cream or liquid) perform only one activity at a time. They require two separate and distinct applications to the hair:

First—the application of a softener or lightener.

Second—the application of a tint or toner.

As a safety precaution, a **skin** or **patch test** must be given before tinting the hair. The hair colorist wears protective gloves during the tint application.

ONE-STEP TINTS (Cream Or Liquid)

One-step tints represent a simplified method of hair coloring. In one application, the hair can be colored permanently **without** requiring pre-shampooing, pre-softening, or pre-lightening.

In most instances, one-step tints contain a lightening agent and a shampoo with an oil base, combined with an aniline derivative tint. When ready for use, 20 volume hydrogen peroxide is added in fixed proportions, according to manufacturer's directions.

A one-step tint is applied on **dry hair only.** If the hair is in an extremely soiled condition and a shampoo is necessary, the hair must be thoroughly dried before the tint is applied. The choice of shades varies from deepest black to lightest blonde.

The advantages of one-step tints are that they:

1. Eliminate time consuming pre-shampooing, pre-softening, or pre-lightening processes.
2. Leave no line of demarcation.
3. Color the hair lighter or darker than the patron's natural color.
4. Blend in grey or white hair to match patron's natural hair shade.
5. Tone down streaks, off-shades, discolorations, and faded hair ends.

SOME GENERAL RULES FOR ONE-STEP COLOR SELECTION

1. To match the natural color of hair and to cover grey hair, select the color closest to the natural shade.
2. To brighten or lighten the hair, and to cover grey hair, select a shade lighter than the natural color. The selected tint must contain enough color to produce the desired shade on grey hair.
3. To darken the hair and cover grey hair, select a color darker than the natural hair color.
4. Study the manufacturer's color chart to learn how to make correct color selections.

HELPFUL SUGGESTIONS

SECTIONING, OUTLINING, AND SUB-DIVIDING

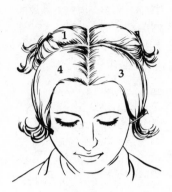

Sectioning the hair in four quarters.

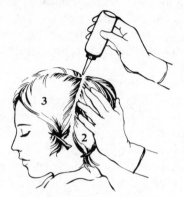

(Optional) Outlining parting with tint for retouch, only if the hair is grey.

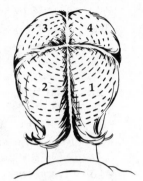

Sub-dividing sections into ¼″ strands.

USING PLASTIC BOTTLE APPLICATOR

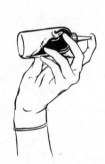

Preparing mixture—shaking gently back and forth.

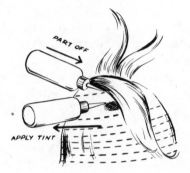

Using plastic bottle with nozzle to part hair and apply tint to ¼″ strand.

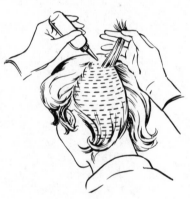

Applying tint to ¼″ strands.

USING BRUSH AS APPLICATOR

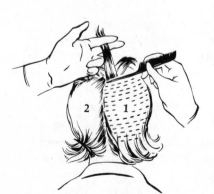

Part each strand with rat-tail comb.

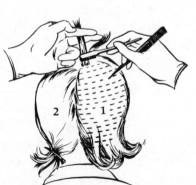

Applying the tint to each strand first on top-side and then the under-side.

STRAND TESTING

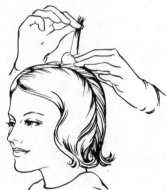

Strand testing for color development.

ONE-STEP TINT FOR VIRGIN HAIR
(Tinting Hair To A Lighter Shade)

Virgin hair is hair that has neither been lightened nor tinted. Hair that has been damaged in any way, such as by permanent waving, chemical straightening, sun, etc., cannot be considered as virgin hair.

The procedure given here for a one-step tint application is in general use today. However, if your instructor's routine varies, follow his/her procedure.

MATERIALS AND IMPLEMENTS

Towels	Applicators:	Selected color tint
Tint cape for patron	Tint brushes	Hydrogen peroxide
Protective gloves	Swab sticks	(20 volume)
Comb	Plastic bottles	Color chart
Glass or plastic bowls	Timer	Acid or normalizing
Record card	Cotton	rinse
Talcum powder	Acid-balanced shampoo	

CONDITIONERS AND COLOR FILLERS

If the hair is damaged, pre-conditioning treatments may be given.

To assure even color, it is advisable to apply color filler to damaged hair. (For more information, see section on **Conditioners and Color Fillers** in this chapter.)

PRELIMINARY STEPS

1. Give preliminary patch test 24 hours before tinting.
2. If the patch test is negative, proceed with the tinting.
3. Examine patron's scalp for irritation or abrasions.
4. Tint may be applied with an applicator bottle or brush.

PREPARATION

1. Assemble all necessary materials and implements.
2. Prepare patron. Protect her clothing with a towel and tint cape. Ask patron to remove her jewelry and glasses.
3. Re-examine the patron's scalp.
4. Select the desired shade of color.
5. Put on protective gloves.
6. Make color strand test.
7. Prepare formula.

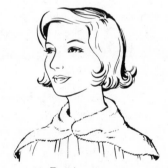

Draping patron.

PROCEDURE

1. Section the hair into four quarters. **If a color filler is used for damaged hair ends, apply it before the tint application. (Be guided by your instructor.)**
2. Select section where grey hair is most prevalent. Where no gray hair is present, select area where the hair is most resistant, usually the crown area.
3. Sub-divide section into ¼" (.625 cm) strands.

4. Pick up a strand of hair and hold it away from the head at the proper angle to expose the scalp area.

5. If color filler was used, apply tint to hair 1" (2.5 cm) from scalp to hair ends. If color filler was **not** used, apply tint to hair 1" from scalp to 1" of hair ends. Then apply tint to hair at scalp area and finally to hair ends.

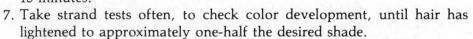

Note: Body heat causes the hair nearest the scalp to process faster. For this reason the tint is applied in the scalp area after the main body of the hair has been done, in order to assure even color processing.

Applying tint 1" from the scalp.

6. Let tint mixture develop for about 15 minutes.

7. Take strand tests often, to check color development, until hair has lightened to approximately one-half the desired shade.

8. Apply tint mixture to scalp area. Be sure that all hair is thoroughly saturated.

9. Leave tint on hair until a strand test indicates that the desired color has developed evenly from the scalp to the ends.

10. Rinse hair with lukewarm water to remove excess color.

11. Remove stains from around hairline, ears, and neck by working in a circular movement with a cotton pledget dipped in left-over tint diluted with shampoo, commercial stain remover, or warm water and a little shampoo.

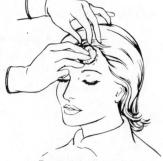

12. Give a mild, acid-balanced (non-strip) shampoo and rinse thoroughly with lukewarm water. Towel dry.

13. Apply a slightly acid rinse or conditioner to restore hair to a more normal condition.

14. Set, dry, and style hair.

15. Fill out record card and file.

Removing tint stains.

CLEANUP

1. Discard all disposable supplies and materials.
2. Close containers tightly; wipe them off, and put them in their proper places.
3. Clean and sanitize implements.
4. Remove stains from tint cape.
5. Tidy up station.
6. Wash and sanitize hands.

TINTING TO DARKER SHADE

When tinting close to, or darker than natural hair color, follow the same preparation and procedure as used for a one-step tint to a lighter shade, with the following exceptions:

1. Select color close to, or darker than, patron's natural hair color.

2. Apply the tint from the scalp area to hair ends.

3. When color has developed evenly from scalp area to hair ends, shampoo and rinse in the usual manner.

TINTING LONG HAIR

The procedure followed for tinting long hair is usually the same as that for shorter hair. Care must be taken to have additional materials on hand to provide for the extra length of hair.

ONE-STEP TINT RETOUCH

To retouch the new growth, follow the same procedure as you would for coloring virgin hair, with the following differences:

1. Apply tint to the new growth only: DO NOT OVERLAP. Check frequently for color development.

2. When the color has almost developed, dilute the remaining tint by adding an acid-balanced shampoo, conditioner, or water, as directed by manufacturer.

3. In order to assure complete and even coverage and color, apply this diluted mixture to the entire head. Gently distribute evenly with the fingertips. Retain for a few minutes. Rinse with warm water to remove excess color.

4. Follow Steps 11 to 15 as for virgin hair tint.

5. Clean up in the usual manner.

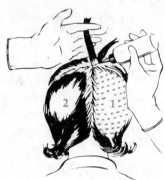

Retouching new growth.

HIGHLIGHTING SHAMPOO TINTS

Highlighting shampoo tints are preparations that combine aniline derivative tints, hydrogen peroxide, and a neutral shampoo base. They are used when a **very slight change** in hair shade is desired. These tints serve to cleanse the hair and highlight its natural color in a single application. (A **patch test** is required.)

Lightening agent. There are some highlighting shampoos that contain just hydrogen peroxide and a shampoo base. By omitting the tint and including only the lightener, color is slightly removed from the hair. (No patch test is required.)

The **method of application** for both the highlighting shampoo tint and the lightening agent is as follows:

Distribute the mixture evenly over the entire head at the shampoo bowl. Retain from 8-15 minutes. Rinse thoroughly.

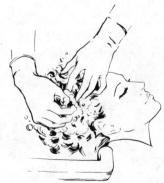

Applying highlighting shampoo tint.

PRE-LIGHTEN OR PRE-SOFTEN

Pre-lighten. If the patron desires a drastic color change that is lighter than her natural color, and wants to completely cover her grey hair, her hair should first be pre-lightened. The pre-lightener is applied in the same manner as for a regular hair lightening treatment.

Select shade from a manufacturer's color chart.

After the pre-lightening has reached the desired shade, the hair is lightly shampooed and towel dried. Then apply the tint in the usual manner.

Pre-soften. If the patron's hair is resistant the hair should be pre-softened in order for it to readily absorb the tint.

Apply the softener from the scalp to the hair ends as in regular lightening and retain it for a few minutes. During this time, little color change takes place, but the hair becomes more receptive to the tint. Do not rinse out the softener. Towel dry and apply tint, as directed by manufacturer.

SAFETY PRECAUTIONS

1. Give a 24-hour patch test before the application of a tint.
2. Do not apply tint if a patch test is positive.
3. Do not apply tint if abrasions are present on the scalp.
4. Use clean applicator bottles, brushes, combs, and towels.
5. Do not brush the hair prior to a tint.
6. Do not apply a tint without reading manufacturer's directions.
7. Take a strand test for color, breakage, and/or hair discoloration.
8. Choose a shade of tint that harmonizes with the patron's general complexion.
9. Use an applicator bottle or bowl (plastic or glass) for mixing the tint.
10. Do not mix tint before you are ready to use it; discard left-over tint.
11. If required, use the correct shade of color filler.
12. Suggest reconditioning treatments for tinted hair.
13. Do not apply tint if metallic or compound dye is present.
14. Take a strand test for correct color shade before applying tint.
15. Use a mild shampoo. If an alkaline or harsh shampoo is used it will strip the color.
16. Do not use water that is too hot; use lukewarm water for removing free color.
17. Protect the patron's clothing by proper draping.
18. Do not permit tint to come in contact with the patron's eyes.
19. Do not overlap during a tint retouch.
20. Fill out a tint record card for each application.
21. Always wash hands before and after serving a patron.
22. Wear gloves to protect the hands.

HAIR LIGHTENING

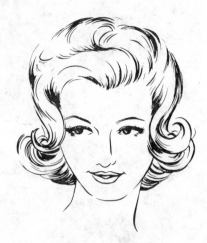

Lightening the hair color, or blonding, is one of the most important and glamorizing services the beauty salon has to offer. Hair colorists prefer to use the professional term "lighteners" rather than "bleaches" for the products that are designed to remove pigment from the hair. When talking to your patrons, you will find that using the term "lightener" has a softer, more pleasing connotation than the harsher term "bleach."

HOW LIGHTENERS ARE USED

Lighteners may be used for two purposes:

1. **As a color treatment,** to lighten the hair to the final shade desired.
2. **As a preliminary treatment,** to prepare the hair for the application of a toner or tint. (This is referred to as **Two-Step Tints**, also called **Two-Process** or **Double-Application Tints**.)
   a) **Toner**—A lightener always is necessary before applying one of the delicate toner shades.
   b) **Tint**—If the patron desires a drastic change to a shade much lighter than her natural shade, the lightener must be used to remove some color before a tint is applied.

EFFECTS OF LIGHTENERS

A lightening product is used to lighten the hair to a desired shade. The hair pigment goes through different changing stages of color as it lightens. The amount of change depends on the pigmentation of the hair and the length of time the lightening agent is left on. For example: A natural head of black hair will go from black to brown, to red, to red-gold, to gold, to yellow, and finally to pale yellow (almost white) stages. The seven stages of lightening are illustrated on the following page.

The hair also becomes more porous during the lightening treatment, a necessary condition to permit penetration of a toner.

Even natural light hair or grey hair must go through the lightening process in order to achieve the necessary degree of porosity for the acceptance of a toner or tint.

HAIR LIGHTENING

SEVEN STAGES IN LIGHTENING HAIR
FROM
DARK HAIR
TO ALMOST WHITE
(PALE YELLOW)

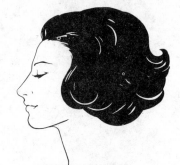

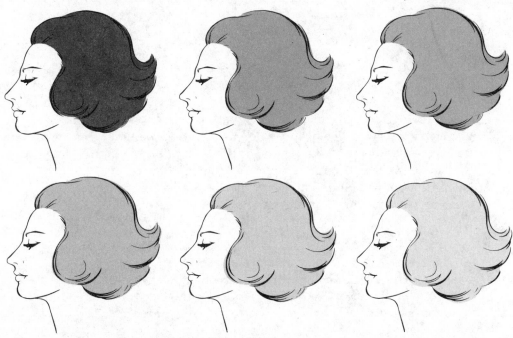

A virgin head of dark hair passes through seven stages before it arrives at the almost white stage. The change in the color depends on the type of lightener chosen and the length of time that it remains on the hair.

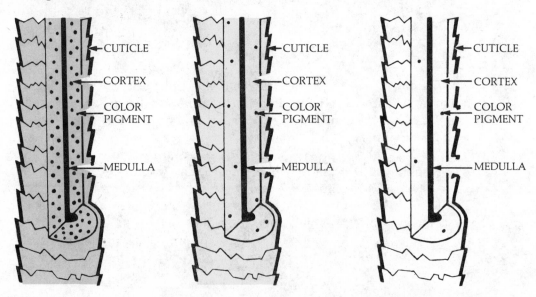

CUTICLE

CORTEX

COLOR
PIGMENT

MEDULLA

CUTICLE

CORTEX

COLOR
PIGMENT

MEDULLA

CUTICLE

CORTEX

COLOR
PIGMENT

MEDULLA

PROBLEMS IN HAIR LIGHTENING

The natural color of hair is determined by its pigment content. Natural hair coloring has either brown or yellow and red pigments, or a mixture of both.

Brown pigment changes to a lighter shade in a few minutes after application of the lightener.

Yellow and **red pigments** are present in diffused form in the cortex of the hair. The diffused **red** pigment creates problems in lightening and tinting. The **diffusion** of the **red** pigment makes it difficult or impossible to completely lighten the pigment without causing great damage to the hair.

Do not promise a patron that her dark hair can be lightened to a very pale blonde shade if she desires to have silver or extremely pale toners applied.

Whatever the reason for lightening, it is important to select the right lightener and the best mixture for the degree of color change desired. To make an **intelligent choice,** follow manufacturer's **literature** and **color charts.**

TYPES OF LIGHTENERS

Lighteners are classified as oil, cream, and powder or paste lighteners.

Oil lighteners are usually mixtures of hydrogen peroxide with a sulfonated oil.

1. **Colored oil lighteners** add temporary color and highlight to the hair as they lighten. The colors contained are **certified** and may be used without a **patch test.** They **remove** pigment and **add** color tones at the same time. Basically, they are **classified** according to their **action** on the hair, namely:
   a) **Gold**—lightens and adds gold highlights.
   b) **Silver**—lightens and adds silvery highlights to grey or white hair and minimizes red and gold tones on other shades.
   c) **Red**—lightens and adds red highlights.
   d) **Drab**—lightens and adds ash highlights. Tones down or reduces red and gold tones.
2. **Neutral oil lightener** removes pigment without adding color tone. It may be used to pre-soften or pre-lighten hair for tint application.

Cream lighteners are the most popular types of lighteners. They are easy to apply, will not run, drip, or dry out. They are easy to control and contain conditioning agents, bluing and thickener, which provide the following benefits:

1. The **conditioning agents** give some protection to the hair.
2. The **bluing agent** helps to drab red and gold tones.
3. The **thickener** gives more control when applying lightener.

Powder or **paste lighteners,** also called **quick lighteners,** contain an oxygen-releasing booster and inert substances for quicker and stronger action.

1. **Paste lighteners** will hold and not run, but will dry out quickly.
2. **Powder lighteners,** mixed into a smooth, creamy paste, do not contain conditioning agents and may dry the hair and irritate the scalp.

ACTION OF HAIR LIGHTENERS

Hair lighteners, depending on manufacturer's directions, can be used:
1. To lighten the entire head of hair for toner application.
2. To lighten hair to a particular shade.
3. To brighten and lighten existing shade.
4. To tip, streak, or frost certain parts of hair.
5. To lighten hair that has already been tinted.
6. To remove undesirable casts and off-shades.
7. To correct dark streaks or spots in lightened or tinted hair.

CHOICE OF HAIR LIGHTENERS

Be guided by the following rules, in addition to manufacturer's directions:
1. Choose a cream lightener (blue base) when pre-lightening for pastel toners, such as blonde, silver, platinum, or biege.
2. Choose a neutral oil lightener to lighten the hair without adding color.
3. Choose an oil lightener (drab series) to avoid red and gold highlights in the natural color of the hair.
4. Choose an oil lightener (red and gold series) to obtain red or gold highlights in the natural color of the hair.
5. Choose a powder lightener for tipping, streaking, or frosting **extremely** resistant hair.

HYDROGEN PEROXIDE

The lightening agent for removing pigment from the hair shaft is hydrogen peroxide. The **active** ingredient of hydrogen peroxide is oxygen gas. To speed the liberation of the oxygen gas, a small amount of **28% ammonia water** is added. However, this leaves the hair with a straw-like appearance, containing reddish or brassy tones. Commercial lightening products now contain substances that modify or prevent these effects.

When properly used, hydrogen peroxide can lighten, soften, and oxidize hair. For the purpose of hair lightening, it is used as a 6% solution, capable of producing 20 volumes of oxygen gas. A weaker strength of peroxide is not suitable for lightening and tinting. The use of a higher strength peroxide, even though it may speed up the lightening action, may be harmful to the hair.

Hydrogen peroxide is available in the form of a liquid, cream, powder, or tablet. The liquid peroxide should be purchased in pint sizes, kept closed when not in use, and stored in a cool, dark, dry place.

Do not permit peroxide to come into contact with **metal.** When liquid peroxide is kept too long, exposed to air, or stored in a warm place, its strength will be weakened. Follow manufacturer's directions when using tablet, powder, cream, or liquid.

USES OF HYDROGEN PEROXIDE

As a **lightening agent,** a hydrogen peroxide solution softens the cuticle of the hair shaft and lightens the shade of the coloring pigment in the cortical layer of the hair.

Lightening makes the hair porous and lighter in color. However, continued use of lighteners will make some hair over-dry and brittle.

As a **softening agent,** hydrogen peroxide softens the cuticle of the hair and makes it more receptive to the penetrating action of an aniline derivative tint. Care must be taken to control the softening process so that the hair is not lightened.

As an **oxidizing agent,** a hydrogen peroxide solution is used in all aniline derivative (penetrating) hair tints. It acts as a developer by liberating oxygen gas, which changes para-phenylene-diamine into a dark-colored compound capable of tinting the hair.

LIGHTENING VIRGIN HAIR

A **preliminary lightening strand test** is necessary to ascertain the length of time a lightening mixture is to be left on the hair. It is also used to help diagnose the condition of the hair.

Preliminary Test Objectives

1. If test shows the hair is not light enough:
   a) Increase strength of mixture, and/or
   b) Increase processing time.
2. If hair strand is too light:
   a) Decrease strength of mixture, and/or
   b) Decrease processing time.
3. Watch strand carefully for reaction to lightening mixture, and for discoloration or breakage. Reconditioning may be required if a negative reaction sets in.
4. If hair is too dark or too resistant, pre-softening may be required.
5. If color and condition are good, proceed with lightening.

A **patch test for toners** must be made 24 hours prior to the application of a **toner.** To save the patron's time, the strand test for lightening should be made the day she has the patch test.

MATERIALS AND IMPLEMENTS

Towels	Comb, clips	Applicator bottle (with
Tint cape	Record card	measurements listed)
Shampoo	Talcum powder	Protective gloves
Cotton	Peroxide (20 volume)	Glass or plastic bowls
Acid or normalizing	Lightening agent	Measuring glass or cup
rinse		Timer

If a paste type lightener is to be used, a brush applicator will be needed.

PROCEDURE

The following general instructions in applying lighteners may be changed by your instructor to conform with manufacturer's directions.

1. Prepare patron. Adjust towel and tint cape to cover and protect patron's clothing.
2. Examine scalp and hair. Do not give a lightening service to a patron with eruptions, abrasions, or inflammation of the scalp. Do not brush or shampoo hair.

3. Section hair into four quarters.

4. Prepare lightening formula and use immediately to prevent deterioration.

5. Put on protective gloves.

6. Apply lightener. If the hair seems resistant or especially dark around the crown, it is advisable to start at the back of the head, so that this region will get more lightening action.

   Apply lightener in 1/8" (.3125 cm) partings. Start about ½-1" (1.25-2.5 cm) from the scalp and extend lightener to a point where the hair shaft shows signs of damage. Apply lightener to both top and underside of hair strand.

7. Continue to apply lightener on both sides of the strand until the entire head is completed. Work mixture into hair with fingers. The hair is more fragile at this point, so **do not comb the lightener through the hair.**

   Keep hair moist with lightener during development. (Preliminary strand test will determine whether or not lightener is brought through the hair ends.)

8. Test for color. Make first strand test about 15 minutes before the time indicated by preliminary strand test. Remove mixture from strand with wet towel or cotton. Dry the strand. If the shade is not light enough, reapply mixture and continue testing frequently until desired shade has almost been developed.

9. Scalp area and hair ends. Towel blot excess lightener. If necessary, prepare a fresh mixture of lightener. Use 1/8" (.3125 cm) partings, and continue as follows:

   a) Apply lightener over the entire scalp area. Avoid overlapping previously lightened hair. Retain lightener for required length of time.

   b) When hair has lightened sufficiently, apply lightener to the hair ends and work through with fingertips.

   c) Pile the hair loosely on top of head. Be guided by your instructor.

10. Remove lightener. When desired shade has been reached, rinse and shampoo hair lightly with cool water. Use a mild shampoo.

11. Dry hair either with towel or under a cool dryer.

12. Examine scalp for abrasions and hair for breakage.
    If scalp is normal, the hair is ready for toner or tint application.

13. Fill out record card and file.

14. Clean up in usual manner.

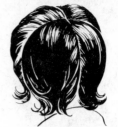

Hair sectioned into four quarters.

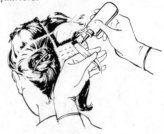

Applying lightener to topside of strand about ½-1" from scalp. (Steps 6 and 7)

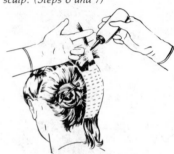

Applying lightener to underside of strand. (Steps 6 and 7)

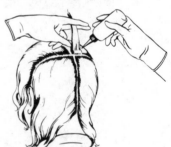

Applying lightener to scalp area. (Step 9)

LIGHTENER RETOUCH

A "lightener retouch" is the term commonly used when a lightener is applied to the new growth only to match the rest of the lightened hair.

As a general rule, black or dark brown hair requires retouch applications more frequently than the lighter shades.

In retouching, the lightener is applied to the **new growth only,** with the following exceptions:

1. If another color is desired.
2. If a lighter shade is desired.
3. If color has become heavy or dull from several applications.

In each case, wait until the new growth is almost light enough or has developed fully. Then bring the **remainder** of the lightener through the hair shaft. One to five minutes is ample time to correct any one of these conditions.

PROCEDURE

The patron's record card should be consulted by the hair colorist as a guide to the lightener to be used and time required for the shade to develop.

A cream lightener is generally used for a lightener retouch because its adhesive quality prevents the overlapping of previously lightened hair.

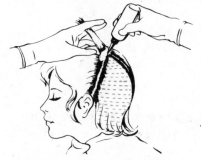
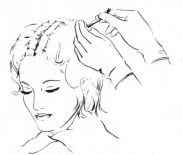
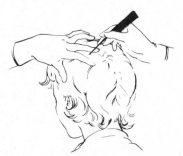

Applying lightener to new growth.   *Strand testing.*   *Checking for complete coverage.*

The **procedure for a lightener retouch** is the same as that for lightening a virgin head of hair, except that the mixture is applied only to the new growth of hair.

CAUTION

Care should be taken not to **overlap** the lightener on to previously lightened or tinted hair.

PRECAUTIONS

1. Give a 24-hour patch test before the lightener application, if a toner is to follow.
2. Drape patron properly to protect her clothing.
3. Examine the scalp before applying a lightener.
4. Do not apply a lightener if irritation, eruptions, or abrasions are present.
5. Use only clean applicator bottles, brushes, sanitized combs, and towels.
6. Always wash your hands before and after serving a patron.
7. Wear gloves to protect your hands.

8. Analyze the condition of the hair and suggest reconditioning treatments, if required.

9. Test for color, breakage, or hair discoloration by giving a strand test prior to hair lightening.

10. Cream or paste lightener must be the thickness of whipped cream to avoid dripping or running, or causing overlapping.

11. Apply lightener to resistant areas first. To insure complete coverage, pick up 1/8" (.3125 cm) sections.

12. Work as rapidly as possible when applying the lightener, to produce a uniform shade without streaking.

13. Take frequent strand tests until the desired shade is reached.

14. After completing the lightener application, check the skin and remove any lightener from these areas.

15. Check and, if necessary, change the towel around the patron's neck. Lightener on the towel will cause irritation if it is allowed to come in contact with the skin.

16. Lightened hair is fragile and requires special care. Use only a very mild shampoo, and rinse with cool water.

17. If a preliminary shampoo is required, do not brush the hair. Avoid irritating the scalp during the shampoo.

18. Never allow lightener to stand; use it immediately. Discard leftover lightener.

19. Cap all bottles to avoid loss of strength.

20. Be sure to read manufacturer's directions before mixing a lightener.

21. Fill out record card after each hair lightening service.

TONERS

Toners are aniline derivative tints, and they are a permanent, penetrating type of hair coloring, requiring a 24-hour **skin** or **patch test.** They consist primarily of pale, delicate colors.

Toners require double applications, and are also known as **Two-Step Tints, Two-Process Tints,** or **Double-Application Tints.**

1. The first application is the lightener.
2. The second application is the toner.

PRE-LIGHTENING FOR TONERS

To achieve the desired toner color, **pre-lightening** is required. Hair should be pre-lightened to gold or pale yellow, depending on the toner color to be used.

Toners penetrate the cuticle and deposit color in the same manner as other permanent tints. They depend on the preliminary lightening to leave the hair both light in color and porous. Some toners (the extreme pale shades) require more pre-lightening than others. The lightener must be left on long enough to achieve the necessary porosity. Coarse, resistant, or dark hair requires longer lightening time than naturally blonde hair.

Although naturally blonde hair may reach the pale yellow stage very quickly, it may **not be porous** enough to permit penetration of the toner. If the required porosity has not developed sufficiently, allow for additional lightening time.

White or grey hair requires a certain amount of pre-lightening to make the hair porous enough to receive a toner. Since white or grey hair is almost decolorized, it needs pre-lightening before the application of a blonde, silver, or pastel shade toner. Pre-lightening is very important when grey hair is a mixture of light and dark strands. Lengthy lightening will not be necessary, but a certain amount of lightening is required to make the hair porous enough to accept the toner.

SELECTING TONER SHADES

The pastel colors, such as silver, ash, platinum and beige, are glamour colors that appeal to many women.

For the patron who wants extremely light and delicately colored hair, the **blonde** colors are the perfect color tones.

For the patron with grey hair and skin tone changes that accompany advancing years, the **lighter silver** tones are flattering.

For the patron desiring extremely pale toner shades of the very light silver, platinum, or beige colors, the hair must be pre-lightened to the **pale yellow,** or almost **white** stage.

Color selection is frequently left to the hair colorist's judgment. Other important factors to be considered are patron's age and complexion.

REMINDERS AND HINTS ON TONERS

Toners are completely dependent upon a proper preliminary lightening treatment, which must leave the hair light and porous enough to receive pale toner shades. A strand test must be made first, and a complete explanation of the possible outcome should be given to the patron.

The possibility may exist that her hair cannot be decolorized enough to achieve the color of her choice without seriously damaging the hair shaft.

If the red and gold pigments have not been eliminated during the lightening process, the patron's choice of toner color may result in a shade with a greenish cast, or the color might not take at all. When this happens, the toner used must be deeper and not as pale or silvery as the patron may have requested.

During the application and development period, toners have quite a different color than the final shade, depending on their basic color. However, when the color has fully developed, the anticipated color will have been achieved. (Example: Ash blonde will have a brownish cast; silver blonde, a bluish cast; and platinum, a violet cast.)

TONER APPLICATION

Preliminary

1. Give a 24-hour patch test before toner application.
2. To determine the final color, give strand test during the same time when you give a patch test.
3. If the patch test is negative and the scalp is normal and without irritation, proceed with the toner service.

Toner Strand Test

1. Mix a small amount of toner with an equal amount of developer. (Be sure to recap bottles immediately.)

2. Apply the mixture to a full strand of lightened hair. Allow color to develop for 15 minutes. Rinse, towel dry, and check color. If color has not developed to desired shade, reapply mixture and check again in 5 minutes. Continue checking until desired shade has been reached.

3. Wash and towel dry. Note the time it took for color to develop, and use this as a guide for giving a toning to the entire head.

MATERIALS AND IMPLEMENTS

In addition to the toner, use the same materials and implements as used for lightening virgin hair.

PREPARATION

1. Arrange all necessary supplies.
2. Prepare patron.
3. Put on protective gloves.
4. Lighten hair to pale yellow (almost white). Then, shampoo hair lightly, rinse thoroughly, and towel dry.
5. Select the desired toner shade.

Prepare formula at room temperature. Pour bottle of toner into applicator bottle or bowl. Add equal amount of developer. If you use an applicator bottle, cover top with gloved hand and turn it over 4-5 times. Do not shake. When using bowl, stir mixture gently for just a few seconds.

PROCEDURE

Wear protective gloves throughout the entire application.

Be sure hair is pre-lightened to the stage necessary for the toner shade to be used.

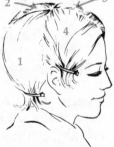

Sectioning the hair into four quarters.

1. Section hair into four quarters, using rat-tail comb or tip of applicator.
2. Starting at the crown of the back right quarter, apply mixture to the scalp area. Make small ¼" (.625 cm) partings. Continue to apply mixture to the other three sections.
3. When application to the scalp area is completed, use comb to distribute and blend mixture through entire strand, applying additional mixture to saturate hair.

CAUTION

Do not comb toner mixture through over-porous hair ends until the last few minutes of developing time. If the ends absorb too much color, dilute remaining mixture with equal amounts of shampoo, conditioner, or water before applying to ends. (Follow manufacturer's recommendation.)

4. Pour additional mixture on hair and blend throughout. Leave hair loose to permit circulation of air, insuring better color development.
5. After 15 minutes, dry a strand of hair and test for color. If desired color has not been reached, recomb more mixture into tested strand. Repeat test frequently with different strand until you reach desired shade.
6. When treatment has been completed, rinse out excess toner thoroughly and shampoo according to manufacturer's recommendation.

7. Towel dry hair.
8. Remove all toner stains from the skin, hairline, ears, and neck.
9. Set, dry, and style hair.
10. Fill out record card and file it.
11. Clean up in the usual manner.

TONER RETOUCH

A toner retouch must be given the same careful consideration as you would give a tint retouch. The new growth must be pre-lightened to the same degree of lightness as was the first toner application. After the lightening process has been completed, the toner is applied as outlined below.

CAUTION

Overlapping the lightener may cause hair damage.

PRELIMINARY STEPS

1. Give patch test before application of toner. Also give strand test.
2. Pre-lighten new growth to stage required for toner.
3. Towel dry hair after lightener has been thoroughly rinsed and shampooed from hair.

PROCEDURE

1. Part hair into 4 sections. Start application at the back of head.
2. Making ¼" (.625 cm) partings throughout, use a plastic applicator bottle or tinting brush to apply the toner mixture to the new growth area only.
3. If hair shaft is holding color from previous treatment, allow the roots to develop to the same degree of color shown by a strand test. Then, using a comb, distribute and blend color through the hair to about 1" (2.5 cm) from the hair ends.
4. Strand test frequently. Reapply mixture to tested strands.
5. When strand test shows color has reached close to the desired shade, work the balance of the mixture through the ends. Should the ends absorb too much color, dilute the toner mixture with an equal amount of shampoo, conditioner or water, as directed by manufacturer.
6. When color is evenly developed, as shown by strand test, thoroughly rinse and shampoo, as recommended by manufacturer.
7. Towel dry hair.
8. Remove toner stains from the skin of hairline, ears, and neck.
9. Set, dry, and style hair.
10. Fill out record card and file.
11. Clean up in the usual manner.

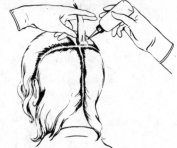

Applying lightener to new growth.

SUMMARY

1. Give 24-hour **patch test** prior to toner application.
2. Do not apply toner if scalp has any irritation, eruptions, or abrasions.
3. Use only non-metallic utensils, such as glass, porcelain, or plastic. **Do not use metallic bowls or dishes.**

4. Always wear protective gloves.
5. For best results, mix ingredients at room temperature immediately before application.
6. For even results, apply toner as rapidly as possible.
7. Remove toner stains from skin with absorbent cotton soaked in mild shampoo and water. **Do not rub.**
8. After a toner application, use a shampoo as directed by manufacturer.
9. Discard leftover toner mixture.
10. Do not give a permanent wave on the same day as toner application.

FROSTING, TIPPING, AND STREAKING

For **partial lightening,** such as in achieving frosting, tipping, and streaking effects, quick lighteners are often advisable.

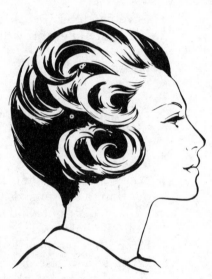

1. **Frosting.** Strands of hair are lightened over various parts of the head. Strands of hair to be lightened are drawn through the holes of a perforated cap with a crochet hook. This procedure is followed to protect the scalp when the lightener is applied. The effect achieved will depend on how many strands of hair are lightened.

2. **Tipping** is similar to frosting. Wisps of hair are lightened in various areas, usually across the front of the head. This produces a contrast with the darker shade of hair. Strands of hair are drawn through holes in a perforated cap with a crochet hook and lightened.

Marbelized streaking.

3. **Streaking.** This is a lightened strand, usually at the front hairline. The width and placement of the lightened strand depend on the "feather" effect to be achieved.

CAP TECHNIQUE FOR FROSTING AND TIPPING

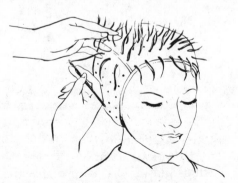

Draw strands through holes with crochet hook.

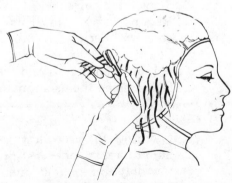

Apply lightener with brush.

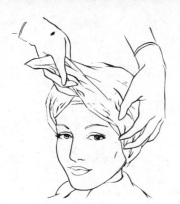

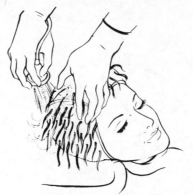

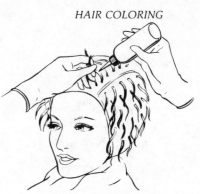

To hasten process, cover the head with aluminum foil or plastic cap.

After hair has sufficiently lightened, remove covering. While cap is still on, shampoo or rinse off lightener and towel dry.

Apply toner in the usual manner.

FROSTING ALL OVER

1. Separate hair (weave).
2. Place aluminum foil underneath hair to be lightened.
3. Apply lightener on both sides of strand.
4. Wrap hair in aluminum foil. Continue this procedure over entire head. Leave ½" (1.25 cm) parting around front hairline.
5. Complete frosting as for cap technique.

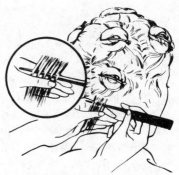

Separating hair (weaving).

STREAKING

Fold and roll up foil.

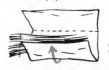

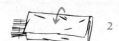

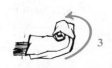

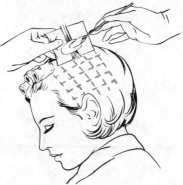

FRONT HAIRLINE STREAKING. *Select 3-4 sections to be streaked. Comb other hair out of way. Apply lightener ½" from scalp. Fold and roll foil. Process and finish as explained on previous page.*

STREAKING ON DARK HAIR. *Section hair to be streaked. Apply lightener ½" from scalp. Fold and roll foil. Process and finish in the usual manner.*

BLONDE-ON-BLONDE EFFECT

The hair to be treated should be light blonde. Section the hair into a checkerboard pattern, as in Fig. 1. Wrap every other section with aluminum foil by folding and rolling up each one. Thirty-forty sections should be sufficient. (Fig. 2)

Apply deepest blonde toner to all unwrapped hair, as in Fig. 3. After the hair has been sufficiently processed, and before removing foils from rolled strands, rinse thoroughly.

Remove foils; towel dry hair; then, apply the lightest toner to the entire head. Shampoo, set, dry, and style hair in the usual manner.

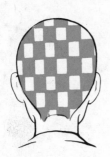

Fig. 1. Checkerboard pattern.

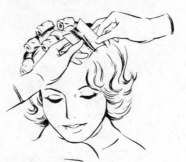

Fig. 2. Rolling up strands not to be lightened with aluminum foil.

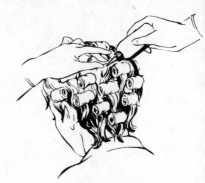

Fig. 3. Applying toner to unwrapped hair.

DAMAGED HAIR

The frequent use of lacquers and hair sprays coats and damages the hair. Damaged hair must be **reconditioned** before it can **successfully** be tinted, lightened, or permanent waved.

Careless application of tints, lighteners, permanent waving solutions, and relaxer to the hair may result in breakage or dry, brittle hair.

The use of either **highly alkaline shampoos** or **soapless oil shampoos,** improper water temperature, improper use of hair dryer, or extreme exposure to the elements may cause hair to become damaged.

Hair may need reconditioning treatments for reasons other than damage resulting from the use of harmful products. Sometimes hair is naturally brittle, thin, and lifeless. Both **neglect** and the **patron's physical condition** may be contributing factors to these conditions.

Hair is considered damaged when it is in one or more of the following conditions:

1. Over-porous.
2. Brittle and dry.
3. Breaks easily.
4. No elasticity.
5. Rough and harsh to the touch.
6. Over-lightened hair that is coarse and spongy and mats easily when wetted.
7. Rejects color or absorbs too much color during tinting.

Any of these hair conditions may create trouble during a tinting, lightening, permanent waving, or hair relaxing treatment. Therefore, damaged hair should receive reconditioning treatments **prior to and after the application of these chemical agents.**

RECONDITIONING PROCEDURE

To restore damaged hair to a more normal condition, commercial products containing lanolin or protein substances should be used.

The reconditioning agent is applied to the hair. If heat is applied, use the heating cap, steamer, or heating lamp according to manufacturer's directions. As to frequency and length of time for each treatment, be guided by your instructor.

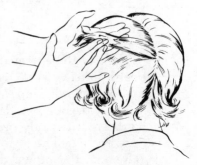

Applying conditioner to the hair.

FILLERS

Fillers are preparations that are available in liquid or cream form. They are used to revitalize, recondition, and correct abused, lightened, tinted, or damaged hair.

There are two general classifications of fillers: conditioner fillers, which are colorless; and color fillers, which range in color shades from platinum to deep brown.

The **conditioner fillers** are used to recondition lightened, tinted, or otherwise damaged hair before beauty salon services. (For further information, consult chapter on **Chemistry**.)

The **color fillers** are applied to abused or damaged hair to equalize porosity and to deposit a base color prior to tinting.

COLOR FILLERS

A color filler is recommended if the hair is in a damaged condition and if there is any doubt that the finished color will be an even shade.

A color filler is applied after hair has been pre-lightened and before the application of a toner or tint. A filler also is used for the patron who has been tinting or lightening her hair and wishes to return to her natural color.

ADVANTAGES OF COLOR FILLERS

1. Deposit color to faded hair shafts and ends.
2. Help hair to hold color.
3. Help to insure a uniform color from the scalp to hair ends.
4. Prevent color streaking.
5. Prevent off-color results.
6. Prevent a dull color appearance.
7. Give more uniform color in a tint back to natural shade.

HOW TO USE COLOR FILLERS

Color fillers may be applied **directly** from their containers to **damaged hair** prior to tinting. Color fillers may be **added** to the tint and applied to **damaged hair ends.** They may be used full strength or may be diluted with water. Be guided by your instructor.

SELECTION OF CORRECT COLOR FILLER

To obtain satisfactory results, select the color filler to match the same basic shade as the toner or tint to be used.

Note: Since manufacturer's directions regarding fillers vary as to color selection, use, and application, be guided by these directions or by your instructor.

REMOVAL OF ANILINE DERIVATIVE TINTS
(With Prepared Commercial Products)

Sometimes it is necessary to remove or partially remove the tint from the hair to correct a previous tinting or to apply a new shade.

Commercial products are used to remove penetrating tints, and are known as tint or color removers. They may contain hydrogen peroxide, acids, sodium hydrosulfite, a mixture of mineral and vegetable oils, or sulfonated oils.

The removal of tints never can be handled mechanically. Each color removal must be treated as an **individual problem** in which nothing can ever be taken for granted.

Chemicals that are sold for the purpose of removing tints always should be used with caution. Follow manufacturer's directions.

PROCEDURE

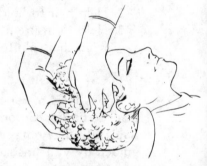

1. Prepare patron.
2. Follow manufacturer's directions about whether or not to shampoo.
3. Section hair into four quarters.
4. Put on protective gloves.
5. Mix preparation in a glass dish. Follow manufacturer's directions for mixing.
6. Start application immediately where the hair is the darkest. (Fig. 1)

Fig. 1. Applying mixture to darkest area.

7. Apply the mixture with a cotton pledget or brush. Saturate the hair thoroughly.
8. After completely covering the hair, strand test immediately, and frequently thereafter.
9. Pile the hair on top of the head. (Fig. 2)
10. If required by manufacturer, apply a warm, damp towel around patron's head, or put on a heating cap. (Fig. 3) Be guided by your instructor.

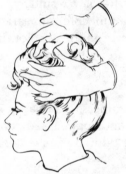

Fig. 2. Piling hair on top of head.

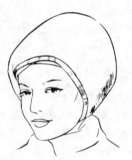

Fig. 3. Hastening the process by putting on a heating cap.

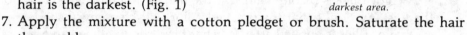

Fig. 4. Shampooing and rinsing thoroughly with cool water.

11. When the color has been removed, shampoo thoroughly, using shampoo and cool water. (Fig. 4) Rinse thoroughly with cool water.

CAUTION

The tint remover must be rinsed thoroughly from the hair; otherwise, its chemical action will continue.

12. Towel dry or thoroughly dry hair under dryer, as required by manufacturer.
13. If color is to be added, proceed with the application of desired shade of tint.
14. If no color is to be applied, set, dry, and style hair in the usual manner.

Note: If the product requires a waiting period before applying tint or other services, be guided by your instructor.

REMOVING COATING DYES

Coating dyes, such as metallic dyes and compound dyes, are coloring agents that do not penetrate, but coat the hair shaft. In removing coating dyes, never guarantee the results, because complete success is not certain. For removing coating dyes be guided by manufacturer's directions or by your instructor.

TINT BACK TO NATURAL COLOR

Each tint back to natural color must be handled as an individual problem. Check the natural shade of the hair next to the scalp.

The determining factors in the selection of the tint shade are:

1. The present condition and color of the hair.
2. The final result desired, which is the original color.

Select an appropriate shade of filler to correspond with the tint to be used. Without the use of an appropriate filler, it will be difficult to obtain a uniform color from the scalp to hair ends, since the hair porosity will vary in degree and area of the head.

Such hair coloring problems require two or more strand tests and guidance by the instructor in color selection and procedure.

PROCEDURE

1. Assemble materials.
2. Prepare patron in the usual manner.
3. Select appropriate tint and color filler, as indicated by the strand test.
4. Shampoo and towel dry the hair, or be guided by your instructor.
5. Section hair into four quarters.
6. If a color filler is required, proceed as directed by your instructor.
7. Re-section hair into four quarters.
8. Sub-divide sections into about ¼" (.625 cm) partings. Apply the tint **as rapidly as possible** to both sides of the hair strand, from scalp to hair ends.
9. Check for complete coverage.
10. Strand test immediately and frequently until desired shade has developed.
11. Give a mild or non-strip shampoo and use a non-strip rinse. Set, dry, and style hair in the usual manner.
12. Fill out record card and file. Clean up work station in the usual manner.

LIGHTENING STREAKED HAIR

Streaks of discoloration often appear on the hair, caused in part by unsuccessful or unskilled lightener application.

To correct streaked hair:

1. Prepare lightening formula as for virgin hair.
2. Apply mixture only to the darker streaks.
3. Work one strand at a time.
4. Allow mixture to remain on hair until all streaks are removed.
5. Shampoo hair.

SPOT LIGHTENING

Because the natural pigmentation of the hair is not distributed evenly, hair often is not lightened evenly from scalp to ends. **Uneven** lightening also may be due to **careless** application of the lightener. When this happens, gold bands or darker streaks may appear. This means that these areas have not been lightened enough. Spot lightening then becomes necessary to insure an even color. Reapply the lightener to these particular areas. Let it remain until these areas have lightened sufficiently to even out the entire head of hair.

LASH AND BROW TINT

An aniline derivative tint **never** should be used for coloring eyebrows or eyelashes; to do so may cause **blindness.** Instead, a harmless coloring agent, such as mascara, should be used.

The **choice of color** is limited to either brown or black. While black is favored in most cases, brown is recommended for very light complexions with blonde hair. Follow the specific directions of manufacturer when applying the coloring agent.

MATERIALS AND IMPLEMENTS

Petroleum jelly (Vaseline)
Lash and brow tinting solutions
  (Solutions No. 1 and No. 2)
Stain remover
Dish of warm, soapy water

Dish of clear, cool water
Towels
Cotton
Paper eye shields
Applicator sticks and eye pads

PREPARATION

1. Follow sanitary measures.
2. Place patron in partially reclining position in facial or shampoo chair at approximately a 45° (.785 rad.) angle. Do not permit her to lie in a straight position, since such a position would permit the tinting solution to enter the eyes more easily.
3. Place a clean towel across her chest.

PROCEDURE

1. Wash lashes and brows with warm, soapy water, using a cotton pledget. Remove all traces of makeup from lashes and brows.
2. Apply petroleum jelly around eyes and on paper shields.
3. Adjust eye shields. Ask patron to look up, adjust shield, and close eye gently. Do the same with the other eye.

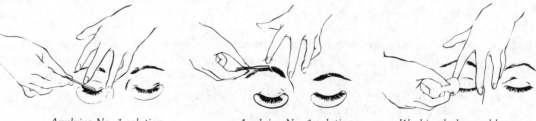

Applying No. 1 solution to lashes. *Applying No. 1 solution to brows.* *Washing lashes and brows.*

4. Apply No. 1 solution to lashes. Moisten cotton-tipped applicator. Touch tip to towel to remove excess moisture. Apply over and under

lashes close to skin. Moisten lashes several times. **Break applicator stick, and discard. Use a fresh applicator stick each time solution is applied.**

5. Apply No. 1 solution to brows, following natural browline. Reapply against natural growth, working solution in thoroughly. **Replace cap on No. 1 solution bottle.** (If bottle caps are interchanged, oxidation starts and the liquids lose their value.)

   Note: *Moisten fresh applicator with stain remover and place on edge of towel for future use. Replace cap on stain remover bottle.*

6. Apply No. 2 solution to lashes and brows in same manner as No. 1 solution. If stain gets on skin, use stain remover immediately. Replace cap on No. 2 bottle.

7. Remove eye shields and wash lashes and brows with cool water, using cotton pledgets.

8. Place moist eye pads over eyelids. Rewash brows with soap and water. Remove eye pads. Place small roll of cotton under lashes and wash them from above with cool water.

9. Remove stains with stain remover. Replace bottle cap.

10. Soothe skin with lotion or cream. Wash the eyes with a boric acid solution.

11. Clean up in the usual manner.

DEFINITIONS PERTAINING TO HAIR COLORING

accelerating (processing) machine: used to shorten the processing time of a lightening or tinting service.

allergy: skin sensitivity to cosmetics, tints, foods, or other substances. In hair coloring, a very small number of patrons may be allergic to aniline derivative tints.

blending: the process of making the color uniform throughout the hair during hair coloring applications or retouches.

certified color: temporary coloring that coats the hair and lasts from one shampoo to another.

coating: the accumulation of residue on the outside of the hair.

color filler: a preparation containing a certified color, used to equalize porosity in over-porous hair so that it can take and hold color evenly.

color testing: method of determining the action of a selected tint on a small strand of hair by washing and drying in order to observe how the color is developing.

conditioner: a cosmetic applied to hair to restore oil, sheen, elasticity, and manageability.

decolorization: the removal of natural or artificial color pigment from the hair.

development time: the time needed to develop the color or the lightener.

developer: an oxidizing agent, such as 20 volume hydrogen peroxide solution. When mixed with a tint, it releases the necessary oxygen gas to develop tint.

frosting, tipping, streaking: techniques for partial lightening of small sections of hair on various parts of the head.

heating cap: used to hasten the coloring process.

highlighting: the brightening effect on the hair accomplished by the application of a tint or the application of a lightener.

idiosyncrasy: an individual peculiarity that makes one susceptible to chemical substances in cosmetics, drugs, and foods.

lift: refers to the degree of lightening. Hair lifted two shades means that hair was made two shades lighter.

line of demarcation: streak caused by overlapping on previously tinted hair.

overlapping: a condition caused in a retouch by having a tint or lightener overlap any part of the previously tinted or lightened hair.

oxidation: a chemical reaction that takes place when peroxide and tinting solution are mixed and applied to the hair.

peroxometer or **hydrometer**: instrument used primarily by chemists to measure the strength of hydrogen peroxide.

plastic cap: cap made of plastic, used to hasten the hair coloring process and other hair treatments.

porosity: the extent to which hair is able to absorb moisture or liquid preparations.

powder or **paste lightener**: a strong, fast-acting product used for special effects and to save time in hair lightening.

pre-lightening: the process of removing partial or total color from the hair before a tinting or toner application.

pre-softening or **softening**: the application of a lightener to soften resistant hair and make it more receptive to the tint.

record card: a written record of patron's hair structure, condition, lightening and tinting color used, and other pertinent information concerning the hair.

resistant hair: hair with poor porosity.

semi-permanent hair coloring: hair coloring that lasts from 4-6 shampoos. Penetrates hair shaft slightly. Contains no peroxide and needs no peroxide to develop color.

sensitivity: a condition in which the skin is highly reactive to a specific chemical. skin reddens or becomes irritated shortly after contact with the chemical. On removal of the chemical the reaction usually subsides.

shampoo-in-color: a commercial product applied according to manufacturer's directions.

skin or **patch test**: a procedure for determining whether or not a person is allergic to an aniline derivative tint.

soap cap: the application of a tint diluted with shampoo. It is worked through the hair like a shampoo.

spot lightening: applying a lightener only to dark areas to even out color.

spot tinting: applying tint to areas insufficiently colored in order to produce even results throughout.

strand test: preliminary test given on a small strand of hair before a coloring or lightening treatment. It is used to pre-determine the mixture and development time required for the treatment. Color development or color testing also is known as **strand testing**.

stripping: a term used to indicate the removal of natural hair pigment, coating, or penetrating tint from the hair.

susceptible: capable of being allergic.

tint back: coloring of the hair back to its natural shade.

tint removal: the use of dye solvent, lightener, or softening treatment to remove an unsatisfactory shade of tint from the hair.

toner: an aniline derivative tint, delicate in shade, that is applied to lightened hair to produce blonde, silver, and pastel shades.

touch-up or **retouch**: the application of coloring or lightener to the new growth of hair.

virgin hair: hair that has neither been lightened nor tinted.

Note: The hair colorist should know whether the hair has been permanently waved or chemically straightened and what, if any, damage resulted thereby.

REVIEW QUESTIONS

HAIR COLORING

1. Define hair tinting.
2. Give four reasons why a patron may wish to have her hair tinted.
3. What knowledge should a cosmetologist have to be successful in the technique of hair coloring?
4. What are the three main groups of hair coloring?
5. What do color rinses contain, and how long do they remain on the hair?
6. What is meant by semi-permanent hair coloring?
7. Which tints are the penetrating type?
8. Name three types of hair coloring that coat the hair.
9. What types of dyes are never used professionally?
10. What type of tints are used professionally to perform most permanent hair coloring?
11. Why do aniline derivative tints remain in the hair until removed by chemicals?
12. State two reasons why aniline derivative tints require a 24-hour patch test.
13. In what two areas is a skin test given?
14. What are two important factors to consider when selecting a color shade?
15. Why should a preliminary strand test be given before the application of a tint?
16. List four conditions that would prohibit the application of an aniline derivative tint.
17. What type of water is used in connection with hair tinting or lightening?
18. What type of tint can be used to lighten and deposit color in the hair in one application?
19. By what other terms are one-step tints known?
20. What is meant by a virgin head of hair?
21. To which part of the hair is a one-step tint retouch applied?
22. What are two purposes of highlighting shampoo tints?
23. When is pre-softening required for a one-step tint?

HAIR LIGHTENING

1. Define hair lightening.
2. When is a two-step tint recommended?
3. By what other terms are two-step tints known?
4. Lightening the hair is usually a preparatory process for which other hair treatment?
5. How does hair lightening affect the porosity of the hair?
6. List three types of commercial lighteners.
7. Why are cream lighteners the most popular with cosmetologists?
8. Why do lightening products contain small quantities of 28% ammonia water?
9. What strength hydrogen peroxide is commonly used?
10. How does hydrogen peroxide act as a lightening agent?
11. What effect does lightening have on the hair?
12. What reaction does hydrogen peroxide have on the hair when used as a softening agent?
13. How does hydrogen peroxide act as an oxidizing agent?
14. What are toners?
15. Why do toners require a 24 hour skin or patch test?
16. Why does white or grey hair require some pre-lightening prior to the application of a toner?
17. To which part of the hair is a lightener retouch applied?
18. On what parts of the hair shaft are frosting, tipping, and streaking usually applied?
19. List seven conditions of the hair that require reconditioning treatments.
20. What are the three purposes for which fillers are used?
21. What are the two general classifications of fillers?
22. What purposes are served by conditioner fillers?
23. When is a color filler recommended?
24. How are color fillers selected to obtain the best results in tinting?
25. Why is it sometimes necessary to remove or partially remove the tint from the hair?
26. How should each color removing treatment be handled?
27. What is meant by a coating dye?
28. List three precautionary measures to follow when tinting hair back to its natural shade.
29. What kind of tint should never be used to color eyebrows and eyelashes?

Chapter 16

CHEMICAL HAIR RELAXING AND CHEMICAL BLOWOUT

CHAPTER LEARNING OBJECTIVES

The student successfully mastering this chapter will know:
1. *What takes place within hair when chemical products are used on it.*
2. *The products used in chemical hair relaxing.*
3. *The basic steps involved in chemical hair relaxing.*
4. *The difference between thio relaxers and sodium hydroxide relaxers.*
5. *Why a strand test is required.*
6. *The methods and techniques employed in chemical hair relaxing.*
7. *Why protective gloves are required.*
8. *Safety precautions that must be used.*
9. *The procedure to be followed when giving a chemical blowout.*

Chemical hair relaxing is the process of permanently rearranging the basic structure of over-curly hair into a straight form. When done professionally, it leaves the hair straight and in a satisfactory condition, to be set into almost any style.

To attain proficiency in chemical hair relaxing, the cosmetologist must acquire the technical knowledge and manipulative skills needed in this specialized branch of cosmetology.

Note: The terms "chemical hair relaxing" and "chemical hair straightening" are used interchangeably to refer to the process of permanently removing waves or curls from hair.

CHEMICAL HAIR RELAXING PRODUCTS

The basic products that are used in chemical hair relaxing are a **chemical hair relaxer**, a **neutralizer**, and a **petroleum cream**, which is used as a protective base to protect the patron's scalp during the sodium hydroxide chemical straightening process.

CHEMICAL HAIR RELAXERS

The two general types of hair relaxers are **sodium hydroxide**, which does not require pre-shampooing, and **ammonium thioglycolate**, which requires pre-shampooing.

Sodium hydroxide (caustic type hair relaxer) has both a softening and a swelling action on hair fibers. As the solution penetrates into the cortical layer, the cross-bonds (sulfur and hydrogen) are broken. The action of the comb, or the hands, in smoothing the hair and distributing the chemical straightens the softened hair.

Manufacturers vary the sodium hydroxide content of the solution from 5-10%, and the pH factor from 10 to higher. In general, the more sodium hydroxide used and the higher the pH, the quicker the chemical reaction will take place on the hair, and the greater the danger will be of hair damage.

When using sodium hydroxide, the cosmetologist must soften the hair within a maximum period of 8 minutes. If the product is left on the hair longer than the required time (as indicated by a strand test), the hair may turn a reddish color, or it may become brittle and break. If the solution is left on the hair longer than 10 minutes, the hair may dissolve. **Because of the high alkaline content of sodium hydroxide, great care must be exercised in its use.**

Ammonium thioglycolate (thio type relaxer). Although ammonium thioglycolate is less drastic in its action than sodium hydroxide, it softens and relaxes over-curly hair in somewhat the same manner.

NEUTRALIZER

The **neutralizer** also is called a **stabilizer** or **fixative.** The neutralizer stops the action of any chemical relaxer that may remain in the hair after rinsing. At the same time, the neutralizer re-forms the cystine (sulfur) cross-bonds in their new position and rehardens the hair.

PROTECTIVE BASE FOR SODIUM HYDROXIDE

The protective base is a petroleum cream that is designed to protect the patron's skin and scalp during the sodium hydroxide chemical straightening process. This protective base also is important during a chemical straightening retouch. It is applied to protect the hair that had been straightened previously, and to prevent over-processing and hair breakage.

The petroleum cream has a lighter consistency than petroleum jelly, and is formulated to melt at body temperature. The melting process assures the complete coverage of the scalp and other protected areas with a thin, oily coating. This helps to prevent burning and/or irritation of the scalp and skin and to protect previously treated hair during the straightening process.

BASIC STEPS

Chemical hair relaxing involves three basic steps: **processing, neutralizing, and conditioning.**

PROCESSING

As soon as the chemical relaxer is applied, the hair begins to soften and to lose its tight curl.

NEUTRALIZING

As soon as the hair has been sufficiently processed, the chemical relaxer is thoroughly rinsed out with warm water, followed by either: 1) a built-in shampoo neutralizer, or 2) a prescribed shampoo and neutralizer.

CONDITIONING

Depending on the patron's needs, the conditioner may be part of a series of hair treatments, or it may be applied to the hair before or after the relaxing treatment.

Most over-curly hair, except virgin hair, is in a damaged condition due to thermal comb or thermal iron treatments, tinting, or lightening. Therefore, conditioning is often necessary to give strength and body to the damaged hair, and to protect it against breakage.

CAUTION

Hair that has had recent tinting, lightening, thermal comb, or thermal iron services should not receive a chemical hair relaxing treatment. Conditioning treatments should be given to restore the hair to a nearly normal condition. Then, if the results of strand tests are favorable, a chemical hair relaxing treatment may be given.

Metallic dye. Hair treated with metallic dyes must not be given a hair relaxing treatment; to do so would damage or destroy the hair.

STRENGTH OF RELAXER

1. **Fine, wooly, tinted** or **lightened hair**—Use mild relaxer.
2. **Normal, medium virgin hair**—Use regular relaxer.
3. **Coarse** or **kinky virgin hair**—Use strong or extra strong relaxer.

ANALYSIS OF PATRON'S HAIR

It is essential that the cosmetologist have a working knowledge of human hair, particularly when giving a relaxing treatment. Recognition of the qualities of hair is achieved by means of visible inspection, feel, and special tests. Before attempting to give a relaxing treatment to over-curly hair, the cosmetologist must judge its texture, porosity, elasticity, and the extent, if any, of damage to the hair. (For more complete information on hair analysis, refer to the chapter on **Permanent Waving.**)

PATRON'S HAIR HISTORY

To help assure consistent satisfactory results, records should be kept of each chemical hair relaxing treatment. These records should include the patron's hair history and the patron's release statement.

The release statement is used to protect the cosmetologist, to some extent, from responsibility for accidents or damages. (For an example of a patron's record card and release statement refer to chapter on **Permanent Waving.**)

Before starting to process the hair, the cosmetologist must be certain of how the patron will react to the relaxer. Therefore, the patron must receive:

1. A thorough scalp and hair examination.
2. A hair strand test.

SCALP EXAMINATION

Inspect the scalp carefully for the presence of eruptions, scratches, or abrasions. To obtain a clearer view of the scalp, part the hair into ½" (1.25 cm) sections. Hair parting may be done with the index and middle fingers, or with the handle of a rat-tail comb. In either case, the cosmetologist must exercise great care not to scratch the scalp. Such scratches may become seriously infected when aggravated by the chemicals in the relaxer.

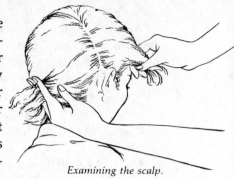

Examining the scalp.

If **scalp eruptions** or **abrasions** are present, do not apply the chemical hair relaxer until the scalp is again in a healthy condition. If the hair is not in a healthy condition, prescribe a series of conditioning treatments to bring it into a more normal condition. Then give a strand test.

STRAND TEST

In order to determine the results to be expected, it is advisable to test the hair for porosity and elasticity. This can be done through the use of one of the following three strand tests:

1. **Finger test** determines the degree of porosity in the hair. Grasp a strand of hair and run it between thumb and index finger of the right hand, from the end toward the scalp. If it ruffles or feels bumpy, the hair is porous and can absorb moisture.

2. **Pull test** determines the degree of elasticity in the hair. Normally, dry, curly hair will stretch about one-fifth its normal length without breaking. Grasp half a dozen strands from the crown area and pull them gently. If the hair appears to stretch, it has elasticity and can withstand the relaxer. If not, conditioning treatments are recommended prior to a chemical relaxing treatment.

3. **Relaxer test.** Application of the relaxer to a hair strand will indicate the reaction of the relaxer on the hair. Take a small section of hair and pull through a slit in a piece of aluminum foil placed as close to the scalp as possible. Apply relaxer to the strand in the same manner as you would apply to the entire head. Allow it to remain on the hair for 2-3 minutes, and then remove it with a piece of dry cotton. If the test is satisfactory, proceed with the treatment. If the hair has not processed sufficiently, repeat the test on another strand and allow a minute or two longer for processing.

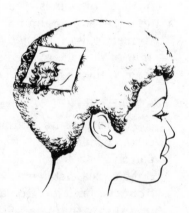

Relaxer strand test.

The area selected for the strand test should be either in the crown or other area where the hair is wiry and resistant.

CHEMICAL HAIR RELAXING PROCESS
(WITH SODIUM HYDROXIDE)

Note: The procedure outlined below is based primarily on products containing **sodium hydroxide.** For this, or any other kind of product, follow manufacturer's directions, and be guided by your instructor.

EQUIPMENT, IMPLEMENTS AND MATERIALS

Chemical relaxer	Protective gloves	Absorbent cotton
Neutralizer or stabilizer	Towels	Neck strip
Shampoo	Rollers	Clips and picks
Shampoo cape	Comb and brush	Hairnet
Protective base	Spatula	End papers
Conditioner—filler	Timer	Cream rinse
Eye pads	Conditioner	Setting lotion
		Record card

PREPARATION

1. Select and arrange the required equipment, implements and materials.
2. Wash and sanitize your hands.
3. Prepare and drape the patron as for a shampoo.
4. Examine and evaluate the scalp and hair.
5. Give a strand test and check results.
6. Do not shampoo hair. (Hair ends may be trimmed after the application of the chemical relaxer.)
7. Have patron sign release card.

PROCEDURE

1. **Section hair.** Part hair into 4-5 sections, as recommended by your instructor.

 FOUR SECTIONS.
Part hair down center from forehead to nape. Part across, starting behind the ear. Extend part from ear to ear.

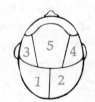 FIVE SECTIONS.
Part across, starting behind the ear. Extend part from ear to ear. Divide front area into 3 sections. Divide back area into 2 sections.

2. **Dry hair.** If moisture or perspiration is present on the scalp, place the patron under a cool dryer for several minutes.

3. **Application of protective base.** Manufacturers recommend the use of a protective base to protect the scalp from the strong chemicals in the relaxer. To apply it properly, part the hair into 4-5 distinct sections. Then subdivide each section into ½-1" (1.25-2.5 cm) partings, to permit thorough scalp coverage.

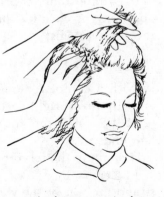

Applying protective base.

225

Apply the base freely to the entire scalp with the fingers. The hairline around the forehead, nape of the neck, and over and around the ears must be completely covered. Complete coverage is important to protect the scalp and hairline from irritation.

APPLYING THE CONDITIONER-FILLER

In many cases a conditioner-filler is required before the chemical relaxer can be used. The conditioner-filler, usually a protein product, is applied to the entire head of hair when dry. It protects over-porous or slightly damaged hair from being over-processed in any part of the hair shaft. It evens out porosity of the hair shaft, and permits uniform distribution and action of the chemical relaxer.

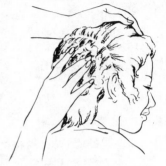

To receive complete benefits from the conditioner-filler, rub it gently into the hair from the scalp to the hair ends, using either the hands or a comb. Then towel dry the hair. Use a cool dryer to completely dry the hair.

Applying conditioner-filler.

CAUTION

Avoid the use of any heat, which could open the pores of the scalp and cause irritation or injury when the relaxer is applied.

APPLYING THE RELAXER

Divide the head into 4-5 sections, in the same manner followed for the application of the protective base.

The processing cream is applied last to the scalp area and hair ends. The body heat will speed up the processing action at the scalp. The hair is in a more porous condition at the ends and may be damaged. In both these areas, less processing time is required, and, therefore, the relaxer is applied last.

There are two methods in general use for the application of the chemical hair relaxer:

1. The Comb Method.   2. The Finger Method.

CAUTION

It is important to protect the patron's eyes with **protective pads** when applying the chemical hair relaxer, and protective gloves must be worn by the cosmetologist.

Comb Method

With a comb, remove a quantity of relaxing cream from the jar. Begin with the back right section of the head. Apply the relaxer, starting ½-1" (1.25-2.5 cm) from the scalp, and comb to within ½" (1.25 cm) of the hair ends.

First apply the relaxer to the top side of the strand. Then, raise the hair in 1" (2.5 cm) sub-sections and apply the relaxer underneath. Flip the completed strand up, out of the way.

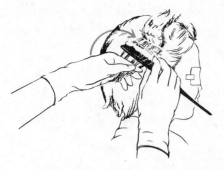

Applying relaxer on top of strand.

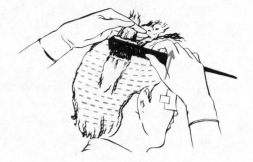

Applying relaxer underneath strand.

Complete the right back area, and moving in a clockwise direction, cover each section of the head in the same manner. Then, go back over the head in the same order, applying additional relaxing cream, if necessary, and combing the relaxer close to the scalp and up to the hair ends. Avoid excessive pressure or stretching of the hair.

Combing the cream through the hair not only spreads the cream, but also stretches the hair gently into a straight position.

STRAND TESTING

While spreading the relaxer, inspect its action by stretching the strands to see how fast the natural curls are being removed. If the action is too fast in any area, direct the patron to the shampoo bowl and rinse the relaxer from that particular section. Then continue the spreading process over the rest of the head, and, finally, to the hair ends.

RINSING OUT RELAXER

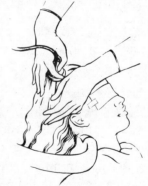

When the hair has been sufficiently straightened, rinse the relaxer out rapidly and thoroughly. The water must be warm, not hot. If the water is too hot, it may burn the patron, cause discomfort because of the very sensitive condition of the scalp, or cause the relaxed hair to revert to its original form. If the water is too cold, it will not stop the processing action. The direct force of the rinse water should be

Rinsing out relaxer.

used to remove the relaxer and avoid tangling the hair. Unless the relaxer is completely removed, its chemical action continues on the hair. The stream of water should be directed from the scalp to the hair ends.

CAUTION

Do not get relaxer or rinse water into the eyes or on unprotected skin. If the relaxer or rinse water accidentally gets into the patron's eyes, wash it out immediately with large quantities of warm water, and take the patron to a doctor without delay. Continue wearing protective gloves until all relaxer has been removed.

SHAMPOOING

Gently work the shampoo (non-alkaline or cream shampoo recommended) into the hair. The hair is very fragile at this point and tangled ends can be broken easily. Use tepid water and avoid firm manipulations, rubbing, or tangling the hair. Keep the hair in a straight position. Relaxed hair requires at least three shampooings at all times.

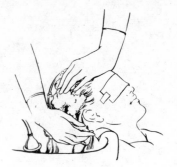

Shampooing the hair.

APPLYING NEUTRALIZER (STABILIZER OR FIXATIVE)

After shampooing the hair, apply a neutralizer. This helps to keep the hair in a relaxed state.

Completely saturate the hair with neutralizer; then comb with a wide-tooth comb, beginning at the nape and working upward toward the forehead.

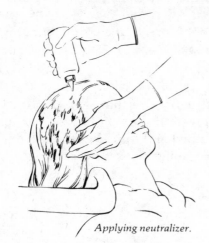

Applying neutralizer.

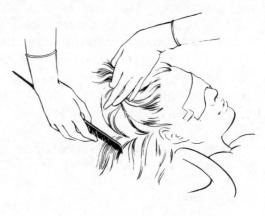

Combing neutralizer through hair.

Use the comb to:
1. Keep the hair straight.
2. Completely saturate the hair with the neutralizer.
3. Remove tangles without too much pulling.

After five minutes, rinse out the neutralizer thoroughly with warm water, and then towel blot. Follow manufacturer's instructions.

Style hair in the usual manner.

Discard used supplies.

Cleanse and sanitize equipment.

Wash and sanitize hands.

Complete hair relaxing record card.

CAUTION

Different products used for relaxing the hair require different methods of handling the hair during the processing and neutralizing period. Always follow manufacturer's directions, and be guided by your instructor.

Hot Thermal Irons

To avoid hair breakage, a lapse of at least 4-6 weeks should be allowed (depending on the length, texture, and thickness of the hair) before hot thermal irons are again used on chemically relaxed hair. Thermal curling with lukewarm heat also can be used to curl chemically relaxed hair. Conditioning treatments should be recommended and the hair dried completely before thermal curling.

APPLYING CONDITIONER

Many manufacturers recommend that you apply a conditioner before setting the hair, to offset the harshness of the sodium hydroxide in the relaxer and to help restore some of the natural oils to the scalp and hair.

Two general types of conditioners are available:

1. **Cream conditioners,** usually lanolin or cholesterol, are applied to the scalp and hair, then carefully rinsed out. The hair is then towel dried. Apply setting lotion; set the hair on large rollers; dry and style the hair in the usual manner.
2. **Protein (liquid) conditioners** are applied to the scalp and hair prior to hairsetting and allowed to remain in the hair to serve as a setting lotion. Set the hair on large rollers, dry, and style in the usual manner.

CAUTION

Because of the fragile condition of the hair, it is advisable to wind the hair on large rollers, without tension.

Finger Method

The finger method of applying the relaxer to the hair is the same as the comb method, except the fingers and palms are used instead of the comb. Everything else is the same. **Wear protective gloves.**

Using your fingers, remove a small quantity of relaxing cream from the jar and lay it on the hair, about ½-1" (1.25-2.5 cm) from the scalp. Gently manipulate the cream through the entire section of hair to about ½" (1.25 cm) from the ends. Make certain that all hair has been covered.

Working in a clockwise direction, repeat the process with the next section, until every section has been covered.

Then, starting with the first section, repeat the procedure, adding relaxer where needed, and also applying relaxer on the hair down to the scalp, but not to the hair ends.

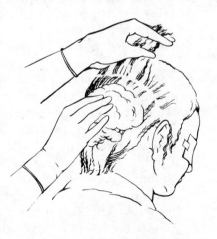

Applying relaxer.

Spreading out the relaxer. Smooth hair gently, as shown in the illustration. The spreading out procedure follows the same pattern that was used in applying the relaxer. There are three specific reasons for this procedure:

1. To be sure the hair is completely covered, from the scalp to the hair ends.
2. To be sure the hair is completely relaxed, from the scalp to the hair ends.
3. To be able to determine how fast the hair is being relaxed.

After spreading the relaxer over the entire scalp area and hair shaft, apply the relaxer to the ends and front hairline.

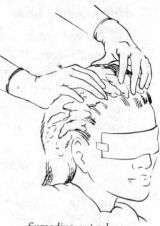

Spreading out relaxer.

SODIUM HYDROXIDE RETOUCH

Follow all the steps for a regular chemical hair relaxing treatment, with one exception: apply the **relaxer only to the new growth.** In order to avoid breakage of previously treated hair, apply a protective cream over the hair that received the earlier treatment, thus avoiding overlapping and damage.

SAFETY PRECAUTIONS

1. Examine the scalp for abrasions; if any are present, do not give a hair relaxing treatment.
2. To be sure a hair relaxing treatment can be given safely, analyze the hair and scalp and give a strand test.
3. Test the elasticity of the hair for its ability to stretch and return to its normal length without breaking. Also, check the porosity of the hair and its ability to absorb moisture.
4. Do not shampoo the hair prior to the application of a sodium hydroxide product.
5. Do not apply a caustic (sodium hydroxide) relaxer over a thio type relaxer.
6. Do not apply a thio type relaxer over a sodium hydroxide type relaxer.
7. Have a thorough understanding of the product being used and its action on the hair. Follow manufacturer's directions carefully.
8. Never use a strong relaxer on fine, wooly hair, as it may cause breakage.
9. Never give a chemical hair relaxing treatment to hair that was recently straightened by a hot thermal comb.
10. Do not relax damaged hair. Suggest a series of conditioning treatments. If hair ends are in a damaged condition, trim them before giving a relaxing treatment.
11. Apply a protective base, to avoid burning or irritating the scalp by the sodium hydroxide relaxer.
12. After the application of the protective base, check carefully to see that the scalp and surrounding skin area have been completely covered. Failure to cover the scalp and skin carefully can result in a burn by the chemicals being used.

13. Wear protective gloves.

14. Protect patron's eyes with protective pads; avoid getting chemicals or rinse water in patron's eyes.

15. Use extreme care when applying the relaxer, to avoid accidentally spreading it on the ears, scalp, or skin.

16. Test the action of the relaxer frequently, to determine how fast the natural curl is being removed.

17. When rinsing the relaxer from the hair, take great care that the water is not too hot. If hot water is used, the hair will revert to its natural curly shape.

18. Be sure to thoroughly remove the relaxer from the hair. Failure to do so will cause the relaxer to continue to process, resulting in hair damage. Direct stream of water from scalp to hair ends.

19. Use a mild shampoo with warm water and gently work it into the hair. Do not give vigorous manipulations.

20. Wear protective gloves until all the relaxer has been removed. When rinsing the shampoo from the hair, always work from the scalp to the ends, to prevent tangling the hair.

21. The application of a neutralizer (stabilizer or fixative) following the shampoo is an important step; it keeps the hair in a relaxed or straightened form.

22. Use a wide-tooth comb and avoid pulling when combing the hair. Avoid scratching the scalp with comb or fingernails.

23. Apply a conditioner to the scalp and hair before setting, to help restore some of the natural oils that have been removed from the scalp and hair by the relaxer.

24. When retouching the new growth, do not allow the relaxer to overlap onto the hair already straightened.

25. Do not use hot irons on chemically relaxed hair.

26. Do not give a hair relaxing treatment to hair treated with a metallic dye.

27. At the completion of each treatment, fill out a record card of the details of the treatment.

28. Always have patron sign a release statement, to protect the cosmetologist and the beauty salon.

CHEMICAL HAIR RELAXING PROCESS (WITH AMMONIUM THIOGLYCOLATE)

Ammonium thioglycolate (also called **thio relaxer**) is the same type of product used in cold waving, with a heavy cream added to the formula in order to keep the hair in a straightened position.

As in cold waving, the relaxer breaks the sulfur and hydrogen bonds, softening and swelling the hair. By the mechanical action of the hands and/or comb, the hair is smoothed and held in a straightened position.

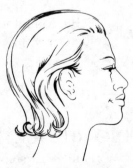

Relaxed hair.

When the hair is straightened, the neutralizer is applied to it (serving the same purpose as the neutralizer in cold waving). It re-forms the sulfur and hydrogen bonds, and rehardens the hair in its newly straightened position.

Manufacturers vary their products according to the texture and condition of the hair. Tinted and lightened hair require a weaker formula.

PROCEDURE

The same precautions must be observed in the use of thio relaxers as in the application of sodium hydroxide products:

1. Prepare the patron in the same manner as previously described.
2. Shampoo the hair with a neutral shampoo. (Be careful not to irritate the scalp.)
3. Towel dry the hair, leaving it slightly damp.
4. Apply scalp conditioner to the scalp only.
5. Prepare neutralizer before applying relaxer.
6. Use protective gloves. Apply relaxer as previously described for sodium hydroxide relaxer.
7. The spreading out and testing procedure is the same as that followed for sodium hydroxide products.
8. When the hair has been sufficiently processed, rinse the relaxer out in a three-step process.
   a) Rinse about 50% of the relaxer from the hair with warm water.
   b) Comb the hair smooth and straight (with the remaining relaxer left in the hair); continue combing for about 5 minutes to rearrange the cystine cross-bonds, leaving the hair in a straight position.
   c) Rinse the remaining relaxer thoroughly from the hair with warm water, keeping the hair smooth and straight while rinsing.
9. After the relaxer has been thoroughly rinsed from the hair, apply the neutralizer as follows:
   a) Pour the prepared neutralizer through the hair and catch it in a plastic bowl.
   b) Repour the neutralizer through the hair and catch it again in a plastic bowl. Repeat this process 6-7 times.
   c) Comb the hair smooth and straight to assure complete neutralizing.
   d) Allow the neutralizer to remain in the hair for at least 5 minutes, in order to assure complete neutralization.
   e) Rinse neutralizer from the hair with lukewarm water and towel blot. Style the hair in the usual manner.

Note: Manufacturers may have different procedures for the final steps. Be guided by your instructor.

CAUTION

Because of the fragile condition of the hair, wind the hair on large rollers, without tension.

THIO RETOUCH

Follow all steps for a regular chemical hair relaxing treatment, with the exception of the **relaxer,** which is applied only to the new growth.

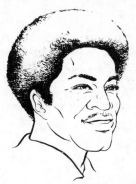
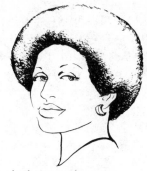

Chemical blowout is the same for both men and women.

CHEMICAL BLOWOUT

To meet the needs of both young and middle-aged salon patrons, great versatility in hairstyling may be achieved with the **chemical blowout.** This technique removes only a small amount of the curl, leaving the hair in a more manageable condition. The chemical blowout serves as a foundation for a variety of hairstyling designs and patterns. A chemical blowout is a combination of chemical hair straightening and hairstyling, which creates a well-groomed style in the Afro-American tradition.

The chemical blowout may be done with either the thio hair relaxer or the sodium hydroxide relaxer. The important consideration with either method is not to over-relax the hair to the point where the blowout process becomes impossible to perform. Usually, when the thio relaxer is used, the hair is shampooed first. When the sodium hydroxide relaxer is used, the hair is shampooed after the hair is relaxed. (Follow manufacturer's or your instructor's directions.)

EQUIPMENT, IMPLEMENTS, AND MATERIALS

The same equipment, implements and materials are used, plus a wide-tooth comb (hair lifter or pick), scissors, clippers, and hand blower.

USING AMMONIUM THIOGLYCOLATE (THIO) FOR CHEMICAL BLOWOUT

PROCEDURE

1. Prepare and drape patron as for a regular hair relaxing treatment.
2. Shampoo hair with a neutral (acid-balanced) shampoo.
3. Towel dry hair, leaving it slightly damp.
4. Apply scalp conditioner to the scalp.
5. Put on protective gloves; apply relaxer in the usual manner.
6. Stop the relaxing procedure by rinsing the relaxer from the hair before it is straightened and while it still shows a wave or curl formation. (Fig. 1)

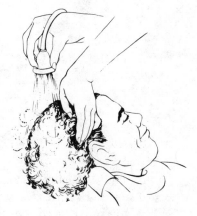

Fig. 1. Rinsing relaxer from the hair.

7. Apply neutralizer.

8. Rinse out neutralizer and towel blot the hair. (Fig. 2)

9. Apply a conditioner to scalp and hair to help restore the natural oils removed by the relaxer.

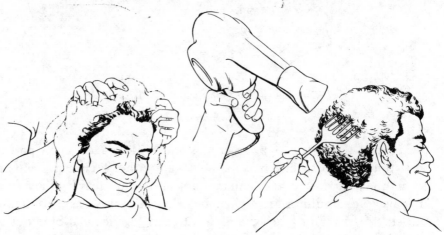

Fig. 2. Towel drying
the hair.

Fig. 3. Hair being lifted with a pick
while being dried.

10. While using an Afro comb (hair lifter or pick) in an upward manner, thoroughly dry the hair with a hand dryer, (Fig. 3). Dry scalp area first towards hair ends. The time permitted for drying depends on the length and thickness of the hair.

11. After the entire head is dried, using the hair lifter and starting at the crown, continue until all the hair has been combed and distributed evenly around the head. (Fig. 4)

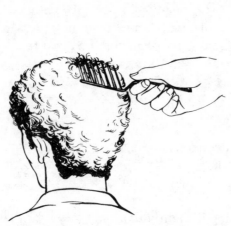

Fig. 4. Distributing hair
with lifter.

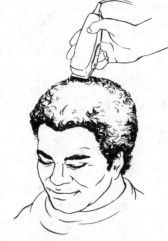

Fig. 5. Shaping hair to
desired style.

12. The dried hair is ready for shaping. Either scissors or clippers may be used. Evenness is very important. Use the shortest hair as a guide for the balance of the head. Visualize the style and length of the hair you have planned for the chemical blowout. (Fig. 5)

13. Start the cutting at the sides. Even out the hair around the head with an electric clipper or scissors while, at the same time, continuing to pick the hair outward from the scalp. The hair must be cut in the direction in which it is to be combed. The object is to achieve a smooth, even cut that is properly contoured. The final cutting should be done only with the scissors, to even out loose or ragged ends only.

14. Outline the hairstyle at the sides, around the ears, and in the nape area, using either the scissors or the clipper.

15. After the hair is cut to the desired style, the finishing touches are applied. Fluff the hair slightly with the lifter, where required, and spray lightly. The lifter or pick is used to improve the smoothness of the style.

CHEMICAL BLOWOUT USING SODIUM HYDROXIDE

Since sodium hydroxide is a very strong chemical that can readily damage the hair, follow manufacturer's directions explicitly.

REVIEW QUESTIONS

CHEMICAL HAIR RELAXING AND CHEMICAL BLOWOUT

1. What is chemical hair relaxing?
2. What are the two types of chemical hair relaxing in general use?
3. Which one of the two types requires pre-shampooing and which one does not?
4. What is the action of a chemical hair relaxer?
5. What is the maximum period of time a sodium hydroxide chemical relaxer should be left on the hair? Why?
6. What chemical compound is required in addition to the chemical relaxing agent?
7. By what other term is neutralizer or stabilizer known?
8. What is the purpose of the base that is applied to the entire scalp and surrounding areas prior to the application of sodium hydroxide relaxer?
9. What hair conditions should prevent treatment with a chemical hair relaxer?
10. What is the purpose of an analysis of the patron's hair prior to applying a chemical relaxer?
11. List four items to consider in a hair analysis.
12. What is the purpose of the patron's record card?
13. Why is it necessary to have the patron sign a release?
14. Why is a scalp examination especially important prior to a chemical hair relaxing treatment?
15. What test should be given the patron before she receives a chemical relaxer treatment?
16. What is the purpose of the strand test in the chemical relaxing procedure?

17. What area of the head is selected for a strand test?
18. After the hair has been treated with a sodium hydroxide relaxer, why should the hair be thoroughly rinsed prior to the application of a shampoo?
19. How should the water be directed when rinsing the chemical relaxer from the hair?
20. What type of shampoo is recommended for hair that has been straightened with a sodium hydroxide relaxer?
21. Why is it important to keep chemically relaxed hair from tangling during a shampoo?
22. Why is the neutralizer necessary in the chemical hair relaxing process?
23. When should the hair be combed after a chemical relaxing treatment?
24. Why should a thermal irons treatment be avoided for 4-6 weeks after a chemical hair relaxing treatment?
25. Why is a scalp and hair conditioner applied after a hair relaxing treatment?
26. Why are large rollers recommended when styling chemically relaxed hair?
27. How is a chemical relaxer retouch given?
28. How is the thio relaxing cream removed from the hair?
29. What is a chemical blowout?
30. How does a chemical blowout differ from a regular chemical hair straightening service?
31. What is the important consideration in giving a chemical blowout?
32. When should the hair be shampooed in a thio relaxing treatment?

Chapter 17

THERMAL HAIR STRAIGHTENING (HAIR PRESSING)

CHAPTER LEARNING OBJECTIVES

The student successfully mastering this chapter will know:

1. *How to recognize and deal with the many differences in hair texture, hair porosity, hair elasticity, and scalp flexibility of patrons who are having their hair pressed.*
2. *The purpose served by hair pressing.*
3. *The products required for successful hair pressing.*
4. *The procedures involved in both soft pressing and hard pressing.*
5. *The safety precautions that must be observed in hair pressing.*
6. *How to handle the special problems that arise in hair pressing.*

Thermal hair straightening (also known as **hair pressing**) is a profitable service and is popular in the beauty salon. When properly done, hair pressing temporarily straightens over-curly or kinky hair. (Permanent hair straightening is covered in the chapter on **Chemical Hair Relaxing.**)

Hair pressing prepares the hair for additional services, such as thermal roller curling and croquignole thermal curling. A good hair pressing is not harmful to the hair, but leaves it in a natural and lustrous condition.

There are two basic methods of hair pressing:

1. **Soft press,** accomplished with a thermal pressing comb.
2. **Hard press,** accomplished with thermal irons over the comb press. A hard press also may be accomplished by a **double comb press.**

CHARACTERISTICS OF HAIR AND SCALP

It is important that the cosmetologist be able to recognize the individual differences in hair texture, hair porosity, hair elasticity, and scalp flexibility. Guided by these observations, the cosmetologist can best determine the right temperature for the pressing comb and what degree of pressure the hair and scalp can tolerate without causing breakage, hair loss, or possible burning of the hair or scalp.

Hair texture refers to the degree of coarseness or fineness of the hair. Variations in individual hair texture are traceable to the following factors:

1. **Diameter of the hair** (coarse, medium, or fine).
   Coarse hair has the greatest diameter. Fine or wooly hair has the smallest diameter.
2. **Feel of the hair** (wiry, soft, silky, or wooly).

The patron's hair texture also depends on whether the hair is dry, oily, grey, tinted, or lightened, and the amount of curliness it has. Careful observation and questioning the patron will help to detect these characteristics.

Coarse, over-curly hair has qualities that make it difficult to press. Coarse hair has the greatest diameter, and during the pressing process it can tolerate more heat and pressure than medium or fine, wooly hair. A microscopic analysis of coarse hair reveals that it consists of the following layers: the cuticle, the cortex, and the medulla.

Medium, curly hair is the normal type of hair cosmetologists deal with in the beauty salon. No special problem is presented by this type of hair, and it is the least resistant to hair pressing. It contains the same layers as coarse, curly hair, but to a lesser degree.

Fine, wooly hair requires special care. To avoid hair breakage, less heat and pressure should be applied than for other hair textures. Only two layers, the cortex and the cuticle, are usually present in fine hair.

Wiry, curly hair may be coarse, medium, or fine. It is recognized by its stiff, hard, glassy feeling. Because of the compact construction of the cuticle cells, it is very resistant to hair pressing, requiring more heat and pressure than other types of hair.

Elasticity is the ability of the hair to stretch and return to its normal length without breaking. Normal hair has its limitations as to the amount of pull or pressure it can withstand. Under normal conditions, the hair can be safely stretched about one-fifth its length.

Hair that has normal elasticity presents a healthy and lustrous appearance. A deficiency in the elasticity of hair causes it to become lifeless and limp. Very little elasticity is left in hair that has been abused by lightening or tinting services. Therefore, hair of this type needs special care during hair pressing.

Hair porosity is the ability of the hair to absorb moisture regardless of whether it is coarse, medium, or fine. After a hair pressing treatment, hair with good porosity returns to its normal curly appearance when it comes into contact with water or moisture.

Scalp. The condition of the patron's scalp may be classified as normal, tight, or flexible.

If the **scalp is normal,** proceed with an analysis of the texture and elasticity of the hair.

If the **scalp is tight** and the hair coarse, to avoid injury to the scalp, press the hair in the direction in which it grows.

The main difficulty with a **flexible scalp** is that the cosmetologist may not apply enough pressure to press the hair satisfactorily.

EXAMINATION OF HAIR AND SCALP

Before the cosmetologist undertakes to press the patron's hair, she should carefully examine the condition of the hair and scalp in order to evaluate the patron's particular needs.

Note: Under no circumstances should hair pressing be given to a patron who has a scalp abrasion, a contagious scalp condition, or a scalp injury.

After examining the patron's hair and scalp, if they are not normal, the cosmetologist may give appropriate advice concerning preliminary corrective treatments. If the hair shows signs of neglect or abuse that was caused by faulty pressing, lightening, or tinting, she should recommend a series of conditioning treatments. Failure to correct dry and brittle hair may result in hair breakage during hair pressing. **Burnt hair strands cannot be conditioned.**

A careful analysis of the patron's hair and scalp should cover the following points:

1. Form of hair (curly or over-curly).
2. Length of hair (long, medium, or short).
3. Texture of hair (coarse, medium, fine, or very fine).
4. Feel of hair (wiry, soft, or silky).
5. Elasticity of hair (normal or poor).
6. Shade of hair (natural, faded, streaked, or grey).
7. Condition of hair (normal, brittle, dry, oily, or damaged).
8. Condition of scalp (normal, flexible, or tight).

RECORD CARD

The patron's hair and scalp record card is useful for present and future hair pressing treatments. It also is advisable to question the patron about any lightener, tint, color restorer (metallic), or other chemical treatment that was used on her hair. This information can be helpful in achieving good hair pressing results.

A record card should include the following:

1. Texture of hair: ☐ Coarse ☐ Medium ☐ Fine ☐ Very fine
2. Condition of hair: ☐ Normal ☐ Dry and brittle ☐ Damaged ☐ Oily
3. History: Chemical process used ☐ Yes ☐ No; Color restorer (metallic) ☐ Yes ☐ No; Lighteners or tints ☐ Yes ☐ No
4. Treatment: ☐ Soft press ☐ Hard press ☐ Roller curls
5. Heat: ☐ High ☐ Medium ☐ Low
6. Conditioning: ☐ Yes ☐ No Name of product . . . .
7. Date . . . . Price . . . .

CONDITIONING TREATMENTS

Effective **conditioning treatments** require the application of special cosmetic preparations to the hair and scalp, thorough brushing, and scalp massage. The use of an infra-red lamp is optional, depending on the type of treatment being given. These treatments usually help get better results from hair pressing.

A **tight scalp** can be rendered more flexible by the systematic use of scalp massage, hair brushing, and direct high-frequency current. The patron will benefit by a better circulation of blood to the scalp.

PRESSING COMBS

There are two types of pressing combs: regular and electric.

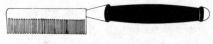

Regular pressing comb.

They are both constructed of either good quality steel or brass. The handle is usually made of wood, which does not readily absorb heat.

Teeth. The space between the teeth of the comb varies with the size and style of the comb. Some combs have more space between the teeth, while others have less.

Size. Pressing combs vary in size; some are short, while others are long.

HEATING COMB

Heat. Depending on their composition, combs vary in their ability to accept and retain heat.

Stoves. Regular pressing combs may be heated on gas stoves or electric heaters.

While the comb is being heated, its teeth should face upward and the handle should be kept away from the fire. After heating the comb to the proper temperature, test it on a piece of light paper. If the paper becomes scorched, allow the comb to cool slightly before applying it to the hair.

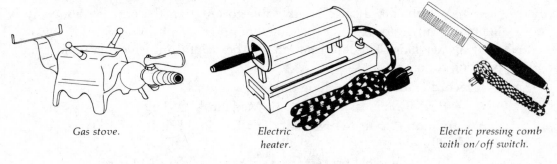

Gas stove.   *Electric heater.*   *Electric pressing comb with on/off switch.*

Electric pressing combs are now available in two forms: one comes with an ON and OFF switch; the other is equipped with a thermostat, which has a control switch that indicates high or low degrees of heat.

CLEANING COMB

The pressing comb will perform more efficiently if it is kept clean and free of carbon.

Wipe the comb clean of loose hair, grease, and dust before and after each use. The intense heat will keep the comb sterile when all loose hair or clinging dirt is removed.

Remove the carbon from the comb by rubbing its outside surface and between its teeth with any one of the following: emery board, fine steel wool pad, or fine sandpaper.

After using any one of these cleaning methods, immerse the metal portion of the comb in a hot soda solution for about one hour; then rinse and dry. The metal will acquire a smooth and shiny appearance.

PRESSING OIL OR CREAM

The application of pressing oil or cream prior to a hair pressing treatment helps prepare the hair for pressing. Both these products have the following beneficial effects:

1. They make hair softer.
2. They prepare and condition hair for pressing.
3. They help prevent hair from burning or scorching.
4. They help prevent hair breakage.
5. They help condition the hair after pressing.
6. They add sheen to pressed hair.

HAIR SECTIONING

Divide the head into four main sections. Then sub-divide these sections into 1-1½" (2.5-3.75 cm) partings. the size of sub-sections depends on the texture and density of the hair.

1. For medium textured hair of average density, use sub-sections of average size.
2. For coarse hair with greater density, use smaller sections in order to assure complete heat penetration and effectiveness.
3. For thin or fine hair with sparse density, use larger sections.

SOFT PRESSING PROCEDURE FOR NORMAL CURLY HAIR

(The following procedure is one of several ways to give a hair pressing treatment and may be changed to meet your instructor's method.)

EQUIPMENT, IMPLEMENTS, AND MATERIALS

Pressing comb	Hairbrush and comb	Spatula
Heating appliance	Brilliantine or pomade	Neck strips
(gas or electric heater)	Shampoo	Thermal irons
Pressing oil	Towels and cape	

PREPARATION

1. Select and arrange required materials.
2. Wash and sanitize hands.
3. Drape patron.
4. Shampoo, rinse, and towel dry patron's hair.
5. Apply pressing oil or cream. (**Note:** *Some cosmetologists prefer to apply pressing oil or cream to the hair after it has been completely dried.*)
6. Dry hair thoroughly.
7. Comb and divide hair into four main sections. Pin up four sections.
8. Place pressing comb in heater.

PROCEDURE

1. Unpin one hair section at a time and sub-divide into small hair sections. Beginning at the right side of the head, work from the front towards the back. (Some cosmetologists prefer to start at the back of the head and work towards the front.)

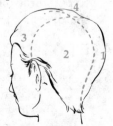

Hair properly sectioned into quarters.

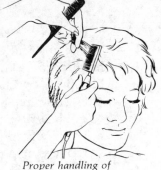

Proper handling of pressing comb.

2. If necessary, apply pressing oil evenly and sparingly over the small hair sections.
3. Test the temperature of the heated pressing comb.
4. Lift the end of a small hair section with the index finger and thumb of the left hand and hold it upward away from the scalp.
5. Hold the pressing comb in the right hand and insert the teeth of the comb into the top side of the hair section.
6. Draw out the pressing comb slightly and make a quick turn so that the hair strand wraps itself partly around the comb. **The back rod of the comb actually does the pressing.**
7. Press the comb slowly through the hair strand until the ends of the hair pass through the teeth of the comb.
8. Press twice on top, reverse the comb, and press once on the bottom side.
9. Bring each completed hair section over to the opposite side of the head.
10. Continue steps 4 to 9 on both sections of the right side of the head; then begin at the back of the left side and work towards the front.

COMPLETION

1. Apply a little brilliantine or pomade to the hair near the scalp and brush it through the hair.
2. If desired, thermal roller or croquignole curling may be given at this time. (The procedures and techniques are found in the chapter on **Thermal Waving, Curling and Blow-Dry Styling.)**
3. Style and comb the hair according to the patron's wishes.
4. Place supplies in their proper places.
5. Sanitize implements and clean equipment.

HARD PRESS

A hard press is recommended when the results of a soft comb press are not satisfactory. The entire comb press procedure is repeated. Pressing oil may be added to hair strands only, if necessary.

A hard press is also known as a **double comb press.**

TOUCH-UPS

Touch-ups are sometimes necessary when the hair regains its curliness due to perspiration, dampness, or other conditions. The process is the same as for the pressing treatment, with the shampoo omitted.

SAFETY PRECAUTIONS

The injuries that may occur in hair pressing are of two types:
1. **Direct injuries** are the immediate results of hair pressing and cause physical damage, such as:
   a) Burnt hair that breaks off.

b) Burnt scalp that causes either temporary or permanent loss of hair.

c) Burns on ears and neck that form scars.

2. **Indirect injuries** are not immediately evident but may subsequently cause physical damage, such as:

a) Skin rash, if the patron is allergic to pressing oil.

b) Progressive breaking and shortening of the hair because of too frequent hair pressings.

In case of burnt scalp, immediately apply 1% gentian violet jelly directly to the burn.

To avoid damage, the hair should not be pressed more than necessary. Good judgment should be used, with consideration always given to the texture of the hair and condition of scalp. The patron's safety is assured only when the cosmetologist observes every precaution and is especially careful during the actual hair pressing. The cosmetologist should avoid using the following:

1. Excessive heat or pressure on the hair and scalp.

2. Too much pressing oil on the hair.

3. Perfumed pressing oil near the scalp if the patron is allergic to it.

RELEASE STATEMENT

A release statement is used for hair pressing, permanent waving, hair tinting, or any other service that may require the cosmetologist's release from responsibility for accidents or damages.

SAMPLE RELEASE

I fully understand that the .... treatment which I have requested, while harmless to normal hair, may be harmful to mine because of its condition as a result of ....

Therefore, I hereby assume all responsibility and risk for any damage that may result, directly or indirectly, from this requested service.

Signature.....................................

Witness..   Date..............

REMINDERS AND HINTS ON SOFT PRESSING

1. Keep the comb clean and free from carbon at all times.

2. Avoid overheating the pressing comb.

3. Test the temperature of the heated comb before applying it to the hair.

4. Adjust the temperature of the pressing comb to the texture and condition of the patron's hair.

5. Use heated comb carefully to avoid burning the skin, scalp, or hair.

6. Prevent the smoking or burning of hair during the pressing treatment by:

a) Drying the hair completely after it is shampooed.

b) Avoiding excessive application of pressing oil over the hair.

7. Use a moderately warm comb to press short hair on the temples and back of the neck.

SPECIAL PROBLEMS

PRESSING FINE HAIR

When pressing fine, wooly hair, follow the same procedure as for normal hair, being careful not to use a hot pressing comb or too much pressure. To avoid hair breakage, give less pressure to the hair near the ends. After completely pressing the hair, style it.

PRESSING SHORT, FINE HAIR

When pressing short, fine hair, extra care must be taken at the hairline. Where the hair is extra short, the pressing comb should not be too hot because the hair is fine and will burn easily; a hot comb also can cause accidental burns, which are very painful and may cause scars. In the event of an accidental burn, immediately apply 1% gentian violet jelly to the burn.

PRESSING COARSE HAIR

In pressing coarse hair, care must be taken that enough pressure is given so that the hair will remain in a straightened condition.

PRESSING TINTED, LIGHTENED, OR GREY HAIR

Tinted, lightened, or grey hair require special care in hair pressing.

Lightened or **tinted hair** may require conditioning treatments, depending on the extent to which it has been damaged. To obtain good results, use a moderately heated pressing comb applied with light pressure.

Avoid **excessive heat** on **grey, tinted,** or **lightened hair,** as the heat may discolor the hair.

REVIEW QUESTIONS

THERMAL HAIR STRAIGHTENING (HAIR PRESSING)

1. What is accomplished by hair pressing?
2. What is a soft press?
3. What is a hard press?
4. Name the layers of coarse hair, starting from the outer layer.
5. What type of hair requires more heat and pressure than other types of hair?
6. What kind of hair has poor elasticity?
7. When should the hair not be pressed?
8. What eight points should the cosmetologist study when analyzing the patron's hair and scalp?
9. Which procedure is followed in a conditioning treatment for the hair and scalp?
10. What supplies are needed for soft hair pressing?
11. What are the main steps in pressing the hair?
12. What important steps follow the hair pressing treatment?
13. What injuries may occur in hair pressing?
14. How is an accidental scalp burn treated?

Chapter 18

THERMAL WAVING, CURLING, AND BLOW-DRY STYLING

CHAPTER LEARNING OBJECTIVES

The student successfully mastering this chapter will know:
1. *The functions of thermal waving and curling in modern hairstyling.*
2. *The various types of thermal curling.*
3. *The parts of thermal irons and how to care for them.*
4. *How to hold and manipulate thermal irons.*
5. *The manipulative techniques in thermal curling and waving.*
6. *The techniques of thermal curling short, medium, and long hair.*
7. *The technique of thermal spiral curling.*
8. *Why blow-dry curling and waving has special appeal to hairstylists and patrons.*
9. *The equipment and supplies needed for blow-dry styling.*
10. *The basic steps for blow-dry curling with a brush.*
11. *The basic steps for blow-dry waving with a comb.*

THERMAL WAVING AND CURLING

The art and technique of using thermal irons for waving and curling were developed in 1875 by a Frenchman, Marcel Grateau. In recognition of his contribution to hairstyling, thermal waving is still known as **marcel waving.**

Thermal waving and **curling** is the art of waving and curling straight or pressed hair with thermal irons, either electrically heated or stove heated, by using special manipulative techniques. Modern, up-to-date implements have contributed to the continued success of these methods of waving and curling hair.

THERMAL IRONS

Thermal irons come in a variety of styles, sizes, and weights. Sizes range from small to jumbo. They come in three different classifications:
1. Conventional (regular) stove heated.
2. Electric self-heated.
3. Electric self-heated, vaporizing.

CAUTION

Electric vaporizing thermal irons must not be used on pressed hair because the moisture from the irons could cause the hair to revert to its natural over-curly form.

Thermal irons must not be used on chemically treated hair; to do so could result in severe hair breakage.

The beginning student should become adept in the use of the conventional type irons before using electric irons. (Always be guided by your instructor.)

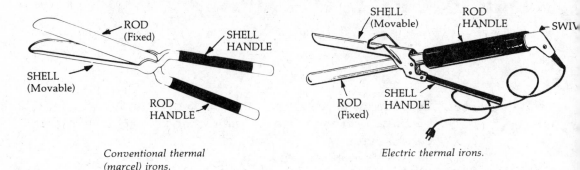

Conventional thermal
(marcel) irons.

Electric thermal irons.

Thermal irons are an important implement in hairstyling. They provide an even heat which may be completely controlled by the cosmetologist. Whether electric irons or stove-heated irons are used, the manipulative techniques are basically the same.

The irons must be made of the best quality steel so that they hold an even temperature during the waving and curling process. The styling portion of the irons are composed of two parts: the rod (prong) and the shell (groove or bowl).

1. The **rod** is a perfectly round solid steel bar.
2. The **shell** is perfectly round with the inside grooved so that the rod can rest in it when the irons are closed.

The edge of the shell nearest the cosmetologist is called the **inner edge;** the one farthest from the cosmetologist is called the **outer edge.**

TEMPERATURE OF THERMAL IRONS

There is no set temperature used for the irons when thermal curling and waving the hair. It depends on the texture of the hair, whether it is fine or coarse, or whether it has been lightened or tinted. Hair that has been lightened or tinted (also white hair) should be curled and waved with lukewarm irons. Coarse hair, as a rule, can stand more heat than fine hair.

TESTING OF THERMAL IRONS

After heating the irons to the desired temperature, test them on a piece of tissue paper. Clamp the heated irons over the tissue and hold for five seconds. If the paper scorches or turns brown, the irons are too hot. Let them cool somewhat before using. It should be noted that fine, lightened, or badly damaged hair can withstand less heat than normal hair.

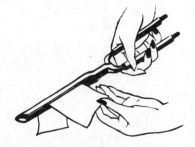

Testing the heat of
thermal irons.

CARE OF THERMAL IRONS

Thermal irons should be kept clean and free from rust and carbon. To remove dirt or grease, wash the irons in a soap solution containing a few drops of ammonia. This cuts the oil and grease that usually adhere to the irons. Fine sandpaper, or steel wool with a little oil, helps to remove rust and carbon. They also polish the irons. Oil the joint of the irons, to permit greater facility in movement.

Tempering. New thermal irons are tempered at the factory in order to hold heat uniformly.

Overheated irons usually lose their temper, and, in most cases, are ruined.

HOLDING THE THERMAL IRONS

Hold the irons in a position that is comfortable and permits complete control. Grasp the handles of the irons in the right hand, far enough away from the joint to avoid the heat. Place the three middle fingers on the back of the lower handle, the little finger in front of the lower handle, and the thumb in front of the upper handle.

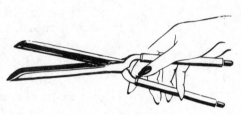

Holding and opening the irons.

COMB USED WITH THERMAL IRONS

The comb should be about 7" (17.5 cm) long, made of hard rubber or another non-flammable substance, and should have fine teeth; fine teeth hold the hair more firmly than coarse teeth.

HOLDING THE COMB

Hold the comb between the thumb and all four fingers of the left hand, with the index finger resting on the backbone of the comb for better control and one end of the comb resting against the outer edge of the palm. This position assures a strong hold and a firm movement.

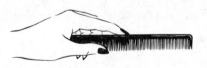

Holding the comb.

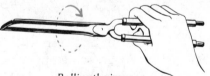

Rolling the irons.

PRACTICING WITH COLD THERMAL IRONS

Since thermal curling and waving is a somewhat difficult operation and uses heated irons, practice with cold irons on a mannequin or hairpiece pinned to a block until the technique is thoroughly mastered.

ROLLING THE THERMAL IRONS

Practice rolling the thermal irons in the hand, first forward, then backward. The rolling movement should be done without any sway or motion in the arm; only the fingers are used to roll the handles in either direction.

(Turn irons away from cosmetologist.)

EXERCISE 1

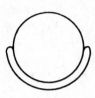 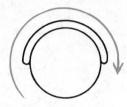 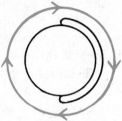

1. Starting position.   *2. One-half turn.*   *3. Full turn.*

EXERCISE 2

1. Insert hair in irons with rod on top (groove facing upward).
2. Turn irons forward for one-half turn (away from you).
3. Turn irons back to starting position.
4. Open irons slightly and slide down 1" (2.5 cm), then clamp.
5. Turn irons backward for full turn (toward you).
6. Turn irons forward to starting position.
7. Release.

THERMAL WAVING with Conventional Thermal (Marcel) Irons

PROCEDURE FOR LEFT-GOING WAVE

Comb the hair thoroughly, following its directional growth. The natural growth will determine whether or not the first wave to be formed will be a

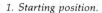

left-going wave or a right-going wave. The procedure given here is for a left-going wave.

Before the wave is begun, comb the hair in a semi-shaping.

1. With the comb, pick up a strand of hair about 2" (5 cm) in width. Insert the irons in the hair with the groove facing upward. (Fig. 1)

One-quarter turn.

2. Close irons and turn them about one-quarter turn forward (away from you). At the same time, draw the hair with the irons about ¼" (.625 cm) to the left, and direct the hair ¼" (.625 cm) to the right with the comb. (Fig. 2)

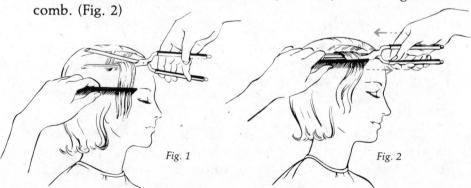

Fig. 1   *Fig. 2*

3. Roll the irons one full turn forward (away from you). (Fig. 3)

   (In doing this, keep the hair uniform with the comb. You will find that the hair has rolled on a slight slant on the prong of the irons.)

   Keep position No. 3 for a few seconds in order to allow the hair to become sufficiently heated throughout.

4. Reverse movement No. 3 by simply unrolling the hair from the irons, bringing them back into their first resting position. (Fig. 4)

   (When this movement is completed, you will find the comb resting somewhat away from the irons.)

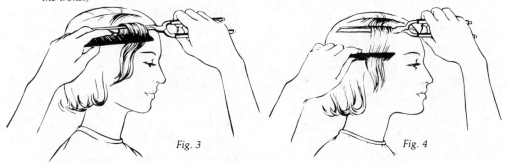

Fig. 3   Fig. 4

5. Open the irons with the little finger and place them just below the ridge, or crest, by swinging the rod of the irons toward you and then closing them. (Fig. 5)

   (The outer edge of the groove should be directly underneath the ridge just produced by the inner ridge.)

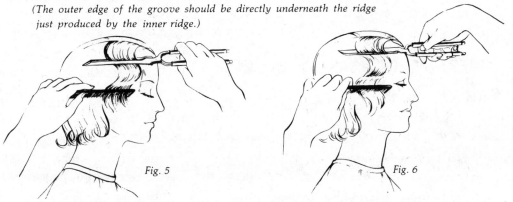

Fig. 5   Fig. 6

6. Keep the irons perfectly still and direct the hair with the comb upward about 1" (2.5 cm), thus forming the hair into a half circle. (Fig. 6)

   (You must remember that, in order to perform movement No. 6 properly, you do not move the comb from the position explained in the footnote of movement No. 5.)

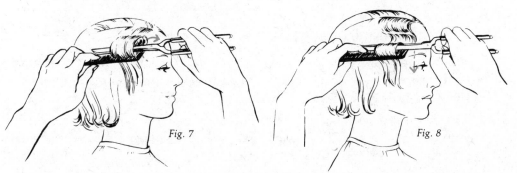

Fig. 7   Fig. 8

7. Without opening the irons, roll them one-half turn forward (from you). (Fig. 7)

   (In this movement, keep the comb perfectly still and unchanged.)

8. Slide the irons down about 1″ (2.5 cm). (Fig. 8)

   (This movement is done by opening the irons slightly [loose grip] and then sliding them down the strand of hair.)

RIGHT-GOING WAVE

After completing movement No. 8, you will find the irons and comb in a position to make the second ridge and the beginning of the right-going wave. For a right-going wave, however, the hair is directed opposite to that of a left-going wave.

JOINING OR MATCHING THE WAVES

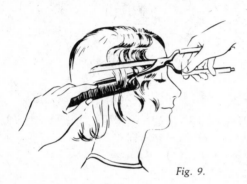

Fig. 9.

After completely waving one strand of hair, wave the next strand to match. While picking up the unwaved hair in the comb, include a small section of the waved strand as a guide to the formation of the new wave. (Fig. 9)

In waving the second strand of hair, be sure that the comb and irons movements are the same as in the first strand of hair; otherwise, the waves will not match.

THERMAL CURLING with Electric Thermal Irons

Thermal curling is the art of creating curls in the hair with the aid of thermal irons and a comb. Since thermal curling requires no setting creams or lotions, it may be used to great advantage for the following:

1. **Straight hair**—permits quick styling. Thermal curling eliminates working with wet hair, use of rollers, and a long hair drying process.

2. **Pressed hair**—permits styling the hair without the danger of its reverting to its former over-curly condition. Thermal curling prepares the hair for any desired style.

3. **Wigs** and **hairpieces**—presents a quick and effective method for their styling.

CURLING IRONS MANIPULATIONS

The following is a series of basic manipulative movements for using heated curling irons. Most other curling irons movements are adaptations or derivations of these basic movements.

The method of holding the irons is a matter of personal preference. The technique used should be the one that gives the cosmetologist the greatest ease, comfort, and facility of movement.

The following illustrations show a grip with only the little finger used for opening the clamp. Some cosmetologists prefer to use the little finger plus the ring finger for this purpose. (See Fig. 8.) Either method is correct.

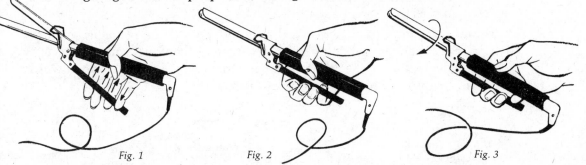

Fig. 1   Fig. 2   Fig. 3

Fig. 1—Use the little finger to open the clamp.

Fig. 2—Use three middle fingers to close the clamp and manipulate irons.

Fig. 3—Shift the thumb to aid in turning and manipulating the irons.

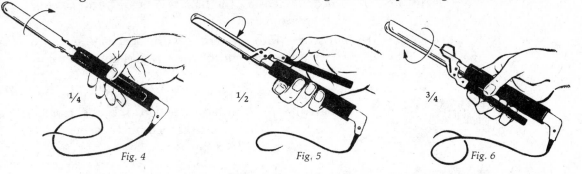

¼   ½   ¾

Fig. 4   Fig. 5   Fig. 6

Fig. 4—Close the clamp and make a one-quarter turn of the irons in a downward direction. A swivel at the base of the shaft handle permits the irons to turn without twisting the electric cord.

Fig. 5—The irons have now made a one-half downward turn and the thumb has been used to ease open the clamp and relax the tension on the hair.

Fig. 6—Use the thumb to continue to turn the irons to three-quarters of a complete turn.

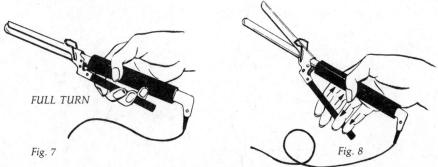

FULL TURN

Fig. 7   Fig. 8

Fig. 7—The irons have made a full turn, and the fingers have been brought back to their original position.

Fig. 8—An alternate method of holding the irons is to use the little finger and the ring finger to open the clamp.

Practice in manipulating the curling irons is recommended to develop proficiency in their use. The following four exercises are designed to help achieve an effective use of the irons.

1. Since it is important to develop a smooth rotating movement, practice turning the irons while opening and closing them at regular intervals. Practice rotating the irons in both directions. Examples: downward (toward you), and upward (away from you). (Fig. 1)

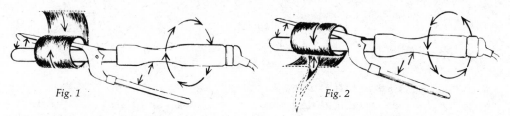

Fig. 1   *Fig. 2*

2. To prevent binding, practice releasing the hair by opening and closing the irons in a quick clicking movement.

3. Practice guiding the hair strand into the center of the curl as you rotate the irons. This exercise results in the end of the strand being firmly in the center of the curl. (Fig. 2)

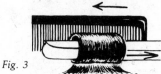

Fig. 3

4. Practice removing the curl from the irons by drawing the comb to the left and the rod to the right. (Fig. 3) Use the comb to protect the patron's scalp from burns.

THERMAL IRONS CURLING METHODS

Today's thermal irons curling methods have improved over the older techniques. The following methods may be changed to conform with your instructor's procedures, which are equally correct:

1. Short hair.
2. Medium length hair.
3. Long hair.
4. Other types of curls.

PREPARATION

1. Comb the hair thoroughly, removing all tangles.
2. Divide head into five sections.
   a) First section, about 2½" (6.25 cm) wide, extends from center of forehead to nape.
   b) Divide two side panels in half, from top parting to neck, to provide four additional sections.
3. Heat thermal irons (large or jumbo size).
4. Sub-divide sections into sub-sections — each approximately ¾ by 2½" (1.875 by 6.25 cm) wide.

(Same procedure is followed for electric irons and stove heated irons.)

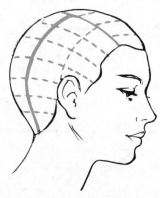

Hair sectioned and sub-divided.

CURLING SHORT HAIR

The base of each curl is formed by sectioning and parting to conform with the size of the curl desired. It is important to consider hair length, density, and texture. The base is usually about 1½-2" (3.75-5 cm) in width and approximately ½" (1.25 cm) in depth.

After sectioning off the base, comb the hair smooth and straight out from the scalp. The hair must be combed smooth in order that the heat and tension are the same for all hair in the section. Loose hairs may result in an uneven and ragged curl.

1. After the irons have been heated to the desired temperature, pick up a strand of hair and comb it up and smooth. With the groove on top, insert the irons about 1" (2.5 cm) from the scalp and hold for a few seconds to form a base. (Fig. 1)

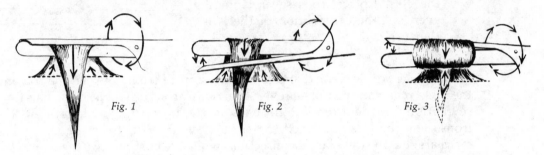

Fig. 1   Fig. 2   Fig. 3

2. Hold the ends of the hair strand with the thumb and two fingers of the left hand, using a medium degree of tension. Turn the irons downward (toward you) with the right hand. (Fig. 2)
3. Open and close the irons rapidly as you turn, to prevent binding. Guide the ends of the strand into the center of the curl as you rotate the irons. (Fig. 3)
4. The result of this procedure will be a smooth, finished curl, with the ends firmly fixed in the center. Remove the curl from the irons. (Fig. 4)

Fig. 4

CURLING MEDIUM LENGTH HAIR

(Using One Loop or Figure 6)

Section and form the base of the curl as previously described.

1. Insert the hair into the open irons at the scalp. Pull the hair over the rod in the direction of the curl and close the shell. Hold irons in this position for about five seconds to heat the hair, and then slide irons up to 1" (2.5 cm) from the scalp. The shell must be on top. (Fig. 1)
2. Turn irons downward ½ revolution; pull the end of the strand over the rod to the left and direct the strand toward the center of the curl. (Fig. 2)

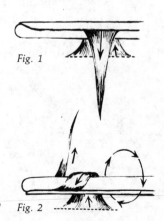

Fig. 1

Fig. 2

3. Complete the revolution of the irons, and continue directing the ends toward the center. (Fig. 3)

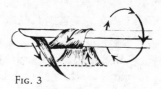

FIG. 3

4. Make another complete revolution of the irons. The entire strand has now been curled with the exception of the ends. Enlarge the curl by opening the shell. Insert the ends of the curl into the opening created between the shell and the rod. (Fig. 4)

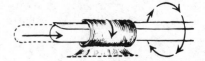

Fig. 4

5. Close the shell and slide irons toward the handles. This technique will move the ends of the strand into the center of the curl. Rotate irons several times, to even out the distribution of the hair in the curl. (Fig. 5)

(During the curling process, use the comb to protect the patron's scalp from burns.)

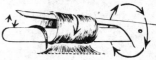

Fig. 5

When the curl is formed and the ends are freed from between the rod and the shell, make one complete revolution of the irons inside the curl. This final revolution is made to smooth the ends and to loosen the hair away from the irons. The comb is then used to help remove the curl from the irons. The irons are drawn slowly in one direction, while the comb draws the hair in the opposite direction. In this way the curl is removed from the irons.

CURLING LONG HAIR

(Using Two Loops or Figure 8)

Section and form the base of the curl as previously described.

1. Insert the hair into the open irons about 1" (2.5 cm) from the scalp. Pull the hair over the rod in the direction in which the curl is to move and close the shell. Hold irons in this position for about five seconds, in order to heat the hair. Hold the strand of hair with a medium degree of tension. (Fig. 1)

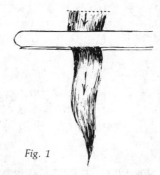

Fig. 1

2. Roll irons under. Click and roll the irons until the groove is facing you. (Fig. 2)

3. With the left hand, pick up the ends of the hair. (Fig. 3)

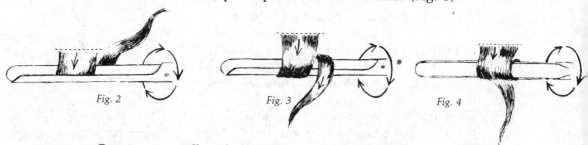

Fig. 2   Fig. 3   Fig. 4

4. Continue to roll and click the irons, keeping them the same distance from the scalp. (Fig. 4)

5 Draw the hair strand toward the point of the irons. (Fig. 5)

6. Draw the strand a little to the right, and, at the same time, push the irons slightly to the left. (Fig. 6)

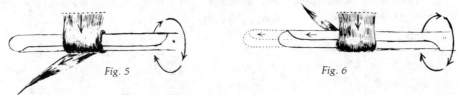

Fig. 5   Fig. 6

7. By pushing irons forward and pushing the hair with the left hand, you form two loops around the closed irons, with the ends of the strand extending out between the loops. (Fig. 7)

8. Roll and click irons under until the ends of the hair disappear. (Fig. 8)

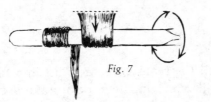
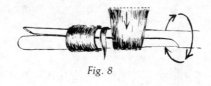

Fig. 7   Fig. 8

9. Rotate irons several times to even out the distribution of the hair in the curl, and to facilitate the movement of the curl off the irons.

OTHER TYPES OF CURLS

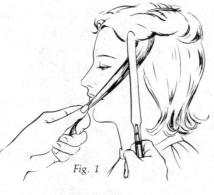

Fig. 1

Spiral curls are hanging curls that are suitable for long hairstyles.

Part the hair into as many sections as there will be curls and comb smooth. Insert the irons at an angle, with the bowl (groove) on top near the base of the strand, and rotate irons until all the hair is wound. Hold the curl in this position for a few seconds, and remove the irons in the usual manner.

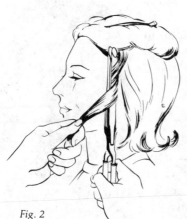
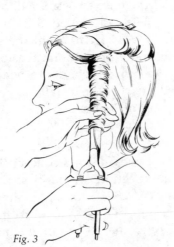
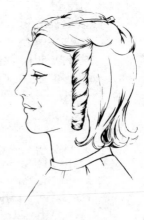

Fig. 2   Fig. 3   Fig. 4

End curls can be used to give a finished appearance to hair ends. Long, medium length, or short hair may be styled with end curls. The hair ends can be turned under or over, as desired.

The position of the curling irons and the direction of their movements will determine whether the end curls will turn under or over.

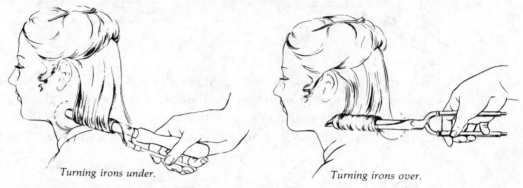

Turning irons under.   *Turning irons over.*

VOLUME THERMAL IRON CURLS

Volume thermal iron curls are used to create volume or lift in a finished hairstyle. The degree of lift desired will determine the type of volume curls to be used.

VOLUME BASE CURLS

Volume base curls provide maximum lift or volume, since the curl is placed very high on its base.

Section off the base in the manner previously described. Hold the curl strand up at a 135° (2.36 rad.) angle. Slide irons over the strand about ½″ (1.25 cm) from the scalp. Wrap the strand over the rod with medium tension. Maintain this position for approximately five seconds, to heat the strand and set the base. Roll the curl in the usual manner, and firmly place it **forward and high on its base.**

FULL BASE CURLS

The full base curl provides a strong curl with full volume. Section off the base as described. Hold the hair strand up at a 125° (2.18 rad.) angle. Slide irons over the hair strand about ½″ (1.25 cm) from the scalp. Wrap the strand over the rod with medium tension. Maintain this position for about five seconds, to heat strand and set the base. Roll the curl in the usual manner, and place it firmly in the **center of its base.**

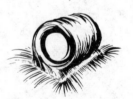

Full base.

HALF BASE CURLS

The half base curl provides a strong curl with moderate lift or volume. Section off the base as described. Hold the hair at a 90° (1.57 rad.) angle. Slide irons over the hair strand about ½″ (1.25 cm) from the scalp. Wrap the strand over the rod with medium tension.

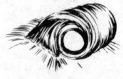

One-half off base.

Maintain this position for about five seconds, to heat strand and set the base. Roll the curl in the usual manner, and place it **half off its base.**

OFF BASE CURLS

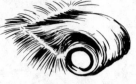

Off base.

The off base curl provides a strong curl with only slight lift or volume. Section off the base as described. Hold the hair at a 70° (1.22 rad.) angle. Slide irons over the hair strand about ½" (1.25 cm) from the scalp. Wrap the strand over the rod with medium tension. Maintain this position for about five seconds, to heat strand and set the base. Roll the curl in the usual manner, and place it **completely off its base.**

HELPFUL HINTS ON THERMAL CURL STYLING

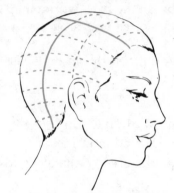

Hair sectioned and sub-divided.

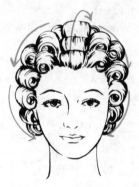

Front view.

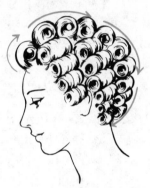

Side view.

Head completely curled with thermal roller curls, also called "style" curls.

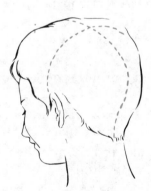

Hair sectioned in quarters.

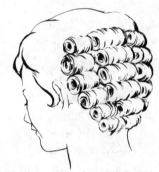

Back of head completely curled.

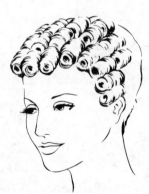

Top and sides of head completely curled.

ARRANGING THE HAIR IN A SUITABLE HAIRSTYLE

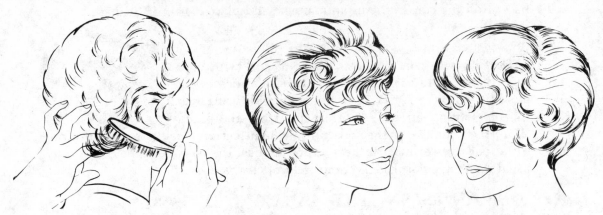

To style the hair into a suitable hairstyle, brush the hair, working up from the neckline. Push the waves and curls into place as you progress over the entire head.

If the hairstyle is to be finished with curls, do the bottom curls last.

SAFETY MEASURES

1. Keep thermal irons clean, and the joint oiled.
2. Use thermal irons only after receiving instruction in their use.
3. Do not overheat the irons, as this may cause the metal to lose its temper.
4. Test the temperature of the irons on tissue paper before placing them on the hair. This will prevent the hair from being burned. Do not inhale the fumes of the irons as they are injurious to the lungs.
5. Do not place the hot irons near the face to test for temperature; a burn of the face may result.
6. Hot irons should not be cooled by twirling them, as they may slip from the hand and become damaged or cause injury.
7. Handle thermal irons carefully, to avoid burning yourself or the patron.
8. Place hot irons in a safe place to cool. Do not leave them where someone may accidentally come in contact with them and be burned.
9. When heating the irons, do not place handles too close to the heater, as the hand may be burned when removing the irons.
10. Make sure the irons are properly balanced in the heater, or they may fall and be damaged or injure someone.
11. Use only hard rubber or non-flammable combs. Celluloid combs must not be used in thermal curling; they are flammable.
12. Do not use metal combs; they may become hot and burn the scalp.
13. Do not use combs with broken teeth. They may break or split the hair, or injure the scalp.
14. Place comb between scalp and thermal irons when curling or waving hair, to prevent burning the scalp.

15. To insure a good thermal curl or wave, clean the hair.
16. If the hair is thick and bulky, thin and taper it first.
17. Never use hot pressing or thermal irons on lightened or tinted hair.
18. Do not allow the hair ends to protrude over the irons; to do so will cause fishhooks, or may cause damage to the hair ends.
19. A first aid kit must be available in case of an accident.
20. Do not use vaporizing thermal irons on pressed hair, as the hair will revert to its original over-curly state.
21. Do not use thermal irons on chemically straightened hair, as they may cause damage to the hair.

BLOW-DRY STYLING

Blow-dry styling, often referred to as a "quick salon service," is basically the technique of drying and styling damp hair in one operation. This technique creates the basic structure of hairstyles without time-consuming setting, drying, and combing out. It helps to develop soft, natural hairstyles with free flowing effects, such as are usually achieved by the use of rollers and curls.

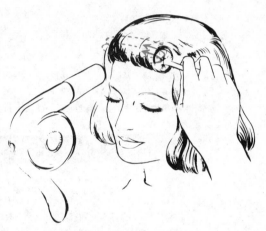

There are two techniques used in blow-dry styling:

1. Blow-dry curling with a brush.
2. Blow-dry waving with a comb.

There are many elaborations of these techniques used by hairstylists in order to achieve special effects or styling objectives. This section will discuss only the two basic techniques. Many additional techniques can be developed with experience and advanced training.

CAUTION

Blow-dry curling and waving should be done with caution on permanently waved hair, relaxed hair, or hair that has been tinted or lightened. This type of hair should be partially towel dried as it easily stretches, which could cause damage.

EQUIPMENT, IMPLEMENTS, AND MATERIALS

The following equipment, implements, and materials are required for blow-dry styling:

Blow dryer (with or without attachments)
Combs (hard rubber or metal)
Shampoo

Styling lotion
Conditioner
Hair spray

THE BLOW DRYER

The blow dryer (without attachments) is an electrical device especially designed for drying and styling the hair in a single operation. Its main parts are a handle, slotted nozzle, small fan, heating element, and controls. When in operation it produces a steady stream of temperature controlled air. The controls permit the stylist to make necessary heat adjustments when operating the blow dryer.

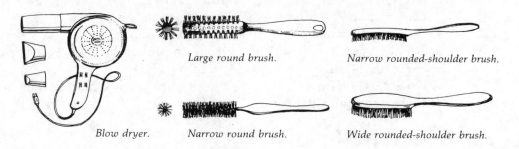

Large round brush.

Narrow rounded-shoulder brush.

Blow dryer.

Narrow round brush.

Wide rounded-shoulder brush.

COMBS AND BRUSHES

Both hard rubber combs and those made of metal are used for blow waving and air waving. Some stylists prefer to use metal combs, since they retain and transmit heat better and thus the hair can be re-styled in the shortest possible time. Combs are available with coarse teeth, half coarse and half fine teeth, and all fine teeth.

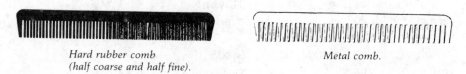

Hard rubber comb
(half coarse and half fine).

Metal comb.

Special narrow synthetic bristle brushes are used in blow-dry styling. It is often easier for the stylist to brush the hair into the desired style with a narrow brush. The smaller the diameter of the brush, the tighter the curl, with better staying qualities.

COSMETICS USED IN BLOW-DRY STYLING

The principal cosmetics used in blow-dry styling include styling lotions, hair and scalp conditioners, and hair sprays.

Styling lotions. Styling lotions are applied to the hair after shampooing in order to make the hair more manageable for blow curling or waving. These lotions have the consistency of a dense liquid and are applied with a plastic squeeze bottle or trigger (pump) action bottle. Styling lotions contain a coating substance which gives blow-dried hair more body and staying qualities.

Hair conditioners. These are used as a corrective treatment for dry and brittle hair. They are used daily or weekly by the patron or immediately prior to the blow-drying service.

Excessive hairstyling by the blow-drying method may cause dryness, split ends, and loss of elasticity. Therefore, it is advisable to use hair conditioners containing a lubricant.

Hair sprays. These are applied to the hair to keep the finished hairstyle in place.

Be guided by manufacturer's directions or by your instructor as to the proper usage of cosmetics on the patron's hair and scalp.

BLOW CURLING WITH ROUND BRUSH

Blow curling is most successful on hair that is naturally curly or has received a permanent wave. The basis for all successful blow styling is the carefully planned hair shaping. In order to properly receive a blow-curling service, hair should be shaped with tapered ends. Successful blow curling is extremely difficult on hair with blunt-cut hair ends.

The following technique is offered as one method of creating a natural-looking, easy-to-wear, informal style with a brush and blower. (Your instructor's methods are equally correct.)

PROCEDURE

1. Shampoo and towel dry the hair.
2. Properly shape the hair leaving tapered ends.
3. Apply styling lotion and/or conditioner.
4. Pre-plan the style. Start at the crown or top of the head, as desired. Section the hair, pick up a wide strand, and comb through. (Fig. 1)
5. Bring the comb out to the hair ends and insert the brush. Brush through the strand, bringing the brush out to the ends.
6. Roll the hair with the brush, making a complete downward turn, away from the face, until the brush rests on the scalp. Maintain this position and start the blower. Direct the blower very slowly through the curl in a back-and-forth movement. (Fig. 2) When the hair section is completely dry, release the brush with a rounded movement.

   Use clippies to secure each curl as it is completed and to hold it in place until it is cooled off.

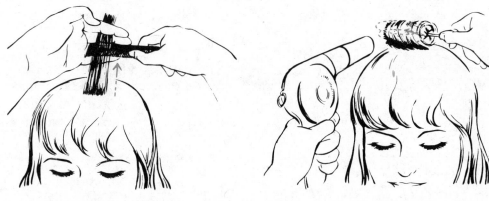

Fig. 1   Fig. 2

7. Continue making curls in the same manner across the crown and back of the head. Clip each curl as completed.

   Shape the neckline curls with a comb, or make pin curls on the nape for a finished, close-to-the-head look.

REMINDERS AND HINTS ON BLOW-DRY STYLING

For successful blow-dry styling it is essential that the hair be in excellent condition.

Permanently waved, chemically relaxed, tinted, or lightened hair should be partially towel dried before being blow-curled or waved. (The hair stretches easily and could be damaged if very wet.)

The hair should be shaped with tapered ends for successful blow-curling or waving.

Remove the excess moisture from the hair with hot air from the blow dryer before starting the styling process.

Styling lotion is important in blow-waving and curling. Comb the hair thoroughly to spread the styling lotion evenly.

Direct the blower slowly through the curls in a back-and-forth movement. Never hold the blower too long in one place. The blower should be directed so that the hot air flows in the same direction as the hair is wound.

To avoid severe scalp burns, direct the hot air away from the patron's scalp, never directly on the scalp.

The hair must be thoroughly cooled before it is combed out. This may be accomplished by switching the dryer to cold and cooling the hair that has been dried.

BRUSHES AND COMBS

The actual styling is performed with the brush or comb. The blow dryer is an implement used for quickly drying the hair while the hair is being styled.

The size of the styling brush used is determined by the style and length of the hair. As a general rule, short hair is styled with a small diameter brush. For medium or longer hair, best results are achieved with large diameter brushes.

To avoid scalp burns, keep heated metal combs away from the scalp.

BLOW DRYER

Make sure that the blow dryer is perfectly clean and free of dirt, grease, hair, etc., before using. Dirt or hair may cause extreme heat and burn hair.

The air intake at the back of the dryer must be kept clear at all times. If this intake is covered and air cannot pass through freely, the element of the dryer may burn out.

BLOW-DRYING THE HAIR

The hot air is directed straight onto the head only for rough drying.

For successful blow-dry styling the air should be directed from the scalp area to the hair ends.

The flow of air is directed to the top half of the brush in a back-and-forth movement. This method acts to deflect the hot air, reduce its heat, and dry the hair nearest the scalp.

Avoid holding the nozzle of the blow dryer too close to the hair for long periods of time. Directing the hot air too close or at the wrong angle can burn or crisp the hair.

In blow-styling it is essential that when the hairstyle is completed the scalp be thoroughly dry. The hairstyle will not hold if the scalp is damp.

Complete the blow-dry styling with a light application of lacquer to give shine and holding power to the hair. However, the soft, natural effects may be destroyed by the use of heavy lacquers.

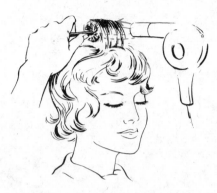

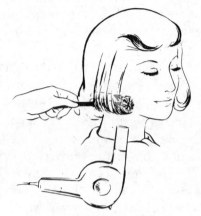

To give the crown hair a slight lift, a small round brush is used. The dryer is kept on the move from side to side along the curl. Secure each curl with clippies as it is completed.

PAGE BOY EFFECT.
Curl hair under.

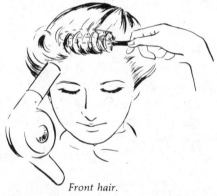

Front hair.

Side hair.

SMOOTH TOP WITH FLIP.
To create a smooth top with flip, the hair ends are lifted by placing brush close to scalp. Rotate brush. As the brush rotates, the hot air is directed to the base within the cupped area.

POPULAR BLOW-DRY STYLES

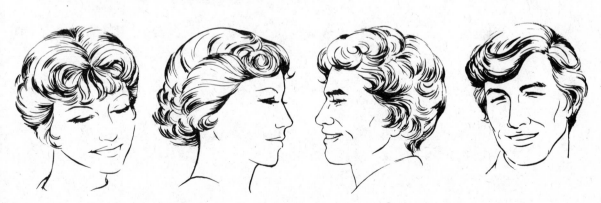

AIR WAVING

Another technique used to create attractive hairstyles without preliminary setting and drying of the hair is by the use of the electric air waver comb and styling comb. Styling the hair with this technique is performed in the same manner as finger waving, using an electric air waver comb and styling comb.

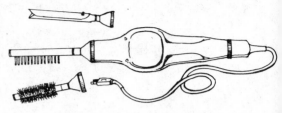

The hair is styled after it has been shaped, shampooed, and towel dried.

Air waver with comb attachment.

To achieve ridges and waves on various parts of the head, the hair must be slightly damp. Apply a light spray of styling lotion to assist in creating the desired hairstyle.

It is important to locate the natural wave formation in the hair. Comb the hair in the direction of the wave desired. This will help to establish the natural hair growth pattern. (Fig. 1) Comb the hair in the direction of the planned hairstyle. Comb the hair with air waver until it is dry enough to hold a wave.

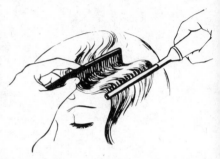

Fig. 1. Combing hair in direction of wave desired.

SHAPING HAIR WITH COMB

1. **Left side part.** Starting at the front section of the head, insert the hand comb into the hair about 1½″ (3.75 cm) from the part. Draw the styling comb towards the back. Insert the air waver under the comb and draw the air waver comb towards the face to form a ridge. Hold both combs in this position until a firm ridge has been formed. (Fig. 2) Continue towards the crown until the entire length of the ridge is completed.

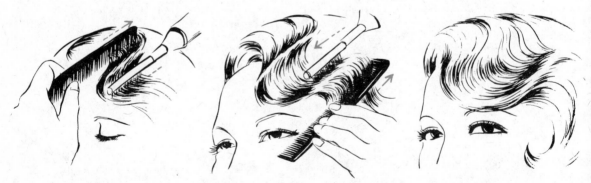

Fig. 2. Forming ridge.   *Fig. 3. Forming second ridge.*   *Fig. 4. Finished style.*

Form the second ridge by starting at the crown and work towards the front. The ridge and shaping is made just the reverse of the first ridge. (Fig. 3)

Support the completed ridgeline with the styling comb while the air waver comb lifts and designs the pattern.

2. **Right side part.** The procedure is exactly the same as that for the left side part, with the exception that the hand comb is held in the right hand and the air waver is controlled by the left hand. However, the waving should start at the crown and work forward towards the face.

A finished wave is formed with the air waver comb and styling comb, taking advantage of the natural waving pattern of the hair. (Fig. 4)

The air waver comb, when used in conjunction with the curling iron, presents many styling opportunities to the stylist. The number of styles and patterns that may be created with these implements working in harmony is only limited by the skill and imagination of the stylist.

SAFETY PRECAUTIONS

1. Styling dryer. Move moderately hot air back and forth on the hair and away from the scalp. Avoid holding the dryer too long in one place.
2. Metal comb. To avoid scalp burns, keep teeth of heated metal comb away from the scalp.
3. In all blow-dry styling it is important that when the curling or waving is completed the scalp must be thoroughly dry. If the ends and the curls are completed, but the scalp is damp, the hairstyle will not hold.

REVIEW QUESTIONS

THERMAL WAVING AND CURLING

1. What is thermal waving and curling?
2. Name the three thermal irons classifications.
3. Why should electric vaporizing thermal irons not be used on pressed hair?
4. What are the two parts of the styling portion of the irons?
5. What degree of heat should be used on lightened, tinted, or white hair?
6. How are the irons tested for desirable temperature?
7. In what position should the irons be held?
8. What type of combs must be used in thermal waving and curling?
9. What are spiral curls?
10. What are end curls used for?
11. What are volume thermal irons curls used for?
12. Why are metal combs not used with thermal irons?
13. How is the comb used to prevent scalp burns?
14. What causes fishhooks on the hair ends in thermal irons curling?

BLOW-DRY STYLING

1. What is blow-dry styling?
2. Name two techniques used in blow-dry styling.
3. What is a blow dryer?
4. What types of combs are used for blow waving and air waving?
5. What are the three principal cosmetics used in blow-dry styling?
6. What is the basis for successful blow styling?
7. How should the hair ends be shaped for blow curling?
8. Why should the teeth of a heated metal comb be kept away from the scalp?
9. What will happen to the style if the ends and curls are completed but the scalp is damp?

Chapter 19

MANICURING

CHAPTER LEARNING OBJECTIVES

The student successfully mastering this chapter will know:
1. *The qualifications of a manicurist.*
2. *The implements and cosmetics used in manicuring.*
3. *How to properly prepare a manicuring table.*
4. *How to hold and use manicuring implements.*
5. *The basic procedure involved in giving a professional manicure.*
6. *The safety rules to follow in giving a manicure.*
7. *The technique involved in the application of artificial nails.*
8. *How to repair damaged and broken nails.*
9. *How to identify nail abnormalities.*
10. *The procedure and benefits of reconditioning nails.*
11. *The procedure for hand and arm massage.*
12. *The theory and practice of pedicuring.*

The ancients regarded long, polished, and colored fingernails as a mark of distinction between aristocrats and common laborers. Manicuring, once considered a luxury for the few, is now a service used by the general public. In fact, many well-groomed women and men use the services of a professional manicurist.

The word **manicure** (man'i-kur) is derived from the Latin "manus" (hand) and "cura" (care), which means the care of the hands and nails. The purpose of a manicure is to improve the appearance of the hands and nails.

If the patron is pleased with a professional manicure, she is more likely to become a regular patron for this service, as well as for other beauty services.

A manicurist should have the following qualifications:
1. Knowledge of the structure of hands, arms, and nails.
2. Knowledge of the composition of the cosmetics used in manicuring.
3. Ability to give a good manicure in an efficient manner.
4. Ability to care for the patron's manicuring problems.
5. Ability to distinguish between disorders that may be treated in the salon and diseases that must be treated by a physician.
6. Ability to please and satisfy patrons.

EQUIPMENT, IMPLEMENTS, COSMETICS, & MATERIALS

The articles used in manicuring that are durable are referred to as **equipment** and **implements**. Cosmetics and materials refer to the **supplies** that are consumed and must be replaced.

EQUIPMENT

Manicuring table and **adjustable lamp.**

Patron's chair and **manicurist's chair** or **stool.**

Cushion [8 x 12″ (20 x 30 cm)], covered with a washable slipcover or sanitized towel, on which the patron rests his or her arm. A towel, folded and covered by a small sanitized towel, may be used instead of the cushion.

Supply tray for holding cosmetics.

Finger bowl (plastic, china, or glass) with removable paper cup for holding warm, soapy water.

Container for clean absorbent cotton.

Electric heater for heating oil when giving a hot oil manicure.

Wet sanitizer container with sterile cotton and 70% alcohol.

Glass containers for cosmetics and accessories.

IMPLEMENTS

Orangewood sticks (2) for loosening cuticle, for working around nail, and for applying oil, cream, bleach, or solvent to the nail and cuticle.

Nail file [7 or 8″ (17.5 or 20 cm) long, thin, and flexible] for shaping and smoothing the free edge of the nail.

Cuticle pusher for loosening and pushing back the cuticle.

Cuticle nippers or **cuticle scissors** for trimming the cuticle.

Nail brush for cleansing the nails and fingertips with the aid of warm, soapy water.

Emery boards (2) for shaping the free edge of the nail with the coarse side, and for beveling the nail with the finer side.

Nail buffer (with removable frame to permit replacement of the chamois cover) for buffing and polishing the nails. (Some states do not permit the use of a nail buffer.)

Fine camel's hair brush for applying lacquer or liquid nail polish. (Camel's hair brush is usually attached to the top of the nail polish bottle.)

Tweezers for lifting small bits of cuticle.

COSMETICS

Nail and hand cosmetics vary in their composition and usage according to the purpose they serve.

Nail cleansers consist of some form of soap, either flaked, beaded, or caked.

Nail polish removers contain organic solvents and are used to dissolve old polish on nails. To offset the drying action of the solvent, oil may be present in the nail polish remover.

MANICURING IMPLEMENTS

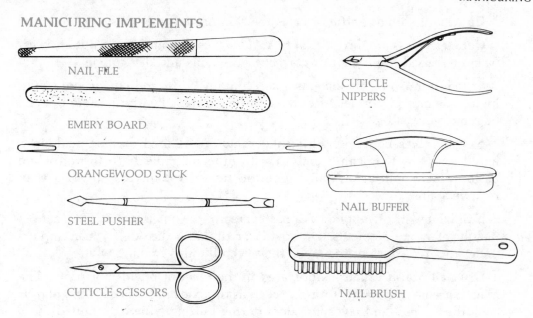

NAIL FILE

CUTICLE NIPPERS

EMERY BOARD

ORANGEWOOD STICK

NAIL BUFFER

STEEL PUSHER

CUTICLE SCISSORS

NAIL BRUSH

PROPER WAY TO HOLD MANICURING IMPLEMENTS

NAIL FILE

*Hold the file firmly
in the right hand,
with the thumb
underneath it for
support and the
other four fingers on
its upper surface.*

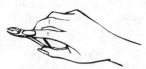

CUTICLE NIPPERS

*Pick up the nippers by the handles.
Place the bent tip of the index finger
over the top of the shank and the
thumb on the side of the handle,
with the remaining fingers over
the opposite handle.*

EMERY BOARD

*It is held in the same manner
as the nail file.*

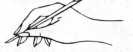

ORANGEWOOD STICK

*It is held in the same manner as in
writing with a pencil.*

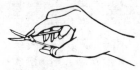

CUTICLE SCISSORS

Held in the same manner as nippers.

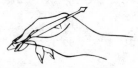

STEEL PUSHER

*It is held in the same manner as in
writing with a pencil. The dull spade
side is used to push back and
loosen the cuticle.*

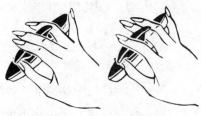

BUFFER

Two ways of holding buffer.

Cuticle oil softens and lubricates the skin around the nails.

Cuticle creams are mixtures of fats and waxes (lanolin, cocoa butter, beeswax, etc.) used to prevent or correct brittle nails and dry cuticle.

Cuticle removers or **solvents** may contain 2-5% sodium or potassium hydroxide plus glycerine. After the cuticle is softened with this liquid, it can be removed easily.

Nail bleaches contain hydrogen peroxide or diluted organic acids in a liquid form, or they can be mixed with other ingredients to form a white paste. When applied over nails, under the free edges, and on fingertips, they remove stains.

Nail whiteners are applied as a paste, cream, or coated string. They consist mainly of white pigments (zinc oxide or titanium dioxide). When applied under the free edges of the nails, they keep the tips looking white.

Dry nail polish usually is prepared in the form of powder or paste. The main ingredient is a mild abrasive, such as tin oxide, talc, silica, or kaolin. It smooths the nail and gives it a gloss during buffing (where permitted).

An **abrasive** is available as a pumice powder and used with a buffer to smooth irregular nail ridges.

Liquid nail polish or **lacquer** is used to color or gloss the nail. It is a solution of nitro cellulose in volatile solvents, such as amyl acetate, together with a plasticiser (castor oil), which prevents too rapid drying. Also present are resin and color.

Nail polish thinner, containing acetone or other solvent, is used to thin out nail polish when it has thickened.

A **base coat** is a liquid product applied before the liquid nail polish. With this application, the nail polish adheres readily to the nail surface. It also forms a hard gloss, which prevents the color in the nail polish from staining the nail tissue.

A **top coat,** or **sealer,** is a liquid applied over the nail polish. This product protects the polish and minimizes its chipping or cracking.

Nail strengtheners are designed to prevent the nails from splitting or peeling. They are applied to the tips of the nails only. They are never applied over polish. The nails must be thoroughly clean, free of oils or creams, and dry. They are applied before the base coat. The product usually contains formaldehyde. **Cuticle shields** are used during the application of nail strengtheners to prevent the product from touching the skin or cuticle.

A **nail dryer** is a solution that protects the nail polish against stickiness and dulling. It can be used either as a spray or brush-on, and it is applied over the top coat or directly on the nail polish.

Powdered alum or **alum solution** is used to stop the bleeding of minor cuts.

Hand creams and **hand lotions** are recommended for overcoming a dry, chapped, or irritated condition of the skin. **Hand creams** are similar in composition to vanishing creams. Other ingredients that may be included are glycerine, cocoa butter, lecithin, or gums. **Hand lotions** are diluted emulsions of stearic acid and water, to which may be added mucilage of quince seed, gum, lanolin, or glycerine.

MATERIALS

Absorbent cotton for application of cosmetics to the nails.

Soap (liquid or any form) for finger bath.

Warm water for finger bath.

Sanitized towel for each patron.

Cleansing tissue for use whenever necessary.

Chamois for replacing soiled chamois on buffer.

Paper cups for replacing used paper cups in finger bowl.

Antiseptic for use in finger bath, and to avoid infection when minor injuries to tissues surrounding the nails occur.

Disinfectant for sanitizing implements, and for disinfecting the manicuring table.

Spatula for removing creams from jars.

Mending tissue paper and **mending liquid** for repairing or covering broken, split, or torn nails.

Perforated adhesive tape for holding compresses on injured nails or tissues, or for covering broken nails.

Scotch tape for repairing or covering broken, split, or torn nails.

70% alcohol is used in a jar sanitizer where implements are kept during a manicure. It is also used to sanitize a patron's fingers before a manicure.

SHAPES OF NAILS

Nails naturally vary greatly in shape, but are usually classified into four general shapes: **square, round, oval,** and **pointed.**

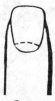
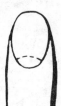
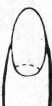
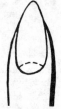

Square   *Round*   *Oval*   *Pointed*

In selecting the nail shape best suited for the patron, consult her wishes and give consideration to the type of fingers she has.

The shape of the nail should conform to that of the fingertips for a more natural effect. In general the oval-shaped nail, nicely rounded at the base, and slightly pointed at the tips, fits most hands. Only a beautiful hand can afford to direct attention to itself by exaggeration of shape and color. Women who perform work with their hands usually require shorter, more round-shaped nails in order to avoid nail breakage and injury.

PREPARATION OF THE MANICURING TABLE

To give a professional manicure, all rules of sanitation must be followed. The table and the manicurist's hands must be perfectly clean. Everything, including containers, bowls, instruments, and materials, must be in perfect order. Do not ask the patron to sit at the table with the remains of the previous manicure in sight. Always clean the table immediately upon completion of a manicure so that it will be ready for the next patron. This will make the manicure more pleasing to the patron, and will put her in a more receptive mood for your advice and suggestions.

PROCEDURE

1. Sponge the manicuring tabletop with a disinfectant.
2. Place a clean towel over the armrest or cushion.
3. Place a bowl of warm, soapy water to the left of the patron.
4. Place the metal implements and orangewood sticks in a jar sanitizer containing cotton saturated with alcohol.
5. Arrange cream jars, lotion bottles, and nail polishes in the order to be used and place them to the left of the manicurist.

MANICURING TABLE SETUP

(Your instructor's manicuring table setup is equally correct.)

1. Towel wrapped armrest
2. Nail file
3. Emery board
4. Alcohol
5. Cotton container
6. Finger bowl
7. Nail brush
8. Wet sanitizer containing manicuring implements
9. Tray with nail polishes

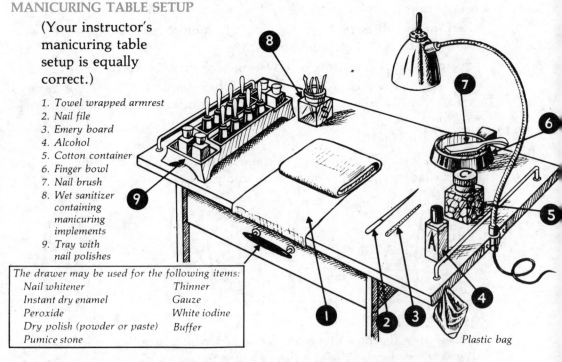

The drawer may be used for the following items:
Nail whitener   Thinner
Instant dry enamel   Gauze
Peroxide   White iodine
Dry polish (powder or paste) Buffer
Pumice stone

Plastic bag

6. Place the nail file (which has been sponged with alcohol) and fresh emery boards to the right of the manicurist.
7. Attach a small plastic bag to the table with scotch tape, on either the right or left side, for waste materials.

The manicuring table drawer always should be clean and neat. Do not use it for waste materials; use the plastic bag.

PROCEDURE FOR A PLAIN MANICURE

PREPARATION

(The routine outlined in this text is one of several ways in which to give a manicure. Whatever routine your instructor outlines for you is equally correct.)

1. Prepare manicuring table as previously outlined.
2. Seat patron.   3. Wash your hands.   4. Examine patron's hands.

CAUTION

Be extremely careful to avoid cutting the patron's skin. However, be prepared to deal with small cuts by having hydrogen peroxide, powdered alum (styptic powder), or alum solution immediately available.

PROCEDURE

1. **Remove old polish.** (Start with the little finger of left hand.) Moisten a pledget of cotton with nail polish remover and press over the nail for a few moments to soften the polish. With a firm movement, bring the cotton from the base of the nail to the tip. Do not smear the old polish into the cuticle or surrounding tissues.

   (An alternate method of removing nail polish is to moisten small pledgets of cotton with nail polish remover and press over old polish on each nail. Then moisten another pledget of cotton with nail polish remover, and use it for removing the small pledgets on the nails. The pressed on pledget acts as a blotter and does not leave a polish smear on the cuticle.)

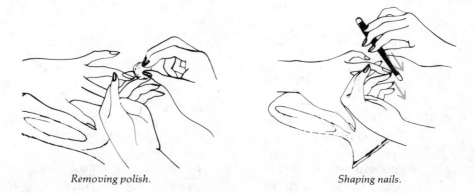

Removing polish.   Shaping nails.

2. **Shape nails.** Discuss with the patron the nail shape best suited for her. File the nails of the **left hand**, starting with the little finger and working towards the thumb, in the following manner:
   a) Hold the patron's finger between the thumb and the first two fingers of the left hand.
   b) Hold the file or emery board in the right hand and tilt it slightly so that filing is confined mainly to the underside of the free edge.
   c) Shape nails into graceful oval tips, never extreme points. Use the file or emery board to shape the nails. File each nail from corner to center, going from right to left and then from left to right. Filing nails with the growth of the nails avoids splitting. Use two short, quick strokes and one long, sweeping stroke on each side of the nail.

   Note: *Never file deep into the corners of the nails. They will look longer and be stronger if permitted to grow out at sides.*

3. **Soften cuticle.** After filing the nails of the left hand, file two nails of the right hand. Then, immerse the left hand into the finger bowl (soap bath) to permit softening of the cuticle. Finish filing the nails of the right hand. Remove the left hand from the finger bowl.

4. **Dry fingertips.** Holding a towel with both hands, carefully dry the left hand, including the area between the fingers. At the same time, gently loosen and push back the cuticle and adhering skin on each nail.

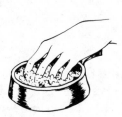

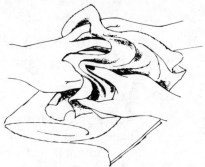

Softening cuticle.

Towel-drying fingertips.

5. **Apply cuticle remover (solvent).** Wind a thin layer of cotton around the blunt edge of an orangewood stick for use as an applicator. Apply cuticle solvent around the cuticle of the left hand.

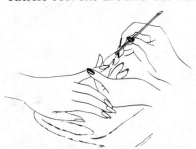

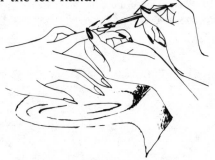

Applying cuticle remover with cotton-tipped orangewood stick.

Loosening dead cuticle with pusher.

6. **Loosen cuticle.** Use the spoon end of the cuticle pusher to gently loosen the cuticle. Keep the cuticle moist while working. Use the cuticle pusher, in a flat position, to remove dead cuticle adhering to the nail without scratching the nail plate. Push the cuticle back with a towel over the index finger.

When using the cuticle pusher and orangewood stick, avoid too much pressure so that live tissue at the root of the nail will not be injured.

7. **Clean under free edge.** Use a cotton-tipped orangewood stick, dipped in soapy water, to clean under free edge, working from the center toward each side, employing gentle pressure.

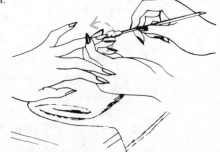

Cleaning under free edge with cotton-tipped orangewood stick.

8. **Trim cuticle.** If necessary, use cuticle nippers to remove dead cuticle, uneven cuticle, or hangnails. In cutting the cuticle, be careful to remove it as a single segment.

9. **When cutting the cuticle of the middle finger of the left hand,** immerse fingers of the right hand into finger bowl (soap bath), while continuing to manicure the left hand.

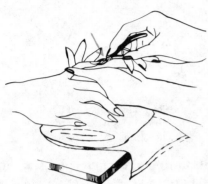

Trimming cuticle with nippers.

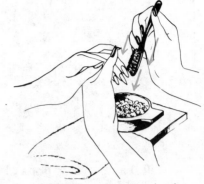

Cleaning nails, using brush in downward movement.

10. **Bleach under free edge.** With a cotton-tipped orangewood stick, apply hydrogen peroxide, or other bleaching preparation, under the free edge of each nail.

   Apply nail whitener under free edge of nails (optional). Use orangewood stick as applicator to apply chalk paste, or use a string treated with nail whitener.

11. **Apply cuticle oil** or **cream** around the sides and base of the nail and massage with the thumb in a rotary movement.

12. **Remove right hand from soap bath.** Manicure the nails and cuticles of right hand as described in Steps 4 through 11.

13. **Cleanse nails.** Brush the nails over the soap bath, using a downward movement, to clean the nails of both hands.

14. **Dry hands and nails thoroughly.**

COMPLETION

1. **Re-examine nails and cuticles.** Carefully re-examine the nails for defects. Use the fine side of an emery board to give the nails a smooth beveled edge. Remove remaining pieces of cuticle.

2. If required, **repair** split or broken nails.

   As an added service, a hand massage or a hand and arm massage may be given at this time.

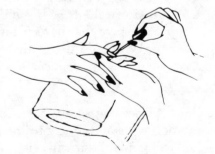

Applying base coat, polish, and seal coat.

3. **Apply base coat.** Apply base coat to the left hand with long strokes, starting with the little finger and working toward the thumb. Allow it to dry until "slick to a light touch."

4. **Apply liquid polish.** Dip the camel's hair brush into the polish and wipe off excess by pressing it gently against the sides of the bottle.

Apply the polish lightly and quickly, using sweeping strokes, from the base to the free edge of the nail, as shown in the illustrations.

(Always keep the polish thin enough to flow freely. If the polish is thick, add a little polish solvent and shake well.)

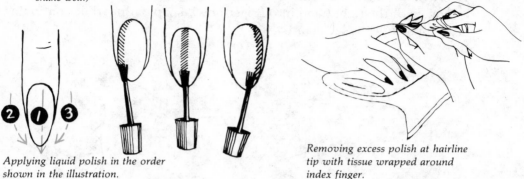

Applying liquid polish in the order shown in the illustration.

Removing excess polish at hairline tip with tissue wrapped around index finger.

5. **Remove excess polish.** Dip a cotton-tipped orangewood stick into nail polish remover. Apply it carefully around the cuticles and nail edges to remove excess polish.

6. **Apply top** or **seal coat.** Apply top coat to the left hand with long strokes, and then apply it to the right hand in the same manner. Brush around and under tips of nails for added support and protection.

   Note: *Top coat application is usually eliminated when liquid polish is sprayed with nail enamel dryer.*

7. **Apply hand lotion.** As an additional service, after the top coat is completely dry, apply hand lotion with light manipulations over the hands, from wrists to fingertips.

FINAL CLEANUP

1. Sanitize used manicuring implements; place them in a cabinet sanitizer.
2. Place used materials (tissues, cotton, emery board, etc.) into closed containers or plastic bag attached to manicuring table.
3. Wipe manicuring table with disinfectant; put everything in order.
4. Clean the tops of nail polish bottles with polish remover.
5. Inspect the manicuring table drawer for cleanliness and order.
6. Wash and dry your hands.

SAFETY RULES IN MANICURING

Observing safety rules in manicuring can be of great help in preventing accidents and injury to the patron or manicurist. The following safety rules will guide the manicurist in protecting the patron:

1. Keep all containers covered and labeled.
2. Hold or move containers with dry hands.
3. Handle sharp-pointed implements carefully, and avoid dropping them.
4. Dull oversharpened cutting edges of sharp implements with an emery board.
5. Bevel a sharp nail edge with an emery board.
6. Do not file too deeply into nail corners.

7. Do not use a sharp, pointed implement to cleanse under the nail.
8. Avoid excessive friction in nail buffing (where permitted).
9. Apply an antiseptic immediately if the skin is accidentally cut.
10. Apply styptic powder or alum solution to stop the bleeding from a small cut. **Never use a styptic pencil.**
11. Avoid pushing the cuticle back too far.
12. Avoid too much pressure at the base of the nail.
13. Do not work on a nail when the surrounding skin is inflamed or contains pus.

INDIVIDUAL NAIL STYLING

SHAPE OF NAILS

For a more natural effect, the shape of the nail should conform to that of the fingertip. A gracefully shaped nail adds beauty to the hands.

Nail shapes may be divided into four types:

1. Oval.
2. Slender tapering (pointed).
3. Square or rectangular.
4. Clubbed (round).

OVAL NAIL

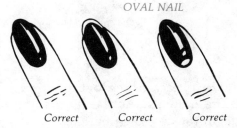

Correct   *Correct*   *Correct*

SLENDER TAPERING (POINTED) NAIL

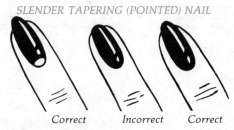

Correct   *Incorrect*   *Correct*

The **oval nail** is the ideal nail shape and can be styled by either covering the entire nail with polish, leaving the free edge white, or leaving the half moon white at the base of the nail.

The **slender tapering nail** is well suited for the thin, delicate hand. The nail should be tapered somewhat longer than usual to enhance the slender appearance of the hand. The nail can be completely polished, or a half moon can be left at the base.

SQUARE OR RECTANGULAR NAIL

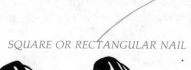
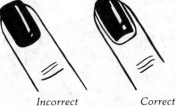

Incorrect   *Correct*

CLUBBED (ROUND) NAIL

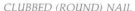
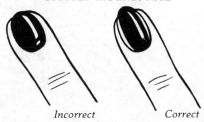

Incorrect   *Correct*

The **square or rectangular nail** should extend only slightly passed the tip of the finger with the nail tip rounded off. The entire nail may be polished with a slight half moon left at the base, and a white margin left at the sides of the nail.

The **clubbed nail** should be slightly tapered and extend just a bit passed the tip of the finger. The entire nail should be polished with a thin white margin left at the sides.

HAND MASSAGE

Include a hand massage with each manicure. It keeps the hands flexible, well-groomed, and smooth.

PROCEDURE

1. Hold the patron's hand in your hand. Place a dab of hand lotion on the back of the patron's hand and spread it to the fingers and wrist.
2. Hold the patron's hand firmly, as in Fig. 1. Bend the hand slowly with a forward and backward movement to limber the wrist. Repeat three times.

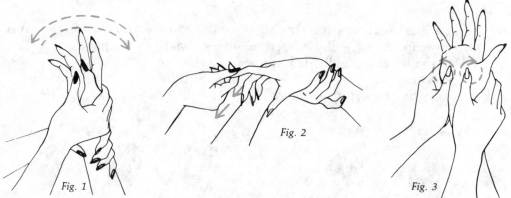

Fig. 1

Fig. 2

Fig. 3

3. Grasp each finger, as in Fig. 2. Gently bend each finger, one at a time, to limber the top of the hand and finger joints. As the fingers and thumb are bent, slide your thumb down towards the fingertips.
4. With the patron's elbow resting on the table, hold the hand upright, as in Fig. 3. Massage the palm of the hand with the cushions of your thumbs, using a circular movement in alternate directions. This movement will completely relax the patron's hand.
5. Rest patron's arm on the table. Grasp each finger at the base, and rotate it gently in large circles, ending with a gentle squeeze of the fingertips, as in Fig. 4. Repeat three times.

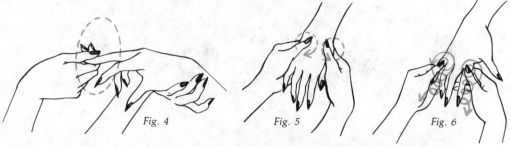

Fig. 4

Fig. 5

Fig. 6

6. Hold the patron's hand as in Fig. 5. Massage the wrist, then top of the hand with a circular movement. Slide back and with both hands wring wrist in opposite direction three times. Repeat movements three times.
7. Finish massage by tapering each finger. Beginning at the base of each finger, rotate, pause, and squeeze with gentle pressure. Then, pull lightly with pressure until tip is reached. (Fig. 6) Repeat three times.
8. Repeat Steps 1 to 7 on other hand.

ELECTRIC MANICURE

The electric manicure is given with the aid of a portable device operated by a small motor. It uses a variety of attachments that perform various operations.

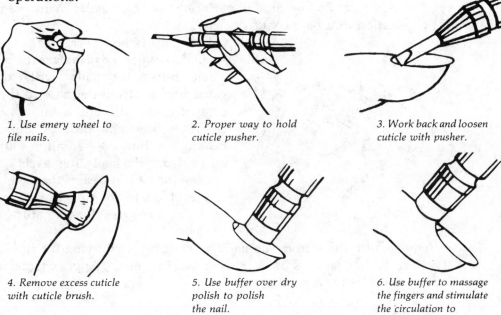

1. Use emery wheel to file nails.

2. Proper way to hold cuticle pusher.

3. Work back and loosen cuticle with pusher.

4. Remove excess cuticle with cuticle brush.

5. Use buffer over dry polish to polish the nail.

6. Use buffer to massage the fingers and stimulate the circulation to the nails.

Before using an electric manicure machine, observe manufacturer's demonstration and follow instructions carefully.

OIL MANICURE

An oil manicure is beneficial for ridged and brittle nails, and for dry cuticles. It also improves the hands by leaving the skin soft and pliable.

PROCEDURE

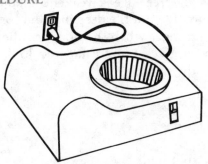

Hot oil manicure heater.

1. Heat vegetable (olive) oil or commercial preparation to a comfortable temperature in an electric heater.
2. Proceed with the manicure to the point where you place the hand in the finger bowl; at that point, have patron place her fingers in the heated oil.
3. Massage the hands and wrists with the oil; then treat the cuticles in the usual manner. Cuticle remover, cuticle oil, or cream are not needed.
4. Remove oil from the hands with warm, damp towel.
5. Wipe each nail carefully with polish remover, to remove all traces of the oil before applying the base coat.
6. Complete as for a plain manicure.

MEN'S MANICURE

Men usually prefer a conservative manicure. File the nails either round or square. Apply a dry polish instead of a liquid polish.

Implements, materials, and supplies are the same as those used for a regular manicure. Follow the same procedure for a regular manicure up to the application of a base coat.

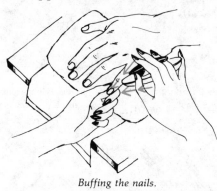

Buffing the nails.

Buff nails (where permitted). Apply a small dab of paste polish over the buffer. Then buff the nails with downward strokes, from the base to the free edge of each nail, until a smooth, clear gloss has been obtained. To prevent a heating or burning sensation, lift the buffer from the nail after each stroke. Buffing the nails increases the circulation of the blood to the fingertips, smooths the nails, and gives them a natural gloss or sheen.

Remove all residue from the nails by washing and drying the fingertips. If a clear liquid enamel is used, buffing is not required. Apply enamel in the same manner as for a regular manicure.

BOOTH MANICURE

A booth manicure is one that is given in the booth and not at the manicuring table. It is usually given while a patron is receiving another service — for example, while a man is having his hair cut or styled.

SPECIAL PROBLEMS

Special problems include unusual nail conditions that should be corrected by the manicurist in order to please the patron.

Nails broken at sides occur when the manicurist removes the corner of the nail out of the nail groove. As a result, the free edge is weakened and the nail cracks and splits at the slightest pressure. Do not file deep into the corners of the nail. Nails appear longer and are stronger when the sides are allowed to grow. This natural line of nail growth gives a more tapered look to the finger, and a longer, slimmer look to the hand.

NAIL REPAIR

Nail repair falls into three general groups:
1. Capping of fragile tips.
2. Repairing of partially broken or split nails.
3. Reattaching tips that are broken off completely.

Capping a fragile tip
1. Tear a wedge-shaped piece of mending tissue the width of the nail at one end and a bit wider at the other.
2. Trim the wide end to fit the nail tip.

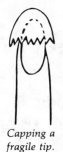

3. Saturate the patch with mending liquid and lay it flat on the nail. The rounded tip should extend about ⅛" (.36 cm) around the free edge of the nail.
4. Smooth patch very lightly with fingertip moistened in polish remover.
5. Have patron turn her palm upward and apply additional mending tissue to exposed edges of tissue. Dip a small orangewood stick into polish remover and use it to turn the tissue inward over the nail edge, pressing firmly to the inner surface of the nail.

Capping a fragile tip.

6. Let the cap dry thoroughly before applying the base coat and polish.

Repairing a split nail

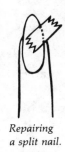

1. Lightly file the split portion of the nail with the fine side of the emery board to help the mending tissue to stick to the nail.
2. Tear a small piece of mending tissue and saturate it with mending liquid until the tissue is transparent.
3. Place saturated tissue over the split area.
4. Tuck the tissue under the nail with orangewood stick. The surface of the patch must be smoothed away from nail edge with cushion of finger moistened in polish remover.

Repairing a split nail.

5. If the split is deep, add a second patch for reinforcement.
6. Dry patch thoroughly before applying the base coat and polish.

Reattaching a broken nail tip

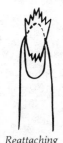

1. Use a thin, flat wisp of cotton saturated with mending liquid. Lay it flat on the nail, extending beyond the broken edge.
2. Fit the broken nail tip in place over saturated cotton.
3. Dip the orangewood stick in remover, and use it to turn ends of cotton back over the nail tip, covering edges of break. Use a very light touch when doing this.
4. Saturate a strip of tissue with mending liquid. Apply diagonally across the nail. If possible, tuck it in at corner beneath stub of nail.

Reattaching a broken nail tip.

5. Smooth surface away from nail edge with fingertip moistened in remover.
6. Allow to dry thoroughly before applying base coat and polish.

CAUTION

Unless the nail repair dries thoroughly before the application of base coat, it will slip, or be rough and uneven.

NAIL WRAPPING

Nail wrapping is used to fortify soft and fragile nails. The procedure used is similar to capping of fragile nail tips.

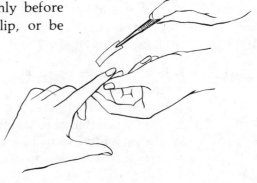

A **fringe of loose skin** left around the nail after a manicure is caused by trimming the cuticle closer than necessary and then rolling back the epidermis. To prevent the occurrence of such loose skin, trim the cuticle only enough to allow a tiny margin of cuticle to remain.

Callous growth at the fingertips can be softened by the application of creams and lotions, and by removing the constant pressure that is causing it. Gentle rubbing with pumice powder also is helpful to start the removing process.

Stains on fingernails may be bleached with prepared nail bleach or peroxide. Slightly damp pumice powder also may be applied and the nails buffed to help remove stains.

ARTIFICIAL NAILS

Clean, attractive hands and nails are an admirable part of a woman's top-to-toe grooming. When a woman cannot grow natural nails of the desired strength and length, she may solve the problem by the application of artificial nails. These may be made of a mixture that builds the nails as it is brushed on or of the press-on type. Artificial nails look natural when properly applied and manicured.

Artificial nails may be used for the following purposes:

1. To conceal broken or damaged nails.
2. To improve the appearance of very short or badly shaped nails.
3. To help overcome the habit of nail biting.
4. To protect a nail or nails against splitting or breakage.

BUILD-ON ARTIFICIAL NAILS

Build-on, also known as **brush-on,** artificial nails are used when one or more nails are to be lengthened. The manicurist should build the type of nail that best conforms to the shape of the patron's fingers and hands.

IMPLEMENTS AND MATERIALS

Regular implements used in manicuring
Instant nail lengthener kit:

Nail forms	Nail lengthener powder
Measuring spoon	Special liquid to dilute powder
Mixing cup	Brushes for application

PROCEDURE

1. Give manicure up to, but not including, application of base coat.
2. Roughen nail surface slightly with emery board.
3. Lightly moisten glue on inside of nail form with a brush and place nail form under the nail. Then press firmly around finger. (Fig. 1)

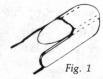

Fig. 1

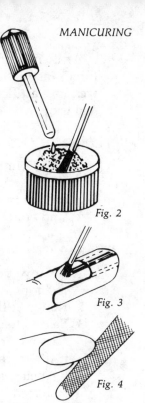

4. Prepare smooth-flowing mixture as directed by manufacturer. (Fig. 2)
5. Brush the mixture on the nail. Start at the base of the nail and continue brushing towards and over the free edge and nail form until desired length is obtained, adding an extra coat over the nail form. Apply it the same way as nail polish. (Fig. 3)
6. Allow the nail to dry and then apply second coat, being careful not to disturb previous coat. Apply third coat if necessary.
7. Wipe off excess mixture on the sides of the nail form; clean the cuticle or sides of the nail with an orangewood stick dipped in polish remover.
8. Allow nail to dry thoroughly for 10-15 minutes.
9. Gently remove the nail form from the nail. File new nail to shape. (Fig. 4)
10. Wash the nail or nails thoroughly. Allow them to dry.
11. Apply a base coat, polish, and top coat or sealer.

Fig. 2

Fig. 3

Fig. 4

REPAIRING BROKEN BUILD-ON NAIL

Prepare mixture. If required, adjust nail form. Apply three coats of mixture to existing nail, with each application extending the tip slightly beyond the previous application. Allow a little drying time between each application.

Let nail dry thoroughly for 10-15 minutes before shaping; then apply polish.

REMOVING BUILD-ON ARTIFICIAL NAILS

Remove nail polish. Saturate cotton pledget with polish remover and apply to the artificial nail. Continue application until the artificial nail has loosened around the cuticle, the tip, and sides of the nail. Continue to loosen the artificial nail very gently with the aid of a metal pusher, until it is removed completely.

SAFETY PRECAUTIONS

1. Clean brush by dipping it into polish remover and wiping it clean.
2. Clean mixing dish by lifting hardened content out with pusher.
3. Make sure bottles are tightly capped when not in use.
4. Do not store product near heat, or use near open flame.
5. Do not apply to injured or inflamed skin.

PRESS-ON ARTIFICIAL NAILS

Models, actresses, saleswomen, and other women whose hands are on display may wear a complete set of press-on artificial nails every day. Women who do other types of work where their hands are not on display may wish to wear artificial nails only for special occasions.

Artificial nails are constructed of either plastic or nylon, and manufacturer's instructions must be followed carefully. Manufacturers advise against wearing artificial nails for more than 48 hours to allow for natural nail growth.

IMPLEMENTS AND MATERIALS

Regular implements and materials used in manicuring plus artificial nails, nail adhesive, and adhesive remover.

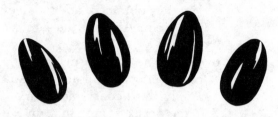

PREPARATION

1. Remove polish from patron's nails, and give a manicure up to, but not including, the application of polish.
2. Roughen the patron's nails by going over them with an emery board.
3. Select the proper nail size for each finger. With a sharp manicuring scissors, trim and then file the artificial nail at the cuticle end so that it fits to the shape of the natural nail. Artificial nails can be flattened by being firmly pressed down before application. They also can be reshaped by being held in warm water for a few seconds and molded to the desired shape.

PROCEDURE

1. Apply a small amount of adhesive evenly on the edges of the patron's nails. Do not apply adhesive on the center of the nails.
2. Apply adhesive on the inside of the artificial nail, excluding tip.
3. Allow the adhesive to dry thoroughly (about 2 minutes).
4. Press artificial nail gently onto the natural nail, with the base touching the cuticle or under it. As each nail is applied, hold it firmly in place for about a minute.
5. Carefully wipe away any excess adhesive from tips and around nails.
6. Allow the artificial nails to dry thoroughly. Advise the patron to avoid disturbing the nails while they are drying.
7. Finish the manicure by applying base coat, polish, and top coat.

REMOVING POLISH

To remove nail polish from nails constructed of **plastic,** use only nail polish remover that has an oily base and does not contain acetone.

Reminder: Polish remover containing acetone will damage plastic artificial nails.

If **nylon**-constructed fingernails have been used, an acetone type of polish remover will not affect them.

REMOVING PRESS-ON ARTIFICIAL NAILS

Apply a few drops of oily nail polish remover around the edge of the nail; then gently lift from the side with an orangewood stick. Do not attempt to pull or twist off the nail, as this could damage or injure the natural nail. Adhesive remover can be used to assist nail remover. It also can be used to remove any surplus adhesive from artificial nails and from natural nails. Artificial nails should be dried carefully and stored in a box. With proper care, they can be reused.

REMINDERS AND HINTS ON ARTIFICIAL NAILS

1. Never apply artificial nails over sore or infected areas.
2. Most manufacturers suggest that artificial nails not be worn for more than 48 hours at a time, in order to allow for natural growth of the nail.
3. Most artificial nail adhesives are flammable, so be cautious with cigarettes, matches, and lighters.
4. When wearing artificial nails, do not subject them to a long period of immersion in water as they might tend to loosen.
5. Do not contaminate the adhesive with oil, cream, or powder.

MANICURE WITH HAND AND ARM MASSAGE

The hand and arm massage is a special service that may be added to the regular manicure. The procedure used is similar to the manicure with hand massage. However, all applications are extended to the forearm, including the elbow.

PROCEDURE

1. Complete hand massage as previously outlined.
2. Place patron's arm on table, palm turned downward, as in Fig. 1. Massage the arm from wrist to elbow, using a slow, circular motion in alternate directions. Repeat three times. Turn patron's palm upward and repeat the same movements three times.

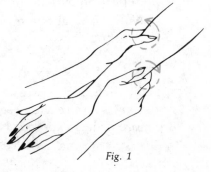

Fig. 1

3. Place your fingers as in Fig. 2. Firmly massage the underpart of the arm to the elbow, using fingers of each hand in alternate crosswise directions. Repeat three times.

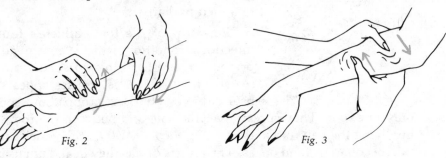

Fig. 2

Fig. 3

4. Place your hands as in Fig. 3. Massage the top of the arm from the wrist to the elbow. Apply thumbs in opposite directions with a squeezing motion. Repeat three times.

5. Cup elbow joint in your hand, as in Fig. 4. Massage the elbow with a circular motion. Repeat three times.

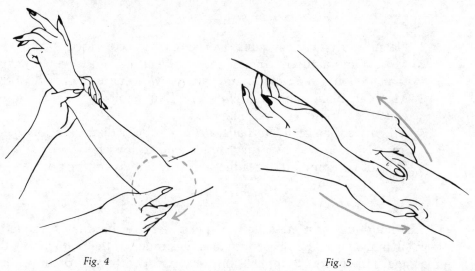

Fig. 4   *Fig. 5*

6. Stroke the arm firmly in opposite directions, from the elbow to wrist as in Fig. 5. Finally, stroke each finger, ending with a gentle squeeze of the fingertips.

7. Repeat Steps 1 to 6 on the other arm.

Note—The above massage manipulations may be extended to include the shoulders.

PEDICURING

Pedicuring is the care of the feet, toes, and toenails. It has become an important salon service because the toes and heels in today's shoe fashions are more or less exposed. Neglected toenails and rough, harsh heels detract

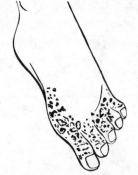

Athlete's foot infection.

from the loveliest of footwear. Foot care not only improves personal appearance, it also adds to the comfort of the feet.

Abnormal foot conditions, such as corns, callouses, and ingrown nails, are best treated by a qualified podiatrist.

Ringworm of the foot (athlete's foot). It is an infectious condition which can spread from one person to another. In acute conditions, deeply seated, itchy, colorless vesicles appear. These appear either singly or in groups, and sometimes on only one foot. They spread over the sole and between the toes, sometimes involving the nail fold and infecting the nail. When the vesicles rupture, the skin becomes red and oozes. The lesions dry as they heal. Fungus infection of the feet is likely to become chronic.

The prevention of infection and the treatment of infection are both accomplished by keeping the skin cool, dry, and clean.

CAUTION

Patrons with athlete's foot (watery blisters and thick white skin between the toes) or other foot infections should not be given a pedicure. They should be referred to a physician for medical help.

EQUIPMENT, IMPLEMENTS, AND MATERIALS

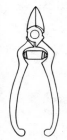

Toenail clippers.

The equipment, implements, and materials required for pedicuring are the same as those for manicuring, with the following additions:

Low stool for cosmetologist or pedicurist.

Ottoman on which to rest patron's foot.

Two basins of warm water, each large enough for foot bath and rinse.

Waterproof apron, or an extra towel, to place over the lap to protect the uniform.

Two towels for drying patron's feet.   **Antiseptic solution.**

Special toenail clippers.   **Cotton pledgets** and **foot powder.**

Witch hazel or other **astringent.**   **Paper towels.**

PREPARATION

1. Arrange required equipment, implements, and materials.
2. Seat patron in facial chair; have patron remove shoes and hose.
3. Place her feet on a clean paper towel on footrest.
4. Wash your hands.
5. Fill the two basins with enough warm water to cover her ankles.
6. Add antiseptic to one basin. Place both feet in bath for 3-5 minutes.
7. Remove feet from basin, rinse feet in second basin, and wipe dry.

PROCEDURE

1. Remove old polish from the nails of both feet. (Fig. 1)
2. File toenails of the left foot with an emery board. File the toenails straight across, rounding them slightly at the corners to conform to the shape of the toes. To avoid ingrown nails, do not file into the corners of the nails. Smooth rough edges with the fine side of an emery board. (Fig.2)

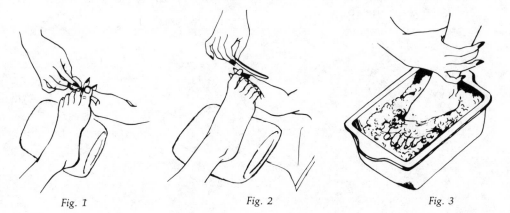

Fig. 1   Fig. 2   Fig. 3

3. Place the left foot in warm, soapy water. (Fig. 3)
4. Shape the nails of the right foot.
5. Remove the left foot from the basin and dry. (Fig. 4)
6. With a cotton-tipped orangewood stick, apply cuticle solvent to the cuticle and under the free edge of each toenail. (Fig. 5)
7. Place the right foot in the bath.
8. Loosen the cuticle gently on the left foot with a cotton-tipped orangewood stick. Keep the cuticle moist with additional lotion or water. Do not use too much pressure. Avoid the use of the metal pusher.
9. Do not cut the cuticle. Only nip a large, ragged hangnail.
10. Rinse the left foot and dry. Massage each toe with cuticle cream or oil.
11. Repeat Steps 5 to 10 on right foot.
12. Scrub both feet in warm, soapy water, rinse, and dry thoroughly.

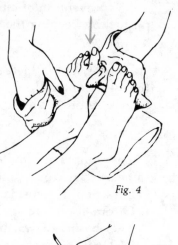

Fig. 4

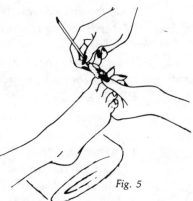

Fig. 5

FOOT MASSAGE

1. Apply lotion or cream over the foot to just above the ankle.
2. Start at the instep of the left foot and apply firm, rotary movements down to the center of the toes. (Fig. 1)
3. Slide the thumbs firmly back to the instep, and repeat same movement.
4. Slide the thumbs back to the hollow of the heel, and repeat same movement.
5. Slide the thumbs back to the base of the foot, and repeat same movement.
6. Start at the heel and work down to the center of the toes. (Fig. 2)
7. Slide firmly back to the heel, and repeat same movement up each side of the foot.

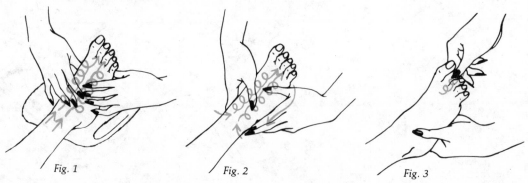

Fig. 1

Fig. 2

Fig. 3

8. Hold one toe in one hand and the heel in the other hand, and apply three rotary movements; do the same with the other toes. (Fig. 3)
9. Slide the right hand to the ankle and the heel of your left hand to the ball of the foot, and apply six firm, rotary movements. (Fig. 4)
10. Change to the right foot and repeat Steps 2 to 9.

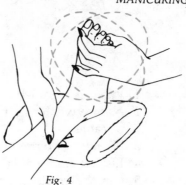

Fig. 4

COMPLETION

1. Remove lotion or cream from both feet with a warm towel.
2. Apply witch hazel or astringent to the feet with a large cotton pledget.
3. Dust lightly with talcum powder.
4. Wipe each toenail with polish remover to remove all traces of lotion or cream.

   Note—Inserting cotton between the toes before application of polish will prevent smearing.
5. Apply a base coat, polish, and seal coat in the same manner as for a manicure.

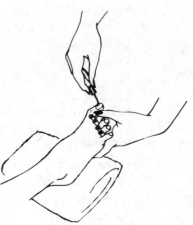

Applying base coat.

6. Cleanup. Clean and sanitize implements, and place in dry sanitizer. Discard used materials. Clean up the booth. Wash your hands.

MISCELLANEOUS TREATMENTS

LEG MASSAGE

The foot massage may be extended up to and over the knee. When massaging from the ankle to the knee, **do not massage over the shinbone and above the knee.** It is advisable to keep the pressure to the muscular tissue on either side of the shinbone. On the calf area of the leg, you may use kneading upward movements up to the underpart of the knee.

REMOVING HAIR FROM LEGS

For complete instructions, see chapter on **Removal of Superfluous Hair.**

HIDING VARICOSE VEINS

Besides recommending the patron with a bad case of varicose veins to a doctor, the pedicurist can suggest the use of a waterproof commercial product for concealing varicose veins disfiguration.

NAILS AND NAIL DISORDERS

The anatomy of the nails and nail disorders are discussed in detail in chapter on **Nails and Nail Disorders.**

REVIEW QUESTIONS

MANICURING

1. What is meant by manicuring?
2. Name two terms that are used to refer to manicuring articles that are durable.
3. Name two terms used to refer to articles that are consumed.
4. List at least five essential implements used in manicuring.
5. List the most commonly used cosmetics in manicuring.
6. Why is a base coat applied before the nail polish?
7. What is the purpose of the top coat, or sealer?
8. Why should the manicuring table be cleaned immediately upon completion of a manicure?
9. When does the manicurist wash her hands for a manicure?
10. For what purposes is powdered alum used?
11. List the important steps in giving a plain manicure.
12. Why should filing be done from the corners to the center of the nail?
13. What is the action of a soap bath?
14. What is the action of a cuticle solvent?
15. What should be done with used manicuring implements?
16. Why is it important to follow safety rules in manicuring?
17. After an accidental cut when manicuring, what do you apply to avoid an infection?
18. What are the four general nail shapes?
19. What is the ideal nail shape?
20. What is the best way to shape the nails for a thin, delicate hand?
21. How should the square or rectangular nail be shaped?
22. How should the clubbed nail be tapered?
23. What is the purpose of the hand massage?
24. What is an electric manicure?
25. For what nail and cuticle conditions are oil manicures recommended?
26. What is a booth manicure?
27. List the three general classifications of nail repair.
28. For what purpose is nail wrapping used?
29. For whom are artificial nails recommended?
30. For what length of time can press-on artificial nails be worn?

PEDICURING

1. What is meant by pedicuring?
2. Which foot conditions should not be treated by the cosmetologist?
3. Why should athlete's foot not be treated in a beauty salon?
4. What are the signs of athlete's foot?
5. How can ingrown toenails be prevented in pedicuring?

Chapter 20

THE NAIL AND
DISORDERS OF THE NAIL

CHAPTER LEARNING OBJECTIVES

The student successfully mastering this chapter will know:
1. *The structure and composition of nails.*
2. *The structures adjoining and affecting nails.*
3. *How nails are nourished.*
4. *How nails grow.*
5. *The various disorders and irregularities of patrons' nails.*
6. *How to recognize diseases of the nails that should not be treated in the beauty salon.*

THE NAIL

The condition of the nail, like that of the skin, reflects the general health of the body. The normal, healthy nail is firm and flexible and appears to be slightly pink in color. Its surface is smooth, curved, and unspotted, without any hollows or wavy ridges.

The **nail,** an appendage of the skin, is a horny, translucent plate that protects the tips of the fingers and toes. **Onyx** (on'iks) is the technical term for nail.

Composition. The nail is composed mainly of **keratin** (ker'ah-tin), a protein substance that forms the base of all horny tissue. The nail is whitish in appearance and allows the pinkish color of the nail bed to be seen. The horny nail plate contains no nerves or blood vessels.

NAIL STRUCTURE

The nails consist of three parts: nail body, nail root, and free edge.

The **nail body,** or **plate,** is the visible portion of the nail that rests upon, and is attached to, the **nail bed.** The nail body extends from the **root** to the **free edge.**

Although the nail plate seems to be one piece, it is actually constructed in layers. The readiness with which nails split, in both their length and thickness, clearly shows this form of structure.

The **nail root** is at the base of the nail and is embedded underneath the skin. It originates from an actively growing tissue known as the **matrix** (ma'triks).

The **free edge** is the end portion of the nail plate that reaches over the fingertip.

STRUCTURES ADJOINING THE NAIL

NAIL BED

The **nail bed** is the portion of the skin upon which the nail body rests. It is supplied with many blood vessels which provide the nourishment necessary for the continued growth of the nail. The nail bed also is abundantly supplied with nerves.

MATRIX

The **matrix** is that part of the nail bed that extends beneath the nail root, and contains nerves, lymph, and blood vessels. The matrix produces the nail as its cells undergo a reproducing and hardening process. The matrix will continue to grow as long as it receives nutrition and remains in a healthy condition.

However, the growth of the nails may be retarded if an individual is in poor health, if a nail disorder or disease is present, or if there is an injury to the nail matrix.

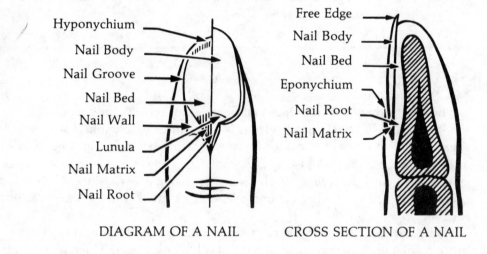

Hyponychium
Nail Body
Nail Groove
Nail Bed
Nail Wall
Lunula
Nail Matrix
Nail Root

Free Edge
Nail Body
Nail Bed
Eponychium
Nail Root
Nail Matrix

DIAGRAM OF A NAIL   CROSS SECTION OF A NAIL

LUNULA

The **lunula** (lu'nu-lah), or **half-moon,** is located at the base of the nail. The area underneath the lunula is the matrix. The light color of the lunula may be due to the reflection of light where the matrix and the connective tissue of the nail bed join.

PARTS SURROUNDING THE NAIL

The **cuticle** (ku'ti-kl) is the overlapping epidermis around the nail. A normal cuticle should be loose and pliable.

The **eponychium** (ep-o-nik'e-um) is the extension of the cuticle at the base of the nail body which partly overlaps the lunula.

The **hyponychium** (hi-po-nik'e-um) is that portion of the epidermis under the free edge of the nail.

The **perionychium** (per-i-o-nik'e-um) is that portion of the cuticle surrounding the entire nail border.

The **nail walls** are the folds of skin overlapping the sides of the nail.

The **nail grooves** are slits, or tracks, on the sides of the nail upon which the nail moves as it grows.

The **mantle** (man'tl) is the deep fold of skin in which the nail root is embedded.

NAIL GROWTH

The growth of the nail is influenced by nutrition, health, and disease. The nail grows forward, starting at the matrix and extending over the tip of the finger.

The average rate of growth in the normal adult is about ⅛" (.3125 cm) per month, growing faster in the summer than in the winter. The nails of children grow more rapidly, whereas those of elderly persons grow more slowly. The nail grows fastest on the middle finger and slowest on the thumb. Although toenails grow more slowly than fingernails, they are thicker and harder.

NAIL MALFORMATION

If the nail is separated from the nail bed through injury, it becomes distorted or discolored. Should the nail bed be injured after the loss of a nail, a badly formed nail will result.

The nails are neither shed automatically nor periodically, as are hairs. If the nail is torn off accidentally, or lost through an infection or disease, it will be replaced only as long as the matrix remains in good condition. Nails lost under such conditions are, on regrowth, frequently badly shaped, due to interference at the base of the nail. Ordinarily, replacement of the nail takes about four months.

VARIOUS SHAPES OF NAILS

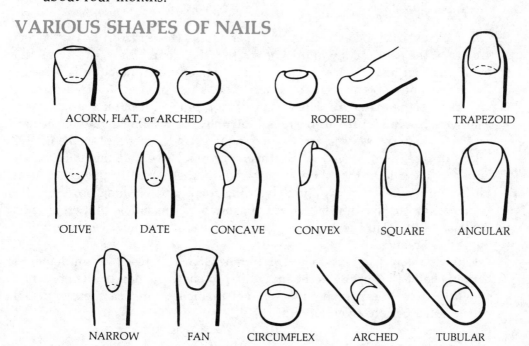

ACORN, FLAT, or ARCHED   ROOFED   TRAPEZOID

OLIVE   DATE   CONCAVE   CONVEX   SQUARE   ANGULAR

NARROW   FAN   CIRCUMFLEX   ARCHED   TUBULAR

NAIL DISORDERS

Diseases of the nail should never be treated by a manicurist. However, she should recognize normal and abnormal nail conditions, and understand the reasons for these conditions. Simple nail irregularities and blemishes come within the province of cosmetology and can be treated by the manicurist. A patron having a nail condition where infection, soreness, or irritation is present should be referred to a physician.

NAIL IRREGULARITIES

Corrugations, or **wavy ridges,** are caused by uneven growth of the nails, usually the result of illness or injury. When giving a manicure to a patron with this condition, carefully buff the nails slightly with pumice powder. This will help to remove or minimize the ridges.

Furrows (depressions) in the nails may run either lengthwise or across the nail. These are usually the result of illness or an injury to the nail cells in or near the matrix. Since these nails are exceedingly fragile, great care must be exercised in giving a manicure. Avoid the use of the metal pusher; use a cotton-tipped orangewood stick around the cuticle.

Leuconychia (lu-ko-nik'e-ah), or **white spots,** appear frequently in the nails, but do not indicate disease. They may be caused by injury to the base of the nail. As the nail continues to grow, these white spots eventually disappear.

Furrows.

Lengthwise depressions.　Crosswise depressions.　Leuconychia.　Onychauxis or hypertrophy.　Onychatrophia.

Onychauxis (on-e-kawk'sis), or **hypertrophy** (hi-per'tro-fi), is an overgrowth of the nail, usually in thickness rather than length. It is usually caused by an internal disturbance, such as a local infection. If infection is present, the nail is not to be manicured. If infection is not present, the nail may be included in the manicure. File it smooth and buff with pumice powder.

Onychatrophia (o-nik-ah-tro'fe-ah), **atrophy,** or **wasting away,** of the nail causes the nail to lose its luster, become smaller, and sometimes shed entirely. Injury or disease may account for this nail irregularity. File the nail smooth with the fine side of the emery board. Advise the patron to protect it from further injury, or from exposure to strong soaps and washing powders.

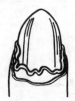
Pterygium.

Pterygium (te-rij'e-um) is a forward growth of the cuticle that adheres to the base of the nail. Use the cuticle nippers carefully to remove the growth. Suggest oil manicures.

Onychophagy (on-e-ko-fa'je), or **bitten nails,** is a result of an acquired nervous habit that prompts the individual to chew the nail or the hardened cuticle. Advise the patron that frequent manicures and care of hardened cuticle often help to overcome this habit.

Onychophagy.

Onychorrhexis (on-e-ko-rek'sis) refers to **split** or **brittle nails.** Among the causes of split nails are injury to the finger, careless filing of the nails, and excessive use of cuticle solvents and nail polish removers. Suggest oil manicures.

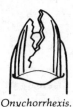

Onychorrhexis.

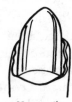

Hangnails.

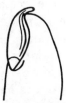

Eggshell nail.

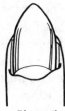

Blue nail.

Hangnail (agnail) is a condition in which the cuticle splits around the nail. Dryness of the cuticle, cutting off too much cuticle, or carelessness in removing the cuticle may result in hangnails. Advise the patron that proper nail care, such as hot oil manicures, will aid in correcting such condition. If not properly cared for, a hangnail may become infected.

Eggshell nails are recognized by the nail plate being noticeably thin, white, and much more flexible than normal nails. The nail plate separates from the nail bed and curves at the free edge. This disorder may be caused by a chronic illness of systemic or nervous origin.

Blue nails may be attributed to poor blood circulation, or a heart disorder. However, a patron with these conditions may receive a regular manicure.

A **bruised nail** will show dark, purplish (almost black or brown) spots in the nail. These are usually due to injury and bleeding in the nail bed. The dried blood attaches itself to the nail and grows out with it. Treat this injured nail gently. Avoid pressure.

Treating cuts. If a cut is accidently inflicted on a patron during a manicure, apply an antiseptic immediately. Do not buff or apply nail polish to the injured finger. To protect against infection, apply a sterile band-aid.

Infected finger. In the case of an infected finger, the patron should be referred to a physician.

NAIL DISEASES

There are several nail diseases that may be met during cosmetology practice. However, any nail disease that shows signs of infection or inflammation (redness, pain, swelling, or pus) must not be treated in a beauty salon. Medical treatment is required for all nail diseases.

Occupation plays an important role in the cause of many nail infections. Infections develop more readily in those who constantly immerse their hands in alkaline solutions. Natural oils are removed from the skin by frequent exposure to soaps, solvents, and other substances. The hands of the cosmetologist are exposed daily to chemical materials. Many of these are harmless, but others have potential dangers. The cosmetologist should safeguard her hands and nails by wearing protective gloves when working with chemicals.

Onychosis (on-i-ko'sis) is a technical term applied to any nail disease.

Onychomycosis (on-e-ko-mi-ko'sis), **tinea unguium** (tin'e-ah ung'gwe-um), or **ringworm of the nails,** is an infectious disease caused by a vegetable parasite. A common form consists of whitish patches that can be scraped off the surface. Another form appears as long yellowish streaks within the nail substance. The disease invades the free edge and spreads toward the root. The infected portion is thick and discolored. In a third form, the deeper layers of the nail are invaded, causing the superficial layers to appear irregularly thin. These infected layers peel off and expose the diseased parts of the nail bed.

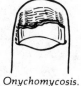

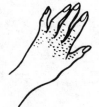

Onychomycosis.

Ringworm (tinea) of the hands is a highly contagious disease caused by a fungus (vegetable parasite). The principal symptoms are papular, red lesions occurring in patches or rings over the hands. Itching may be slight or severe.

Most cases of dermatitis of the hands resemble tinea, but are actually a contact dermatitis, plus a staphylococcic infection. Only a physician can determine this condition.

Tinea unguium.

Ringworm of the foot (athlete's foot). In acute conditions, deep, itchy, colorless vesicles appear. These appear singly, in groups, and sometimes on only one foot. They spread over the sole and between the toes, perhaps involving the nail fold and infecting the nail. When the vesicles rupture, the skin becomes red and oozes. The lesions dry as they heal. Fungus infection of the feet is likely to become chronic.

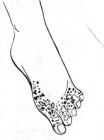

Athlete's foot.

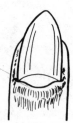

Paronychia.

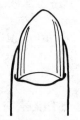

Onychocryptosis.

Both the prevention of infection and beneficial treatment are accomplished by keeping the skin cool, dry, and clean.

Paronychia (par-o-nik'e-ah), or **felon,** is an infectious and inflammatory condition of the tissues surrounding the nails. This condition is traceable to bacterial infection.

Onychia is an inflammation of the nail matrix, accompanied by pus formation. Improper sanitization of nail implements and bacterial infection may cause this disease.

Onychocryptosis (on-ik-o-krip-to'sis), or **ingrown nails,** may affect either the finger or toe. In this condition, the nail grows into the sides of the flesh and may cause an infection. Filing the nails too much in the corners and failing to correct hangnails are often responsible for ingrown nails.

Onychoptosis (on-e-kop-to'sis) is the periodic shedding of one or more nails, either in whole or in part. This condition may follow certain diseases, such as syphilis.

Onychoptosis.

Onycholysis (on-e-kol'i-sis) is a loosening of the nail, without shedding. It is frequently associated with an internal disorder.

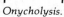

Onycholysis.

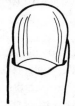

Onychophyma.

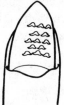

Onychophosis.

Onychogryposis.

Onychophyma (on-e-ko-fi'mah) denotes a swelling of the nail.

Onychophosis (on-e-ko-fo'sis) refers to a growth of horny epithelium in the nail bed.

Onychogryposis (on-e-ko-gri-po'sis) pertains to enlarged and increased curvature of the nails.

REVIEW QUESTIONS

THE NAIL

1. Describe the appearance of a healthy nail.
2. What are nails?
3. What is the main function of the nail?
4. What is the technical term for nail?
5. Of what is the nail composed?
6. Describe the structure of the nail plate.
7. Locate the following:
   - a) nail root
   - b) nail body
   - c) free edge
   - d) nail bed
8. What part of the nail contains the nerve and blood supply?
9. What three factors retard the growth of the nail?
10. Where does the formation of the nail occur?
11. How does the nail receive its nourishment?
12. Where is the lunula located?
13. What gives lunula the half-moon, whitish appearance?
14. Where is the eponychium found?
15. Define the following:
    - a) cuticle
    - b) mantle
    - c) nail groove
16. What is the hyponychium?
17. Define perionychium.
18. What two factors promote the growth of the nail?
19. Where does nail growth start and in which direction does it continue?
20. What is the average growth of the nail in the normal adult?
21. If a healthy nail is torn off, will it be replaced by a new one?

NAIL DISORDERS

1. Should an infected fingernail be given a manicure?
2. What may cause wavy ridges?
3. Match the following:
   a) leuconychia
   b) onychauxis
   c) onychophagy
   d) atrophy
   e) pterygium

   1) cuticle adhering to base of nail
   2) wasting away of nail
   3) bitten nails
   4) white spots in nail
   5) hypertrophy
4. List 12 abnormal conditions of the nails that do not prohibit a manicure.
5. What is the technical name for split or brittle nails?
6. What treatment would you recommend for brittle nails?
7. What are hangnails? Give their cause.
8. How are hangnails treated?
9. How is an accidental cut treated during a manicure?
10. Define onychosis.
11. What parasite causes ringworm of the nails?
12. What parasite causes ringworm of the hands?
13. What are the signs of athlete's foot (ringworm of the foot)?
14. What causes a paronychia condition?
15. Define onychia.
16. How is paronychia identified?
17. What toenail disease is identified by inflammation of the matrix accompanied by a pus formation?
18. What is the technical term for ingrown nails?
19. Match the following:
    a) onycholysis
    b) onychophyma
    c) onychoptosis

    1) swelling of nail
    2) periodic shedding of nail
    3) loosening of nail

Chapter 21

THEORY OF MASSAGE

CHAPTER LEARNING OBJECTIVES

The student successfully mastering this chapter will know:
1. *The purpose of massage.*
2. *The manipulations used in massage, and their beneficial results.*
3. *The various types of massage movements, and how they are applied.*
4. *The motor nerve points of the face and neck.*
5. *The physiological effects of massage.*

Massage is used to exercise facial muscles, maintain muscle tone, and stimulate circulation. Cosmetologists give massages to their patrons to help them keep their skin fresh and muscles firm.

To master massage techniques, a cosmetologist must have a knowledge of anatomy and physiology, and considerable practice in performing the various movements.

Massage involves the application of external manipulations to the head and body. This is accomplished manually or with the use of electrical appliances, such as therapeutic lamps, high-frequency current, facial steamers, heating caps, scalp steamers, and vibrators.

Areas of massage. The cosmetologist's services are limited to only certain areas of the body, namely:

Scalp	Upper chest and back
Face, neck, and shoulders	Hands and arms

CAUTION

Do not give a massage when certain conditions exist, such as a heart condition, high blood pressure, inflamed and swollen joints, or glandular swelling. Nor should you give a massage when abrasions of the skin, skin disorders, or broken capillaries are evident.

Qualifications. To inspire confidence in a patron, it is important that you give a massage with a firm, sure touch. To do this, you must develop:

Strong flexible hands	Self-control
A quiet temperament	The use of psychology

Keep your hands soft by using creams, oils, and lotions. Bevel nails smooth to prevent your scratching the patron's skin. Your wrists and fingers should be flexible, and palms firm, warm, and dry.

Cream, ointment, or oil should be applied to permit better hand movements and prevent drag or damage to the patron's skin.

HOW MANIPULATIVE MOVEMENTS ARE ACCOMPLISHED

Every massage treatment combines one or more of the basic movements. Each manipulation is applied in a definite way for a particular purpose. It is used according to the patron's condition and the desired results. The result of a massage treatment will depend on the amount of pressure, the direction of movement, and the duration of each type of manipulation. **Direction of movement is from the insertion of a muscle toward its origin.**

The **origin** of a muscle is the fixed attachment of one end of that muscle to a bone or tissue.

The **insertion** is the attachment of the opposite end of the muscle to another muscle, or to a movable bone or joint.

CAUTION

Massaging a muscle in the wrong direction (from its origin to its insertion) could result in the loss of resiliency and the sagging of the skin and muscles.

BASIC MANIPULATIONS USED IN MASSAGE

Effleurage (Stroking Movement)

Effleurage (ef-loo-rahzh). This is a light, continuous movement applied with the fingers and palms in a slow and rhythmic manner. No pressure is used. The palms are used **over large surfaces,** while the cushions of the fingertips are used **over small surfaces** (around the eyes). Effleurage is frequently applied to the forehead, face, scalp, back, shoulders, neck, chest, arms, and hands for its soothing and relaxing effects.

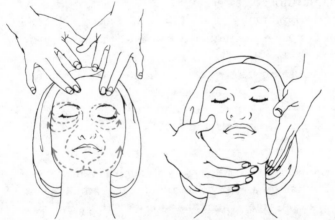
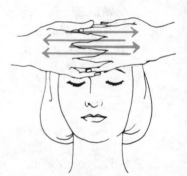

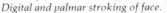
Digital and palmar stroking of face.   *Digital stroking of forehead.*

Position of fingers for stroking. Curve the fingers slightly, with just the cushions of the fingertips touching the skin. Do not use the end of the fingertips for massage movements. Fingertips cannot control the degree of pressure. In addition, the free edges of the fingernails are likely to scratch the skin.

Position of palms for stroking. Hold the whole hand loosely, keep the wrist and fingers flexible, and curve the fingers slightly to conform to the shape of the area being massaged.

Petrissage (Kneading Movement)

Petrissage (pe-tre-sahzh). Grasp the skin and flesh between the fingers and palm of the hand. As the tissues are lifted from their underlying structures, they are squeezed, rolled, or pinched with a **light, firm pressure**. This movement invigorates the part being treated and is usually limited to back, shoulder, and arm massage.

Purpose of kneading. The pressure should be light but firm. When grasping and releasing the fleshy parts, the movements must be in rhythm, never jerky. Kneading movements give deeper stimulation to the muscles, nerves, and skin glands, and improve the circulation.

Digital kneading of the cheeks can be achieved by light pinching movements.

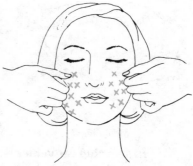

Digital kneading of cheeks.

Fulling, a form of petrissage, is used mainly in massage of the arms. With the fingers of both hands grasping the arm, a kneading movement is applied over the flesh. The kneading movement must be used with light pressure on the underside of the patron's forearm, and between the shoulder and elbow.

Friction (Deep Rubbing Movement)

Friction (frik'shun). This movement requires pressure on the skin while it is being moved over the underlying structures. Use your fingers or palms. Friction has a marked influence on the circulation and glandular activity of the skin.

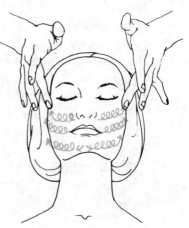

Circular friction on face.

Circular friction movements are usually used on the scalp, arms, and hands. **Light** circular friction movements are usually used on the face and neck.

Chucking, rolling, and **wringing** are variations of friction and are used principally to massage the arms and legs.

The **chucking movement** is accomplished by grasping the flesh firmly in one hand and moving the hand up and down along the bone, while the other hand keeps the arm or leg in a steady position.

The **rolling movement** requires that the tissues be compressed firmly against the bone and twisted around the arm or leg. Both hands of the cosmetologist are active as the flesh is twisted down the arm in the same direction.

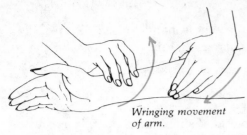

Wringing movement
of arm.

Wringing is a vigorous movement in which the cosmetologist's hands are placed a little distance apart on both sides of the arm or leg. While the hands are worked downward, the flesh is twisted against the bones in opposite directions.

Percussion or Tapotement Movement

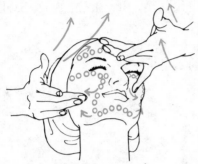

Digital tapping on face.

Percussion (per-kush'un), or **tapotement** (tah-pot-man'), consists of tapping, slapping, and hacking movements. This form of massage is the most stimulating. It should be applied with care and discretion.

In facial massage, use only **light digital tapping.** In tapping, the fingertips are brought down against the skin in rapid succession. The fingers must be flexible, to create an even force over the area being massaged.

In **slapping movements,** flexible wrists permit the palms to come in contact with the skin in light, firm, and rapid slapping movements. One hand follows the other. With each slapping stroke (which must be nothing more than a firm, light, and quick contact with the skin) the flesh is slightly lifted.

For **hacking movements,** use the wrists and outer edges of the hands. Both the wrists and fingers must move in fast, light, firm, flexible motions against the skin in alternate succession. **Hacking** and **slapping movements** are used mainly to massage the back, shoulders, and arms.

Percussion movements tone the muscles and impart a healthy glow to the part being massaged.

Vibration (Shaking Movement)

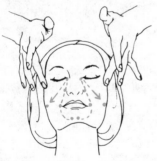

Vibratory movement of face.

Vibration (vi-bra'shun). This movement is accomplished by rapid muscular contractions in the arms of the cosmetologist, while the balls of the fingertips are pressed firmly on the point of application. It is a highly stimulating movement, and should be limited to only a few seconds duration on any one spot. Muscular contractions also can be produced by the use of a mechanical vibrator.

Joint Movements

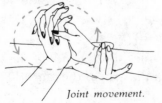

Joint movement.

Joint movements are restricted to the massage of the arm, hand, and foot. These movements are applied either with or without resistance. (For information on joint movements, see chapter on **Manicuring.**)

MOTOR NERVE POINTS OF THE FACE AND NECK

In order to obtain the maximum benefits from a facial massage, the cosmetologist must consider the motor nerve points which affect the underlying muscles of the face and neck.

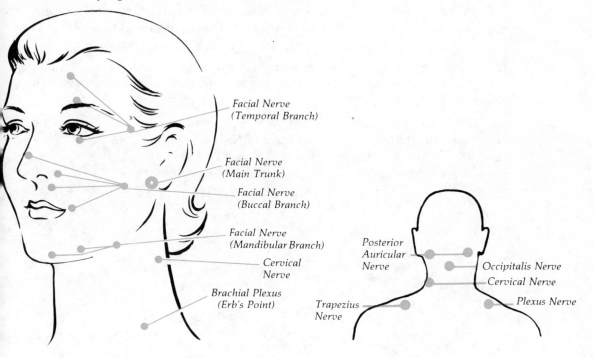

Facial Nerve
(Temporal Branch)

Facial Nerve
(Main Trunk)

Facial Nerve
(Buccal Branch)

Facial Nerve
(Mandibular Branch)

Cervical
Nerve

Brachial Plexus
(Erb's Point)

Posterior
Auricular
Nerve

Occipitalis Nerve

Cervical Nerve

Plexus Nerve

Trapezius
Nerve

PHYSIOLOGICAL EFFECTS OF MASSAGE

To obtain proper results from a scalp or facial massage, the cosmetologist must have a thorough knowledge of all the structures involved: muscles, nerves, and blood vessels.

Every muscle and nerve has a **motor point.** The location of motor points varies among individuals due to differences in body structures. However, a few manipulations on the right motor points will induce relaxation at the beginning of the massage treatment.

Skillfully applied massage directly or indirectly influences the structures and functions of the body. The immediate effects of massage are first noticed on the skin. The part being massaged responds by increased circulation, secretion, nutrition, and excretion.

The following beneficial results may be obtained by proper facial and scalp massage:

1. The skin and all its structures are nourished.
2. Fat cells in the subcutaneous tissue are reduced.
3. The skin is rendered soft and pliable.
4. The circulation of the blood is increased.
5. The activity of the skin glands is stimulated.
6. The muscle fiber is stimulated and strengthened.
7. The nerves are soothed and rested.
8. Pain is sometimes relieved.

Relaxation is achieved through light but firm, slow rhythmic movements, or very slow, light hand vibrations over the motor points for a short time. Another technique is to pause briefly over the motor points, using light pressure.

Body tissues are stimulated by movements of moderate pressure, speed, and time, or by light hand vibrations of moderate speed and time.

Body contours or fatty tissues are reduced by firm kneading, or by fast, firm, and light slapping movements over a fairly long period of time. Moderately fast hand vibrations with firm pressure also will accomplish this reduction.

The frequency of facial or scalp massage depends on the condition of the skin or scalp, the age of the patron, and the condition to be treated. As a general rule, normal skin or scalp can be kept in excellent condition with the help of a weekly massage, accompanied by the proper home care.

REVIEW QUESTIONS

THEORY OF MASSAGE

1. For what purpose is massage used?
2. What is meant by massage?
3. Which electrical appliances are used with facial, scalp, or body massages?
4. List three body conditions when massage should not be given.
5. Which three qualifications should a cosmetologist possess?
6. Give the technical and common names for five types of massage movements.
7. Describe the origin of a muscle.
8. Describe the insertion of a muscle.
9. In which direction should a muscle be massaged?
10. What is the effect of massaging the muscle in the wrong direction?
11. What kind of massage movements produce a soothing effect?
12. Describe the following movements: a) chucking; b) rolling; c) wringing.
13. What are the effects of massage on: a) skin; b) muscle fibers; c) fat cells; d) blood circulation; e) nerves, and f) pain?
14. How often may a massage be given to a patron with a normal skin or scalp?

Chapter 22

FACIALS

CHAPTER LEARNING OBJECTIVES

The student successfully mastering this chapter will know:
1. *The physical and psychological effects of a facial.*
2. *What materials and equipment are required for facial treatments.*
3. *The beneficial effects of a facial.*
4. *The procedure and manipulative skills required to give a facial.*
5. *The various types of corrective facials given in the beauty salon.*
6. *The variety and purpose of cosmetics used in facial treatments.*
7. *When to give an acne treatment.*
8. *Ingredients used in masks and packs.*
9. *The beneficial effects of masks and packs.*
10. *How to apply masks and packs.*
11. *How to remove masks and packs.*

Receiving a professional facial is one of the most enjoyable and relaxing services available to the beauty salon patron. Those individuals who have participated in this very restful or stimulating experience do not hesitate to return for repeat facials. When received as a regular periodic service, facials result in very noticeable improvement in the patron's skin tone, texture, and appearance.

Facial treatments can be developed into a profitable service. The patron's hairstyle may be beautiful, but if the face it frames is covered with an unattractive skin, the effect of the hairstyle will be lost.

The cosmetologist does not treat skin diseases. However, she must be able to recognize the various skin ailments that she cannot attempt to treat; she must also know when to advise the patron to see her doctor for treatment.

Facial treatments fall under two categories:
1. **Preservative**—maintaining the health of the facial skin by using correct cleansing methods, increasing circulation, relaxing the nerves, and activating the skin glands and metabolism through massage.
2. **Corrective**—correcting some facial skin conditions, such as dryness, oiliness, blackheads, aging lines, and minor conditions of acne.

Facial treatments are beneficial for:

1. Cleansing the skin.
2. Increasing circulation.
3. Activating glandular activity.
4. Relaxing the nerves.
5. Maintaining muscle tone.
6. Strengthening weak muscle tissue.
7. Correcting certain skin disorders.
8. Helping prevent the formation of wrinkles and aging lines.
9. Softening and improving skin texture and complexion.
10. Giving a youthful feeling.

PLAIN FACIAL

The patron enjoys the relaxation and stimulation from massage, the soothing effects of creams and lotions, and finally the application of an attractive makeup. Facials may be given as often as once a week, except where otherwise indicated.

PREPARATION

The facial booth should be located in the quietest area in the school or salon. From the moment the patron enters the booth, help her to relax by talking to her quietly and gently. Perform all work as noiselessly as possible.

All creams and packs should be removed from their containers with a spatula; never dip your fingers into any of the products used.

Everything that is to be used for the facial should be set out and arranged in an orderly manner.

EQUIPMENT, IMPLEMENTS, AND MATERIALS

Cleansing lotion	Talcum powder	Witch hazel
Cleansing cream	Head covering or	Makeup tray
Massage cream	headband	Tissue strips
Astringent lotion	Cotton pads	Lubricating oil
Skin freshener	Clean sheet and/or	High-frequency
(Milder astringent)	salon gown	machine and
Antiseptic solution	Safety pins	other apparatus
Infra-red lamp	Towels	Sponges
Cleansing tissues	Spatulas	Cotton swabs
Absorbent cotton	Facial steamer	

PROCEDURE

The information given here may be changed to conform with your instructor's routine.

1. **Prepare the patron.**
   a) Greet the patron and put her at ease by saying something complimentary. Be sincere.
   b) Ask the patron to remove her earrings and neck jewelry and place them in her purse.
   c) Help the patron remove her dress or blouse and carefully hang it up.

d) When seated in the facial chair, remove the patron's shoes and place booties on her feet.

e) Wash your hands.

f) Place a clean towel across the back of the facial chair. At no time should the patron's bare shoulders touch the chair.

g) Protect the patron's hair by fastening a headband lined with tissue around her hair.

There are several types of head coverings on the market. Some types are of a turban design; others are designed with elastic, similar to a shower cap. They are generally made of either cloth or paper towels. Draping the head with a towel is done in the following manner:

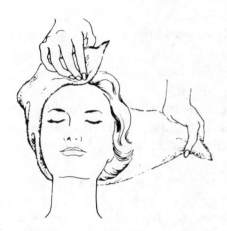 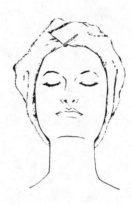

1. Fold the towel lengthwise from one of the top corners to the opposite lower corner, and place it over the headrest with the fold facing down. Place the towel on the headrest before the patron enters the facial area. When the patron is in a reclining position, the back of head should rest on the towel, so that one side of the towel can be brought up to the center of the forehead to cover the hairline.

2. With the other hand, bring the other side of the towel over the center and cross it over.

3. Use a regular bobby pin to hold the towel in place. Check to be sure that all strands of hair are tucked under the towel, earlobes are not bent, and the towel is not wrapped too tightly.

(For paper towel procedure, be guided by your instructor.)

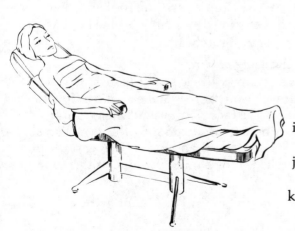

h) Remove lingerie straps from the patron's shoulders and adjust the towel, draping it across her chest and the middle of her back.

(Alternate method): If patron is given a strapless gown to wear, tuck the shoulder lingerie straps into the top of the gown.

i) Adjust the headrest, then lower the facial chair to a reclining position.

j) Cover the patron with a clean sheet or other suitable covering.

k) Wash your hands.

2. **Analyze the skin.**
   a) Remove makeup to determine:
      1. If the skin is dry.
      2. If the skin is oily.
      3. If comedones or acne are present.
      4. If broken capillaries are visible.
      5. If the skin texture is soft and velvety, or harsh and rough.
      6. The skin's color and fine lines.
   b) This analysis will determine:
      1. The choice of cream to use in massage.
      2. The amount of pressure to use in massage movements.
      3. The areas that need extra attention.
      4. If special lubricating oil is needed around the eyes and/or throat.
      5. The type of astringent to use.
      6. The color of makeup to apply.

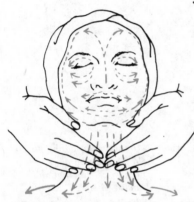

Spreading cream over the face, neck, chest, and back.

3. **Apply cleansing cream.**
   a) Remove a little cleansing cream from the jar with a spatula. Blend the cream with the fingers to soften it. (Remove lipstick and eye makeup very carefully.)
   b) Apply cream over the face, using both hands. Start at the chin and, with a sweeping movement, spread cream to the end of the jaw, from the base of the nose to the temples, along the side of the nose up over the bridge, between the brows, and across the forehead to the temples.
   c) Take additional cleansing cream and blend. Smooth down the neck, chest, and back with long, even strokes.
   d) Starting at the center of the forehead, go lightly around the eyes to the temples and back to the center of the forehead.
   e) Slide the fingers down the nose to the upper lip, smooth to the temples and the forehead, lightly down to the chin, then firmly up the jawline to the temples and forehead.

4. **Remove cleansing cream.**
   a) Remove cream with cleansing tissues or warm, moist towel. Start at the forehead and follow the contour of the face. Remove all the cream from one area before proceeding to the next. Finish with the neck, chest, and back. (If eyebrows are to be arched, they should be done at this time.)

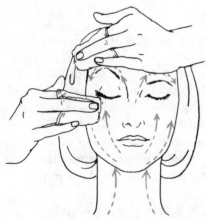

Removing cleansing cream with tissues or with a warm, moist towel.

5. **Steam the face** (optional).
   a) Steam the face mildly with warm, moist towels, or with a facial steamer.

6. **Apply massage cream.**

   a) Select a massage cream for the patron's skin type. Apply it in the same manner as the cleansing cream to face, neck, shoulders, and chest.

   (Use a lanolin or hormone cream for dry skin, but a cold cream will do for an oily skin.)

   b) If needed, apply special lubricating oil around the eyes and neck.

7. **Give facial manipulations** (either before or during exposure to infra-red lamp).

   a) Cover the patron's eyes with cotton pads moistened with witch hazel.

   b) Place the lamp at a comfortable distance.

   c) Expose face to infra-red rays for 3-5 minutes.

   d) Massage face as described on next page.

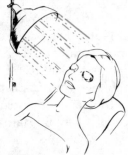

Exposing the face to an infra-red lamp.

8. **Remove massage cream.**

   a) Remove cream with tissues or warm, moist towels in the same manner as followed for removing cleansing cream.

9. **Apply astringent lotion.**

   a) Sponge the face with cotton pledgets moistened with astringent lotion.

10. **Apply foundation and makeup.**

11. **Completion.**

    a) Return the facial chair to an upright position.

    b) Remove the protective head covering.

    c) Remove the protective towel and body covering.

    d) Assist the patron with her garments and shoes.

12. **Cleanup.**

    a) Discard all disposable supplies and materials.

    b) Close containers tightly, clean them, and put them in their proper places.

    c) Place used towels in appropriate container.

    d) Tidy up the booth. Return unused cosmetics to the dispensary.

    e) Wash and sanitize your hands.

REMINDERS AND HINTS IN FACIAL MASSAGE

1. Try to get the patron to relax.
2. Provide quiet atmosphere; speak softly.
3. Maintain a clean, orderly arrangement of supplies.
4. Follow systematic procedure.
5. If your hands are cold, warm them before touching the patron.
6. Make sure your fingernails are not too long or pointed.

FACIAL MANIPULATIONS

In giving facial manipulations, you must remember that an even tempo, or rhythm, induces relaxation. Do not remove your hands from the patron's face once the manipulations have been started. Should it become necessary to remove your hands, feather them off, and then gently replace them with feather-like movements.

Note: Each instructor may have developed her own routine in giving manipulations. The following illustrations merely show the different movements that may be used on the various parts of the face, chest, and back. (Follow your instructor's routine.)

Massage movements are usually directed towards the **origin** of a muscle, in order to avoid damage to muscular tissues.

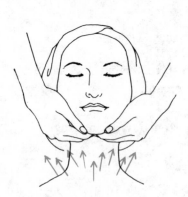

1. CHIN MOVEMENT.
Lift the chin, using a slight pressure.

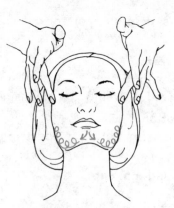

2. LOWER CHEEKS.
Using a circular movement, rotate from chin to ears.

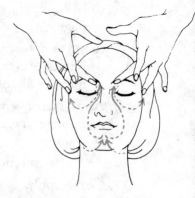

3. MOUTH, NOSE, AND CHEEK MOVEMENTS.
Follow diagram.

Note: Many facial specialists prefer to start massage manipulations at the chin, while others prefer to start at the forehead. Both are correct. Be guided by your instructor.

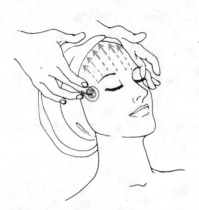

4. LINEAR MOVEMENT OVER FOREHEAD.
Slide fingers to temples; rotate with pressure on upward stroke; slide to left eyebrow; then stroke to hairline across forehead and back.

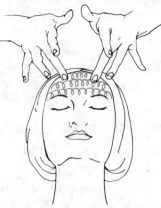

5. CIRCULAR MOVEMENT OVER FOREHEAD.
Starting at eyebrow line, work across middle of forehead, and then towards the hairline.

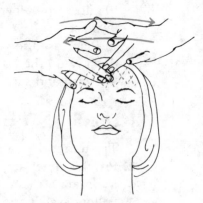

6. CRISS-CROSS MOVEMENT.
Start at one side of forehead and work back.

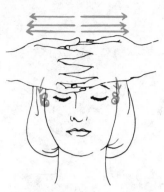

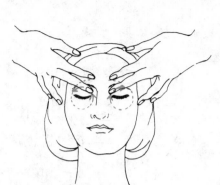

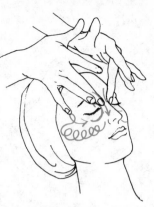

7. STROKING (HEADACHE) MOVEMENT.
Slide fingers to center of forehead; then draw fingers, with slight pressure, toward temples, and rotate.

8. BROW AND EYE MOVEMENT.
Place middle fingers at inner corner of eyes and index fingers over brows. Slide to outer corners of eyes, under eyes, and back to inner corners.

9. NOSE AND UPPER CHEEK MOVEMENT.
Slide fingers down nose. Apply rotary movement across cheeks to temples, and rotate gently. Slide fingers under eyes and back to bridge of nose.

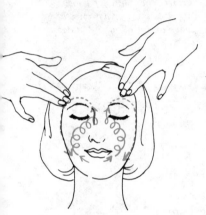

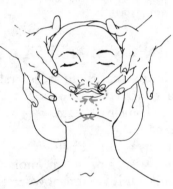

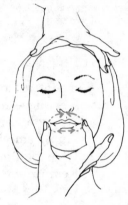

10. MOUTH AND NOSE MOVEMENT.
Apply circular movement from corners of mouth up sides of nose. Slide fingers over brows and down to corners of mouth.

11. LIP AND CHIN MOVEMENT.
Draw fingers from center of upper lip, around mouth, going under lower lip and chin.

12. (OPTIONAL MOVEMENT.)
Hold head with left hand; draw fingers of right hand from under the lower lip, around mouth, to center of upper lip.

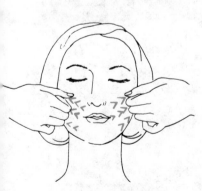

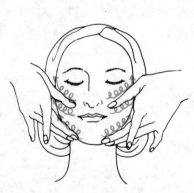

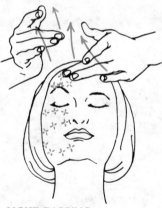

13. LIFTING MOVEMENT OF CHEEKS.
Proceed from the mouth to ears, and then from nose to top part of ears.

14. ROTARY MOVEMENT OF CHEEKS.
Massage from chin to ear lobes, from mouth to middle of ears, and from nose to top of ears.

15. LIGHT TAPPING MOVEMENT.
Work from chin to earlobe, mouth to ear, nose to top of ear, and then across forehead. Repeat on other side.

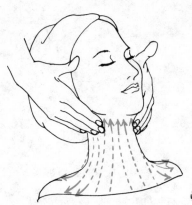

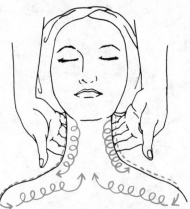

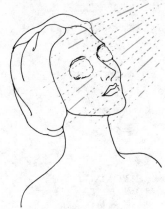

16. STROKING MOVEMENT OF NECK.
Apply light upward strokes over front of neck. Use heavier pressure on sides of neck in downward strokes.

17. CIRCULAR MOVEMENT OVER NECK AND CHEST.
Starting at back of ears, apply circular movement down side of neck, over shoulders, and across chest.

18. INFRA-RED LAMP (OPTIONAL).
Protect eyes with eye pads; adjust lamp over patron's face; leave on for about 5 minutes.

CHEST, BACK, AND NECK MANIPULATIONS (OPTIONAL)

Some instructors prefer to treat these areas first before starting the regular facial. A suggested procedure is as follows:

1. Apply and remove cleansing cream.
2. Apply emollient cream.
3. Give manipulations as outlined below.
4. Remove cream with tissues or warm, moist towel.
5. Dust the back lightly with talcum powder and smooth.

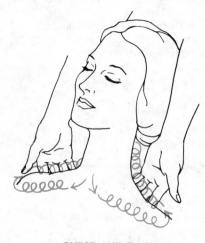

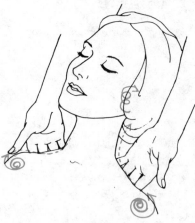

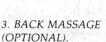

1. CHEST AND BACK MOVEMENT.
Use rotary movement across chest and shoulders, then to spine. Slide fingers to base of neck. Rotate 3 times.

2. SHOULDERS AND BACK MOVEMENT.
Rotate shoulders 3 times. Glide fingers to spine, then to base of neck. Apply circular movement up to back of ear, and then slide fingers to front of earlobe. Rotate 3 times.

3. BACK MASSAGE (OPTIONAL).
To stimulate and relax patron, use thumbs and bent index fingers to grasp the tissue at the back of the neck. Rotate 6 times. Repeat over shoulders and back to the spine.

SPECIAL PROBLEMS

FACIAL FOR DRY SKIN

A dry skin is caused by an insufficient flow of sebum (oil) from the sebaceous glands. The facial for dry skin helps correct the dry condition of the skin. It may be given with or without an electrical current. For more effective results, the use of electrical current is recommended.

PROCEDURE WITH INFRA-RED RAYS

1. Prepare the patron as for a plain facial.
2. Apply cleansing cream; remove with tissues or with warm, moist towel.
3. Sponge the face with cleansing lotion (for dry skin).
4. Apply massage cream.
5. Apply lubricating oil, or eye cream, over and under the eyes.
6. Apply lubricating oil over the neck.
7. Cover the patron's eyes with cotton pads moistened with witch hazel or boric acid solution.
8. Expose the face and neck to infra-red rays for not more than 5 minutes.
9. Give manipulations 3-5 times.
10. Remove massage cream and oil with tissues or with a warm, moist towel.
11. Apply skin lotion suitable for dry skin.
12. Blot face with tissues or towel.
13. Apply a base foundation and makeup suitable for the patron's skin tones.
14. Complete and clean up as for a plain facial.

CAUTION

For dry skin, avoid using lotions that contain a large percentage of alcohol. Read manufacturer's directions.

PROCEDURE WITH GALVANIC CURRENT

The procedure for giving a dry skin facial with galvanic current is similar to the procedure for giving a dry skin facial with infra-red rays, with a few changes:

1. Repeat Steps 1-3 of the Procedure with Infra-red Rays.
2. Apply negative galvanic current for 3-5 minutes, to open the pores.
3. Repeat Steps 4-11 of the Procedure with Infra-red Rays.
4. Apply positive galvanic current 3-5 minutes, to close the pores.
5. Repeat Steps 12-14 of the Procedure with Infra-red Rays.

DRY, SCALY SKIN FACIAL WITH INDIRECT HIGH-FREQUENCY CURRENT

1. Follow Steps 1-8 of the Procedure with Infra-red Rays.

2. Give manipulations, using the indirect method of applying high-frequency current, for not more than 7 minutes.
3. Apply 2-3 cold towels to the face and neck.
4. Sponge the face and neck with skin freshener (milder astringent).
5. Apply a base foundation and makeup suitable for the patron's skin tones.
6. Complete and clean up as for a plain facial.

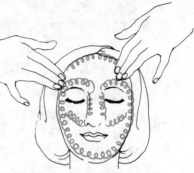

High-frequency indirect method. Patron holds electrode.

FACIAL FOR OILY SKIN AND BLACKHEADS (COMEDONES)

An oily skin and/or blackheads (**comedones**) are caused by a hardened mass of sebum formed in the ducts of sebaceous glands.

Note: For appropriate diet to minimize an oily skin and blackheads, the patron should be guided by her medical doctor.

PROCEDURE

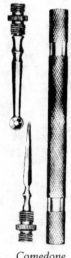

Comedone extractor.

1. Prepare the patron as for a plain facial.
2. Apply cleansing cream; remove it with warm, moist towel. If the skin is extremely oily, it may be washed with warm water and a medicated soap.
3. Apply cleansing lotion for an oily skin.
4. Reapply cleansing cream and steam the face with 3-4 moist, warm towels, or steam the face with the facial steamer, to open the pores.
5. Cover the fingertips with tissues and gently press out blackheads. Do not press so hard as to bruise skin tissue. Blackheads also may be removed with a sanitized comedone extractor.
6. Sponge the face with an antiseptic.
7. Cover the patron's eyes with pads moistened with witch hazel or boric acid solution.
8. Apply blue light over the bare skin for not more than 3-5 minutes.
9. Apply massage cream suitable for this condition.
10. Give manipulations.
11. Remove cream with warm, moist towel.
12. Moisten a pledget of cotton with an astringent lotion. Apply it to the face and neck with upward and outward movements, to close the pores.
13. Blot excess moisture with tissues.
14. Apply a base foundation and suitable makeup.
15. Complete and clean up as for a plain facial.

TREATMENT FOR WHITEHEADS (MILIA)

Milia, or whiteheads, is a common skin disorder, caused by the formation of sebaceous matter within or under the skin. It usually occurs in skin of fine texture. The surface openings may be so small that the sebum cannot exude. As a result, it collects in small, hardened, round, pearly-white formations under the skin.

This condition may be treated under the supervision of a dermatologist.

FACIAL FOR ACNE

Since acne is a disorder of the sebaceous glands, it requires medical direction. If the patron is under medical care, the role of the cosmetologist is to work closely with the patron's physician and carry out his instructions as to the kind and frequency of treatment.

Under medical direction, the cosmetologist must limit the cosmetic treatment of acne to the following measures:

1. Reducing the oiliness of the skin by local applications.
2. Removing blackheads with a sanitized comedone extractor.
3. Cleansing the skin.
4. Using special medicated preparations.
5. Suggesting a regulated diet.

EQUIPMENT, IMPLEMENTS, AND MATERIALS

Acne cream or ointment	Facial glass electrode
Acne lotion	Medicated soap
Antiseptic	Skin toner
Cleansing cream	Cotton mask
Medicated cleansing lotion	High-frequency apparatus and accessories
Towels	Other supplies used in a plain facial
Astringent lotion for oily skin	

PROCEDURE

1. Prepare the patron as for a plain facial.
2. Cleanse the face with medicated soap and warm water.
3. Apply acne cream or ointment over the face and neck.
4. Apply high-frequency current with direct application over the affected parts for not more than 5 minutes.
5. Remove the acne cream or ointment with tissues or warm, moist towel.
6. Saturate a thin cotton mask with acne lotion. Apply the mask to the face and affected parts, then resaturate with acne lotion if necessary. Retain for 10 minutes.
7. Remove the mask and blot residue with a cool, wet towel.
8. Saturate cotton pledgets with astringent lotion, and apply with a light blotting movement.
9. Moisten a piece of cotton with an antiseptic lotion and touch each pimple (acne).
10. Apply lipstick only, unless a medicated foundation lotion is used.
11. Complete and clean up as for a plain facial.

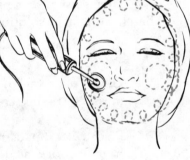

Applying high-frequency current with facial electrode.

CAUTION

Avoid the use of regular facial makeup.

DIET FOR ACNE

Modern studies show that acne may be due to hereditary and environmental factors. It can be aggravated by emotional stress and faulty diet. Acne is not believed to be caused by any particular food or drink, but foods high in fats, starches and sugars tend to worsen the condition. The patron should consult a physician for a prescribed diet. A well balanced diet, drinking plenty of water, and following healthful personal hygiene habits are recommended.

PACKS AND MASKS

Face packs and masks are popular in the beauty salon. They can be used as part of a facial or applied as a separate treatment.

Pack facials are recommended for normal and oily skin, and are usually applied directly to the skin. On the other hand, **mask** facials are recommended for dry skin, and are applied to the skin with the aid of gauze layers or masks.

PACK FACIALS

Clay and lemon packs are usually recommended for normal or oily skins.

A bleach pack can be used to reduce the visibility of freckles. However, it may take as many as five applications before any improvement is noticed.

EQUIPMENT, IMPLEMENTS, AND MATERIALS

All items used for a plain facial, plus witch hazel, boric acid solution, and facial packs.

PROCEDURE

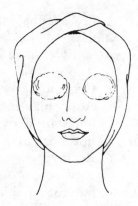

1. Give a plain facial, including removal of massage (tissue) cream, after manipulations.
2. Place cotton pads moistened with witch hazel or boric acid solution over eyes.
3. Apply chosen pack—either clay, lemon, or bleach. Keep it away from the nose, eyes, and mouth.

Pack applied, and eyes protected.

Note: *If a bleach pack is used, protect the eyebrows with emollient cream.*

4. Allow the pack to remain on the skin until dry. (Follow manufacturer's directions.)
5. Remove the pack carefully with a warm steamed towel.
6. Apply an astringent and pat dry.
7. Apply makeup.

There are various commercial packs available. Follow manufacturer's directions as to their preparation and application.

EGG PACK

A prepared egg facial pack is recommended to cleanse the pores and tighten the skin. It should be used only on skin tough enough to withstand its drawing power. An egg pack should be left on the face 3-5 minutes. However, if the patron feels any discomfort, the pack should be removed immediately with a moist, warm towel. After removing the pack, apply skin lotion and dry the face. Finish as for a plain facial.

HOT OIL MASK FACIAL

A hot oil mask facial is usually recommended for dry skin and for skin inclined to wrinkle. The mask is applied directly to the skin with the aid of gauze layers. Openings are provided for the mouth, eyes, and nostrils.

EQUIPMENT, IMPLEMENTS, AND MATERIALS

All items used for a plain facial, plus the following:

Scissors	Hot oil preparation
2 sections of gauze or prepared	Hot oil heater
gauze facial mask	Red dermal lamp

Formulas for a hot oil mask may contain prepared olive oil and massage oil, or equal parts of massage cream and massage oil may be used. The mixture is heated in a small container. A gauze facial mask is prepared by cutting openings with scissors for the mouth, nose, and eyes.

Various commercial masks are now available. Follow manufacturer's directions as to their preparation and application.

PROCEDURE

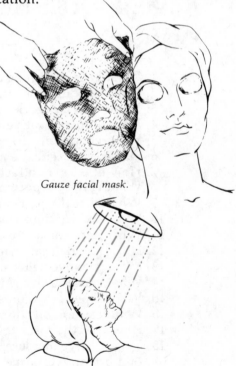

Gauze facial mask.

Red dermal lamp.

1. Give a plain facial, including the removal of massage cream.
2. Cover the eyes with eye pads moistened with witch hazel or boric acid solution.
3. Moisten gauze facial mask with warm oil and place on face, starting at the throat.
4. Place a red dermal lamp or infrared ray lamp about 24" (60 cm) from the patron's face.
5. Allow the patron to rest 5-10 minutes under the lamp.
6. Remove the gauze facial mask.
7. Apply additional massage or moistening cream.
8. Give facial manipulations.
9. Remove cream with a warm steamed towel.
10. Apply an astringent lotion and then apply makeup.

Various commercial masks are now available. Follow manufacturer's directions as to their preparation and application.

FIFTEEN REASONS WHY A PATRON MAY FIND FAULT WITH A FACIAL

A patron may find fault with the cosmetologist giving her a facial for the following reasons:

1. Offensive body odor, foul breath, or tobacco odor.
2. Harming or scratching the skin.
3. Excessive or rough massage.
4. Getting facial creams into eyes.
5. Using towels that are too hot.
6. Breathing into the patron's face.
7. Not being careful or sanitary.
8. Not showing interest in the patron's skin problems.
9. Carelessness in removing cream, leaving a greasy film behind the ears, under the chin, or in other areas.
10. Not permitting the patron to relax, either by talking or being tense while giving facial manipulations.
11. Being disorganized, and going frequently for supplies.
12. Heavy, rough, or cold hands.
13. Lack of rhythm in facial manipulations.
14. Massaging muscles in the wrong direction.
15. Exerting too much pressure on the face.

REVIEW QUESTIONS

FACIALS

1. What benefits can be achieved by a patron who receives regular facials?
2. What conditions of the skin may not be treated by a cosmetologist?
3. Name two categories under which facial treatments fall.
4. How do preservative treatments maintain the health of the facial skin?
5. What conditions do corrective treatments help?
6. Name six specific benefits of facial treatments.
7. How often may a facial generally be given?
8. What is the purpose of draping the patron's head before a facial?
9. Why must the patron's skin be analyzed before a facial?
10. What six decisions does skin analysis help the cosmetologist to make?
11. What implement is used to remove cream from a jar?
12. How should facial manipulations be given to induce relaxation in a patron?
13. Massage movements are usually directed toward what part of the muscle?
14. What causes a dry skin?
15. What types of lotion should be avoided when treating dry skin?
16. What causes comedones?
17. How does the cosmetologist close the pores when giving an oily skin facial?
18. To what five measures must a cosmetologist limit her cosmetic treatment of a patron with acne?
19. For what type of skin are packs recommended?
20. For what type of skin are masks recommended?
21. When are the following facial packs used?
    a) bleach pack; b) clay pack; c) lemon pack; d) egg pack.
22. For what type of skin is a hot oil mask facial used?

Chapter 23

FACIAL MAKEUP

CHAPTER LEARNING OBJECTIVES

The student successfully mastering this chapter will know:
1. *The composition of facial cosmetics.*
2. *How to recognize the various facial types.*
3. *The procedure of makeup application.*
4. *How to minimize facial defects by the use of corrective makeup.*
5. *The proper makeup application for the various facial types.*
6. *The kinds of makeup cosmetics and their purposes.*
7. *The proper corrective makeup for the eyes, lips, and cheeks.*
8. *The technique for properly shaping the eyebrows.*
9. *The safety precautions to be exercised in the application of makeup.*

Makeup is applied to the face for the purpose of improving its appearance. The main objective of a makeup application is to emphasize good facial features and to minimize defects. There is no fixed pattern for applying facial makeup. In practicing this art, the cosmetologist must carefully analyze each patron's face and consider her individual needs.

The professional who applies makeup must take into consideration the structure of the patron's face, the inter-relationships of color, and the basic principles of optical illusions. Makeup is used to create shadow and light, and to develop the illusion of facial beauty. The appearance of beauty can be achieved by properly coordinating facial makeup, hairstyle, and clothing colors.

PREPARATION

Makeup is usually applied after a facial massage. If it is applied just before a comb-out, remove rollers and clips.

Sit or stand in back of, or slightly to one side of, the patron to administer this service. However, if necessary, move to the front of the patron, to ease or facilitate the makeup application.

Note: Wash and sanitize your hands. All items used for applying and removing makeup must be sanitized.

Products must be removed from containers with a sanitized spatula or clean applicator.

DRAPING

Before applying makeup, properly drape the patron to protect her skin, hair, and clothing, and have her recline in a facial chair with her head slightly raised.

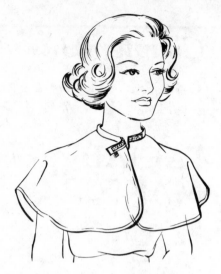

IMPLEMENTS AND MATERIALS

Appropriate cleansing cream or lotion
Tissues
Cotton pads
Cosmetic sponges
Cotton pledgets
Astringent lotion or skin freshener
Moisturizer or other products for use under the foundation
Cream, liquid, or cake foundation
Shading and highlighting cosmetics for facial contouring and corrective makeup
Spatulas
Disposable towels
Disposable cotton or felt-tipped applicators

Disposable cotton puffs
Draping sheets and towels
Headband or turban
Liquid, cream, or powdered cheek color (rouge)
Face powder
Eye colors and eye shadow
Eyebrow pencils
Eyeliner (cake or liquid)
Mascara (cream or dry)
Eye makeup applicators and brushes
Lip colors (a variety of colors)
Lip color applicators (brushes and pencils)

COSMETICS USED IN FACIAL MAKEUP

FOUNDATION FOR MAKEUP

Probably no single item of makeup is as important as the foundation. Its proper application creates a pleasing facial contour, evens out skin color, provides a base for color harmony, conceals minor imperfections, and protects the skin from soil, wind, and weather. As many as three different foundation colors may be used at the same time in a corrective makeup application.

Skin tones determine the color of the foundation base. Skin tones are generally classified as follows: white, ivory, cream, pink, florid, sallow, olive, tan, brown, and ebony.

Choice of foundation color. In choosing the foundation color for light skin, a shade darker than the natural skin tone is usually desirable to impart color. When the skin is dark, match the foundation to the natural skin tone. Selecting the correct foundation color is of extreme importance to the success of the entire makeup application.

For either a sallow or pale skin tone, a rosy foundation and powder generally will give the desired glow.

For a florid skin tone, a biege foundation and powder will soften the reddish tone.

For all other skin tones (fair, medium, or dark), select the depth of foundation and powder to blend with the lightness or darkness of the skin tone.

Note: Too light a foundation makes the face look pale and artificial. A little foundation goes a long way. Using too much of it is undesirable as it gives the skin a pasty appearance.

Selecting the right foundation. Liquid and cream foundations are the most widely used, and they give a slight sheen to the skin. Water based or cake foundations give a matte (dull) finish.

1. **Cream foundation** gives the most natural look and a longer lasting makeup. It is formulated for both dry and oily skin types.
2. **Liquid (lotion) foundation** is a color suspended in an emulsion of delicate light oil. For quick and effective blending, apply it on one skin area at a time, using long, smooth strokes.
3. **Cake foundation** adds color, gives a smooth and velvety look, and helps conceal minor skin discoloration. It is applied with a moistened pad. Cake foundation is effective for an oily skin. To prevent drying, apply a moisturizer to dry skin before applying cake makeup.

Skin blemishes can be hidden with the aid of:

1. **Stick foundation.** Makeup in stick form is particularly useful in the covering or masking of minor skin blemishes. The advantage of a stick is that it can easily be applied to a small blemish to give a relatively thick film coverage.
2. **Blemish masking creams** are similar to the pigmented foundation creams.

FACE POWDERS

Face powders improve the overall attractiveness of the skin by concealing skin blemishes, toning down excessive coloring, gloss, or shine, enhancing the natural skin coloring, and adding delicate scent. Modern powders make the skin soft and velvety to the touch.

Face powders come in cake or powdered form, in a wide variety of shades, and in different weights. Light and medium weights may be used on dry and normal skin. Use a heavy weight powder on oily skin. Face powder should be selected to blend with the color tone of the skin.

Generally, the selected shade of face powder may be the same shade as the foundation, or a shade lighter. However, a powder that is darker than the foundation may be used when deeper color is desired.

Translucent (colorless) powder blends with all foundations and will not turn color when applied.

The purpose of **cheek color** is to give a soft glow of color to the face. It aids in creating better facial contours by minimizing imperfect features.

Cheek color should coordinate with, or be the same color as, the lip color. However, cheek color that is a shade lighter than the lip color generally is more desirable than a darker shade. The color on the cheeks should be less vivid in broad daylight than in artificial light. Bright colors call attention to that area of the face and the makeup begins to look artificial.

There are four types of cheek color: liquid, cream, dry, and brush on.

1. **Liquid cheek color** blends well and is suitable for all skin types. Apply it over the foundation before powdering the face.
2. **Cream cheek color** closely resembles pigmented foundation creams and cream makeup. Cream cheek color is generally preferred for dry and normal skin.
3. **Dry (compact) cheek color** imparts a matte (dull) finish. If well formulated, it blends harmoniously with the facial makeup.
4. **Brush-on powdered cheek color** is easy to use and is applied with a special cosmetic brush.

Lip color adds color to the lips and helps to correct the shape of the mouth. Artistry and a keen sense of fashion are essential in selecting the appropriate lip color shade or tint. Also to be considered is whether the prevailing fashion calls for a light or dark lip color, and whether a thin or thick film application is desirable.

The basic tints and shades of lip color are blue-red, yellow-red, orange, and true red. All shades and tints of lip color originate from these basic colors.

Lip color is available in stick, cream, and liquid form.

EYE MAKEUP

Eye colors and shadows are produced in pastel blue, pastel turquoise, lavender-mauve, grey, blue, pastel green, metallic silver, metallic blue, and shades of chestnut, beige, and brown.

Eye color or **shadow,** when applied to the upper lids, complements the eyes by making them look brighter and more expressive. As a general rule, the eye color or shadow should match the color of the eyes, or be a shade lighter. The eye color or shadow should be more subtle for daytime wear, whereas the colors or shadows for evening wear can be more sophisticated.

Eye colors and shadows are available in stick, cream, and cake form.

Eyeliners are intended for application to the eyelids, close to the lashes. They are made in shading tones, and may either be in pencil, cake, or liquid form, packaged with a small semi-stiff applicator brush. Color shades correspond to those for eye colors and shadows, but they are more intense. The eyeliner should be the same color as the mascara.

Eyebrow pencils are used to modify the natural outline of the eyebrows, usually after tweezing, and to heighten the effect. They may be used to darken the eyebrows, to fill in where the brow is thin or devoid of hair, and to correct misshapen brows. Eyebrow pencils cannot be sanitized. Brush-on brow color comes in powdered form and is applied with a brush. Cream, liquid and cake eyebrow colorings are other types that may be applied with a brush.

Mascara is available in liquid, cake, and cream form. Mascara colors come in black, brown, and a variety of other tints and shades. When applied to the eyelashes, mascara makes them look fuller and longer. It also can be used to darken the eyebrows.

Mascara and eyebrow pencil colors should be the same or color co-ordinated. Usually, the lashes look better when darker than the brows.

PROCEDURE FOR APPLYING A PROFESSIONAL MAKEUP

(The procedure given here may be changed to conform with your instructor's preferred routine.)

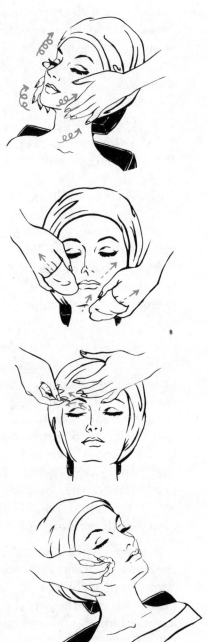

1. **Apply cleansing cream or lotion.** Remove a small quantity of cleanser from the container with a spatula and place it in the palm of the left hand, or apply a dab of lotion to an applicator. With the fingertips of the right hand, place dabs of cleanser on the forehead, nose, cheeks, chin, and neck. Spread the cleanser over the face and neck with light upward and outward circular movements.

2. **Remove the cleanser** with tissue mitts or moistened cotton pads, using an upward and outward motion. Be especially gentle around the eyes. If necessary, apply cleanser a second time, to remove heavy makeup or color on the eyes and lips.

3. **Eyebrows.** Eyebrow arching is a complete service in itself. The procedure for arching is given in another section of this chapter. However, you may remove a few straggly hairs before a facial makeup by tweezing the hair in the same direction in which it grows.

4. **Apply astringent lotion or skin freshener (toner).** For oily skin, apply astringent lotion; for dry skin, apply a skin freshener (mild astringent). Moisten a cotton pad with the lotion and pat it lightly over the entire face and under the chin and neck. Blot off excess moisture with tissues or a cotton pad.

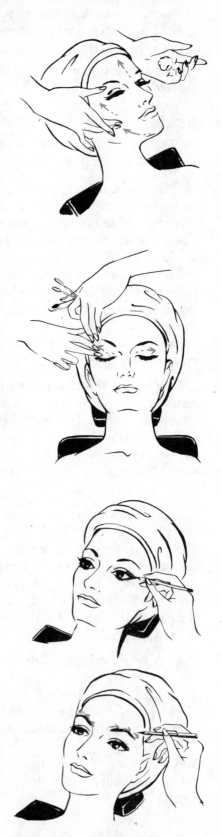

5. **Apply foundation.** Select the appropriate type and color of foundation. Test for color by blending the foundation on the patron's jawline. Place a small amount of the foundation in the palm of your hand. With the tips of your fingers, apply sparingly and evenly over the entire face and around the neckline. Use gentle upward and outward motions. Blend carefully near the hairline, and remove excess foundation with a cosmetic sponge or cotton pledget. When a moisturizer is needed, apply it in the same way, but before applying the foundation.

6. **Apply eye color** (or **shadow**). Select color to match or complement the eyes. Apply color lightly on the upper lid and softly blend outward with the color applicator or the fingertips. Shade a prominent puffy area beneath the brow, or highlight a small space between the eyelid and the brow. Eye color may be selected to complement the color of the clothing. For example, blue eye color may be worn with a blue dress.

7. **Apply eyeliner.** Eyeliner is used to make the eyes look larger and lashes appear thicker. Select cake or liquid liner in a color to harmonize with the mascara you will apply. Pull eyelid taut, and gently draw a very fine line along the entire lid, as close to the lashes as possible. If eyeliner pencil is used, the point should be fine and care should be taken to avoid injury or discomfort to the patron.

8. **Apply eyebrow makeup.** Brush the brows in place. With light feathery strokes, apply color with a fine pointed pencil. Brush the brows carefully. Excess color can be removed with a cotton-tipped swab.

9. **Apply mascara.** Ask the patron to open her eyes wide. Put a small amount of cream mascara on a clean brush. Apply the mascara to the upper lashes by brushing gently upward and outward on the underside of the lashes. Gently brush a small amount of mascara on the lower lashes. When applying moistened dry mascara, or the applicator wand type, use according to manufacturer's directions.

10. **Apply cheek color (rouge).** Cheek color is sometimes applied after the application of foundation and before powdering. Dry powdered cheek color is brushed on following the application of powder. Select the appropriate type and color. Have the patron smile, to raise the cheeks. Apply liquid or cream cheek color with a sanitized applicator, and blend carefully upward and outward toward the temples.

11. **Apply powder.** Following the application of foundation, apply powder with a sanitary cotton puff or a cosmetic sponge. Press it over the face and whisk the excess away with a powder brush or puff. A moistened cosmetic sponge may be pressed lightly over the finished makeup.

12. **Apply lip color (lipstick).** Lip color is removed from its container with a sanitized spatula. The lips are first outlined with a sanitized applicator such as a brush or pencil. Rest the ring finger on the patron's chin, to steady your hand. Ask the patron to relax her lips and part them slightly. Brush on the lip color. Ask the patron to stretch her lips in a slight smile, to enable you to smooth the lip color in any small crevices. After the lip color application, blot the lips with a tissue.

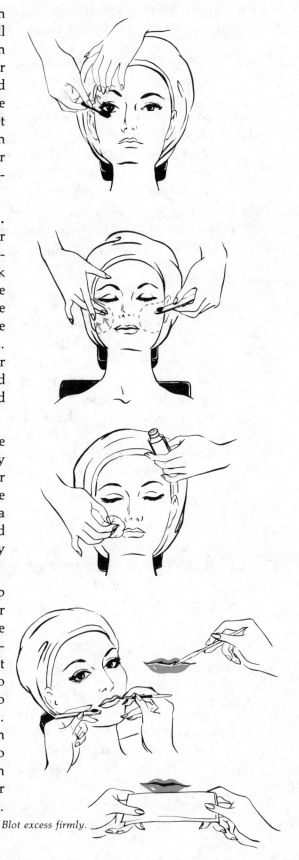

Blot excess firmly.

MAKEUP TECHNIQUES
FOR THE BLACK WOMAN

When applying makeup to any face, many of the same techniques are used. The skin is analyzed and given a facial for its specific condition, and makeup is selected to enhance the coloring of the patron's skin, eyes, and hair. Most cosmetic manufacturers offer a full range of makeup colors and some manufacturers specialize in makeup for black women.

Before applying makeup, thoroughly cleanse the face, use an appropriate astringent, and apply a moisturizer, if moisture is lacking.

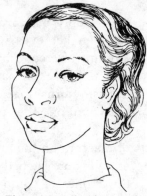

1. The purpose of makeup is to enhance the individual beauty of the patron. A personalized makeup will add to her sense of confidence in selecting and applying her makeup.

FOUNDATION

When selecting a foundation for black skin, color is important. Black skin generally requires less foundation coverage because the same imperfections that are quite visible on a light skin are harder to see on a dark skin. When selecting a foundation, the color should be tried on the jawline and blended to be sure it is compatible with the individual's personal coloring. An ashy look should be avoided.

POWDER

Translucent powder is preferred, but a tinted powder may be used if it does not change color when applied over the foundation.

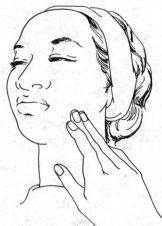

2. It is important to select a makeup base or foundation that gives radiance to the natural skin tone and covers small imperfections. Translucent powder may be used to tone down too much sheen.

CONTOUR SHADING
AND HIGHLIGHTING

Shading and highlighting of the facial features with makeup for corrective purposes, or to enhance certain features, may be done as effectively on dark skins as on light. However, shading will not be prominent on dark skins, but highlighting will create interesting planes on the face when applied to the cheeks and center of the nose.

3. Cheek color should be applied high on the cheekbones. Deeper colors are usually the most flattering. Be especially cautious of cheek colors that are light pink or orange.

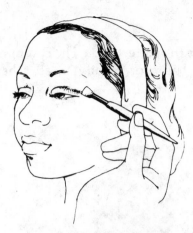
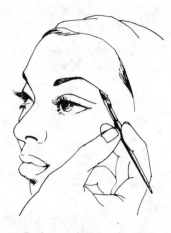
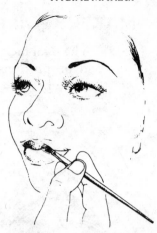

4. Pastel colors in eye makeup that look right on a light skin will often be too pale and washed out on a dark skin. Eye shadow should be deeper and brighter in color.

5. Eyebrows that are already dark should not be darkened with a harsh, black pencil. A dark brown or brown-black pencil or brush-on color will be softer and more natural looking.

6. Foundation can be applied over the lips, and then a lipline drawn slightly inside the natural ridge of the lips and color filled in. Any attempt to make a full mouth appear smaller may look too contrived and should be avoided.

7. Many exciting color combinations in makeup are available for black women. Artistic makeup can enhance every woman's beauty and increase her poise.

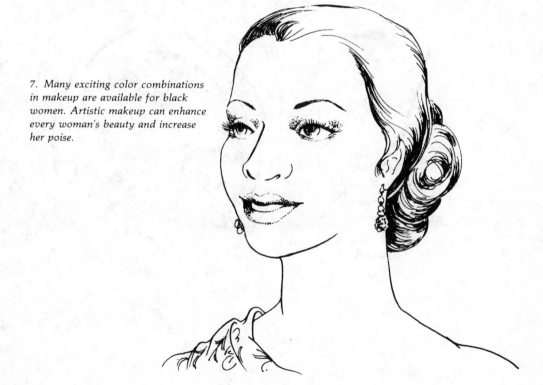

MAKEUP FOR FACIAL TYPES

The **oval facial type** is generally accepted as the perfect face. The contours and proportions of the oval face form the basis for modifying all other facial types.

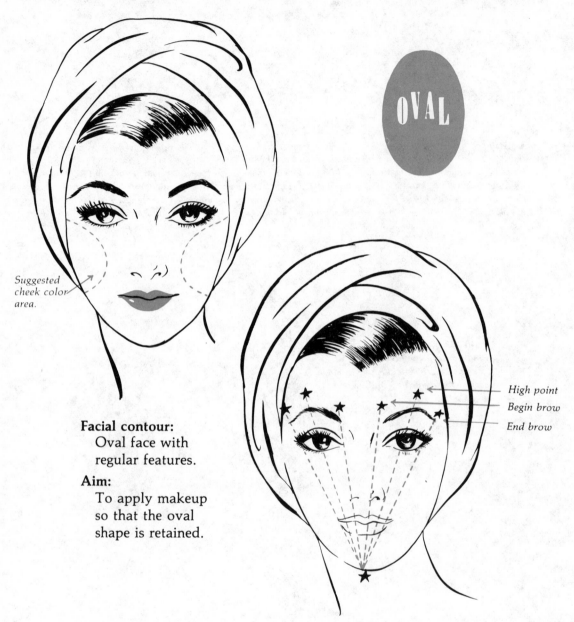

Suggested cheek color area.

OVAL

High point
Begin brow
End brow

Facial contour:
Oval face with regular features.

Aim:
To apply makeup so that the oval shape is retained.

MAKEUP SUGGESTIONS

Cheeks: Apply cheek color on cheekbones in a triangular fashion. Blend color upward and outward toward the temples, no higher than the outer corners of the eyes.

Eyebrows: They should frame the eyes in a soft, natural arch.

Lips: Accentuate the natural bowline of the upper lip. Outline the lower lip so that it appears slightly fuller than the upper lip.

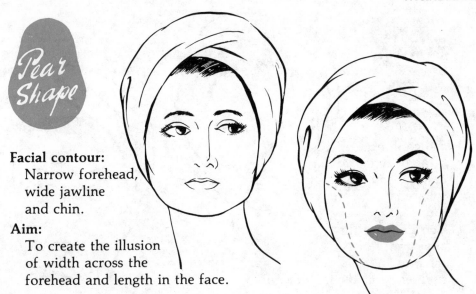

Facial contour:
Narrow forehead,
wide jawline
and chin.

Aim:
To create the illusion
of width across the
forehead and length in the face.

MAKEUP SUGGESTIONS

Cheeks: Apply color to cheekbones and extend the color downward along the jawline to create the illusion of slenderness. Shading or a darker foundation can be applied to a wide jawline or double chin to slenderize the width of the face.

Eyebrows: They should retain a natural slightly high arch.

Lips: Apply lip color to accent both the upper and lower lips.

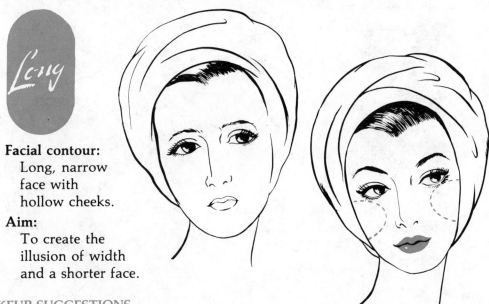

Facial contour:
Long, narrow
face with
hollow cheeks.

Aim:
To create the
illusion of width
and a shorter face.

MAKEUP SUGGESTIONS

Cheeks: Apply cheek color on cheekbones no higher than the outer corners of the eyes and no lower than the tip of the nose.

A shading cosmetic or darker foundation can be applied to the chin and forehead to create the illusion of width to the face.

Eyebrows: They should retain a natural arch.

Lips: Apply lip color to give the illusion of fullness and width to the lips.

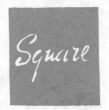

Square

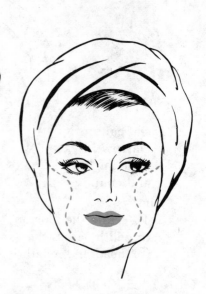

Facial contour:
Straight forehead
hairline and
square jaw.

Aim:
To slenderize the
appearance of
the face and offset the
squareness of the features.

MAKEUP SUGGESTIONS

Cheeks: Apply color to the cheekbones, extending the color downward on the jawline. A shading cosmetic or a darker foundation can be applied to the heavy area of the jaw to create the illusion of slenderness.

Eyebrows: A rounded arch will create softness which detracts from the squareness of the jawline.

Lips: Apply lip color to create fullness and width to offset the squareness of the jawline.

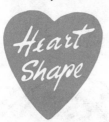

Heart Shape

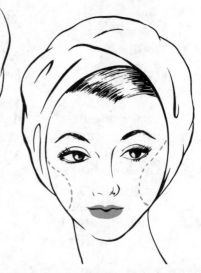

Facial contour:
Wide forehead
and narrow chinline.

Aim:
To minimize the width
across the forehead and
increase the width across
the jawbone line.

MAKEUP SUGGESTIONS

Cheeks: To minimize the width of the forehead and cheeks, apply cheek color high on the cheekbones, extending the color to the temples. A shading cosmetic or darker foundation can be applied to the forehead to minimize its width.

Eyebrows: They should not be spaced widely. Allow about the length of one eye between brows. Arch high, but retain a natural look.

Lips: When applying lip color, follow the natural contour of the lips.

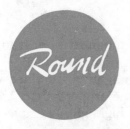

Round

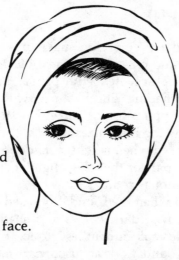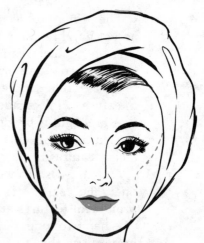

Facial contour:
Round hairline and round chinline.

Aim:
To slenderize the appearance of the face.

MAKEUP SUGGESTIONS

Cheeks: The round face will appear longer and narrower if cheek color is applied high on the cheekbones, extending toward the temples. The color can be blended downward along the sides of the face and at least ½" (1.25 cm) outward from the nose. A shading cosmetic or darker foundation can be applied to the jawline under the cheeks to create the illusion of slenderness.

Eyebrows: Follow the natural contour of the eyebrow, avoiding a high rounded arch.

Lips: Outline lips and fill in color, avoiding excessive fullness.

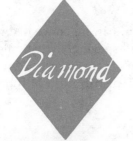

Diamond

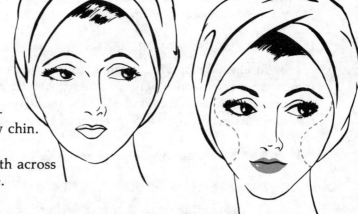

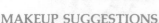

Facial contour:
Narrow forehead, extreme width through the cheekbones, and narrow chin.

Aim:
To reduce the width across the cheekbone line.

MAKEUP SUGGESTIONS

Cheeks: Apply color on the heavy area of the cheekbones. Extend the color no higher than the outer corners of the eyes and no lower than the wider part of the face. A lighter foundation can be applied to the chin and forehead to create the illusion of width or fullness to the face.

Eyebrows: Since the forehead is narrow, brows should not be spaced widely. Allow about the width of one eye between the brows. Follow the natural arch.

Lips: Follow the natural contour of the lips, but avoid exaggerated fullness.

CORRECTIVE MAKEUP

The primary objective of corrective makeup is to minimize poor features, accent good features, and create the optical illusion of an oval face.

Facial features can be accented with proper highlighting, subdued with correct shadowing or shading, and balanced with the proper hairstyle.

A basic rule for the application of makeup is that highlighting emphasizes a feature, while shadowing minimizes it.

A **highlight** is produced when a lighter shade than the original foundation is used on a particular part of the face. Highlights bring out the parts of the facial features to be emphasized.

A **shadow** is formed when the foundation used is darker than the original one. The use of shadows (dark colors and shades) minimizes or subdues prominent features and makes them less noticeable.

When two tones of foundations are used, care must be taken to blend them properly so that there will be no line of demarcation.

Color harmony can be achieved when the makeup tones flatter the color of the eyes, hair, and skin. To determine what is best for each patron, the makeup artist must:

1. Analyze the color of the patron's skin, hair, and eyes.
2. Examine the front and profile views of her facial features.
3. Select and apply those makeup highlights and/or shades that will produce the desired corrective results.

CONCEALING WRINKLES WITH FOUNDATION CREAM

Age lines and wrinkles, due to dryness of the skin, can be concealed with foundation cream. Foundation cream should be used sparingly. It should be applied evenly, in a light outward circular motion over the entire surface of the face. Care should be taken to remove any heavy distribution of foundation cream in lines and wrinkles of the face.

CORRECTIVE MAKEUP FOR FOREHEAD

Low forehead. Applying a lighter foundation cream to the forehead gives it a broader appearance between the brows and hairline.

Bulging forehead. Applying a darker foundation over the prominent area gives an illusion of fullness to the rest of the face and minimizes the bulging forehead.

With a suitable hairstyle, attention can be drawn away from the forehead.

CORRECTIVE MAKEUP FOR NOSE AND CHIN

Large or protruding nose. Apply a darker foundation on the nose, and use a lighter foundation on the cheeks at the sides of the nose. This will create fullness in the cheeks, making the nose appear smaller. Avoid placing the cheek color close to the nose.

Short and flat nose. Apply a lighter foundation down the center of the nose, stopping at the tip. This will make the nose appear longer and larger. If the nostrils are wide, apply a darker foundation to both sides of the nostrils.

Broad nose. Use a darker foundation on the sides of the nose and nostrils. Avoid carrying this dark tone into the laugh lines, as it will accentuate them. The foundation must be carefully blended to avoid visible lines.

Protruding chin and receding nose. Shadow the chin with a darker foundation, and highlight the nose with a lighter foundation.

Receding chin (small chin). Highlight the chin by using a lighter foundation than the one used on the face.

Sagging double chin. Use a darker foundation on the sagging portion, and use a natural skin tone foundation on the face.

CORRECTIVE MAKEUP FOR JAWLINE AND NECK

The neck and jaws are just as important as the eyes, cheeks, and lips. When applying makeup, carry the foundation cream down below the neckline of the patron's dress, to prevent the appearance of a line of demarcation.

Broad jaws. Apply a darker shade of foundation over the heavy area of the jaws, starting at the temples. This will minimize the lower part of the face, and create an illusion of width to the upper part of the face.

Narrow jawline. Highlight the jawline by using a lighter foundation than the one used on the rest of the face.

Round, square, or **triangular face.** Apply a darker shade of foundation over the prominent area of the jawline. By creating a shadow over this area, an illusion of ovalness is created.

Small face—short and thick neck. Use a darker foundation on the neck than the one used on the face. This will make the neck appear thinner.

Long, thin neck. Apply a lighter foundation on the neck than the one used on the face. This will create fullness and counteract the long, thin appearance of the neck.

CORRECTIVE MAKEUP FOR EYES

The eyes are very important features of correct facial balance. The right eye makeup, therefore, is essential for corrective facial makeup. Creating the proper optical illusion, with reference to the appearance of the eyes, will make a great contribution to the overall facial appearance being developed. Eyes can be made to appear larger or smaller by the use of eye colors and/or shadows.

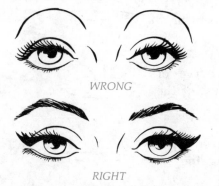

WRONG

RIGHT

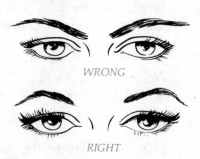

WRONG

RIGHT

Round eyes can be lengthened by extending the shadow beyond the outer corners of the eyes.

Close-set eyes. For eyes that are set too close together, apply shadow lightly up from the outer edges of the eyes and a highlighting cosmetic at the inner corners of the eyes.

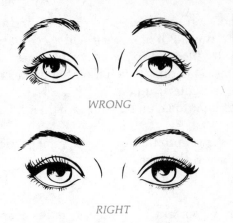

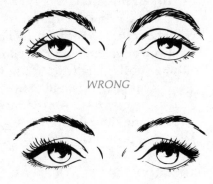

WRONG   *WRONG*

RIGHT   *RIGHT*

Bulging eyes can be minimized by blending the shadow carefully over the prominent part of the upper lid, carrying it lightly to the line of the brow. Use dark shadow, as in illustration. Avoid high, rounded eyebrows.

Heavy-lidded eyes. Shadow evenly and lightly across the lid from the edge of the eyelash line to the small crease in the eye socket, as seen in this illustration.

Small eyes can be made to appear larger by extending the shadow or eye color slightly above, beyond, and below the eyes.

Eyes set too far apart. For eyes that are set too far apart, use shadow on the upper inner side of the eyelid.

Deep-sunken eyes. Use very little shadow on the lids nearest the temples, and leave untouched the part next to the nose and inner corners of the eyes.

Dark circles under eyes. Apply a lighter foundation cream, blending it into the dark area.

Puffy eyes. Apply a darker shade of foundation to the puffy area.

CORRECTIVE MAKEUP FOR LIPS

Thin lower lip. Use a lip color pencil to extend the curve of the lower lip to balance with the size of the upper lip.

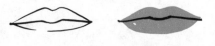

Thin upper lip. Build up the curve of upper lip to balance with the fullness of the lower lip.

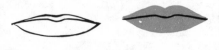

Thin lips. Increase the size of both upper and lower lips with a gentle, curving line.

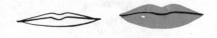

Small mouth. Build out the sides of the upper and lower lips, and extend the corners of the mouth.

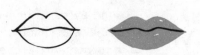

Drooping corners. Build up the upper lip at the corners of the mouth.

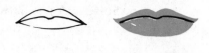

Large, full lips. Keep lip color inside the lipline. A lighter color can be applied to the lips, and then a deeper color brushed on the center of both lips.

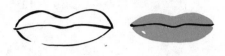

Mouth too oval. Use a lip color pencil to draw a slight indent (Cupid's bow) on the upper lip.

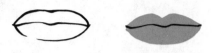

Sharp-pointed Cupid's bow. Use a lip color pencil to soften the sharp peaks of the lips. Fill in the Cupid's bow with lip color; widen the sides of both upper and lower lips.

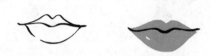

Uneven lips. Use a lip color pencil to correct the uneven lines of the lips. Fill in areas, as shown in the illustration.

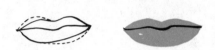

EYEBROW ARCHING

Correctly shaped eyebrows have a marked effect on the beauty and contour of the face.

The natural arch of the eyebrow follows the bony structure, or the curved line of the orbit (eye socket). Most people have a disorderly growth of hairs both above and below the natural line. These hairs should be removed, to give a clean-cut and attractive appearance.

Because of the sensitivity of the skin around the eyes, some patrons cannot tolerate tweezing. For them, shaving or a wax depilatory may be used. How to apply a wax depilatory will be found in the chapter on **Removal of Superfluous Hair.**

IMPLEMENTS, SUPPLIES, AND MATERIALS

Emollient cream	Eyebrow brush	Astringent lotion
Cotton pledgets	Towel	Antiseptic lotion
Cleansing tissue	Tweezers	Eyebrow pencil

PROCEDURE FOR GIVING AN EYEBROW ARCH

1. **Prepare patron.** Seat the patron in a facial chair in a reclining position, as for a facial massage. Or, seat her in a half-upright position and work from the side.
2. **Select type of arch.** Discuss with the patron the type of eyebrows suitable for her facial characteristics.
3. **Cover patron's eyes** with cotton pledgets moistened with witch hazel or a boric acid solution.
4. **Brush eyebrows** with a small brush, to remove powder and scaliness.

5. **Soften brows.** Saturate two pledgets of cotton or a towel with hot water and place over the brows. Allow to remain on the brows long enough to soften and relax eyebrow tissue. Brows and surrounding skin may be softened by rubbing emollient cream into them.

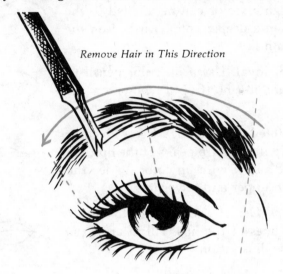

Remove Hair in This Direction

6. **Remove hairs between brows.** When tweezing, stretch the skin taut with the index finger and thumb (or index and middle finger) of the left hand. Grasp each hair individually with tweezers, and pull with a quick motion in the direction in which the hair grows. Sponge tweezed area frequently with cotton moistened with an antiseptic lotion, to avoid infection. Hairs between the brows and above the browline are tweezed first, as the area under the browline is much more sensitive.

7. **Remove hairs from above the eyebrow line.** Brush hair downward. Shape the upper section of one eyebrow, then shape the other. Sponge area with antiseptic frequently.

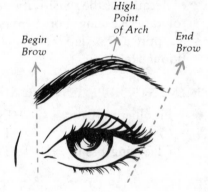

Begin Brow   *High Point of Arch*   *End Brow*

8. **Remove hairs from under eyebrow line.** Brush hairs upward. Shape the lower section of one eyebrow, then shape the other. Sponge the area with an antiseptic.

(Optional: Apply emollient cream and massage brows. Remove cream with tissues.)

9. **Apply an astringent.** After the tweezing has been completed, sponge the brows and surrounding skin with an astringent, to contract the skin.

10. **Apply brow makeup.** Brush brows, placing the hair in its normal position. Use eyebrow pencil where necessary.

The eyebrows should be treated about once a week.

THE USE OF THE EYEBROW PENCIL

When a patron wants to correct misshaped eyebrows, remove all unnecessary hairs, then instruct her in the use of the eyebrow pencil, until the necessary hairs have grown in again.

When there are spaces in the brow devoid of hair, the spaces can be filled in with hair-like strokes with an eyebrow pencil. Use the eyebrow brush to soften the pencil marks.

When the arch is too high, remove the superfluous hair from the top of the brow, and fill in the lower part with eyebrow pencil. **Where the arch is too low,** remove the superfluous hair from the lower part of the brow, and build up the shape of the brow by means of the eyebrow pencil.

High forehead. The eyebrow arch may be slightly elevated to detract from the high forehead. Avoid giving the patron a surprised look.

CORRECTIVE PLACING AND SHAPING OF THE EYEBROWS

Low forehead. A low arch gives more height to the very low forehead.

Wide-set eyes. The eyes can be made to appear closer together by extending the eyebrow lines to the inside corners of the eyes. However, care must be taken to avoid giving the patron a frowning look.

Close-set eyes. To make the eyes appear farther apart, widen the distance between them; also slightly extend the brows outward.

Round face. Arch the brows high to make the face appear narrower. Start on a line directly above the inside corner of the eye and extend to the end of the cheekbone.

Long face. The illusion of a shorter face can be created by making the eyebrows almost straight. Do not extend the eyebrow lines farther than the ends of the eyes.

Triangular face. To offset the narrow forehead, arch the eyebrows slightly on the ends only. Start the lines directly above the inside corners of the eyes and continue to the ends of the cheekbones.

Square face. The face will appear more oval if there is a high arch on the ends of the eyebrows. Begin the lines directly above the corners of the eyes and extend the lines outward.

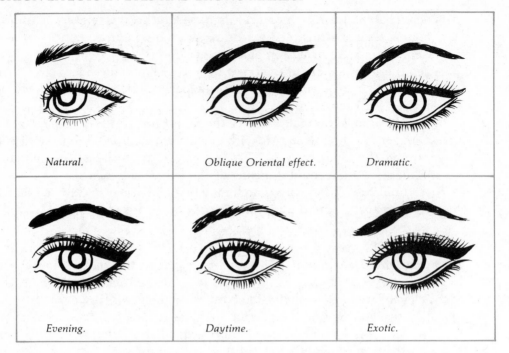

Natural.

Oblique Oriental effect.

Dramatic.

Evening.

Daytime.

Exotic.

MAKEUP COSMETICS

Cosmetics	Forms Available	Uses
Face Powder	Cake or powder	Takes shine from face. Helps makeup to set. Gives face matte (dull) finish.
Foundation (Clear or Tinted)	Cream, liquid, cake	Base for makeup.
Lip Color (Lipstick)	Stick, cream, liquid	Gives color and sheen to lips.
Cheek Color (Rouge)	Cream, dry, liquid, brush on	Gives cheeks soft, warm glow.
Mascara	Cake, cream, liquid	Adds color to eyelashes.
Eyeliner	Cake, pencil, liquid	Emphasizes eyes.
Eye Shadow	Stick, cream, cake	Adds color to eyelids.
Eyebrow Color	Pencil or powder	Defines eyebrows by drawing fine lines in eyebrow area.
Astringent Skin Freshener	Liquid or cream	Closes pores of oily skin.
Moisturizer	Emulsion or thick cream	Helps retain moisture in the skin.

SAFETY PRECAUTIONS

1. Wash and sanitize your hands before and after a makeup application, or after touching any object unrelated to the procedure.
2. Properly drape patron (for her protection).
3. Sanitize all brushes after each use.
4. Use only sanitized brushes and implements.
5. Do not get lotions, antiseptics, astringents, or eye makeup into patron's eyes.
6. Sharpen eyebrow and eyeliner pencils after each use.
7. Discard all disposable items, such as sponges, after each use.
8. After each use, wash and sanitize all linens that touch patron's skin.
9. Use spatula to remove creams from containers.
10. Keep fingernails round and smooth, to avoid scratching patron.
11. Use salt shaker type of container for powder.
12. Pour all lotions from bottle containers.
13. Do not apply liquid or cream lip color directly on patron's lips. Use a brush.
14. Use an antiseptic on tweezed area, to avoid infection.
15. Protect patron's hair and skin from direct contact with facial chair.

REVIEW QUESTIONS

FACIAL MAKEUP

1. What is the purpose of facial makeup?
2. Why is the foundation or base important in facial makeup?
3. What effect does using a foundation that is too light have on the appearance of the face?
4. Name three types of foundations.
5. What type of foundation may be used for:
   a) oily skin?
   b) dry skin?
6. Which two cosmetics are used to hide skin blemishes?
7. List the four ways in which face powders improve the overall attractiveness of the skin.
8. What is the purpose to be achieved by using cheek color?
9. Name four types of cheek color.
10. What is the special beneficial feature of each of the following cheek colors:
    a) liquid?
    b) cream?
    c) dry (compact)?
    d) brush-on (powdered)?

11. For what two reasons is lip color used?
12. What are the four basic tints and shades of lip color?
13. Where should eyeliners be applied?
14. To which parts are the following eye makeups applied:
    a) eye shadow?
    b) mascara?
    c) eyebrow pencil?
15. What effect is created when using:
    a) eye shadow?
    b) mascara?
    c) eyebrow pencil?

EYEBROW ARCHING

1. Why is eyebrow arching important?
2. What is the correct way to tweeze the brow hair when arching?
3. During arching the brows, why is an antiseptic applied to tweezed areas?
4. After tweezing the brows, why is an astringent applied?
5. How often should eyebrows be treated?
6. How can spaces in the eyebrow devoid of hair be filled in?

Chapter 24

FALSE EYELASHES

CHAPTER LEARNING OBJECTIVES

The student successfully mastering this chapter will know:
1. *The reason for using false eyelashes.*
2. *The two types of false eyelashes.*
3. *How to select the proper eyelashes.*
4. *How to apply and remove strip eyelashes.*
5. *The meaning of eye tabbing.*
6. *The procedure for affixing and removing semi-permanent eyelashes.*
7. *How to deal with problem eyelash conditions.*
8. *The safety precautions to be followed in the application of false eyelashes.*

A beautifully made up face requires the proper application of cosmetics that will harmonize with the natural coloring of the skin. It also requires the formation and shaping of eyelashes that coordinate with and enhance the overall facial appearance. When the natural eyelashes are not long enough or thick enough to completely satisfy the patron, false lashes are applied.

There are two basic types of false eyelashes in general use. They are:
1. Strip eyelashes.
2. Semi-permanent individual eyelashes (eye tabbing).

APPLYING STRIP EYELASHES

Strip eyelashes are available in a variety of types, sizes, and textures. They may be made of either human hair or synthetic fibers. Synthetic fiber eyelashes are made with a permanent curl and do not react to changes in weather conditions.

EQUIPMENT, IMPLEMENTS, AND MATERIALS

Wet sanitizer to sanitize metal implements

Strip eyelashes	Lash adhesive	Eye makeup remover
Tweezers	Tissues	(clear)
Cotton swabs	Adhesive tray	Manicure table
Eyelash brush	Eyelid and eyelash	Adjustable light (goose-
Hand mirror	cleaner	neck lamp)
Manicure scissors	Eyelash remover	Lounge style chair

PROCEDURE

1. Wash and sanitize your hands.
2. Check to see that all required supplies and sanitized implements are on hand.
3. Place the patron in the lounge style chair with her head at a comfortable working height.
4. Be certain that the patron's face is well lighted. However, for the patron's comfort, don't shine the light directly into her eyes.
5. If the patron has not already done so, remove all eye makeup. If the eyelashes are not entirely clean, the adhesive will not adhere properly.
6. If the patron wears contact lenses, they must be removed before starting to apply the lashes.
7. Brush patron's lashes to make sure that they are clean and free from foreign matter. Brushing also separates lashes.
8. Discuss with the patron the length of eyelashes desired and the effect she hopes to achieve. Try to create an effect that makes the patron's eyelashes fuller, more attractive, yet not unnatural looking.
9. Always work from behind the patron, except when applying bottom lashes.
10. Carefully remove the eyelash strip from a package.
11. Follow manufacturer's directions very carefully.
12. **Start with the upper lash.** If the lash is too long to fit the curve of the upper lid, the outside edge should be trimmed. With your fingers, bend the lash into a horseshoe shape. This makes it more flexible so it will fit the contour of the eyelid. (Fig. 1)

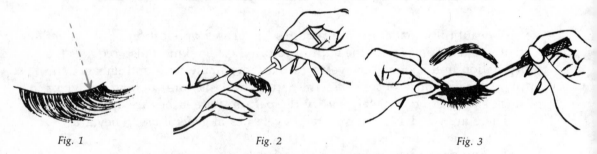

Fig. 1   Fig. 2   Fig. 3

13. **Feather the lash.** This is done by nipping into it with the points of your scissors, which creates a more natural look.
14. **Apply a thin strip of lash adhesive** to the base of the lash and allow a few seconds for setting. (Fig. 2)
15. **Apply the lash.** Start with the shorter (inside) part of the lash, and place it in a position midway between the inside corner of the eye where the curve of the iris begins. Position the rest of the lash as close to the patron's own lash as possible. The rounded end of a lashliner brush may be used to press the lash on. (Fig. 3) The line is usually drawn on before the application of the lash and retouched after the lash is in place. (Fig. 4)
16. **Apply bottom lash.** Lash adhesive is used in the same manner as in the application of the upper lash. The lash is placed on top of the lower lash. A shorter lash is placed toward the center of the eye, and a longer one, toward the outer edge.

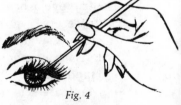

Fig. 4

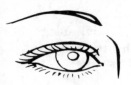 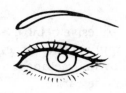 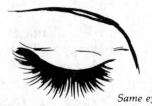 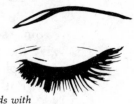

Sparse eyelashes.

*Same eyelids with
false eyelashes attached.*

REMOVING FALSE STRIP EYELASHES

There are commercial preparations, such as pads saturated with specially prepared lotions, to facilitate the removal of false eyelashes. The lash base also may be softened by the application of a face cloth saturated with warm water and a gentle face soap or cleanser. Hold the pad or cloth over the eyes for a few seconds to soften the adhesive. Starting from the inner corner of the lashline, gently pull the lash. Cotton tipped swabs may be used to remove makeup and adhesive remaining on the lid.

APPLYING SEMI-PERMANENT INDIVIDUAL EYELASHES (EYE TABBING)

Eye tabbing is the technique of attaching individual, synthetic eyelashes to a patron's own eyelashes. Synthetic fibers are used in the manufacture of false eyelashes because they can be easily curled.

Because the synthetic lashes are attached to the patron's own and become part of them, they last as long as the natural eyelashes, about 6-8 weeks. Hence, they are referred to as "semi-permanent eyelashes." However, due to the fact that natural lashes fall out regularly (a few each week), taking the attached false lashes with them, the false lashes should be filled in by periodic visits to the beauty salon.

The wearers of semi-permanent false eyelashes can participate in all normal activities with the same freedom as with natural eyelashes. Semi-permanent eyelashes will not come off when showering or participating in athletic exercises.

EQUIPMENT, IMPLEMENTS, AND MATERIALS

Wet sanitizer to sanitize metal implements

Tweezers
Cotton swabs
Eyelash brush
Hand mirror
Adhesive tray
Eyelash remover
Adhesive container
Eye makeup remover (clear)
Manicure table
Adjustable light (gooseneck lamp)
Makeup or facial chair

Manicure scissors
Tissues
Trays of eyelashes
Eyelash adhesive
Eyelid and eyelash cleaner

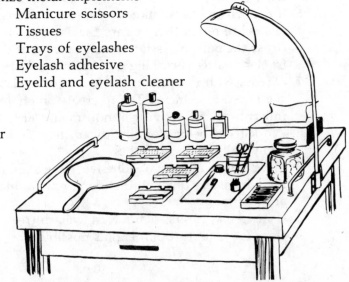

ALLERGY TEST

Since some women are allergic to the adhesive being used, it is advisable to give the patron an allergy test before applying the lashes. This test may be accomplished by either one of the following methods:

1. Put a drop of the adhesive behind one ear; or
2. Attach a single eyelash to each eyelid.

In either case, if there is no reaction within 24 hours, it is safe to proceed with the application.

LENGTHS OF FALSE LASHES

False lashes usually come in three lengths: short, medium, and long. Some manufacturers have developed a fourth length, extra short.

These different lengths are used by themselves or in combination, in order to achieve certain planned effects.

1. A natural effect is created by using the short lashes with a few medium size lashes intermingled with the short ones.
2. A more luxurious effect, enhancing the appearance of the patron's own eyelashes, can be achieved by using a mixture of short and medium length lashes with a few long ones added for glamor.
3. A very glamorous or high styling effect is achieved by using only long lashes.
4. The extra short lashes are used on lower lashes or in combination with others to achieve special effects.

PROCEDURE FOR UPPER LASHES (TOP)

1. Wash and sanitize your hands.
2. Check to see that all required supplies and sanitized implements are on hand.
3. Place the patron in the makeup chair with her head at a comfortable working height.
4. Make sure that the patron's face is well lighted. However, for the patron's comfort, make sure that the light does not shine directly into her eyes.
5. If the patron has not already done so, remove all eye makeup. If the eyelashes are not entirely clean, the adhesive will not adhere properly.
6. Brush the patron's lashes to make sure that they are clean and free from foreign matter. Brushing also separates lashes.
7. Discuss with the patron the length of eyelashes desired and the effect she hopes to achieve. Try to create an effect that makes the eyelashes fuller, more attractive, yet not unnatural looking.
8. Work from behind or slightly to the side of the patron, except when applying the bottom lashes.
9. Place a small amount of adhesive in the adhesive container. The adhesive used dries very quickly; therefore, only a small quantity should be used at one time.
10. Using the tweezers, remove an eyelash from the tray. Hold the lash as close to the butt (bulb) end as possible. (Fig. 1)

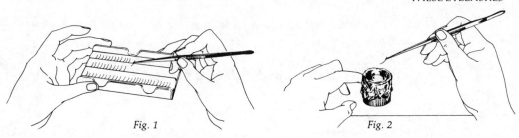

Fig. 1 Fig. 2

11. When the lash is free from the tray, move the tweezer past the center of the lash.

12. Brush the under side of the individual lash over the adhesive. (Fig. 2) **Note:** *To form an adhesive container, place a small piece of aluminum foil over the open end of a bottle cap.*

13. Only a very small amount of adhesive is needed. If too much adhesive is picked up, brush off the excess with your fingertip.

14. If the patron wears glasses, place the first lash in the center of the lid. Have the patron put her glasses on. If the lash touches the glass, it is too long and a shorter length must be selected. If the lash does not touch, it may be used. (Fig. 3)

15. It is important to remember that the lash is held in the tweezers at exactly the same angle that it will be placed on the natural lash.

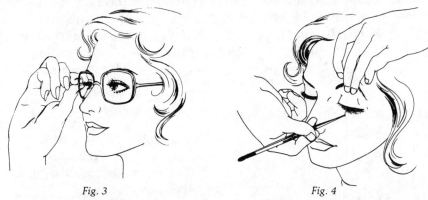

Fig. 3 Fig. 4

16. If you are right handed you will start applying lashes at the outer corner of the left eye, applying the lashes side by side until you reach the inner corner of the left eye. This method will prove to be the most efficient and time saving. The first 2-3 lashes applied to the outer corner and the last 2-3 lashes applied to the inner corner of the eye should be short, to give a gradual, more natural buildup to the lashes.

17. Start the application procedure by brushing the adhesive from the under side of the individual lash onto the top side of the patron's natural lash. Transfer the adhesive to the entire length of the natural lash starting at the base (the part closest to the lid) and brushing out to the tip.

18. The individual lash is placed on top of the natural lash, as close to the eyelid as possible without actually touching the lid. (Fig. 4) For efficient performance, the tweezer must be kept free of adhesive.

19. Start the application of lashes to the other eye by applying the individual lashes to the inside corner of the eye and continue placing the lashes side by side until reaching the outer corner of the eye.

20. For the inside corner of the eye it may be necessary to use the thumb of the free hand to gently extend the eyelid and hold it taut. This exposes the natural inside corner of the eye and permits the placing of the artificial eyelash properly. (Fig. 5)

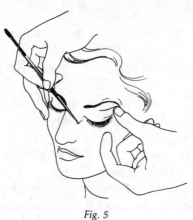

Fig. 5

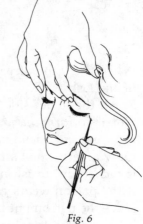

Fig. 6

21. When necessary, the same technique is applied when attaching the outside corner lashes. (Fig. 6)
22. When attaching lashes in the corners of the eyes, the upper and lower lashes must be kept separated for several seconds to permit the adhesive to dry and prevent the eyelids from sticking together.
Note: *If you are left handed, follow the above procedure, but start at the outer corner of the right eye and work toward the left.*

PROCEDURE FOR BOTTOM LASHES (LOWER)

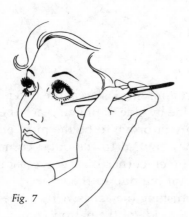

Fig. 7

The application of bottom (lower) lashes requires a different technique.

1. The patron is required to sit up and face the cosmetologist.
2. The patron looks upward with eyes wide open. (Fig. 7)
3. Use only short lashes.
4. The procedure for picking up adhesive and applying bottom lashes is the same as for the upper lashes.
5. Have the patron hold her eyes open for a few extra seconds to permit the adhesive to dry.
6. More adhesive is used in the application of lower lashes in order to assure a more lasting application.

CAUTION

Patrons should be advised that the natural oils from the eyelids tend to dissolve the adhesive. As a result, the lower false lashes will not stay on as long as the upper lashes. Lower lashes will begin to fall off about one week after application.

PROBLEMS

OILY EYELIDS

Due to the oil secreted by the eyelids, the false lashes have great difficulty in staying on the natural eyelashes. The oil dissolves the adhesive and the lashes fall off.

Use the same technique as for lower lashes. Apply more adhesive. Make sure that the adhesive is spread over the entire length of the natural eyelash, and hold the lash in place several additional seconds to permit the adhesive to dry.

Generally, the false lashes will not hold as long on patrons with oily eyelids.

SPARSE EYELASHES

A special technique is required for those patrons with sparse eyelashes. The gaps must be filled in to develop full and luxurious eyelashes.

PROCEDURE

1. Instead of applying the false lash to the top of the natural lash, apply it to both sides of the natural lash.
2. Angle the lash slightly inward. This technique fills in all the gaps.
3. Then a second set of eyelashes is cemented on top of the first set of lashes.
4. The second set of lashes also is angled inwardly, effectively closing any gaps that may exist.

Thus, patrons with very sparse eyelashes will have full, luxurious, beautiful eyelashes.

REMOVING FALSE INDIVIDUAL LASHES

If it is necessary to remove false eyelashes, do not, under any circumstances, attempt to pull them off. Pulling off the false eyelashes also will pull out the natural eyelashes.

Have the patron sit directly in front of you. To protect her eyes, place an eye pad, shield, or tissue under her eyelashes, with the eyes closed. Saturate a small, soft brush or cotton swab with eyelash remover. Gently brush or swab the eyelash until the adhesive dissolves and the lash can be removed.

REMINDERS AND HINTS ON APPLYING FALSE EYELASHES

1. Do not cement one false eyelash to two natural eyelashes.
2. Do not touch the eyelids with tweezer or any other implement.
3. Work with clean tweezers at all times.
4. Be careful when working around patron's eyes.
5. Immediately clean dried adhesive from tweezers with adhesive remover.
6. Patron must sit up straight and face cosmetologist when adhesive remover is being used.
7. Do not get any chemical into patron's eyes.

REVIEW QUESTIONS

FALSE EYELASHES

1. What are the two basic types of false eyelashes?
2. What advantages do synthetic fiber eyelashes have?
3. What is the application of semi-permanent individual eyelashes called?
4. How long do individual synthetic eyelashes last?
5. What great advantage do the wearers of semi-permanent false eyelashes enjoy?
6. Why is it necessary to give an allergy test before attaching semi-permanent individual eyelashes?
7. Where are the extra short lashes usually used?
8. Why do oily eyelids present a problem in the application of false eyelashes?
9. What technique is used to make false eyelashes adhere to oily eyelids?
10. How are sparse eyelashes filled in?
11. Why should you not pull off false eyelashes?

Chapter 25

SUPERFLUOUS
HAIR REMOVAL

CHAPTER LEARNING OBJECTIVES

The student successfully mastering this chapter will know:
1. *The two general classifications of superfluous hair removal.*
2. *The techniques involved in the two methods of permanent hair removal.*
3. *Methods of temporary hair removal, and the techniques of each.*

ELECTROLYSIS

Superfluous hair is not a new problem. It has plagued individuals from time immemorial, and throughout the ages they have sought ways and means to disguise or get rid of it. Unwanted hair is a problem that vitally concerns many men and women.

Today, there are two types of hair removal:

    1. Permanent.   2. Temporary.

There are several means of temporary hair removal which will be discussed in another section of this chapter. This section will cover the permanent hair removal method called **electrolysis** (e-lek-trol'i-sis).

Unwanted hair could not be removed permanently until 1875, when Dr. Charles E. Michel, an ophthalmologist, used an electric current directed through a thin wire to remove ingrowing eyelashes. When he found that the lashes did not grow back, he suggested that this method could be used for removing unwanted hair from the face. A few dermatologists adopted its use, but the process was so slow and tedious that it could not be used to any great extent.

In 1916, the multiple needle machine was developed and electrolysis became a practical aid to beauty. The demand for treatments grew slowly at first, and then more rapidly when the shortwave method was introduced. This newer method was much faster, requiring less time to clear an area. Permanent removal of heavy growths on large areas, such as arms and legs, then became practical.

Electrolysis is the process of removing hair permanently by means of electricity. The term "electrolysis" has become synonymous with both the multiple needle galvanic method and the more modern single needle short-wave method.

Electrologist (e-lek-trol'o-jist) is a person trained to give electrolysis treatments for permanent hair removal.

Hypertrichosis (hi-per-trik-o'sis) is a growth of hair in excess of the normal. It is a Greek word, combining **hyper** (meaning "over") and **tricho** (meaning "hair").

Hirsuties (her-su'shi-ez) is excessive hairiness.

Hirsutism (her'sut-izm) is the presence of excess hair on areas where it is not normally expected.

The following terms are synonymous with shortwave electrolysis:
Thermolysis (ther-mol'i-sis)
Diathermy (di'ah-ther-me)
High-frequency (hi fre'quen-se)

GENERAL INFORMATION

The importance of training. The electrologist is dealing with a woman's skin, and an inefficient or unskilled operator could cause irreparable damage. Therefore, every electrologist must be thoroughly trained, both in the theory and in the practice of electrolysis. This means that she must use live models to practice on, under the direct supervision of a licensed instructor, until she has been properly certified and is confident of her skill.

Machines. Shortwave machines have many safety factors. They are automatically timed and F.C.C. (Federal Communications Commission) approved. Pain is reduced to a minimum by the rapid shut off of current.

Areas that may be treated. Lips, chin, cheeks, arms, legs, body, eyebrows, hairline, and underarms may receive electrolysis treatments.

Areas that may not be treated. Do not treat the eyelids, inside the ears, nostrils, or moles. Do not treat diabetic patrons or those getting hormone treatments without written permission from a doctor.

Causes of unwanted hair. No one knows the exact cause. Authorities agree, however, that heredity has something to do with it, as unwanted hair often seems to run in families and appears to be more common in certain races. Glandular disturbances also are known to influence hair growth.

METHODS OF PERMANENT HAIR REMOVAL

Two methods of permanent hair removal are the **galvanic multiple needle method** and the more advanced **shortwave method**.

1. The galvanic method destroys the hair by decomposing the papilla (the source of nourishment for the hair).

2. The shortwave method destroys the hair by coagulating the papilla through the use of heat.

SHORTWAVE METHOD

Note—Since the shortwave method is the one extensively used, its procedure is given here.

The **shortwave** is the quicker method of permanent hair removal and the one most generally used. In fact, the overwhelming majority of all permanent hair removal treatments today are performed by the shortwave method. Only one needle is used, but it is a much finer needle than those used in the galvanic method.

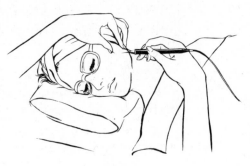

Inserting needle in shortwave method.

EQUIPMENT, IMPLEMENTS, AND MATERIALS

Everything needed for a shortwave treatment should be ready and at hand. Here is a checklist of essential equipment and supplies:

Shortwave machine
Fluorescent magnifying light
Treatment chair and ottoman
   for patron
Cotton pads

Antiseptic lotion
Sunglasses to protect patron's eyes
After-treatment lotion
Antiseptic powder

PREPARATION OF PATRON

Seat the patron comfortably in a reclining position. Place a clean towel or facial tissue under her head, and have another tissue handy for disposal of hairs as you remove them. Adjust the position of the operating arm of the machine to approximately 6-8" (15-20 cm) above the area to be worked on. Sanitize the area to be treated, using a cotton pad saturated with a good antiseptic. Use only **sanitized tweezers** and **needle.**

PREPARING MACHINE

Turn machine to "ON." Adjust machine according to manufacturer's instructions.

Turn **timer control** to "automatic." (See chart provided with machine.)

Turn **time and intensity control** knob to "O," as a starting point.

Plug in foot pedal and place it in a comfortable position.

Adjust operator's stool to the desired height.

SHORTWAVE MACHINE

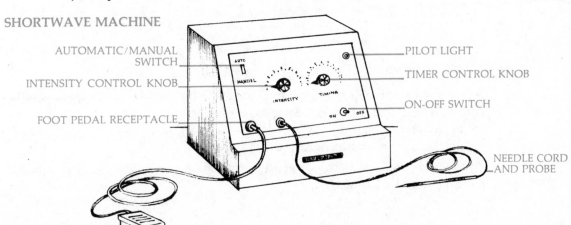

AUTOMATIC/MANUAL SWITCH

INTENSITY CONTROL KNOB

FOOT PEDAL RECEPTACLE

PILOT LIGHT

TIMER CONTROL KNOB

ON-OFF SWITCH

NEEDLE CORD AND PROBE

The quicker the current is shut off, the less sensation the patron will feel. Therefore, the timer should be set at the shortest time interval, usually "O" for **fine hair,** "½" for **medium hair,** and "1" for **heavy hair.** When the need arises to use more current, increase the intensity up to 10 before increasing time to ½.

A good shortwave machine is F.C.C. approved.

It is automatically timed, thus eliminating human failure or the necessity for the electrologist to keep close watch on the time.

The depth of insertion will vary according to the coarseness of the hair, usually from ⅛-¼" (.3125-.625 cm).

INSERTING NEEDLE INTO FOLLICLE

Most hair grows at an angle to the surface of the skin. You insert the needle on the underside of the hair and slide it slowly into the follicle alongside the hair root.

Needle inserted correctly.

After you have inserted the needle, depress the foot pedal. The current goes on and shuts off automatically. Never depress the foot pedal while you are inserting the needle. Remove the needle and lift the hair out gently with tweezers. If it does not glide out easily, reinsert the needle a second time, repeating the procedure outlined above. If the hair still does not glide out easily, remove it forcibly with tweezers and treat again during subsequent treatments.

In making insertions, it is important to observe carefully the **angle or slant of the hair follicle** before you insert the needle. The slant of follicles varies from 15-90° (.26-1.6 rad.). Hairs that have been tweezed grow in all directions. Some follicles are curved, and for this reason the needle point is rounded. Do not force the needle into the follicle because the side or wall of the follicle might be pierced and the current would not reach the papilla.

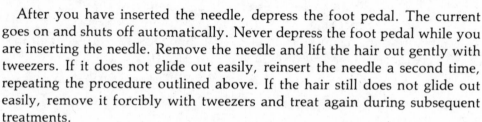

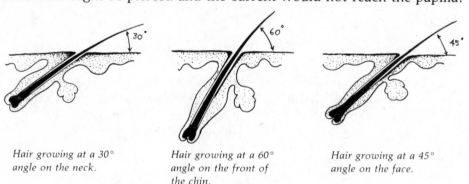

Hair growing at a 30° angle on the neck.

Hair growing at a 60° angle on the front of the chin.

Hair growing at a 45° angle on the face.

AFTER-TREATMENT PROCEDURE

After the treatment is completed, turn the machine off. Saturate a pad of cotton with a special after-treatment lotion and press it gently on the area worked upon. This cools and soothes the skin and closes the pores from which the hair has been removed.

When the lotion has dried, gently press on an antiseptic powder, using a piece of sterile cotton.

REGROWTH

It takes from 8-13 weeks for the hair to grow from the papilla to the surface of the skin. When a patron has been tweezing regularly, the hair tweezed one week is not the hair she tweezed the preceding week, but hair that she tweezed many weeks before. Due to distorted follicles (sometimes caused by tweezing or waxing, sometimes due to natural causes), it is not always possible to destroy the papilla with the first treatment, and the hair will grow again. Additional treatment will be required for permanent removal. The regrowth will vary; it is usually not more than 10% in virgin hair, but may be as much as 20% or 25% in cases of distorted follicles.

REMINDERS AND HINTS ON ELECTROLYSIS

1. Patrons should be told that sometimes, after a treatment on legs or arms, tiny scabs may appear. These soon drop off, leaving the skin in a normal, healthy condition. Application of a special after-treatment lotion will hasten the healing process.
2. Hands, implements, and the area to be treated must be very carefully sanitized.
3. Never remove hairs from areas where the skin shows signs of eruption, abrasion, or inflammation.
4. Do not remove hairs from warts or moles.
5. Never use force when inserting the needle.
6. Do not treat hairs that are too close together. Work checkerboard fashion. Needles placed too close together may result in pitting.
7. Do not treat children.
8. Instruct the patron on how to care for her skin after treatment. Advise the patron not to pick or tamper with her skin.
9. Remind patron that some follicles have multiple hairs, and what may appear to be a regrowth is a dormant hair starting to grow from the same follicle opening.

ELECTRIC TWEEZER METHOD

Another method for the removal of superfluous hair that is being used in salons uses an electrically charged tweezer. This technique is known by various commercial names, depending on the manufacturer of the machine.

The electrically charged tweezer is used to grasp a single strand of hair. The hair is used as a dielectric* material to transfer thermal radio frequency energy to the germinal matrix of the hair root for at least 30 seconds. It is claimed that the germinal matrix is caused to detach from the papilla, allowing the hair to slide out easily.

The process of clearing any area of hair is slow, as no more than two hairs can be removed per minute.

----

* *Dielectric is a term applied to a non-conducting material that transmits electric effects by induction, but not by conduction.*

TEMPORARY METHODS

SHAVING

Shaving is usually recommended when the annoying hairs cover a large area, such as in the armpits and on the arms and legs. A shaving cream is applied before shaving.

An **electric razor** may also be used. The application of a pre-shaving lotion helps to reduce any irritation.

TWEEZING

Tweezing is commonly used for shaping the eyebrows and for removing undesirable hairs from around the mouth and chin. (The procedure for tweezing the eyebrows will be found in the chapter on **Facial Makeup**.)

HAIR LIGHTENING

To lessen the visibility of superfluous hair, you can lighten it by applying an oil bleach mixed with two parts of peroxide.

Procedure

1. Apply the mixture thoroughly to the hair with a tint brush or swab.
2. Repeat the application to keep the lightener wet until the hair has lightened to the desired shade. Lightening time varies from 15-50 minutes, depending on the color and texture of the hair. Dark, coarse hair takes more time than fine, lanugo hair, which is softer and lighter.
3. Remove lightener.
4. Apply an emollient cream.

DEPILATORIES

Depilatories also belong to the group of temporary methods for the removal of superfluous hair. There are **physical** (wax) and **chemical** types of depilatories.

Hot Wax

The wax type of depilatory is applied either heated or cold, as recommended by manufacturer. It may be applied over such parts of the body as the cheeks, chin, upper lip, nape area, arms, and legs.

Procedure

1. Remove clothing from the part to be treated and seat the patron in a comfortable position.
2. Wash the skin area with a mild soap and water. Rinse thoroughly and dry.
3. Spread talcum powder over the skin surface.
4. Melt wax in a double boiler on a stove.
5. Test temperature and consistency of heated wax by applying a little of it on your arm.

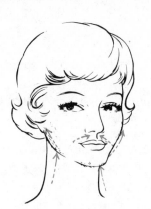

Superfluous hair.

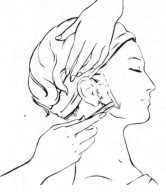

Spread wax downward.

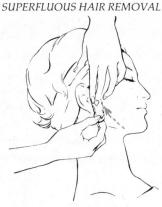

Pull wax off upward.

6. Spread warm wax evenly over the skin surface with a spatula or fingertips, following the same direction as the hair growth.
7. Allow the wax to cool and harden.
8. Quickly pull off the adhering wax against the direction of hair growth.
9. Gently massage treated area.
10. Dust off remaining powder from the skin.
11. Apply an emollient cream or antiseptic lotion to the area treated.

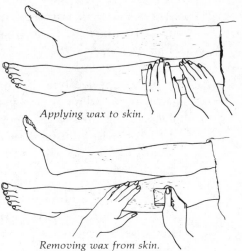

Applying wax to skin.

Removing wax from skin.

Safety Precautions

1. To prevent burns, test temperature of heated wax before applying it to patron's skin.
2. Keep wax from running into the patron's eyes or over any areas where it is not wanted.
3. Do not use a wax depilatory under the arms, over warts, on moles, abrasions, irritated or inflamed skin.

Cold Wax

For those patrons who cannot tolerate heated wax, a cold wax method of hair removal also is available. This technique has all the advantages of hot wax, with the wax available in a ready-to-use form. It removes the hair in the same manner as warm wax, but needs no heating or special equipment.

The cold wax is applied at room temperature. Using a spatula, evenly spread a thin coat of wax in the direction of hair growth. A strip of cellophane or cotton cloth is used to firmly press down the wax so that it adheres correctly. The skin is held taut with one hand while the other hand takes a firm hold on the wax strip, and with one fast movement pulls off the strip against the hair growth. This movement removes the wax together with the hair adhering to it.

Chemical Depilatories

Chemical depilatories, available as a cream, paste, or powder mixed with water into a paste, are generally used to remove hair from the legs.

A **skin test** is advisable to determine whether the individual is sensitive to the action of this type of depilatory.

To give such a test, select a hairless part of the arm, apply a portion of the depilatory according to manufacturer's directions, and leave it on skin from 7-10 minutes. If at the end of this time there are no signs of redness or swelling, the depilatory can be used with safety over a large area of the skin.

Procedure

The cream or powder depilatory is used as follows:

1. The cream type is applied directly from the container, while the powder type is mixed to form a smooth paste according to the directions of manufacturer.
2. After the skin has been cleansed and dried, a thick layer of the depilatory is applied over the area where the hair is to be removed.
3. The surrounding skin is protected with vaseline.
4. Depending on the thickness of the hair, the depilatory is kept on the hair for 5-10 minutes.
5. Then, the depilatory and hair are washed off with warm water.
6. Finally, the skin is patted dry and cold cream is applied.

REVIEW QUESTIONS

SUPERFLUOUS HAIR REMOVAL

1. What are the two categories of hair removal?
2. What is electrolysis?
3. What three terms are synonymous with shortwave electrolysis?
4. How is pain kept at a minimum when the shortwave machine is used?
5. Which areas can be treated by electrolysis?
6. What are the known causes of superfluous hair?
7. Name two methods for removing unwanted hair permanently?
8. How does each of the two methods remove hair permanently?
9. Which is the quicker of the two methods of permanent hair removal?
10. What factor determines the depth of the needle insertion?
11. In what degrees can the angle or slant of the hair follicle vary?
12. Name three temporary ways in which superfluous hair may be removed.
13. For which parts of the face is tweezing most suitable?
14. Name two types of depilatories.
15. On which six parts of the body may heated wax be used?
16. Name three important safety precautions to observe when using wax.
17. For which patron is cold wax used?
18. Name three forms in which chemical depilatories are available.
19. Why should you give a patron a skin test before applying a chemical depilatory?

Chapter 26

CELLS

The student successfully mastering this chapter will know:
1. *The functions of human cells.*
2. *The structure and composition of cells.*
3. *The growth and reproduction of cells.*
4. *The meaning and process of metabolism.*
5. *The functions of body tissues, organs, and systems.*

To develop a general knowledge of how to care for the scalp, skin, hair, and nails, you must have a thorough understanding of the health, growth, and repair of these areas, as well as how they function. It is, therefore, important for cosmetologists to study and understand the major parts of the body upon which they render services or apply treatments.

The body is composed of cells, tissues, organs, and systems. It is made up of one-fourth solid matter and three-fourths liquid.

CELLS

Cells are the basic units of all living things, which include humans, animals, plants, and bacteria. Every part of the body is composed of cells, which differ from each other in size, shape, structure, and function.

A cell is a minute (mi-nut') portion of living substance containing **protoplasm** (pro'to-plazm), which is a colorless, jelly-like substance in which food elements and water are present. The two main parts of the cell are:
1. **Nucleus** (nu'kle-us) (dense protoplasm)—found in the center and plays an important part in the reproduction of the cell.
2. **Cytoplasm** (si'to-plazm) (less dense protoplasm)—found outside the nucleus and contains food materials necessary for the growth, reproduction, and self-repair of the cell.

STRUCTURE OF THE CELL

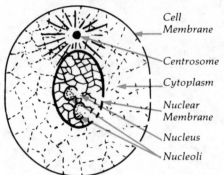

Cell Membrane

Centrosome

Cytoplasm

Nuclear Membrane

Nucleus

Nucleoli

The cell consists of protoplasm and contains the above essential parts.

The protoplasm of the cells contains the following important structures:

Nucleus (dense protoplasm)—found in the center, which plays an important part in the reproduction of the cell.

Cytoplasm (less dense protoplasm)—found outside of the nucleus and contains food materials necessary for the growth, reproduction, and self-repair of the cell.

Centrosome (sen'tro-som)—a small, round body in the cytoplasm, which also affects the reproduction of the cell.

Cell membrane encloses the protoplasm. It permits soluble substances to enter and leave the cell.

CELL GROWTH AND REPRODUCTION

As long as the cell receives an adequate supply of food, oxygen and water, eliminates waste products, and is favored with proper temperature, it will continue to grow and thrive. However, if these requirements are not fulfilled, and the presence of toxins (poisons) or pressure is evident, then the growth and the health of the cells are impaired. Most body cells are capable of growth and self-repair during their life cycle.

In the human body, when a cell reaches maturity, reproduction takes place by indirect division. This is a process in which a series of changes occur in the nucleus before the entire cell divides in half. Remember that the nucleus is surrounded by a thinner form of protoplasm, called cytoplasm, which supplies the food materials necessary for growth and reproduction.

DIAGRAM ILLUSTRATING INDIRECT DIVISION OF THE HUMAN CELL

1

2

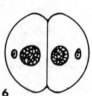

3

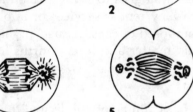

4   5   6

METABOLISM

Metabolism (me-tab'o-lizm) is a complex chemical process whereby the body cells are nourished and supplied with the energy needed to carry on their many activities.

There are two phases to metabolism:

1. **Anabolism** (an-ab'o-lizm)—the building up of cellular tissues. During anabolism, the cells of the body absorb water, food, and oxygen for the purpose of growth, reproduction, and repair.

2. **Catabolism** (kah-tab'o-lizm)—the breaking down of cellular tissues. During catabolism, the cells consume what they have absorbed in

order to perform specialized functions, such as muscular effort, secretions, or digestion.

Cells have various duties. They create and renew all parts of the body; they assist in blood circulation by carrying food to the blood and waste matter from the blood; and they control all body functions.

TISSUES

Tissues are composed of groups of cells of the same kind. Each tissue has a specific function and can be recognized by its characteristic appearance. Body tissues are classified as follows:

1. **Connective tissue** serves to support, protect, and bind together other tissues of the body. Bone, cartilage, ligament, tendon, and fat tissue are examples of connective tissue.
2. **Muscular tissue** contracts and moves various parts of the body.
3. **Nerve tissue** carries messages to and from the brain, and controls and coordinates all body functions.
4. **Epithelial** (ep-i-the'le-al) **tissue** is a protective covering on body surfaces, such as the skin, mucous membranes, linings of the heart, digestive and respiratory organs, and glands.
5. **Liquid tissue** carries food, waste products, and hormones by means of the blood and lymph.

ORGANS

Organs are structures containing two or more different tissues that are combined to accomplish a specific function.

The most important organs of the body are: the brain, which controls the body; the heart, which circulates the blood; the lungs, which supply oxygen to the blood; the liver, which removes toxic products of digestion; the kidneys, which excrete water and other waste products; and the stomach and intestines, which digest food.

SYSTEMS

Systems are groups of organs that cooperate for a common purpose, namely the welfare of the entire body. The human body is composed of the following important systems:

Skeletal (skel'e-tal) **system**—bones.

Muscular (mus'ku-lar) **system**—muscles.

Nervous (ner'vus) **system**—nerves.

Circulatory (ser'ku-lah-to-re) **system**—blood supply.

Endocrine (en'do-krin) **system**—ductless glands.

Excretory (eks'kre-to-re) **system**—organs of elimination.

Respiratory (re-spir'ah-to-re) **system**—lungs.

Digestive (di-jes'tiv) **system**—stomach and intestines.

Reproductive (re-pro-duk'tiv) **system**—reproducing.

The **skeletal system** is the physical foundation or framework of the body. The function of the skeletal system is to serve as a means of protection, support, and locomotion.

The **muscular system** covers, shapes, and supports the skeleton. Its function is to produce all the movements of the body.

The **nervous system** controls and coordinates the functions of all the other systems, and makes them work harmoniously and efficiently.

The **circulatory system** consists of a closed system of vessels, such as arteries, veins and capillaries, which carry blood from the heart to all parts of the body, and then back to the heart. This system supplies body cells with food materials, and also carries away waste products.

The **endocrine system** is composed of a group of specialized glands, which can either benefit or adversely affect the growth, reproduction, and health of the body.

The **excretory system,** which includes the kidneys, liver, skin, intestines and lungs, purifies the body by the elimination of waste products.

The **respiratory system,** whose most important organs are the trachea (windpipe), bronchial tubes and lungs, supplies the body with oxygen and removes carbon dioxide.

The **digestive system** changes food into a soluble form, suitable for use by the cells of the body.

The **reproductive system** performs the function of reproducing and perpetuating the human race.

All these systems are closely interrelated and dependent upon each other. While each forms a unit specially designed to perform a specific function, that function cannot be performed without the complete cooperation of some other system or systems.

REVIEW QUESTIONS
CELLS

1. What is a cell?
2. In what four ways do cells differ from each other?
3. Of what substance are cells composed?
4. Name the two main structures found in the protoplasm.
5. What is the function of: a) nucleus; b) cytoplasm?
6. How does a human cell reproduce?
7. What is metabolism?
8. Name two phases of metabolism.
9. What activities occur during the anabolism or construction process of the cells?
10. What activities occur during the catabolism or destructive process of the cells?
11. What are tissues?
12. List five classifications of body tissues.
13. What is an organ?
14. Which organ circulates the blood in the human body?
15. Which organ supplies oxygen to the blood?
16. What are systems?
17. Name nine body systems.
18. Which system is the physical framework of the body?
19. Which system covers, shapes, and supports the skeleton?
20. Which system controls and coordinates the functions of all other systems in the body?
21. To what system do the arteries, veins, and capillaries belong?

Chapter 27

THE SKIN AND DISORDERS OF THE SKIN

CHAPTER LEARNING OBJECTIVES

The student successfully mastering this chapter will know:
1. *The structure and composition of the skin (histology).*
2. *How the skin is nourished and what factors are involved in giving the skin its color, elasticity, and texture.*
3. *The nerves and glands that are contained in the skin.*
4. *The functions of the skin.*
5. *The definitions of important terms relating to skin disorders.*
6. *The various types of skin lesions encountered in the beauty salon.*
7. *The disorders of the sebaceous and sudoriferous glands.*
8. *Which skin disorders may be handled in the beauty salon and which should be referred to a physician.*
9. *The noncontagious infections of the skin and various pigmentations encountered.*

THE SKIN

The skin is the largest and one of the most important organs of the body. The scientific study of the skin and scalp is important to the cosmetologist because it forms the basis for an effective program of skin care, beauty services, and scalp treatments. The cosmetologist with a thorough understanding of skin, its structure and functions will be in a better position to give patrons professional advice on scalp, facial, and hand care.

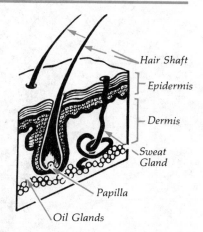

Hair Shaft

Epidermis

Dermis

Sweat Gland

Papilla

Oil Glands

A **healthy skin** is slightly moist, soft and flexible, possesses a slightly acid reaction, and is free from any disease or disorder. Its **texture** (feel and appearance) ideally is smooth and fine grained. A **good complexion** is an indication of the fine texture and healthy color of the skin.

The skin varies in thickness, being thinnest on the eyelids and thickest on the palms and soles. Continued pressure over any part of the skin may cause it to thicken and develop into a callous.

The skin of the scalp is constructed similarly to the skin elsewhere on the human body. However, the scalp has larger and deeper hair follicles to accommodate the longer hair of the head.

ONE SQUARE INCH OF SKIN CONTAINS:

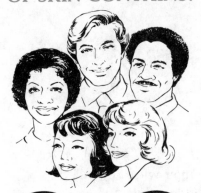

19,500 sensory cells
at the ends of nerve fibers

65 hairs

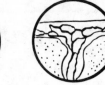

13 sensory
apparatuses for cold

78 sensory apparatuses
for heat

78 yards of
nerves

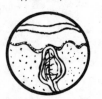

160-165 pressure apparatuses
for the perception of
tactile stimuli

19-20 yards of
blood vessels

1,300 nerve endings to
record pain

95-100 sebaceous
glands

650 sweat glands

9,500,000 cells

DIAGRAM OF A SECTION OF THE SCALP

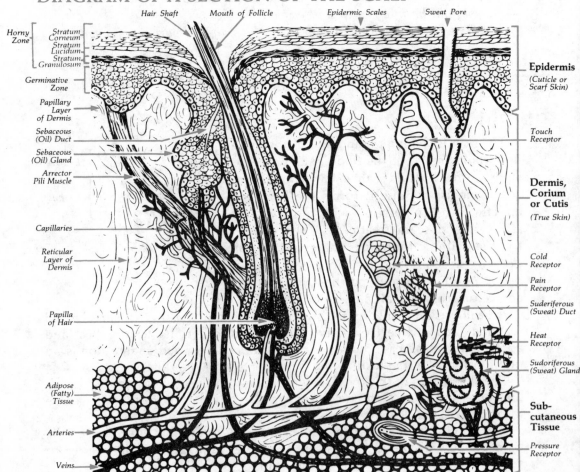

Hair Shaft
Mouth of Follicle
Epidermic Scales
Sweat Pore

Horny Zone
Stratum Corneum
Stratum Lucidum
Stratum Granulosum
Germinative Zone
Papillary Layer of Dermis
Sebaceous (Oil) Duct
Sebaceous (Oil) Gland
Arrector Pili Muscle
Capillaries
Reticular Layer of Dermis
Papilla of Hair
Adipose (Fatty) Tissue
Arteries
Veins

Epidermis
(Cuticle or Scarf Skin)

Touch Receptor

Dermis, Corium or Cutis
(True Skin)

Cold Receptor
Pain Receptor
Suderiferous (Sweat) Duct
Heat Receptor
Sudoriferous (Sweat) Gland

Sub-cutaneous Tissue

Pressure Receptor

HISTOLOGY OF THE SKIN

The skin contains two main divisions: the epidermis and the dermis.

1. The **epidermis** (ep-i-der'mis) is the outermost layer of the skin. This layer is commonly called the **cuticle** (ku'ti-kl), or **scarf skin.**

2. The **dermis** (der'mis) is the underlying, or inner layer, of the skin. It is also called the **derma, corium** (ko're-um), **cutis** (ku'tis), or **true skin.**

The **epidermis** is the outer layer of skin that forms a protective covering of the body. It contains no blood vessels, but has many small nerve endings. The epidermis contains the following layers:

1. The **stratum corneum** (stra'tum kor'ne-um), or horny layer, is the outer layer of the skin. Its scale-like cells are continually being shed and replaced by underneath cells coming to the surface. These cells contain **keratin** (ker'ah-tin), a protein substance. The overlapping cells are covered by a thin layer of oil which helps make the stratum corneum almost waterproof.

2. The **stratum lucidum** (lu'si-dum), or clear layer, consists of small transparent cells through which light can pass.

3. The **stratum granulosum** (gran-u-lo'sum), or granular layer, consists of cells that look like distinct granules. These cells are almost dead and undergo a change into a horny substance.

*4. The **stratum germinativum** (jer'mi-na-tiv-um), formerly known as the **stratum mucosum** (mu-ko'sum), is composed of several layers of differently shaped cells. The deepest layer is responsible for the growth of the epidermis. It also contains a dark skin pigment, called **melanin** (mel'ah-nin), which protects the sensitive cells below from the destructive effects of excessive ultra-violet rays of the sun or of an ultra-violet lamp.

The **dermis** is the true skin. It is a highly sensitive and vascular layer of connective tissue. Within its structure are found numerous blood vessels, lymph vessels, nerves, sweat glands, oil glands, hair follicles, arrector pili muscles, and papillae. The dermis consists of two layers: the papillary, or superficial layer, and the reticular, or deeper layer.

1. The **papillary** (pap'i-la-re) **layer** lies directly beneath the epidermis. It contains small cone-shaped projections of elastic tissue that point upward into the epidermis. These projections are called **papillae** (pah-pil'e). Some of these papillae contain looped **capillaries** (cap'i-la-res); others contain nerve fiber endings, called **tactile corpuscles** (tak'til kor'pus-ls). This layer also contains some of the melanin skin pigment.

2. The **reticular** (re-tik'u-lar) **layer** contains the following structures within its network:

   a) Fat cells.
   b) Blood vessels.
   c) Lymph vessels.
   d) Oil glands.
   e) Sweat glands.
   f) Hair follicles.
   g) Arrector pili muscles.

Stratum germinativum also is referred to as the basal or Malpighian layer.

†**Subcutaneous** (sub-ku-ta'ne-us) **tissue** is a fatty layer found below the dermis. This tissue is also called **adipose** (ad'i-pos), or **subcutis** (sub-ku'tis), tissue and varies in thickness according to the age, sex, and general health of the individual. It gives smoothness and contour to the body, contains fats for use as energy, and also acts as a protective cushion for the outer skin. Circulation is maintained by a network of arteries and lymphatics.

HOW THE SKIN IS NOURISHED

Blood and lymph supply nourishment to the skin. As they circulate through the skin, the blood and lymph contribute essential materials for growth, nourishment, and repair of the skin, hair, and nails. In the subcutaneous tissue are found networks of arteries and lymphatics that send their smaller branches to hair papillae, hair follicles, and skin glands. The capillaries are quite numerous in the skin.

NERVES OF THE SKIN

The skin contains the surface endings of many nerve fibers. They are:
1. Motor nerve fibers, which are distributed to the arrector pili muscles attached to the hair follicles.
2. Sensory nerve fibers, which react to heat, cold, touch, pressure, and pain.
3. Secretory nerve fibers, which are distributed to the sweat and oil glands of the skin. These nerves regulate the excretion of perspiration from the sweat glands and control the flow of sebum to the surface of the skin.

SENSORY NERVES OF THE SKIN

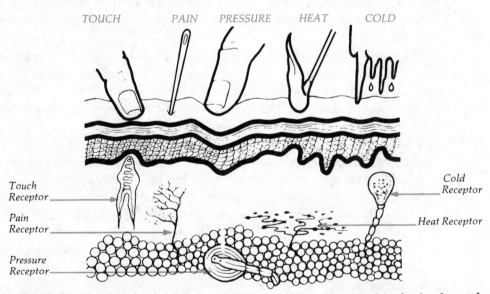

Sense of touch. The papillary layer of the dermis provides the body with the sense of touch. Nerves supplying the skin register basic types of sensations, namely: touch, pain, heat, cold, pressure, or deep touch. Nerve endings are most abundant in the fingertips. **Complex sensations,** such as vibrations, seem to depend on the sensitivity of a combination of these nerve endings.

---

†*Some histologists regard the subcutaneous tissue as a continuation of the dermis.*

SKIN ELASTICITY

The **pliability of the skin** depends on the elasticity of the dermis. For example, healthy skin regains its former shape almost immediately after being expanded.

Aging skin. The aging process of the skin is a subject of vital importance to everyone. Perhaps the most outstanding characteristic of the aged skin is its loss of elasticity.

SKIN COLOR

The **color of the skin,** whether fair, medium, or dark, depends in part on the blood supply to the skin, and primarily on the **melanin,** or coloring matter, that is deposited in the stratum germinativum and the papillary layers of the dermis. The pigment's color varies in different people. The distinctive color of the skin is a hereditary trait and varies among races and nationalities.

THE GLANDS OF THE SKIN

The skin contains two types of duct glands that extract materials from the blood to form new substances.

1. The **sudoriferous** (su-dor-if'er-us), or **sweat, glands** excrete sweat.
2. The **sebaceous** (se-ba'shus), or **oil, glands** secrete sebum.

The **sweat glands** (tubular type) consist of a coiled base, or **fundus** (fun'dus), and a tube-like duct which terminates at the skin surface to form the **sweat pore.** Practically all parts of the body are supplied with sweat glands, which are more numerous on the palms, soles, forehead, and in the armpits.

BODY HAIR AND FOLLICLE
Body hair (lanugo) with multiple oil (sebaceous) glands.

The sweat glands regulate body temperature and help to eliminate waste products from the body. Their activity is greatly increased by heat, exercise, emotions, and certain drugs.

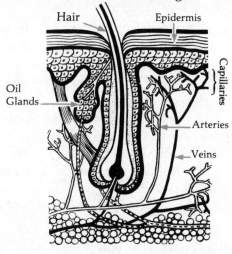

SCALP HAIR, FOLLICLE AND OIL GLANDS

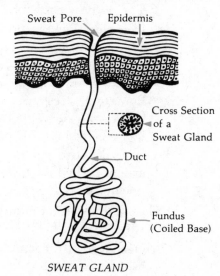

SWEAT GLAND

The excretion of sweat is under the control of the nervous system. Normally, 1-2 pints (.47-.95 l) of liquids containing salts are eliminated daily through the sweat pores in the skin.

The **oil glands** (saccular type) consist of little sacs whose ducts open into the hair follicles. They secrete **sebum** (se'bum), which lubricates the skin and preserves the softness of the hair. With the exception of the palms and soles, these glands are found in all parts of the body, particularly in the face.

Sebum is an oily substance produced by the oil glands. Ordinarily, it flows through the oil ducts leading to the mouths of the hair follicles. However, when the sebum becomes hardened and the duct becomes clogged, a **blackhead** is formed. Cleanliness is of prime importance in keeping the skin free of blemishes.

FUNCTIONS OF THE SKIN

The principal functions of the skin are protection, sensation, heat regulation, excretion, secretion, and absorption.

1. **Protection.** The skin protects the body from injury and bacterial invasion. The outermost layer of the epidermis is covered with a thin layer of sebum, thus rendering it waterproof. It is resistant to wide variations in temperature, minor injuries, chemically active substances, and many microbes.

2. **Sensation.** Through its sensory nerve endings, the skin responds to heat, cold, touch, pressure, and pain. Extreme stimulation of a sensory nerve ending produces pain. A minor burn is very painful, but a deep burn that destroys the nerves may be painless. Sensory endings, responsive to touch and pressure, are situated near hair follicles.

3. **Heat regulation.** The healthy body maintains a constant internal temperature of about 98.6° Fahrenheit (37° Celsius). As changes occur in the outside temperature, the blood and sweat glands of the skin make necessary adjustments in their functions. Heat regulation is a function of the skin, the organ that protects the body from the environment. The body is cooled by the evaporation of sweat.

4. **Excretion.** Perspiration from the sweat glands is excreted from the skin. Water lost by perspiration carries salt and other chemicals with it.

5. **Secretion.** Sebum is secreted by the sebaceous glands. Excessive flow of oil from the oil glands may produce **seborrhea** (seb-o-re'ah). Emotional stress may increase the flow of sebum.

6. **Absorption** is limited, but it does occur. Female hormones, when an ingredient of a face cream, may enter the body through the skin and influence it to a minor degree. Fatty materials, such as lanolin creams, are absorbed largely through hair follicles and sebaceous gland openings.

The skin has an immunity responsiveness to many things that touch it or gain entry into it.

Appendages of the skin are hair, nails, and sweat and oil glands.

DISORDERS OF THE SKIN

This information has been compiled to help the cosmetologist become familiar with certain common skin and scalp disorders with which she may come into contact in the beauty salon. There are few disorders of the skin or scalp that logically come within the province of the cosmetologist.

The cosmetologist must be prepared to recognize certain skin conditions and must know how to act properly with relation to them. Some skin and scalp disorders may be treated in cooperation with, and under the supervision of, a physician. Medicinal preparations, available only by prescription of a physician, for scalp, skin, or hair disorders must be applied in accordance with the directions of the physician.

Any patron with a skin condition that the cosmetologist does not recognize to be a simple disorder should be referred to a physician.

The most important thing to know is that a patron who has an inflammatory **skin disorder,** which may or may not be infectious, should not be served in the beauty salon. The cosmetologist should be able to recognize these conditions and to suggest that proper measures be taken to prevent more serious consequences.

Thus, the cosmetologist safeguards her own health, as well as the health of the **public.**

DEFINITIONS PERTAINING TO SKIN DISORDERS

Listed below are a number of important terms which should be familiar to the cosmetologist in order that she properly understands the subject of skin, scalp, and hair disorders.

Dermatology (der-mah-tol'o-je)—the study of the skin, its nature, structure, functions, diseases, and treatment.

Dermatologist (der-mah-tol'o-jist)—a skin specialist.

Pathology (pa-thol'o-je)—the study of disease.

Trichology (tri-kol'o-je)—the study of the hair and its diseases.

Etiology (e-te-ol'o-je)—the study of the causes of disease.

Diagnosis (di-ag-no'sis)—the recognition of a disease by its symptoms.

Prognosis (prog-no'sis)—the foretelling of the probable course of a disease.

LESIONS OF THE SKIN

A lesion is a structural change in the tissues caused by injury or disease. There are three types: primary, secondary, and tertiary. The cosmetologist is concerned with primary and secondary lesions only.

Knowing the principal skin lesions helps the cosmetologist to distinguish between conditions that may or may not be treated in a beauty salon.

Symptom is a sign of disease. The symptoms in diseases of the skin are divided into two groups:

1. **Subjective** refers to symptoms that can be felt, as itching, burning, or pains.
2. **Objective** refers to symptoms that can be seen, as pimples, pustules, or inflammation.

Macule (mak'ul)—a small, discolored spot or patch on the surface of the skin, neither raised nor sunken, as freckles.

Papule (pap'ul)—a small, elevated pimple in the skin, containing no fluid, but which may develop pus.

Wheal (whel)—an itchy, swollen lesion that lasts only a few hours. (Examples: hives, or the bite of an insect, such as a mosquito.)

Tubercle (tu'ber-kl)—a solid lump larger than a papule. It projects above the surface or lies within or under the skin. It varies in size from a pea to a hickory nut.

Tumor (tu'mer)—an external swelling, varying in size, shape, and color.

Vesicle (ves'i-kl)—a blister with clear fluid in it. Vesicles lie within or just beneath the epidermis. (Example: Poison ivy produces small vesicles.)

Bulla (bul'ah)—a blister containing a watery fluid, similar to a vesicle, but larger.

Pustule (pus'tul)—an elevation of the skin having an inflamed base, containing pus.

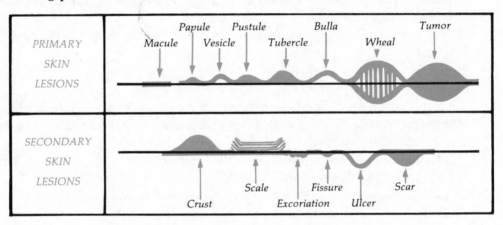

DEFINITIONS PERTAINING TO SECONDARY LESIONS

The secondary lesions are those in the skin that develop in the later stages of disease. These are:

Scale—an accumulation of epidermal flakes, dry or greasy. (Example: abnormal or excessive dandruff.)

Crust (scab)—an accumulation of serum and pus, mixed perhaps with epidermal material. (Example: the scab on a sore.)

Excoriation (eks-ko're-a'shun)—a skin sore or abrasion produced by scratching or scraping. (Example: a raw surface due to the loss of the superficial skin after an injury.)

Fissure (fish'ur)— a crack in the skin penetrating into the derma, as in the case of chapped hands or lips.

Ulcer (ul'ser)—an open lesion on the skin or mucous membrane of the body, accompanied by pus and loss of skin depth.

Scar (cicatrix) (si-ka'triks)—likely to form after the healing of an injury or skin condition that has penetrated the dermal layer.

Stain—an abnormal discoloration remaining after the disappearance of moles, freckles or liver spots, sometimes apparent after certain diseases.

DEFINITIONS PERTAINING TO DISEASE

Before describing the diseases of the skin and scalp so that they will be recognized by the cosmetologist, it is well to understand what is meant by disease.

Disease is any departure from a normal state of health.

Skin disease—any infection of the skin characterized by an objective lesion (one that can be seen) which may consist of scales, pimples, or pustules.

Acute disease—one manifested by symptoms of a more or less violent character and of short duration.

Chronic disease—one of long duration, usually mild but recurring.

Infectious (in-fek'shus) **disease**—one due to pathogenic germs taken into the body as a result of contact with a contaminated object or lesion.

Contagious disease—one that is communicable by contact.

Note:—The terms "infectious disease," "communicable disease," and "contagious disease" are often used interchangeably.

Congenital disease—one that is present in the infant at birth.

Seasonal disease—one that is influenced by the weather, as prickly heat in the summer, and forms of eczema, which are more prevalent in cold weather.

Occupational disease (such as dermatitis)—one that is due to certain kinds of employment, and is caused by coming in contact with cosmetics, chemicals, or tints.

Parasitic disease—one that is caused by vegetable or animal parasites, such as pediculosis or ringworm.

Pathogenic disease—one produced by disease-causing bacteria, such as staphylococcus and streptococcus, pus-forming bacteria.

Systemic disease—due to under- or over-functioning of the internal glands. It may be caused by faulty diet.

Venereal disease—a contagious disease commonly acquired by contact with an infected person during sexual intercourse.

Epidemic—the manifestation of a disease that attacks simultaneously a large number of persons living in a particular locality. Infantile paralysis, influenza, virus, or smallpox are examples of epidemic-causing diseases.

Allergy—a sensitivity that certain persons develop to normally harmless substances. Skin allergies are quite common. Contact with certain types of cosmetics, medicines, and tints, or eating certain foods, all may bring about an itching eruption, accompanied by redness, swelling, blisters, oozing, and scaling.

Inflammation—a skin disorder characterized by redness, pain, swelling, and heat.

There are several common disorders of the sebaceous (oil) glands which the cosmetologist should be able to identify and understand.

Comedones (kom-e-donz), or **blackheads,** are worm-like masses of hardened sebum, appearing most frequently on the face, forehead, and nose.

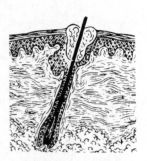

Blackheads accompanied by pimples often occur in youths between the ages of 13 and 20. During the adolescent period, the activity of the sebaceous glands is stimulated, thereby contributing to the formation of blackheads and pimples.

When the hair follicle is filled with an excess of oil from the sebaceous gland, a blackhead forms and creates a blockage at the mouth of the follicle. Should this condition become severe, medical attention is necessary.

Blackhead (plug of sebaceous matter and dirt) forming around mouth of hair follicle.

To treat blackheads, the skin's oiliness must be reduced by local applications of cleansers, and the blackheads removed under sterile conditions. Thorough skin cleansing each night is a very important factor. Cleansing creams and lotions often achieve better results than common soap and water.

Milia (mil'e-ah), or **whiteheads,** is a disorder of the sebaceous (oil) glands caused by the accumulation of sebaceous matter beneath the skin. This may occur on any part of the face, neck and, occasionally, on the chest and shoulders. Whiteheads are associated with fine-textured, dry types of skin.

Acne (ak'ne) is a chronic inflammatory disorder of the sebaceous glands, occurring most frequently on the face, back, and chest. The cause of acne is generally held to be microbic, but predisposing factors are adolescence and disturbance of the digestive tract. Acne, or common pimples, is also known as **acne simplex** or **acne vulgaris.**

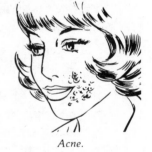

Acne.

Acne appears in a variety of different types, ranging from the simple (non-contagious) pimple, to serious, deep-seated skin conditions. It is always advisable to have the condition examined and diagnosed by a physician before any service is given in the beauty salon.

Seborrhea (seb-o-re'ah) is a skin condition caused by an excessive secretion of the sebaceous, or oil, glands. An oily or shiny condition of the nose, forehead, or scalp indicates the presence of seborrhea. On the scalp, it is readily detected by the unusual amount of oil on the hair.

Asteatosis (as'te-ah-to'sis) is a condition of dry, scaly skin, characterized by absolute or partial deficiency of sebum, due to senile changes (old age) or some bodily disorders. In local conditions, it may be caused by alkalis, such as those found in soaps and washing powders.

Rosacea (ro-za'se-a), formerly called **acne rosacea,** is a chronic inflammatory congestion of the cheeks and nose. It is characterized by redness, dilation of the blood vessels, and the formation of papules and pustules. It is usually caused by poor digestion and over-indulgence in alcoholic beverages. It also may be caused by over-exposure to extreme climate, faulty elimination, and hyperacidity. It is usually aggravated by eating and drinking hot, highly spiced, or highly seasoned foods or drinks.

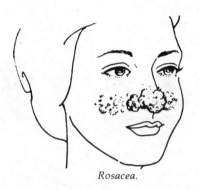

Rosacea.

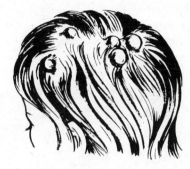

Steatoma.

Steatoma (ste-ah-to'mah), or **sebaceous cyst,** is a subcutaneous tumor of the sebaceous gland. Its contents consist of sebum, and its size ranges from a pea to an orange, and usually occurs on the scalp, neck, and back. A steatoma is sometimes called a **wen.**

DEFINITIONS PERTAINING TO DISORDERS OF SUDORIFEROUS (SWEAT) GLANDS

Bromidrosis (brom-id-ro'sis), or **osmidrosis** (oz-mi-dro'sis)—foul-smelling perspiration, usually noticeable in the armpits or on the feet.

Anidrosis (an-i-dro'sis), or **lack of perspiration**—often a result of fever or certain skin diseases. It requires medical treatment.

Hyperidrosis (hi-per-i-dro'sis), or **excessive perspiration**—caused by excessive heat or general body weakness. The most commonly affected parts are the armpits, joints, and feet. Medical treatment is required.

Miliaria rubra (mil-e-a're-a roob'ra) (**prickly heat**)—an acute, inflammatory disorder of sweat glands, characterized by an eruption of small red vesicles, and accompanied by burning and itching of skin. It is caused by exposure to excessive heat.

DEFINITIONS PERTAINING TO INFLAMMATIONS

Dermatitis (der-mah-ti'tis)—a term used to denote an inflammatory condition of the skin. The lesions come in various forms, such as vesicles or papules.

Eczema (ek'ze-mah)—an inflammation of the skin, of acute or chronic nature, presenting many forms of dry or moist lesions. It is frequently accompanied by itching or by a burning sensation. All cases of eczema should be referred to a physician for treatment. Its cause is unknown.

Psoriasis (so-ri'ah-sis)—a common, chronic, inflammatory skin disease whose cause is unknown. It is usually found on the scalp, elbows, knees, chest, and lower back, rarely on the face. The lesions are round, dry patches covered with coarse, silvery scales. If irritated, bleeding points occur. It is not contagious.

Herpes simplex (hur'pez sim'pleks)—a virus infection of unknown origin, commonly called **fever blisters.** It is characterized by the eruption of a single, or group, of vesicles on a red swollen base. The blisters usually appear on the lips, nostrils, or other part of the face, and rarely last more than a week. Indigestion may be one of the causes.

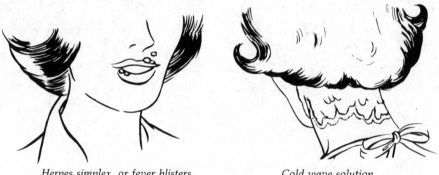

Herpes simplex, or fever blisters, involving the lips and nostrils.

Cold wave solution inflammation.

Occupational disorders in cosmetology—abnormal conditions resulting from contact with chemicals or tints in the course of performing services in the beauty salon. Some individuals may develop allergies to ingredients in cosmetics, antiseptics, cold waving lotions, and aniline derivative tints, which may cause eruptive skin infections known as **dermatitis venenata** (ven-e-na'tah). It is important that cosmetologists employ protective measures, such as the use of rubber gloves or protective creams whenever possible.

DEFINITIONS PERTAINING TO PIGMENTATIONS OF THE SKIN

In abnormal conditions, **pigment** may come from inside or outside the body.

Abnormal colors are seen in every skin disorder and in many systemic disorders. Pigmentation is observed when certain drugs are being taken internally.

Tan—caused by excessive exposure to the sun.

Lentigines (len-tij'i-nez) (singular, **lentigo**), or **freckles**—small yellow to brown colored spots on parts exposed to sunlight and air.

Stains—abnormal brown skin patches, having a circular and irregular shape. Their permanent color is due to the presence of blood pigment. They occur during aging, after certain diseases, and after the disappearance of moles, freckles, and liver spots. The cause of these stains is unknown.

Chloasma (klo-az'mah)—characterized by increased deposits of pigment in the skin. It is found mainly on the forehead, nose, and cheeks. Chloasma is also called **moth patches** or **liver spots.**

Naevus (ne'vus)—commonly known as **birthmark.** It is a small or large malformation of the skin due to pigmentation or dilated capillaries.

Leucoderma (lu-ko-der'mah)—abnormal white patches in the skin, due to congenital defective pigmentation. It is classified as:

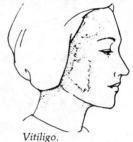

Vitiligo (vit-i-li'go)—an acquired condition of leucoderma, affecting the skin or the hair. The only treatment is a matching cosmetic color, making it less conspicuous.

Albinism (al'bin-izm)—congenital absence of melanin pigment in the body, including the skin, hair, and eyes. The silky hair is white. The skin is pinkish white and will not tan.

Vitiligo.

DEFINITIONS PERTAINING TO HYPERTROPHIES (NEW GROWTHS)

Keratoma (ker-ah-to'mah), or **callous**—an acquired, superficial, round, thickened patch of epidermis, due to pressure friction on the hands and feet. If the thickening grows inward, it is called a **corn.**

Mole—a small, brownish spot, or blemish, on the skin. Moles are believed to be inherited. They range in color from pale tan to brown or bluish black. Some moles are small and flat, resembling freckles, while others are more deeply seated and darker in color. Large, dark hairs often occur in moles. Any change in a mole requires medical attention.

CAUTION

Do not treat or remove hair from moles.

Verruca (ve-roo'kah)—technical term for **wart.** It is caused by a virus and is infectious. It can spread from one location to another, particularly along a scratch in the skin.

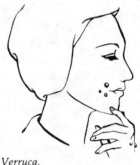

Verruca.

REVIEW QUESTIONS

THE SKIN

1. Briefly describe a healthy skin.
2. What does a good complexion indicate?
3. Name the two main divisions of the skin.
4. Locate the epidermis and give its main function.
5. Name the four layers of the epidermis.
6. Which epidermal layer is continually being shed and replaced?
7. Which epidermal layer consists of small, transparent cells?
8. Which epidermal layer starts to undergo a change into a horny substance?
9. Which layer of the epidermis is responsible for its growth?
10. What type of tissue is the dermis?
11. Name the two layers of the dermis.

12. Which structures are found in the papillary layer?
13. Which structures are found in the reticular layer?
14. What is the function of the subcutaneous tissue?
15. How is the skin nourished?
16. Name three types of nerve fibers found in the skin.
17. To which structures in the skin are the motor nerve fibers distributed?
18. To what five sensations will the sensory nerves of the skin react?
19. What nerve fibers in the skin regulate and control the excretion of perspiration and the flow of sebum?
20. Which part of the body is most abundantly supplied with nerve endings?
21. What is meant by pliability of the skin?
22. What is the characteristic of aged skin?
23. What determines the color of the skin?
24. Where is the coloring matter of the skin found?
25. What determines the distinctive color of the skin?
26. Name two types of duct glands that are found in the skin.
27. Describe the structure of the sweat glands.
28. Where are sweat glands found?
29. What is the function of the sweat glands?
30. Name four ways of increasing the activity of the sweat glands.
31. What regulates the temperature of the body?
32. Describe the structure of the oil glands.
33. Which substance is secreted by the oil glands?
34. What is the chief function of sebum?
35. Where are the oil glands found?
36. What are the six important functions of the skin?
37. What is the normal temperature of the human body?
38. Name one cosmetic that the skin can absorb in small amounts.
39. Name the four appendages of the skin.

DISORDERS OF THE SKIN

1. Why is it necessary that the cosmetologist be very careful before trying to deal with a skin disorder in the beauty salon?
2. What should a cosmetologist do if she does not recognize a skin disorder that may or may not be infectious?
3. Why should the cosmetologist refuse to treat a patron with an infectious or contagious disease?
4. Define dermatology.
5. What is a dermatologist?
6. What is a lesion?
7. What is the difference between objective and subjective lesions? Give one example of each.
8. Name eight primary lesions of the skin.
9. Name seven secondary lesions of the skin.
10. Define disease.
11. What are the common terms for: a) comedones; b) milia?
12. What causes the formation of comedones?

13. Define acne.
14. Which of the following terms apply to disorders of the sebaceous (oil) glands?
    Milia, acne, bromidrosis, anidrosis, comedones, seborrhea, hyperidrosis.
15. Briefly describe: bromidrosis, anidrosis, hyperidrosis, and miliaria rubra.
16. Define dermatitis.
17. Define eczema.
18. What is the characteristic appearance of psoriasis?
19. On which five parts of the body is psoriasis usually found?
20. Define herpes simplex. What is it commonly called?
21. Where do fever blisters usually occur?
22. Define dermatitis venenata. Name two hair services that may cause dermatitis venenata.
23. What are freckles, and what causes them?
24. What are the common names for chloasma?
25. What is the common name for naevus?
26. Define: a) leucoderma; b) vitiligo.
27. Define albinism.
28. What is the technical term for callous?
29. What is a mole?
30. What is the technical term for a wart?

Chapter 28

THE HAIR AND DISORDERS OF THE SCALP AND HAIR

CHAPTER LEARNING OBJECTIVES

The student successfully mastering this chapter will know:
1. *The composition and divisions of the hair.*
2. *The different structures within the hair root and hair follicle.*
3. *The important facts about sebum.*
4. *The facts relating to hair structure, growth, and distribution.*
5. *The theories relating to the life and replacement of hair.*
6. *The meaning of hair texture, porosity, density, and elasticity.*
7. *The causes of the changes in hair color.*
8. *The various types of dandruff and their treatment.*
9. *Which scalp and hair diseases may be treated in the beauty salon.*
10. *How to recognize the various forms of alopecia.*
11. *The various contagious diseases of the scalp and hair.*
12. *How to recognize the hair disorders seen in the beauty salon.*

HAIR

Hair is an **appendage** (ah-pen'daj) of the skin. It is a slender, thread-like outgrowth of the skin and scalp of the human body. There is no sense of feeling in hair, due to the absence of nerves.

The study of hair, technically called **trichology** (tri-kol'o-je), is of paramount importance to cosmetologists because hair is what they primarily deal with. The chief purposes of hair are **adornment** and **protection** of the head from heat, cold, and injury.

To keep hair healthy and beautiful, proper attention must be given to its care and treatment. Knowledge and **analysis** (ah-nal'i-sis) of the patron's hair, tactful suggestions for its improvement, and sincere interest in maintaining its health and beauty should be the concern of every cosmetologist.

Abuse of hair by harmful cosmetic applications or faulty hair services can cause the hair structure to become weakened or damaged.

COMPOSITION OF HAIR

Hair is chiefly composed of a **protein** (pro'te-in), called **keratin** (ker'ah-tin), which is present in all horny growths, such as nails, claws, and hoofs. The chemical compostion of hair varies with its color.

The average hair is composed of: carbon, 50.65%; hydrogen, 6.36%; nitrogen, 17.14%; sulfur, 5.0%; and oxygen, 20.85%.

DIVISIONS OF HAIR

Full grown human hair is divided into two principal parts: the hair root and hair shaft.

1. The **hair root** is that portion of the hair structure located beneath the skin surface. This is the portion of the hair enclosed within the follicle.
2. The **hair shaft** is that portion of the hair structure extending above the skin surface.

STRUCTURES ASSOCIATED WITH HAIR ROOT

Structures closely associated with the hair root are the hair follicle, hair bulb, and hair papilla.

The **hair follicle** (fol'i-kl) is a tube-like depression, or pocket, in the skin or scalp that encases the **hair root**. For every hair there is a follicle, which varies in depth depending on the thickness and location of the skin.

One or more oil glands are attached to each hair follicle.

The funnel-shaped mouths of hair follicles are breeding places for germs and for the accumulation of sebum and dirt.

The follicle does not run straight down into the skin or scalp, but is set at an angle so that the hair above the surface has a natural flow to one side. This natural flow is sometimes called the **hair stream** of the scalp. Since the angles run according to areas set by nature, hair emerges from the scalp slanting in a given direction.

The **hair bulb** is a thickened, club-shaped structure forming the lower part of the hair root. The lower part of the hair bulb is hollowed out to fit over and cover the hair papilla.

The **hair papilla** (pa-pil'a) is a small cone-shaped elevation located at the bottom of the hair follicle which fits into the hair bulb. Within the hair papilla is a rich blood and nerve supply, which contributes to the growth and regeneration of the hair. It is through the papilla that nourishment reaches the hair bulb. The papilla has the ability to produce hair cells. As long as the papilla functions, the hair will grow. New hair cells cannot be formed nor can the hair grow without the papilla. If the papilla is healthy and well nourished, it will produce a new hair.

STRUCTURES CONNECTED TO HAIR FOLLICLES

The **arrector pili** (ah-rek'tor pi'li) is a small involuntary muscle attached to the underside of a hair follicle. Fear or cold contracts it, causing the hair to stand up straight, giving the skin the appearance of "gooseflesh." Eyelash and eyebrow hairs lack arrector pili muscles.

CROSS SECTION
OF HAIR

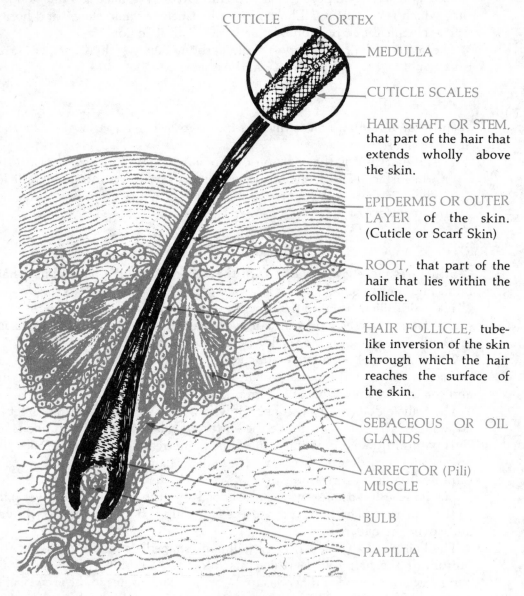

CUTICLE   CORTEX

MEDULLA

CUTICLE SCALES

HAIR SHAFT OR STEM, that part of the hair that extends wholly above the skin.

EPIDERMIS OR OUTER LAYER of the skin. (Cuticle or Scarf Skin)

ROOT, that part of the hair that lies within the follicle.

HAIR FOLLICLE, tube-like inversion of the skin through which the hair reaches the surface of the skin.

SEBACEOUS OR OIL GLANDS

ARRECTOR (Pili) MUSCLE

BULB

PAPILLA

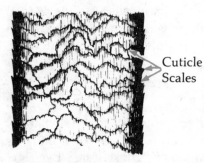

Cuticle Scales

MAGNIFIED VIEW OF HAIR CUTICLE

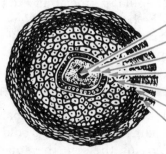

Medulla of Hair
Cortex of Hair
Cuticle of Hair
Inner or Epidermic Coat
Outer or Dermic Coat
Inner Root Sheath
Outer Root Sheath

CROSS SECTION OF THE HAIR AND FOLLICLE

Sebaceous (se-ba′shus), or **oil, glands** consist of little sacular structures situated in the dermis. Their ducts are connected to hair follicles. Secretion of an oily substance, **sebum** (se′bum), gives luster and pliability to the hair and keeps the skin surface soft and supple. However, the sebaceous glands frequently become troublemakers. By overproducing, they bring on a common form of oily dandruff.

The **production of sebum** is influenced by five factors: diet, blood circulation, emotional disturbances, stimulation of endocrine glands, and drugs.

Diet exerts an influence on the general health of the hair. The overeating of sweet, starchy, and fatty foods may cause the sebaceous glands to become overactive and secrete too much sebum.

Blood circulation. The hair derives its nourishment from the blood supply, which, in turn, depends on the foods eaten for certain elements. In the absence of necessary foods, the health of the hair may be affected.

Emotional disturbances are linked with the health of the hair through the nervous system. Healthy hair may be an indication of a healthy body.

Endocrine (en′do-krin) **glands.** The secretions of the endocrine glands influence the health of the body. Any disturbance of these glands may affect the health of the body and, ultimately, the health of the hair.

Certain drugs, such as hormones, if taken without a doctor's advice, may adversely affect the hair's ability to receive permanent waving and other hair services.

HAIR STRUCTURE

Shapes of hair. As a rule, hair has one of three general shapes. As it grows out, hair assumes the shape, size, and direction of the follicle. A **cross-sectional view** of the hair under the microscope reveals that:

1. Straight hair is usually round. (Fig. 1)
2. Wavy hair is usually oval. (Fig. 2)
3. Curly or kinky hair is almost flat. (Fig. 3)

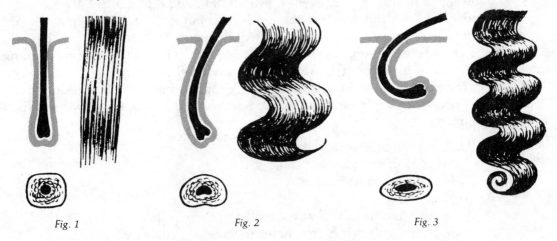

Fig. 1   Fig. 2   Fig. 3

There is no strict rule regarding cross-sectional shapes of hair. Oval, straight, and curly hair have been found in all shapes.

The **structure of the hair** is composed of cells arranged in the following three layers:

1. **Cuticle** (ku'ti-kl), the outside horny layer, is composed of transparent, overlapping, protective scale-like cells, pointing away from the scalp towards the hair ends. Chemicals raise these scales so that solutions can enter into the hair cortex. The cuticle protects the inner structure of the hair.

2. **Cortex** (kor'teks), the middle or inner layer, which gives strength and elasticity to the hair, is made up of a fibrous substance formed by elongated cells. This layer contains the pigment that gives the hair its color.

3. **Medulla** (me-dul'ah), the innermost layer, is referred to as the pith, or marrow, of the hair shaft, and is composed of round cells. The medulla may be absent in fine and very fine hair.

HAIR DISTRIBUTION

Hair is found all over the body, except on the palms, soles, lips, and eyelids.

There are three types of hair on the body:

1. **Long hair** protects the scalp against the sun's rays and injury, gives adornment to the head, and forms a pleasing frame for the face. **Soft long hair** also grows in the armpits of both sexes and on the faces of men.

2. **Short** or **bristly hair,** such as the eyebrows and eyelashes, adds beauty and line of color to the face. **Eyebrows** divert sweat from the eyes. The **eyelashes** help protect the eyes from dust particles and light glare.

3. **Lanugo** (la-nu'go) **hair** is the fine, soft, downy hair of the cheeks, forehead, and nearly all other areas of the body. It helps in the efficient evaporation of perspiration.

HAIR GROWTH

Hair cycle. If the hair is normal and healthy, each individual hair goes through a steady cycle of events: **growth, fall,** and **replacement.** The average growth of healthy hair on the scalp is about ½" (1.25 cm) per month. The rate of growth of human hair will differ on specific parts of the body, between sexes, among races, and with age. Scalp hair also will differ among individuals in **strength, elasticity,** and **waviness.**

The growth of scalp hair occurs more rapidly between the ages of 15-30, but declines sharply between 50-60. Scalp hair grows faster on women than on men.

Hair growth also is influenced by:
1. Seasons of the year.
2. Nutrition and hormones.
3. Health.

Climatic conditions will affect the hair in the following ways:
1. Moisture will deepen the natural wave.
2. Cold air will cause the hair to contract.
3. Heat will cause the hair to swell or expand and absorb moisture.

Hair growth is not increased by any of the following:

1. Close clipping, shaving, trimming, cutting, or singeing have no effect on the rate of hair growth.
2. The application of ointments or oils will not increase hair growth. They act as lubricants to the hair shaft, but do not feed the hair.
3. Hair does not grow after death. The flesh and skin contract, thus giving the appearance of some growth.
4. Singeing the hair will not seal in the natural oil.

Normal hair shedding. A certain amount of hair is shed daily. This is nature's method of making way for new hair. The average daily shedding is estimated at 50-80 hairs. Hair loss beyond this estimated average indicates some scalp or hair trouble.

Eyebrows and **eyelashes** are replaced every 4-5 months.

REPLACEMENT OF HAIR

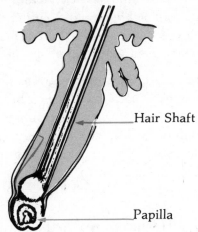

Hair Shaft

Papilla

1. At an early stage of shedding, the hair shows its separation from the papilla.

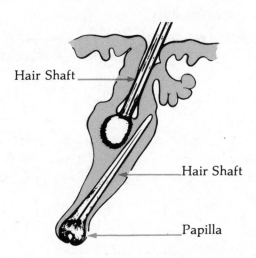

Hair Shaft

Hair Shaft

Papilla

2. At a later stage of the hair shedding, you will note a new hair growing from the same papilla.

Hair depends on the papilla for its growth. As long as the papilla is not destroyed, the hair will grow. If the hair is pulled out from the roots, it will nevertheless grow again, but should the papilla be destroyed, it will never grow again.

In human beings, new hair replaces old hair in the following ways:

1. The bulb loosens and separates from the papilla.
2. The bulb moves upward in the follicle.
3. The hair moves slowly to the surface, where it is shed.
4. The new hair is formed by cell division, which takes place at the root of the hair around the papilla.

LIFE AND DENSITY OF HAIR

The exact life span of hair has not been agreed upon. The average life of hair will range from **2-4 years.** Other factors, such as sex, age, type of hair, heredity, and health, have a bearing on the duration of hair life.

The average area for a head is about 120 square inches (780 cm²). There is an average of 1000 hairs to a square inch (6.5 cm²).

The number of hairs on the head varies with the color of the hair:

Blonde	140,000	Black	108,000
Brown	110,000	Red	90,000

COLOR OF HAIR

The **natural color of hair,** its strength and texture, mainly depend on heredity. To be successful in giving hair lightening and tinting services, the cosmetologist must understand the color and distribution of hair pigment. The cosmetologist also must understand hair texture, porosity, and elasticity.

The cortex contains coloring matter, minute grains of **melanin** (mel'ah-nin), or pigment. The source of pigment has not been definitely settled. It is probably derived from the color-forming substances in the blood, as is all pigment of the human body. The color of hair, light or dark, depends on the color and on the amount of grains of pigment it contains.

GREYING OF HAIR

Grey hair is caused by the absence of hair pigment in the cortical layer. It is really mottled hair — spots of white or whitish yellow scattered about in the hair shafts. Normally, grey hair grows out in this condition from the hair bulb. Greying does not take place after the hair has grown.

In most cases, the greying of hair is a result of the natural aging process in humans, and it is not related to the hair's texture or growth. Greying also can happen as a result of some serious illness or nervous shock. An early diminishing of the pigment brought on by emotional tensions also may cause the hair to turn grey.

Premature greying of hair in a young person is usually the result of a defect in pigment formation occurring at birth. Often it will be found that several members of a family are affected with premature greyness.

HAIR DEFINITIONS AND TECHNICAL TERMS

Hirsuties (her-su'shi-ez), or **hypertrichosis** (hi-per-tri-ko'sis), means hairiness, or superfluous hair. It is recognized by the growth of hair in unusual amounts or locations, as on the faces of women.

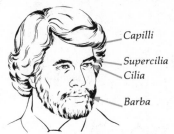

Capilli
Supercilia
Cilia
Barba

Technical terms given to hair on the head and face:
Barba (bar'bah)—the face.
Capilli (kah-pil'i)—the head.
Cilia (sil'e-ah)—the eyelashes.
Supercilia (su-per-sil'e-ah)—the eyebrows.

An **albino** (al-bi'no) is a person born with white hair, the result of an absence of coloring matter in the hair shaft, accompanied by no marked pigment coloring in the skin or irises of the eyes.

Definitions of Directional Hair Growth

Whorl

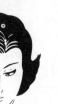

Cowlick

Hair stream—Hair sloping in the same direction is known as hair stream, which is a result of the follicles sloping in the same direction. Two such streams, sloping in opposite directions, form a **natural parting** of the hair.

Whorl—Hair that forms in a swirl effect, as in the crown, is called a whorl.

Cowlick—A tuft of hair standing up is known as a cowlick. Cowlicks are usually noticeable at the front hairline. However, they may be located on other parts of the scalp. In styling, cowlicks must be considered, and the hair styled accordingly.

HAIR ANALYSIS

Much of the cosmetologist's time is taken up with servicing and styling patrons' hair. For this reason, it is important that the cosmetologist be able to recognize the condition of a patron's hair, as well as distinguish the type of hair to be serviced.

CONDITION

Hair knowledge and skill in ascertaining the condition of the hair can be acquired by constant observation and practice in the use of the senses of sight, touch, hearing, and smell.

1. **Sight.** Observing the hair will immediately give you some knowledge about its condition. Sight contributes approximately 15 percent to hair analysis, with the sense of touch the final determining factor.
2. **Touch.** Unless cosmetologists develop to their full capacity the sense of touch in relation to hair, they cannot give professional hair services to patrons. When the sense of touch is fully developed, fewer mistakes are made in judging the hair.
3. **Hearing.** Listen to what the patron tells you about her hair, health problems, reaction to cosmetics, and medications she may be taking. You will be in a better position to analyze the condition of her hair accurately.
4. **Smell.** Unclean hair and certain scalp disorders will create an odor. If the patron generally has good health, you might recommend that she keep her scalp clean by shampooing regularly.

TEXTURE, POROSITY, AND ELASTICITY

Besides condition, the other important qualities by which human hair is judged are: **texture** (teks'tur), **porosity** (po-ros'i-te), and **elasticity** (e-las-tis'i-te).

TEXTURE

Hair texture refers to the degree of coarseness or fineness of the hair which may vary on different parts of the head. Variations in hair texture are due to:

1. **Diameter of the hair,** whether coarse, medium, fine, or very fine. Coarse hair has the greatest diameter; very fine hair has the smallest.
2. **Feel of the hair,** whether harsh, soft, or wiry.

Usually cuticle scales of **coarse hair** are closely overlapped and raised away from the hair shaft, which is responsible for the **hygroscopic** (hi-gro-skop'ik) quality (ability to absorb moisture) of coarse hair.

Medium hair is the normal type most commonly met in the beauty salon. This type of hair does not present any special problem.

Fine or **very fine hair** requires special care. Its microscopic structure reveals that only two layers, the cortex and cuticle, are present.

Wiry hair, whether coarse, medium, or fine, has a hard, glassy finish caused by the cuticle scales lying flat against the hair shaft. It takes longer to permanent wave, tint, or lighten this type of hair.

POROSITY

Hair porosity is the ability of the hair to absorb moisture regardless of whether the hair is coarse, medium, fine, or very fine.

Good porosity—hair with the cuticle layer raised from the hair shaft can absorb a fair or normal amount of moisture or chemicals.

Moderate porosity (normal hair)—the average type of hair met in the beauty salon is less porous than hair with good porosity.

Usually hair with good or moderate porosity presents no problem when receiving hair services, whether permanent waving, hair tinting, or lightening.

Poor porosity (resistant hair)—hair with the cuticle layer lying close to the hair shaft usually absorbs the least amount of moisture. Hair with poor porosity requires thorough analysis and strand tests before the application of hair cosmetics.

Extreme porosity—poor condition (tinted, lightened, or damaged hair)—hair that has been made extremely porous by continuous or faulty treatments.

ELASTICITY

Hair elasticity is the ability of hair to stretch and return to its original form without breaking. Hair with normal elasticity is springy and gives a live and lustrous appearance. Normal dry hair is capable of being stretched about one-fifth its length; it will spring back when released. However, wet hair can be stretched 40-50% of its length. Porous hair will stretch more than hair with poor porosity. Hair may be classified as having good elasticity, normal elasticity, or poor elasticity. (For additional information on hair elasticity see chapter on **Cold Waving.**)

DISORDERS OF THE SCALP

Just as the skin is continually being shed and replaced, the uppermost layer of the scalp is being cast off all the time. Ordinarily, these horny scales are loose and fall off freely. The natural shedding of these horny scales should not be mistaken for dandruff.

DANDRUFF

Dandruff consists of small, white scales that usually appear on the scalp and hair. It is also known by the medical term of **pityriasis** (pit-e-ri'ah-sis).

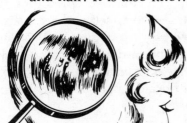

Light dandruff.

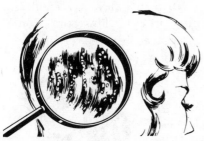

Heavy dandruff.

Long neglected, excessive dandruff may lead to baldness.

A **direct cause** of dandruff is the excessive shedding of the epithelial cells. Instead of growing to the surface and falling off, the horny scales accumulate on the scalp.

Indirect or **associated causes** of dandruff are a sluggish condition of the scalp, occasioned by poor circulation, infection, injury, lack of nerve stimulation, improper diet, and uncleanliness. Contributing causes are the use of strong shampoos and insufficient rinsing of the hair after a shampoo.

The two principal types of dandruff are:

1. **Pityriasis capitis simplex** (ka-pee'tis sim' plex)—dry type.
2. **Pityriasis steatoides** (ste-ah-toy'dez)—a greasy or waxy type.

Pityriasis capitis simplex (dry dandruff) is characterized by an itchy scalp and small white scales, which are usually attached in masses to the scalp, or scattered loosely in the hair. Occasionally, they are so profuse that they fall to the shoulders. Dry dandruff is often the result of a sluggish scalp caused by poor circulation, lack of nerve stimulation, improper diet, emotional and glandular disturbances, or uncleanliness. **Treatment:** Frequent scalp treatments, use of mild shampoos, regular scalp massage, daily use of antiseptic scalp lotions, and applications of scalp ointments may help correct this condition.

Pityriasis steatoides (greasy or waxy type of dandruff) is a scaly condition of the epidermis. The scales become mixed with sebum, causing them to stick to the scalp in patches. The associated itchiness causes the person to scratch the scalp. If the greasy scales are torn off, bleeding or oozing of sebum may follow. Medical treatment is advisable.

SUMMARY

The nature of dandruff is not clearly defined by medical authorities. It is generally believed to be of infectious origin. Some authorities hold that it is due to a specific microbe.

However, from the cosmetologist's point of view, both forms of dandruff are to be considered contagious and may be spread by the use of common brushes, combs, and other articles. Therefore, the cosmetologist must take the necessary precautions to sanitize everything that comes into contact with the patron.

ALOPECIA

Alopecia (al-o-pe'she-ah) is the technical term for any abnormal form of loss of hair.

The natural falling out of the hair should not be confused with alopecia. When hair has grown to its full length, it comes out by itself and is replaced by a new hair. The natural shedding of hair occurs most frequently in spring and fall. On the other hand, the hair lost in alopecia does not come back, unless special treatments are given to encourage hair growth.

Certain hairstyles, such as ponytail and tight braids, may be contributing factors to constant hair loss or baldness.

Alopecia senilis (se-nil'is) is the form of baldness occurring in old age. This loss of hair is permanent.

Alopecia prematura (pre-mah-tu'rah) is the form of baldness, beginning any time before middle age with a slow thinning process. This condition is caused by the first hairs falling out and being replaced by weaker ones.

Alopecia areata (ar-e-a'tah) is the sudden falling out of hair in round patches, or baldness in spots, sometimes caused by anemia, scarlet fever, typhoid fever, or syphilis. Affected areas are slightly depressed, smooth, and very pale, due to a decreased blood supply. Patches may be round or irregular in shape, and they may vary in size from ½" (1.3 cm) to 2-3" (5.1-7.6 cm) in diameter. In most conditions of alopecia areata, the nervous system has been subjected to some injury. Since the flow of blood is influenced by the nervous system, the affected area also is poorly nourished.

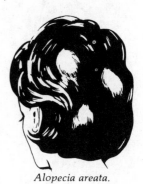

Alopecia areata.

Alopecia may appear in a variety of different forms, caused by many abnormal conditions. Sometimes an alopecia condition may be improved by proper scalp treatments.

CONTAGIOUS DISORDERS

Vegetable Parasitic Infections

Tinea (tin'e-ah) is the medical term for **ringworm**. Ringworm is caused by **vegetable parasites.** All forms are contagious. **Tinea** is transmissible from one person to another. The disease is commonly carried by scales or hairs containing fungi. Shower baths, swimming pools, and unsanitized articles also are sources of transmission.

Ringworm starts with a small, reddened patch of little blisters. Several such patches may be present. Any ringworm condition should be referred to a physician.

Tinea capitis (kap'i-tis) (ringworm of the scalp) is a contagious, vegetable parasitic disease of the scalp, characterized by red papules, or spots, at the opening of the hair follicles. The patches spread and the hair becomes brittle and lifeless. It breaks off, leaving a stump, or falls from the enlarged open follicles.

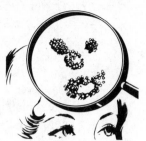

Tinea capitis.

Tinea favosa (fa-vo'sah), also called **favus** (fa'vus) or **honeycomb ringworm,** is an infectious growth caused by a vegetable parasite. It is characterized by dry, sulfur-yellow, cup-like crusts on the scalp, called **scutula** (skut'u-lah), which have a peculiar mousy odor. Scars from favus are bald patches that may be pink or white and shiny. It is very contagious and should be referred to a physician.

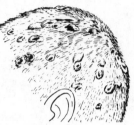

Favus.

Animal Parasitic Infections

Scabies (itch) is a highly contagious, animal parasitic skin disease, caused by the itch mite. Vesicles and pustules may form from the irritation of the parasites, or from scratching the affected areas.

Pediculosis (pe-dik-u-lo'sis) **capitis** is a contagious condition caused by the head louse (animal parasite) infesting the hair of the scalp. As the parasites feed on the scalp, itching occurs and the resultant scratching may cause an infection.

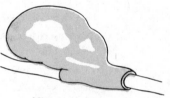

Nit.

The head louse is transmitted from one person to another by contact with infested hats, combs, brushes, or other personal articles.

To kill head lice, advise patron to apply larkspur tincture, or other similar medication, to the entire head before retiring. The next morning, she should shampoo with germicidal soap. Treatment should be repeated as necessary. Never treat a head lice condition in the beauty salon.

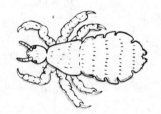

Head louse.

Staphylococci Infections

Furuncle (fer-un'kl), or **boil,** is an acute staphylococci infection of a hair follicle which produces constant pain. A furuncle is the result of an active inflammatory process, limited to a definite area and subsequently producing a pustule perforated by a hair.

Carbuncle (kar'bun-kl) is the result of an acute staphylococci infection, and is larger than a furuncle. It should be referred to a physician.

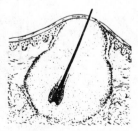

Furuncle (boil).

DISORDERS OF THE HAIR

NON CONTAGIOUS DISORDERS

Canities (kah-nish'i-ez) is the technical term for grey hair. Its immediate cause is the loss of natural pigment in the hair. It may be either of two types:

1. **Congenital canities** exists at or before birth. It occurs in albinos and occasionally in persons with perfectly normal hair. A patchy type of congenital canities may develop either slowly or rapidly, according to the cause of the condition.
2. **Acquired canities** may be due to old age; it may be premature in early adult life.

Causes of acquired canities may be worry, anxiety, nervous strain, prolonged illness, various wasting diseases, and heredity.

Ringed hair. Alternate bands of grey and dark hair.

Hypertrichosis (hi-per-tri-ko'sis), or **hirsuties,** means superfluous hair; an abnormal development of hair on areas of the body normally bearing only downy hair.   **Treatment:** Tweeze or remove by depilatories, electrolysis, shaving, or epilation.

CAUTION

Do not treat small pigmented areas.

Trichoptilosis (trik-op-ti-lo'sis) is the technical name for **split hair ends.** **Treatment:** The hair should be well oiled to soften and lubricate the dry ends. The ends also may be removed by cutting.

Trichorrhexis nodosa (trik-o-rek'sis no-do'sah), or **knotted hair,** is a dry, brittle condition with the formation of nodular swellings along the hair shaft. The hair breaks easily and shows a brush-like spreading out of the fibers of the broken-off hair. Softening the hair with ointments may prove beneficial.

Monilethrix (mon-il'e-thriks) is the technical term for **beaded hair.** The hair breaks between the beads or nodes. Scalp and hair treatments may be beneficial.

Fragilitas crinium (frah-jil'i-tas krin'e-um) is the technical term for **brittle hair.** The hairs may split at any part of their length. Hair treatments may be given.

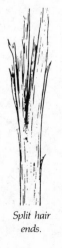

Split hair
ends.

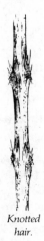

Knotted
hair.

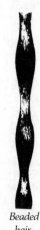

Beaded
hair.

REVIEW QUESTIONS

HAIR

1. Define hair.
2. Why is the study of hair important to the cosmetologist?
3. What are the main purposes of hair?
4. What kind of treatment may cause the hair structure to become weakened?
5. Give the name of the protein found in hair.
6. Name the two parts into which the length of the hair is divided.
7. What is the hair root?
8. What is the hair shaft?
9. What is the hair follicle?
10. What is meant by hair stream?
11. For what foreign bodies are the mouths of hair follicles favorite breeding places?
12. What is the hair bulb?
13. What is the hair papilla?
14. What is the function of the papilla?
15. How does the hair receive its nourishment?
16. What muscle and gland are attached to the hair follicle?
17. What causes "gooseflesh?"
18. What function is performed by the oil glands for hair?
19. List five factors that influence the production of sebum.
20. What determines the size and shape of the hair?
21. Name three general shapes of hair.
22. Name three layers found in hair.
23. Which hair layer serves to protect its inner structure?
24. Which hair layer contains coloring matter?
25. Which layer is sometimes missing in very fine hair?
26. Which parts of the body do not contain any hair?
27. Briefly describe the appearance of lanugo hair.
28. What is the function of lanugo hair?
29. What is meant by hair cycle?
30. What is the average rate of growth of hair on the head?
31. List three ways in which climatic conditions will affect the hair.
32. What is the average number of hairs shed daily?
33. Briefly explain the hair replacement process.
34. What is the average life span of scalp hair?
35. About how many hairs are there on a head of: a) blonde hair; b) brown hair; c) black hair; d) red hair?
36. What is melanin?
37. What causes the hair to turn grey?
38. What is an albino?
39. What is a: a) cowlick; b) whorl?
40. Name the four senses used when analyzing the hair.
41. Name the four important qualities by which hair is judged.

42. Define hair texture.
43. Define hair porosity.
44. Define hair elasticity.
45. To what extent can normal hair be stretched: a) when dry; b) when wet?

DISORDERS OF THE SCALP AND HAIR

1. How is dandruff recognized?
2. What is a direct cause of dandruff?
3. List six conditions that may be the cause of dandruff.
4. Give the medical term for: a) dandruff; b) dry type of dandruff; c) greasy or waxy type of dandruff.
5. What is meant by alopecia?
6. Is the ordinary falling out of hair considered a disease? Explain.
7. At what times of the year does the shedding of hair occur most frequently?
8. What is alopecia senilis?
9. Define alopecia prematura.
10. What is alopecia areata?
11. What is the common term for tinea?
12. What is the cause of tinea?
13. How is tinea transmitted from one person to another?
14. What is the common name for pediculosis capitis? Should this condition be treated by the cosmetologist?
15. What is a furuncle?
16. What is the technical term for grey hair?
17. Give several causes of grey hair.
18. What is meant by ringed hair?
19. Briefly describe the following: a) trichoptilosis; b) hypertrichosis.
20. What is another term for hypertrichosis?
21. Give the medical terms for: a) knotted hair; b) beaded hair.
22. What is meant by fragilitas crinium?

Chapter 29

ANATOMY

CHAPTER LEARNING OBJECTIVES

The student successfully mastering this chapter will know:

1. *The structure and functions of the human body.*
2. *Why a basic understanding of the various organs and systems and how they function will help to improve the professional skill of the cosmetologist.*
3. *The many tissues, organs, and systems of the human body and how they function.*
4. *How the malfunction of a body system or organ can affect cosmetology services.*
5. *The effect of the various organs and systems on the general health of the patron.*

Anatomy (ah-nat'o-me) and **physiology** (fiz-e-ol'o-je) are subjects of considerable importance in the practice of cosmetology. Knowledge of the structure and functions of the human body forms the scientific basis for the proper application of cosmetic services. A basic understanding of these subjects will help to improve the professional skill of the cosmetologist. He or she will then know which cosmetic service is best for a patron's condition, and how to adjust and control it for best results.

Anatomy is the study of the organs and systems of the body, such as muscles, bones, and arteries. The cosmetologist is basically concerned with those parts being treated in the salon, such as the head, face, neck, arms, and hands.

Histology (his-tol'o-je), or **microscopic** (mi-kro-skop'ik) **anatomy,** is the study of the minute structure of the various parts of the body. The cosmetologist is particularly concerned with the histology of the skin and its appendages (hair, nails, and sweat and oil glands).

Physiology is the study of the functions or activities performed by the various parts of the body.

The names of bones, muscles, arteries, veins, and nerves are seldom used in the beauty salon. However, an understanding of body structures will help make you more proficient in performing many of the salon services. (For example, facials and hand and arm massage.)

THE SKELETAL SYSTEM

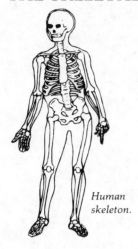

Human skeleton.

The **skeletal** (skel'e-tal) **system** is the physical foundation of the body. It is composed of differently shaped bones united by movable and immovable joints.

Bone is the hardest structure of the body. It is composed of fibrous tissues firmly bound together, consisting of about one-third animal matter and two-thirds mineral matter.

The scientific study of bones, their structure and functions, is called **osteology** (os-te-ol'o-je). **Os** is the technical term for bone.

The following are the functions of bone:
1. To give shape and strength to the body.
2. To protect organs from injury.
3. To serve as attachments for muscles.
4. To act as levers for all bodily movements.

BONES OF THE SKULL

The **skull** is the skeleton of the head. It is an oval, bony case that shapes the head and protects the brain. The skull is divided into two parts: the cranium, consisting of 8 bones, and the skeleton of the face, consisting of 14 bones.

The following bones are involved indirectly in connection with scalp and facial manipulations: *(The bones are numbered to correspond with the bones shown on the illustration.)*

EIGHT BONES OF THE CRANIUM

1. **Occipital** (ok-sip'i-tal) **bone** forms the lower back part of the cranium.
2. **Two parietal** (pah-ri'e-tal) **bones** form the sides and top (crown) of the cranium.
3. **Frontal** (frun'tal) **bone** forms the forehead.
4. **Two temporal** (tem'po-ral) **bones** form the sides of the head in the ear region (below the parietal bones).
5. **Ethmoid** (eth'moid) **bones** are light and spongy bones between the eye-sockets and form part of the nasal cavities.
6. **Sphenoid** (sfe'noid) **bone** joins together all the bones of the cranium.
(The ethmoid and sphenoid bones are not affected by massage.)

FOURTEEN BONES OF THE FACE

7. **Two nasal** (na'sal) **bones** form the bridge of the nose.
8. **Two lacrimal** (lak'ri-mal) **bones** are small fragile bones located at the front part of the inner wall of the eyesockets.
9. **Two zygomatic** (zi-go-mat'ik), or **malar, bones** form the prominence of the cheeks.
10. **Two maxillae** (mak-sil'e) are the upper jawbones which join to form the whole upper jaw.
11. **Mandible** (man'di-bl) is the lower jawbone, and is the largest and strongest bone of the face. It forms the lower jaw.

DIAGRAM OF THE CRANIUM, FACE, AND NECK BONES

Facial bones affected by massage: 7—Nasal bones; 9—Zygomatic bones; 10—Maxillae bones; 11—Mandible bones.

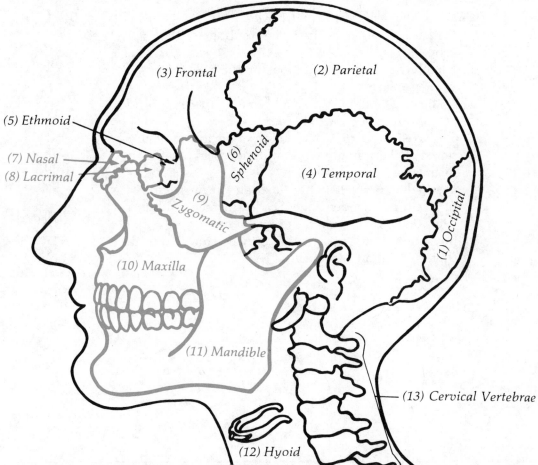

Facial bones that do not appear on the illustration are: **Two turbinal** (tur'bi-nal) **bones** which are thin layers of spongy bone on either of the outer walls of the nasal depression. **Vomer** (vo'mer) is a single bone that forms part of the dividing wall of the nose. **Two palatine** (pal'ah-tin) **bones** form the floor and outer wall of the nose, roof of the mouth, and floor of the orbits.

BONES OF THE NECK

12. **Hyoid** (hi'oid) **bone,** a "U" shaped bone, is located in the front part of the throat, and is referred to as the "Adam's apple."
13. **Cervical vertebrae** (ser'vi-kal ver'te-bre) form the top part of the spinal column located in the neck region.

BONES OF THE CHEST (THORAX)

Thorax (tho'raks), or **chest,** is an elastic bony cage made up of the breast bone, the spine, the ribs, and connective cartilage. It serves as a protective covering for the heart, lungs, and other delicate internal organs. This framework is held in place by 24 ribs, 12 on each side.

BONES OF THE SHOULDER, ARM, AND HAND

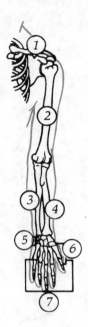

1. **Shoulder.** Each side of the shoulder is made up of one clavicle and one scapula, forming the back of the shoulder.

Bones of the arm, wrist, and hand:

2. **Humerus** (hu'mer-us) is the largest bone of the upper arm.

3. **Ulna** (ul'nah) is the large bone on the little finger side of the forearm.

4. **Radius** (ra'de-us) is the small bone on the thumb side of the forearm.

5. The **wrist**, or **carpus** (kar'pus), is a flexible joint composed of eight small, irregular bones, held together by ligaments.

6. The **palm**, or **metacarpus** (met-ah-kar'pus), consists of five long, slender bones, called metacarpal bones.

7. The **fingers**, or **digits** (dij'its), consist of three **phalanges** (fah-lan'jez) in each finger, and two in the thumb, totaling 14 bones.

REMINDER

WHY YOU SHOULD KNOW ANATOMY

The names of bones, muscles, arteries, veins, and nerves are seldom used in the routine of the beauty salon. However, an understanding of body structures will determine why certain steps are required in giving facial, hand and arm massage; facial makeup; hair shaping and hairstyling.

THE MUSCULAR SYSTEM

The **muscular** (mus'ku-lar) **system** covers, shapes, and supports the skeleton. Its function is to produce all movements of the body.

Myology (mi-ol'o-je) is the study of the structure, functions, and diseases of the muscles.

No outward sign of human life is more distinctive than that of **muscular** movement.

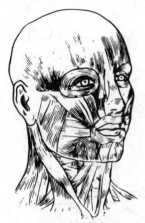

The muscular system consists of over 500 muscles, large and small, comprising 40-50% of the weight of the human body.

Muscles are contractile fibrous tissue on which the various movements of the body depend for their variety and action. The muscular system relies upon the skeletal and nervous systems for its activities.

There are three kinds of muscular tissues:

1. **Striated** (striped) or voluntary, which are controlled by the will, such as those of the face, arms, and legs.

2. **Non-striated** (smooth) or involuntary, which function without the action of the will, such as those of the stomach and intestines.

3. **Cardiac** (heart muscle) which is the heart itself, and is not duplicated anywhere else in the body.

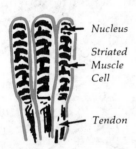
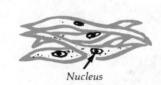
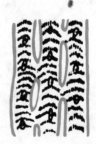

STRIATED (STRIPED) MUSCLE CELLS

NON-STRIATED (SMOOTH) MUSCLE CELLS

CARDIAC (HEART) MUSCLE CELLS

ORIGIN, INSERTION, AND BELLY OF MUSCLES

When a muscle contracts and shortens, one of its attachments usually remains **fixed** and the other one **moves**.

Origin of a muscle is the term applied to the more **fixed** attachment, such as muscles attached to bones or to some other muscle. Muscles attached to bones are usually referred to as **skeletal muscles.**

Insertion of a muscle is the term applied to the more **movable** attachment, such as muscles attached to a movable muscle, to a movable bone, or to the skin.

Belly of a muscle is the part between the origin and the insertion.

STIMULATION OF MUSCLES

Muscular tissue may be stimulated by any of the following:
Chemicals (certain acids and salts)
Massage (hand massage and electric vibrator)
Electric current (high-frequency and faradic current)
Light rays (infra-red rays and ultra-violet rays)
Heat rays (heating lamps and heating caps)
Moist heat (steamers or moderately warm steam towels)
Nerve impulses (through the nervous system)

DIAGRAM OF THE MUSCLES OF THE HEAD, FACE, AND NECK

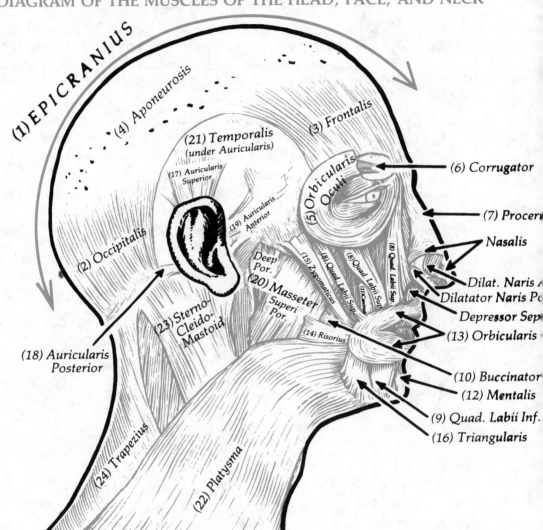

MUSCLES AFFECTED BY MASSAGE

The cosmetologist is concerned with the **voluntary muscles** of the head, face, neck, arms, and hands. It is essential to know where these muscles are located, and what they control. Pressure in massage is usually directed **from the insertion to the origin.**

(The muscles are numbered to correspond with the muscles shown on the illustrations.)

MUSCLES OF THE SCALP

1. **Epicranius** (ep-i-kra'ne-us), or **occipito-frontalis** (ok-sip'i-to-fron-ta'lis), is a broad muscle that covers the top of the skull. It consists of two parts: (2) the **occipitalis** (ok-sip-i-ta'lis), or back part, and (3) the **frontalis** (fron-ta'lis), or front part. Both are connected by a tendon (4) **aponeurosis** (ap-o-nu-ro'sis). The frontalis raises the eyebrows, draws the scalp forward, and causes wrinkles across the forehead.

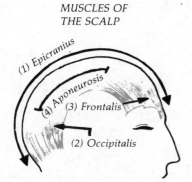

MUSCLES OF THE SCALP

(1) Epicranius
(4) Aponeurosis
(3) Frontalis
(2) Occipitalis

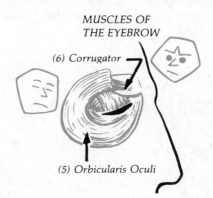

MUSCLES OF THE EYEBROW

(6) Corrugator
(5) Orbicularis Oculi

MUSCLES OF THE EYEBROW

5. **Orbicularis oculi** (or-bik-ù-la'ris ok'ü-li) completely surrounds the margin of the eyesocket and closes the eye.
6. **Corrugator** (kor'u-ga-tor) muscle is beneath the **frontalis** and **orbicularis oculi,** and draws the eyebrow down and in. It produces vertical lines, and is the muscle used for **frowning.**

MUSCLES OF THE NOSE

7. The **procerus** (pro-se'rus) covers the bridge of the nose, depresses the eyebrow, and causes wrinkles across the bridge of the nose.

(The other nasal muscles are small muscles around the nasal openings which contract and expand the openings of the nostrils.)

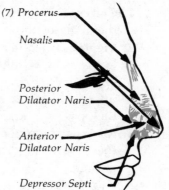

(7) Procerus
Nasalis
Posterior Dilatator Naris
Anterior Dilatator Naris
Depressor Septi

8. **Quadratus labii superioris** (kwod-ra'tus la'be-i su-pe-re-or'is) consists of three parts. It surrounds the upper part of the lip, raises and draws back the upper lip, and elevates the nostrils, as in expressing **distaste.**

9. **Quadratus labii inferioris** (in-fe-re-or'is) surrounds the lower part of the lip. It depresses the lower lip and draws it a little to one side, as in the expression of **sarcasm.**

10. **Buccinator** (buk'se-na-tor) is the muscle between the upper and lower jaws. It compresses the cheeks and expels air between the lips, as in **blowing.**

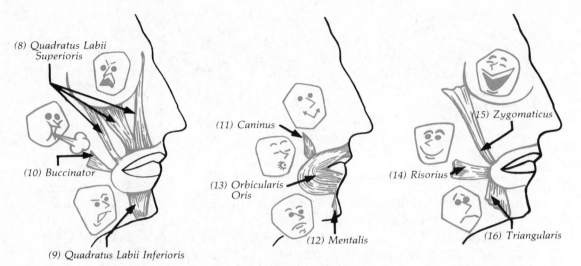

(8) Quadratus Labii Superioris

(10) Buccinator

(9) Quadratus Labii Inferioris

(11) Caninus

(13) Orbicularis Oris

(12) Mentalis

(15) Zygomaticus

(14) Risorius

(16) Triangularis

11. **Caninus** (ka-ni'nus) lies under the quadratus labii superioris. It raises the angle of the mouth, as in **snarling.**

12. **Mentalis** (men-ta'lis) is situated at the tip of the chin. It raises the lower lip, causing wrinkling of the chin, as in **doubt** or **displeasure.**

13. **Orbicularis oris** (or-bik-u-la'ris o'ris) forms a flat band around the upper and lower lips. It compresses, contracts, puckers, and wrinkles the lips, as in **kissing** or **whistling.**

14. **Risorius** (ri-so're-us) extends from the masseter muscle to the angle of the mouth. It draws the corner of the mouth out and back, as in **grinning.**

15. **Zygomaticus** (zi-go-mat'i-kus) extends from the zygomatic bone to the angle of the mouth. It elevates the lip, as in **laughing.**

16. **Triangularis** (tri-ang-gu-la'ris) extends along the side of the chin. It draws down the corner of the mouth.

MUSCLES OF THE EAR

Three muscles of the ear are practically functionless:

17. **Auricularis** (au-rik-ū-la'ris) **superior** is above the ear.

18. **Auricularis posterior** is behind the ear.

19. **Auricularis anterior** is in front of the ear.

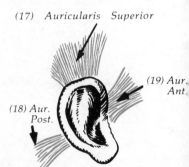

(17) Auricularis Superior

(19) Aur. Ant.

(18) Aur. Post.

MUSCLES OF MASTICATION

20. **Masseter** (mas-e'ter) and (21) **temporalis** (tem-po-ra'lis) are muscles that coordinate in opening and closing the mouth, and are referred to as **chewing** muscles.

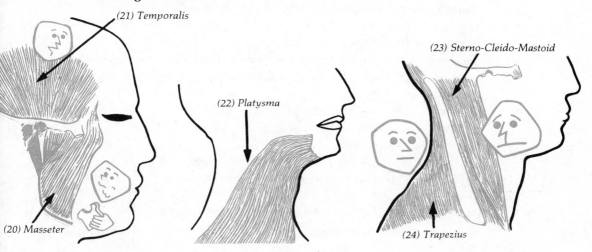

(21) Temporalis

(22) Platysma

(23) Sterno-Cleido-Mastoid

(20) Masseter

(24) Trapezius

MUSCLES OF THE NECK

22. **Platysma** (plah-tiz'mah) is a broad muscle that extends from the chest and shoulder muscles to the side of the chin. It depresses the lower jaw and lip, as in the expression of **sadness**.

23. **Sterno-cleido-mastoid** (ster'no-kli'do-mas'toid) extends from the collar and chest bones to the temporal bone in back of the ear. It rotates the head, and it bends the head, as in **nodding**.

MUSCLES THAT ATTACH ARMS TO BODY

The principal muscles that attach the arms to the body and permit movements of the shoulders and arms are:

24. **Trapezius** (tra-pe'ze-us) and (25) **latissimus dorsi** (la-tis'e-mus dor'si) which cover the back of the neck and upper and middle region of the back. They rotate the shoulder blade and control the swinging movements of the arm.

26. **Pectoralis** (pek-tor-al'is) **major** and **pectoralis minor** cover the front of the chest. They also assist in swinging movements of the arm.

27. **Serratus anterior** (se-ra'tus an-te're-or) assists in breathing and in raising the arm.

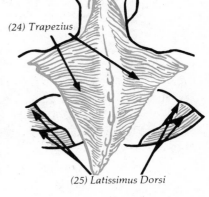

(24) Trapezius

(25) Latissimus Dorsi

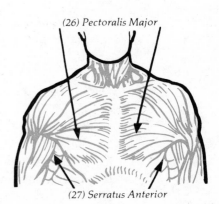

(26) Pectoralis Major

(27) Serratus Anterior

The principal muscles of the shoulder and upper arm are:

1. **Deltoid** (del'toid)—the large, thick triangular shaped muscle that covers the shoulder and lifts and turns the arm.
2. **Biceps** (bi'seps)—the two-headed and principal muscle in the front of the upper arm. It lifts the forearm, flexes the elbow, and turns the palm downward.
3. **Triceps** (tri'seps)—the three-headed muscle of the arm that covers the entire back of the upper arm and extends the forearm forward.

The forearm is made up of a series of muscles and strong tendons. The cosmetologist is concerned with the following:

4. **Pronators** (pro-na'tors)—the most important of the group, turn the hand inward, so that the palm faces downward.
5. **Supinators** (su-pi-na'tors)—turn the hand outward and the palm upward.
6. **Flexors** (flek'sors)—bend the wrist, draw the hand up, and close the fingers toward the forearm.
7. **Extensors** (eks-ten'sors)—straighten the wrist, hand, and fingers to form a straight line.

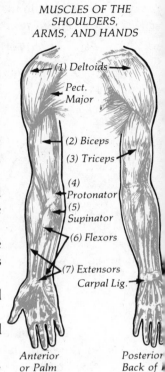

Anterior or Palm

Posterior Back of

MUSCLES OF THE HAND

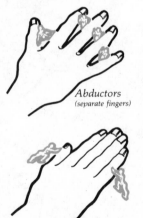

Abductors (separate fingers)

Adductors (draw fingers together)

The hand has many small muscles overlapping from joint to joint, imparting flexibility and strength. When the hands are properly cared for, these muscles will remain supple and graceful. They close and open the hands and fingers.

Abductor (ab-duk'tor) and **adductor** (a-duk'tor) muscles—located in the thumb and fingers, at the base of the digits. The abductor muscles separate the fingers and the adductor muscles draw them together.

THE NERVOUS SYSTEM

Neurology (nu-rol'o-je) is the branch of anatomy that deals with the nervous system and its disorders.

The **nervous** (ner'vus) **system** is one of the most important systems of the body. It controls and coordinates the functions of all the other systems and makes them work harmoniously and efficiently. Every square inch of the human body is supplied with fine fibers which we know as **nerves.**

The main purposes in studying the nervous system are to understand:

1. How the cosmetologist administers scalp and facial services for the patron's benefit.
2. What effects these treatments have on the nerves in the skin and scalp, and on the body as a whole.

DIVISIONS OF THE NERVOUS SYSTEM

The principal parts that compose the nervous system are the brain and spinal cord and their nerves. Generally, the nervous system is composed of three main divisions:

1. The **cerebro-spinal** (ser-e'bro-spi'nal), or **central,** nervous system.
2. The **peripheral** (pe-rif'er-al) nervous system.
3. The **sympathetic** (sym-pa-thet'ik), or **autonomic** (aw-to-nom'ik), nervous system.

The **cerebro-spinal nervous system** consists of the brain and spinal cord. The following are its functions:

1. Controls consciousness and all mental activities.
2. Controls voluntary functions of the five senses: seeing, smelling, tasting, feeling, and hearing.
3. Controls voluntary muscle actions, such as all body movements and facial expressions.

The **peripheral nervous system** is made up of the sensory and motor nerve fibers that extend from the brain and spinal cord and are distributed to all parts of the body. Its function is to carry messages to and from the central nervous system.

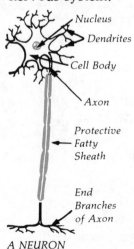

A NEURON OR NERVE CELL

Nucleus
Dendrites
Cell Body
Axon
Protective Fatty Sheath
End Branches of Axon

The **sympathetic nervous system** is related structurally to the cerebro-spinal (central) nervous system, but its functions are independent of the will. (The sympathetic nervous system also is referred to as the **autonomic nervous system,** meaning self-controlled.)

The sympathetic nervous system is very important in the operation of the internal body functions, such as breathing, circulation, digestion, and glandular activities. Its main purpose is to regulate these internal operations, keeping them in balance and working properly.

Nerve Cells and Nerves

A **neuron** (nu'ron), or **nerve cell,** is the structural unit of the nervous system. It is composed of a **cell body** and long and short fibers called **cell processes** (pros'e-sez).

The cell body stores energy and food for the cell processes, which convey the nerve impulses throughout the body. Practically all the nerve cells are contained in the brain and spinal cord.

Nerves are long, white cords made up of fibers (cell processes) that carry messages to and from various parts of the body. Nerves have their origin in the brain and spinal cord, and distribute branches to all parts of the body, which furnish both sensation and motion.

TYPES OF NERVES

Sensory nerves, called **afferent** (af'er-ent) **nerves,** carry impulses or messages from sense organs **to the brain,** where sensations of touch, cold, heat, sight, hearing, taste, smell, and pain are experienced.

Motor nerves, called **efferent** (ef'er-ent) **nerves,** carry impulses **from the brain** to the muscles. The transmitted impulses produce movement.

Mixed nerves contain both sensory and motor fibers. Many nerves are mixed nerves.

Sensory nerves are situated near the surface of the skin. Motor nerves are in the muscles. As impulses pass from the sensory nerves to the brain and back over the motor nerves to the muscles, a complete circuit is established and movement of the muscles results.

Reflex (re'fleks) is an autonomic response to a stimulus that starts with a nerve impulse which travels through the spinal cord to the brain, then back to the muscle. (Example: the quick removal of the hand from a hot object.) A reflex act does not have to be learned.

The Brain and Spinal Cord

The **brain** is the largest mass of nerve tissue in the body and is contained in the cranium. The weight of the average brain is 44-48 ounces (1232-1344 g). It is considered to be the central power station of the body, sending and receiving telegraphic messages. Twelve pairs of cranial nerves originate in the brain and reach various parts of the head, face, and neck.

The **spinal cord** is composed of masses of nerve cells, with fibers running upward and downward. It originates in the brain, extends down to the lower extremity of the trunk, and is enclosed and protected by the spinal column.

Thirty-one pairs of spinal nerves, extending from the spinal cord, are distributed to the muscles and skin of the trunk and limbs.

Some of the spinal nerves supply the internal organs controlled by the sympathetic nervous system.

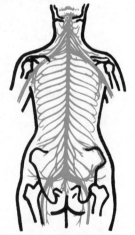

Spinal cord.

Fatigue and Nourishment

Worry or excessive mental or muscular work can cause **fatigue,** resulting in an accumulation of waste products. Weariness, irritability, poor complexion, and dull eyes may be signs of nervous exhaustion.

An adequate energy reserve is dependent upon proper food, exercise, and oxygen. Rest and relaxation help renew depleted energy resources.

Appropriate **massage manipulations** can help relieve fatigue. When giving manipulations, the cosmetologist should always pause over nerve centers.

Nourishment for the nerves is received through blood vessels, lymph spaces, and lymphatics found in the connective tissue surrounding them.

Stimulation to the nerves causes muscles to contract and expand. Heat on the skin causes relaxation; cold causes contraction.

Nerve stimulation may be accomplished by any of the following:

Chemicals (certain acids or salts)

Massage (hand massage or electric vibrator)

Electric currents (high-frequency and faradic current)

Light rays (infra-red and ultra-violet rays)

Heat rays (heating lamps and heating caps)

Moist heat (steamers or moderately warm steam towels)

CRANIAL NERVES

There are 12 pairs of cranial (kra'ne-al) nerves, all connected to a part of the brain surface. They emerge through openings on the sides and base of the cranium, and reach various parts of the head, face, and neck. They are classified as motor, sensory and mixed nerves, containing both motor and sensory fibers.

The cranial nerves are named numerically, according to the order in which they arise from the brain, and also by names that describe their nature or function.

First—Olfactory (ol-fak'to-re) (sensory) controls the sense of smell.

Second—Optic (op'tik) (sensory) controls the sense of sight.

Third—Oculomotor (ok-u-lo-mo'tor) (motor) controls the motion of the eye.

Fourth—Trochlear (trok'le-ar) (motor) controls the motion of the eye.

Fifth—Trigeminal (tri-jem'i-nal), or trifacial (tri-fa'shal), (sensory-motor) controls the sensations of the face, tongue, and teeth.

Sixth—Abducent (ab-du'sent) (motor) controls the motion of the eye.

Seventh—Facial (fa'shal) (sensory-motor) controls motion of the face, scalp, neck, ear, and sections of the palate and tongue.

Eighth—Acoustic (ah-koos'tik), or auditory (aw'di-to-re), (sensory) controls the sense of hearing.

Ninth—Glossopharyngeal (glos-o-fah-rin'je-al) (sensory-motor) controls the sense of taste.

Tenth—Vagus (va'gus), or pneumogastric (nu-mo-gas'trik), (sensory-motor) controls motion and sensations of the ear, pharynx, larynx, heart, lungs, esophagus, etc.

Eleventh—Accessory (ak-ses'o-re) (motor) controls the motion of neck muscles.

Twelfth—Hypoglossal (hi-po-glos'al) (motor) controls the motion of the tongue.

NERVES OF INTEREST TO THE COSMETOLOGIST

The three cranial nerves that are of interest to the cosmetologist in giving facial and scalp treatments are: The fifth cranial (trigeminal or trifacial), seventh cranial (facial), eleventh cranial (accessory).

Also of interest to the cosmetologist is the spinal (cervical) nerve, which originates in the spinal cord and is involved in scalp and neck massage.

The **fifth cranial, trifacial,** or **trigeminal nerve** is the largest of the cranial nerves. It is the chief sensory nerve of the face, and the motor nerve of the muscles of mastication. It consists of three branches: **ophthalmic, mandibular,** and **maxillary.**

The following are the important branches of the fifth cranial nerve that are affected by massage:

1. **Supra-orbital** (su′prah-or′bi-tal) **nerve** affects the skin of the forehead, scalp, eyebrow, and upper eyelid.
2. **Supra-trochlear** (su′prah-trok′le-ar) **nerve** affects the skin between the eyes and upper side of the nose.
3. **Infra-trochlear** (in′fra-trok′le-ar) **nerve** affects the membrane and skin of the nose.

DIAGRAM OF THE NERVES OF THE HEAD, FACE, AND NECK

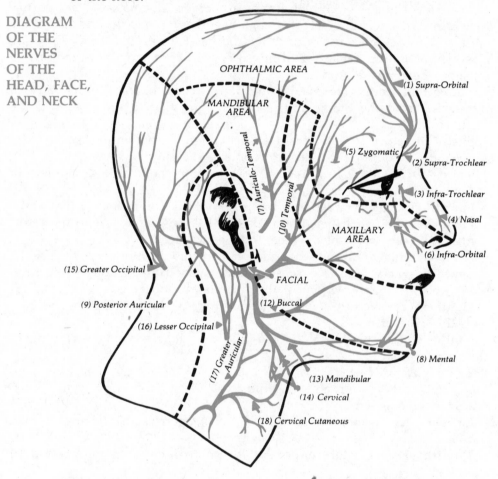

4. **Nasal** (na′zal) **nerve** affects the point and lower side of the nose.
5. **Zygomatic** (zi-go-mat′ik) **nerve** affects the skin of the temple, side of the forehead, and upper part of the cheek.
6. **Infra-orbital** (in′frah-or′bi-tal) **nerve** affects the skin of the lower eyelid, side of the nose, upper lip, and mouth.
7. **Auriculo-temporal** (aw-rik′u-lo-tem′po-ral) **nerve** affects the external ear and skin above the temple, up to the top of skull.
8. **Mental** (men′tal) **nerve** affects the skin of the lower lip and chin.

The **seventh (facial) cranial nerve** is the chief motor nerve of the face. It emerges near the lower part of the ear; its divisions and their branches supply and control all the muscles of facial expression, and extend to the muscles of the neck.

Of all the branches of the facial nerve, the following are the most important:

9. **Posterior auricular** (pos-ter'ior aw-rik'u-lar) **nerve** affects the muscles behind the ear at the base of the skull.
10. **Temporal** (tem'po-ral) **nerve** affects the muscles of the temple, side of forehead, eyebrow, eyelid, and upper part of the cheek.
11. **Zygomatic** (zi-go-mat'ik) **nerve (upper and lower)** affects the muscles of the upper part of the cheek.
12. **Buccal** (buk'al) **nerve** affects the muscles of the mouth.
13. **Mandibular** (man-dib'ular) **nerve** affects the muscles of the chin and lower lip.
14. **Cervical** (ser'vi-kal) **nerve** (branch of the facial nerve) affects the side of the neck and the platysma muscle.

Eleventh (accessory) **cranial nerve** (spinal branch) affects the muscles of the neck and back (not shown on illustration).

Cervical nerves originate at the spinal cord, and their branches supply the muscles and scalp at the back of the head and neck, as follows:

15. **Greater occipital** (ok-sip'i-tal) **nerve,** located in the back of the head, affects the scalp as far up as the top of the head.
16. **Smaller (lesser) occipital nerve,** located at base of the skull, affects the scalp and muscles of this region.
17. **Greater auricular** (aw-rik'u-lar) **nerve,** located at side of the neck, affects the external ear, and the area in front and back of the ear.
18. **Cervical cutaneous** (ku-ta'ne-us), or **cutaneous colli** (co'li), **nerve,** located at side of the neck, affects the front and side of the neck as far down as the breastbone.

NERVES OF THE ARM AND HAND

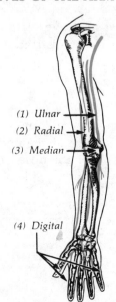

(1) Ulnar
(2) Radial
(3) Median
(4) Digital

The principal nerves supplying the superficial parts of the arm and hand are:

1. The **ulnar** (ul'nar) **nerve** (sensory-motor)—with its branches, supplies the little finger side of the arm and the palm of the hand.
2. The **radial** (ra'de-al) **nerve** (sensory-motor)—with its branches, supplies the thumb side of the arm and the back of the hand.
3. The **median** (me'de-an) **nerve** (sensory-motor)—a smaller nerve than the ulnar and radial nerves. With its branches, supplies the arm and hand.
4. The **digital** (dij'i-tal) **nerves** (sensory-motor)—with its branches, supplies all fingers of the hand.

THE CIRCULATORY SYSTEM

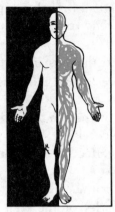

The **circulatory** (ser'ku-lah-to-re), or **vascular** (vas'ku-lar), **system** is vitally related to the maintenance of good health. The vascular system controls the circulation of the blood through the body in a steady stream by means of the **heart** and the blood vessels (the **arteries** [ar'ter-ez], **veins**, and **capillaries** [kap'i-la-rez]).

The vascular system is made up of two divisions:

1. The **blood-vascular** (blud vas'ku-lar) **system**, which comprises the heart and blood vessels (arteries, capillaries, and veins) for the circulation of the blood.

2. The **lymph-vascular** (limf vas'ku-lar), or **lymphatic** (lim-fat'ik), **system**, consisting of lymph glands and vessels through which the lymph circulates.

These two systems are intimately linked with each other. Lymph is derived from the blood and is gradually shifted back into the bloodstream.

THE HEART

The **heart** is an efficient pump. It keeps the blood moving within the circulatory system.

The heart is a muscular, conical-shaped organ, about the size of a closed fist. It is located in the chest cavity, and is enclosed in a membrane, the **pericardium** (per-i-kar'de-um). The **vagus** (tenth cranial nerve) and nerves from the **sympathetic nervous system** regulate the heartbeat. Generally, the heart beats about 72-80 times a minute.

The interior of the heart contains four chambers and four valves. The ·upper thin-walled chambers are the **right atrium** (a'tre-um) and **left atrium**. The lower thick-walled chambers are the **right ventricle** (ven'tri-kl) and **left ventricle. Valves** allow the blood to flow in only one direction. With each contraction and relaxation of the heart, the blood flows in, travels from the **atria** (a'tre-ah) to the ventricles, and is then driven out, to be distributed all over the body. Atrium is also called **auricle** (aw'ri-kl).

BLOOD VESSELS

The arteries, capillaries, and veins are tube-like in construction. They transport blood to and from the heart and to various tissues of the body.

Arteries are thick-walled muscular and elastic tubes that carry **pure** blood from the heart to the capillaries.

Capillaries are minute, thin-walled blood vessels that connect the smaller arteries to the veins. Through their walls, the tissues receive nourishment and eliminate waste products.

CROSS SECTION OF A VEIN

Veins are thin-walled blood vessels that are less elastic than arteries. They contain cup-like valves to prevent back flow, and carry impure blood from the various capillaries back to the heart. Veins are located closer to the outer surface of the body than the arteries.

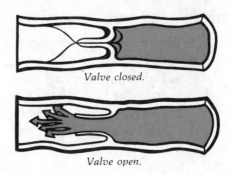

Valve closed.

Valve open.

DIAGRAM OF THE HEART

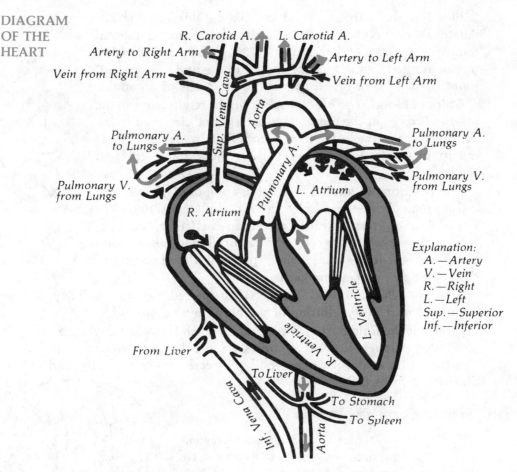

R. Carotid A. L. Carotid A.
Artery to Right Arm
Vein from Right Arm
Sup. Vena Cava
Aorta
Artery to Left Arm
Vein from Left Arm
Pulmonary A. to Lungs
Pulmonary A.
Pulmonary A. to Lungs
Pulmonary V. from Lungs
L. Atrium
Pulmonary V. from Lungs
R. Atrium
L. Ventricle
From Liver
R. Ventricle
To Liver
To Stomach
To Spleen
Inf. Vena Cava
Aorta

Explanation:
A.—Artery
V.—Vein
R.—Right
L.—Left
Sup.—Superior
Inf.—Inferior

CHIEF FUNCTIONS OF THE BLOOD

The following are the primary functions of the blood:

1. To carry water, oxygen, food, and secretions to all cells of the body.
2. To carry away carbon dioxide and waste products to be eliminated through the lungs, skin, kidneys, and large intestine.
3. To help to equalize the body temperature, thus protecting the body from extreme heat and cold.
4. To aid in protecting the body from harmful bacteria and infections, through the action of the white blood cells.
5. To clot the blood, thereby closing injured minute blood vessels and preventing the loss of blood.

THE CIRCULATION OF THE BLOOD

The blood is in constant circulation, from the moment it leaves until it returns to the heart. There are two systems that take care of this circulation:

1. **Pulmonary** (pul'mo-na-re) **circulation** is the blood circulation that goes from the heart to the lungs to be purified, and then returns to the heart.
2. **General circulation** is the blood circulation from the heart throughout the body and back again to the heart.

THE BLOOD

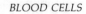
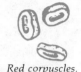

Blood is the nutritive fluid circulating through the circulatory system. It is a sticky, salty fluid, with a normal temperature of 98.6° Fahrenheit (37° Celsius), and it makes up about one-twentieth of the weight of the body. From 8-10 pints (3.76-4.7 l) of blood fill the blood vessels of an adult.

Red corpuscles.

Color of blood. The blood itself is bright red in color in the arteries (except in the pulmonary artery) and dark red in the veins (except in the pulmonary vein). This change in color is due to the gain or loss of oxygen as the blood passes through the lungs.

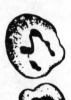

Composition of blood. The blood is composed of one-third cells (red and white corpuscles and blood platelets) and two-thirds plasma. The function of **red corpuscles** (red blood cells) is to carry oxygen to the cells. **White corpuscles** (white blood cells), or **leucocytes** (lu'ko-sits), perform the function of destroying disease causing germs.

White corpuscles.

Platelets.

Blood platelets are much smaller than the red blood cells. They play an important part in the **clotting of the blood** over a wound.

Plasma is the fluid part of the blood in which the red and white blood cells and blood platelets flow. It is straw-like in color. About nine-tenths of the plasma is water, and it carries food and secretions to the cells, and carbon dioxide from the cells.

THE LYMPH-VASCULAR SYSTEM

The **lymph-vascular** (limf-vas'ku-lar) **system**, also called **lymphatic system**, acts as an aid to the venous system, and consists of lymph spaces, lymph vessels, lymph glands, and **lacteals** (lak'te-alz).

Lymph is a colorless, watery fluid that circulates through the lymphatic system and is derived from the plasma of the blood, mainly by filtration.

The lymph acts as a middleman between the blood and the tissues. It carries nourishment from the blood to the cells, and removes waste material from the cells.

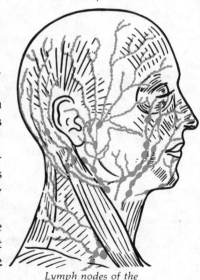

Lymph nodes of the head, face, and neck.

ARTERIES OF THE HEAD, FACE, AND NECK

The **common carotid** (kah-rot'id) **arteries** are the main sources of blood supply to the head, face, and neck. They are located on either side of the neck and divide into internal and external carotid arteries. The **internal division** of the common carotid artery supplies the brain, eyesockets, eyelids, and forehead, while the **external division** supplies the superficial parts of the head, face, and neck.

The **external carotid artery** subdivides into a number of branches which supply blood to various regions of the head, face, and neck. Of particular interest to the cosmetologist are the following arteries:

(The arteries are lettered and numbered to correspond with the arteries shown on the illustration.)

A. **Facial artery (external maxillary)** (mak'si-ler-e) supplies the lower region of the face, mouth, and nose. Some of its branches are:

1. **Submental** (sub-men'tal) **artery**—supplies the chin and lower lip.
2. **Inferior labial** (la'be-al) **artery**—supplies the lower lip.
3. **Angular** (ang'u-lar) **artery**—supplies the side of the nose.
4. **Superior labial artery**—supplies the upper lip, septum, and wing of nose.

DIAGRAM OF
THE ARTERIES
OF THE
HEAD, FACE,
AND NECK

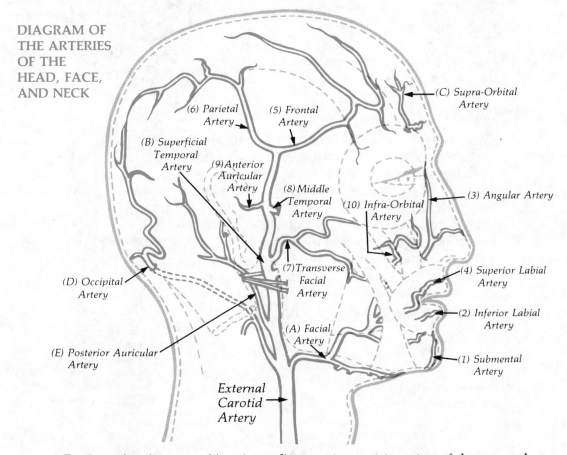

B. **Superficial temporal** (tem'po-ral) **artery** is a continuation of the external carotid artery, which supplies muscles, skin, and scalp to front, side, and top of head. Some of its important branches are:

5. **Frontal** (frun'tal) **artery**—supplies the forehead.

6. **Parietal** (pah-ri'e-tal) **artery**—supplies the crown and side of head.

7. **Transverse** (trans-vers') **facial artery**—supplies the masseter.

8. **Middle temporal** (tem'por-al) **artery**—supplies the temples.

9. **Anterior auricular** (aw-rik'u-lar) **artery**—supplies the anterior part of the ear (partially shown on illustration).

C. The **supra-orbital** (su'prah-or'bi-tal) **artery**, branch of the internal carotid artery—supplies part of the forehead, the eyesocket, eyelid, and upper muscles of the eye.

10. **Infra-orbital** (in'frah-or'bi-tal) **artery**—originates from the internal maxillary artery, and it supplies the muscles of the eye.

D. **Occipital** (ok-sip'i-tal) **artery**—supplies the back of the head, up to the crown.

E. **Posterior auricular** (aw-rik'u-lar) **artery**—supplies the scalp, back and above the ear, and skin behind the ear.

VEINS OF THE HEAD, FACE, AND NECK

The blood returning to the heart from the head, face, and neck flows on each side of the neck in two principal veins: the **internal jugular** and **external jugular.** The most important veins of the face and neck are parallel to the arteries and take the same names as the arteries.

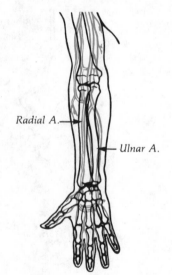

External Jugular

Posterior External Jugular

Internal Jugular

BLOOD SUPPLY FOR THE ARM AND HAND

The **ulnar** (ul'nar) and **radial** (ra'de-al) **arteries** are the main blood supply for the arm and hand. The **ulnar artery** and its numerous branches supply the little finger side of the arm and the palm of the hand.

The **radial artery** and its branches supply the thumb side of the arm and the back of the hand.

The important **veins** are located almost parallel with the arteries and take the same names as the arteries. While the arteries are found deep in the tissues, the veins lie nearer to the surface of the arms and hands.

Radial A.

Ulnar A.

THE ENDOCRINE SYSTEM

Glands are specialized organs that vary in size and function. The blood and nerves are intimately connected with the glands. The nervous system controls the functional activities of the glands. The glands have the ability to remove certain constituents from the blood and to convert them into new compounds.

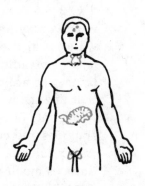

There are two main sets of glands:

1. One group is called the **duct glands**, possessing canals that lead from the gland to a particular part of the body. Sweat and oil glands of the skin and intestinal glands belong to this group.

    (Information on sweat and oil glands can be found in the chapter on **The Skin and Disorders of the Skin.**)

2. The other group, known as **ductless glands**, has its secretions thrown directly into the bloodstream, which in turn influences the welfare of the entire body.

THE EXCRETORY SYSTEM

The **excretory** (eks'kre-to-re) **system,** including the kidneys, liver, skin, intestines and lungs, purifies the body by the elimination of waste matter.

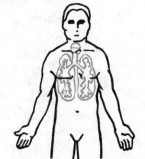

Kidneys

Each plays the following part in the excretory system:

1. The **kidneys** excrete urine.
2. The **liver** discharges bile pigments.
3. The **skin** eliminates perspiration.
4. The **large intestine** evacuates decomposed and undigested food.
5. The **lungs** exhale carbon dioxide.

Bladder

Metabolism of the cells of the body forms various toxic substances which, if retained, would have a tendency to poison the body.

THE RESPIRATORY SYSTEM

The **respiratory** (re-spir'ah-to-re) **system** is situated within the chest cavity, which is protected on both sides by the ribs. The **diaphragm** (di'ah-fram), a muscular partition that controls breathing, separates the chest from the **abdominal** (ab-dom'i-nal) region.

The **lungs** are spongy tissues composed of microscopic cells into which the inhaled air penetrates.

These tiny air cells are enclosed in a skin-like tissue. Behind this, the fine capillaries of the vascular system are found.

With each **respiratory** cycle, an exchange of gases takes place. During **inhalation** (in-ha-la'shun), oxygen is absorbed into the blood, while carbon dioxide is expelled during **exhalation** (eks-ha-la'shun). Oxygen is required to change food into energy.

Oxygen is more essential than either food or water. Although a man or woman may live more than 60 days without food, and a few days without water, if air is excluded for a few minutes, death ensues.

Nose breathing is healthier than mouth breathing because the air is warmed by the surface capillaries, and the bacteria in the air are caught by the hairs that line the **mucous** (mu'cus) membranes of the nasal passages.

The rate of breathing depends on the activity of the individual. Muscular activities and energy expenditures increase the body's demands for oxygen. As a result, the rate of breathing is increased. A person requires about three times as much oxygen when walking than when standing.

Abdominal breathing is of value in building health. **Costal breathing** involves light, or shallow, breathing of the lungs, without action of the diaphragm. Abdominal breathing means deep breathing, which brings the diaphragm into action. The greatest exchange of gases is accomplished with abdominal breathing.

THE DIGESTIVE SYSTEM

The **digestive** (di-ges'tiv) **system** changes food into **soluble** (sol'yu-bl) form, suitable for use by the cells of the body. Digestion is started in the mouth and completed in the small intestine. From the mouth, the food passes down the **pharynx** (far'inks) and the **esophagus** (e-sof'ah-gus), or food pipe, and into the stomach. The food is completely digested in the small intestine. The large intestine (colon) stores the refuse for elimination through the rectum. The complete digestive process of food takes about nine hours.

Digestion is the process of converting food into a form that can be assimilated by the body.

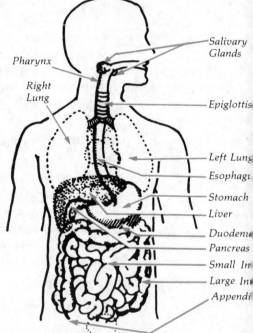

Diagram illustrating the human alimentary canal with its principal digestive glands.

Responsible for the chemical changes in food are the **enzymes** (en'zymz) present in the digestive secretions. **Digestive enzymes** are chemicals that change certain kinds of food into a form capable of being used by the body.

Intense emotions, excitement, and fatigue seriously disturb digestion. On the other hand, happiness and relaxation promote good digestion.

REVIEW QUESTIONS

ANATOMY

1. Why is knowledge of anatomy and physiology of considerable importance in the practice of cosmetology?
2. What is anatomy?
3. With what five parts of the body is the cosmetologist basically concerned?
4. What is histology?
5. With what parts of the body is the cosmetologist primarily concerned in the study of histology?
6. What are the four appendages of the skin?
7. What is physiology?

THE SKELETAL SYSTEM

Bones of the Skull

1. What is the hardest structure of the body?
2. List four functions of the bones.
3. Define skull.
4. Into how many parts is the skull divided? Name them.
5. The cranium consists of how many bones?
6. List the skull bones affected by scalp massage.
7. Locate the occipital bone.
8. Locate the parietal bones.
9. Which bone forms the forehead?
10. What bones are located in the ear region?
11. Which bone joins together all the cranial bones?
12. How many bones are found in the face?
13. List the facial bones affected by facial massage.
14. What is formed by the maxillae?
15. Which bony structure is formed by the mandible?
16. Which bones form the prominence of the cheeks?
17. Where is the hyoid bone located?
18. Locate the cervical vertebrae.
19. What is the bony chest cage called?

Bones of the Shoulder, Arm, and Hand

1. Name the two bones found in the shoulder.
2. Name the bones of the: a) upper arm; and b) the two bones of the forearm.
3. How many bones are found in the: a) wrist; b) palm; and c) fingers of the hand?
4. What is another name for the wrist?
5. What are the bones in the palm of the hand called?
6. What is the technical name for the fingers of the hand?
7. Where are the phalanges located?

THE MUSCULAR SYSTEM

1. Define muscle.
2. What are the important functions of the muscles of the body?
3. Name three kinds of muscular tissue.

4. Distinguish between voluntary and involuntary muscles.
5. Upon which two systems of the body is the muscular system dependent for its activities?
6. Briefly define: a) origin of muscle; b) insertion of muscle.
7. Name seven sources capable of stimulating muscular tissue.

Muscles of the Head, Face, and Neck

1. Locate the scalp muscle and name its two parts.
2. What is the function of the frontalis?
3. Which muscle surrounds the eyesocket?
4. Name the muscle of the eyebrow.
5. Which muscle covers the bridge of the nose?
6. Which muscle forms a flat band around the upper and lower lips?
7. Which muscle depresses the lower jaw and lip?
8. Which muscles cover the back of the neck?

Muscles of the Shoulder, Arm, and Hand

1. Name the three principal muscles of the upper arm and shoulder.
2. Name four types of muscles found in the forearm.
3. Distinguish between the functions of the pronator and supinator muscles.
4. Distinguish between the flexor and extensor muscles.

THE NERVOUS SYSTEM

1. Give two reasons why the cosmetologist should study the nervous system.
2. What are the three principal parts that make up the nervous system?
3. Name the three main divisions of the nervous system.
4. Name the three main functions of the cerebro-spinal nervous system.
5. Explain the peripheral system and what its function is.
6. Name the main function of the sympathetic (autonomic) nervous system.
7. What is a neuron?
8. What is a neuron, or nerve cell, composed of?
9. Define nerves.
10. Name two kinds of nerves that are found in the body.
11. What is the other name for: a) sensory nerves, and b) motor nerves?
12. What is the function of sensory nerves?
13. What is the function of motor nerves?
14. Give an example of a reflex.
15. How many pairs of cranial nerves are there? Spinal nerves?
16. What are three causes of fatigue?
17. List six agents by which nerve stimulation may be accomplished.
18. Which three cranial nerves are the most important in the massaging of the head, face, and neck?

Nerves of the Head, Face, and Neck

1. Which is the largest cranial nerve?
2. What is the function of the fifth, or trifacial, nerve?
3. Which cranial nerve controls the muscles of facial expression?
4. Which branches of the trifacial nerve affect the following regions?
   a) forehead
   b) lower side of nose
   c) skin of lower eyelid and upper lip
   d) skin of lower lip
   e) skin above temple
   f) skin of upper part of cheek
5. Which region of the head is affected by the greater occipital nerve?
6. Which cranial nerve affects the neck muscles?
7. Which branches of the facial nerve affect the following regions or muscles?
   a) muscle of side of forehead
   b) muscle of chin and lower lip
   c) platysma muscle
   d) muscle behind ear
   e) mouth muscles
   f) muscles of upper part of cheek

Nerves of the Arm and Hand

1. Name and locate the principal nerves of the arm and hand.
2. Which nerves affect the fingers?

THE CIRCULATORY SYSTEM

1. Why is it necessary for the cosmetologist to understand the functions of the circulatory system?
2. What is the function of the heart?
3. Name three kinds of vessels found in the vascular system.
4. Which blood vessels carry pure blood from the heart to the body?
5. What two blood vessels do capillaries connect?
6. What is the function of the veins?
7. Which two systems take care of blood circulation throughout the body?
8. What is the normal temperature of blood?
9. What is the composition of blood?
10. What is the composition of blood plasma?
11. What is the most important function of the red blood cells?
12. What is a function of the white blood cells?
13. What is lymph?
14. From what source is lymph derived?
15. List the important functions of lymph.

Blood Vessels of the Head, Face, and Neck

1. Which main arteries supply blood to the entire head, face, and neck?
2. Name two main divisions of the common carotid arteries.
3. Which branches of the common carotid arteries supply the cranial cavity?
4. Which branches of the common carotid arteries supply blood to the skin and muscles of the head and face?
5. Give the common name for the external maxillary artery.
6. Name the artery that supplies the chin.
7. Which artery supplies the forehead?
8. Name the arteries that supply the: a) upper lip; b) lower lip.
9. What part of the head does the parietal artery supply? Frontal artery?
10. Name five branches of the superficial temporal artery.
11. What part of the head does the occipital artery supply?
12. What artery supplies that part of the scalp that is in back of and above the ear?
13. Name the artery that supplies the eye muscles.
14. Name the principal veins by which the blood from the head, face, and neck is returned to the heart.

Blood Circulation of Arm and Hand

1. Name the principal arteries supplying the arm and hand.
2. Which artery supplies the little finger side of the arm and palm of the hand?
3. Which artery supplies the thumb side of the arm?

GLANDS AND OTHER SYSTEMS

1. What two main types of glands are there in the human body?
2. Name the five important organs of the excretory system.
3. Describe a respiratory cycle.
4. Name the important organs of the digestive system.

Chapter 30

ELECTRICITY AND
LIGHT THERAPY

CHAPTER LEARNING OBJECTIVES

The student successfully mastering this chapter will know:
1. *The nature of electricity.*
2. *Forms of electricity.*
3. *Electrical measurements.*
4. *The different types of currents.*
5. *The benefits to be derived from the various currents.*
6. *The various types of electrical equipment available for use in the beauty salon.*
7. *Safety practices when using electricity.*
8. *The meaning of the term "light therapy."*
9. *How light disperses when passed through a prism.*
10. *How light rays are produced.*
11. *The effects of ultra-violet rays.*
12. *The benefits that can be derived from infra-red rays.*

ELECTRICITY

The beneficial effects of electricity have long been recognized to be of value in the practice of cosmetology. Electricity can be a valuable tool, provided it is used intelligently and safely. It is used to supply light and heat and to operate electrical appliances. It is essential to the operation of a modern beauty salon.

Although the exact nature of electricity is not thoroughly understood, its generating sources and effects are known. It is generally believed that electricity is a form of energy, which, when in motion, produces **magnetic**, **chemical**, and **heat** effects.

An **electric current** is the movement of electricity along a conductor.

An **electric wire** is composed of twisted fine metal threads (conductor) covered with rubber or silk (insulator or nonconductor).

A **conductor** is a substance that readily transmits an electric current. Most metals, carbon, the human body, and watery solutions of acids and salts are good conductors of electricity.

Electrodes, composed of good conductors, serve as points of contact when electricity is applied to the body.

A **nonconductor** or **insulator** is a substance that resists the passage of an electric current, such as rubber, silk, dry wood, glass, cement, or asbestos.

FORMS OF ELECTRICITY

Two forms of electricity are used, namely:
1. **Direct current** (DC) is a constant and even-flowing current, traveling in one direction.
2. **Alternating current** (AC) is a rapid and inter-rupted current, flowing first in one direction and then in the opposite direction.

If necessary, one type of current can be changed to the other type by means of a converter or rectifier.

A **converter** is an apparatus used to convert direct current into an alternating current. A **rectifier** is used to change an alternating current to a direct current.

A **complete circuit of electricity** is the entire path traveled by the current from its generating source through various conductors (wire, electrode, or body) and back to its original source.

A **fuse** is a safety device that prevents the overheating of electric wires. It will blow out when the circuit is overloaded with too many connections on one wire or when faulty equipment is used. To reestablish the circuit, disconnect apparatus before inserting a new fuse.

The **circuit breaker** has largely replaced the fuse in modern electrical wiring. This device has all the safety features offered by the fuse and is much easier to handle.

The circuit breaker does not require replacement every time it is set off. It is a switch device that automatically clicks off at the first indication of trouble in the circuit. When the trouble is corrected the switch is simply reset and all the safety factors are restored.

ELECTRICAL MEASUREMENTS

Electrical measurements are expressed in terms of the following units:

A **volt** (V) is the unit of **pressure** which forces the current forward.

An **ampere** (am'par) (A) is the unit of **current flow** (strength).

An **ohm** (O) is the unit of **resistance** to the flow of current.

If we increase the voltage applied to the circuit, the electron flow becomes stronger. Reducing the voltage makes the current weaker.

If we leave the voltage the same, increasing the resistance will make the current weaker. Reducing the resistance naturally allows more current to flow.

Instead of the ampere, which is too strong, the **milliampere** (mil-e-am'par), 1/1000th part of an ampere, is used for facial and scalp treatments. The **milliamperemeter** (mil-e-am'par-me'ter) is an instrument for measuring the rate of flow of an electric current.

GALVANIC CURRENT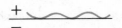

The **galvanic** (gal-van'ik) current is a constant and direct currrent (DC) rectified to a safe, low voltage level. Chemical changes are produced when this current is passed through certain solutions containing acids or salts. Chemical effects also are produced when a galvanic current is passed through the tissues and fluids of the body.

Test for polarity. Polarity means the opposite poles in an electric current. Before applying the galvanic current, the cosmetologist should know which is the positive and which is the negative pole. Most electrical appliances now have a polarity indicator. If necessary, polarity can be tested as follows:

1. Separate the tips of two conducting cords and immerse them into a glass of salt water. Turn the selector switch of the appliance to the galvanic current. As the water is decomposed, more active bubbles will accumulate at the negative pole than at the positive pole.

2. Place the tips of two conducting cords on two pieces of moistened litmus paper. The paper under the positive pole will turn red, while the paper under the negative pole will turn blue.

The effects of the positive pole on the body are just the opposite of those produced by the negative pole.

Positive Pole (Anode)	Negative Pole (Cathode)
Produces acidic reaction.	Produces alkaline reaction.
Soothes nerves.	Stimulates nerves.
Decreases blood supply.	Increases blood supply.
Hardens tissues.	Softens tissues.

The **positive pole** may be used:

1. To close the pores after finishing a facial treatment.
2. To decrease redness, as in mild acne.
3. To prevent inflammation after comedone and blemish treatment.
4. To force acid pH solutions, such as astringents, into the skin.

The **negative pole** may be used to:

1. Stimulate the circulation of blood to dry skin and scalp.
2. Force alkaline pH solution into the skin (a process that softens and liquifies grease deposits which are accumulations of sebum in the hair follicles).

Note: *Do not use the negative galvanic current over skin with either broken capillaries or a pustular acne condition, or on a patron with high blood pressure.*

How applied. The effects of the galvanic current are experienced by the patron as the current passes through her.

The **active electrode,** applied by the cosmetologist, is connected to the particular pole whose action is desired.

The **inactive electrode** is held by the patron and is connected to the other pole.

Both the active and inactive (positive and negative) poles must be in use to complete the circuit through the patron. Both the active and inactive carbon (ball and cylinder) electrodes must be lightly wrapped in a moistened cotton pledget.

Example: To close the pores, the ball electrode, which would be active, is wrapped in cotton moistened with astringent. The cylinder electrode (inactive), held by the patron, is wrapped in cotton moistened with water. After good contact is established with the two electrodes, the current is slowly turned on to the desired strength. At the end of the treatment, the current is slowly reduced before breaking contact with the patron.

PHORESIS

Chemical solutions can be forced into the unbroken skin by means of a galvanic current. This process is called **phoresis** (fo-re'sis). **Cataphoresis** (kat-uh-fo-re'sis) is the use of the positive pole to introduce a positive charged substance (an acid pH astringent solution) into the skin. **Anophoresis** (an-uh-fo-re'sis) is the use of the negative pole to force a negatively charged substance (an alkaline pH solution) into the skin.

FARADIC CURRENT

The **faradic** (fa-rad'ik) current is an alternating and interrupted current capable of producing a mechanical reaction without a chemical effect. It is used principally to cause muscular contractions.

When the faradic current is applied to the body, the muscles are toned, circulation is improved, and metabolism is increased. The faradic current may be used during scalp and facial manipulations.

How applied. Two electrodes are required to complete the faradic circuit. The cosmetologist wears a wrist electrode with a moistened pad, while the patron holds a carbon electrode wrapped in damp absorbent cotton. Before turning on the current, contact is established with the patron's forehead. During treatment the current is applied with the fingertips. At the completion of the treatment, the current is slowly turned off before breaking contact with the patron.

It is just as important to know when to use the faradic current as when not to use it. The massage action of the faradic current is beneficial because it invigorates the part being treated.

CAUTION

Do not use the faradic current if it causes pain or discomfort, or if the face is very florid. If the patron has many gold-filled teeth, or if she has any indication of high blood pressure, broken capillaries, or a pustular condition of the skin, treatment with faradic current should not be given.

Benefits derived from the use of the faradic current are as follows:

1. Improves muscle tone.
2. Promotes removal of waste products.
3. Increases circulation of the blood.
4. Relieves congested blood.
5. Increases glandular activity.
6. Stimulates hair growth.

SINUSOIDAL CURRENT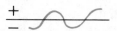

The **sinusoidal** (si-nus-oid'al) current, which resembles the faradic current in many respects, may be used during scalp and facial manipulations. It is an alternating current that produces mechanical contractions in muscles. The manner of application is the same as for the faradic current, requiring an electrode on the cosmetologist's wrist, while the patron holds the carbon electrode.

The sinusoidal current has the following **advantages:**

1. It supplies greater stimulation, deeper penetration, and less irritation than the faradic current.
2. It soothes the nerves, and penetrates into the deeper muscle tissue.
3. It is best suited for the nervous type of patron.

Do not use the sinusoidal current if the face is very flushed, or if the patron has broken capillaries in the skin, high blood pressure, or any pustular condition of the skin.

CAUTION

The faradic and sinusoidal currents are never used longer than 15-20 minutes on a patron.

HIGH-FREQUENCY CURRENT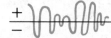

The **high-frequency** (fre'kwen-se) current is characterized by a high rate of oscillation.

Of chief interest to the cosmetologist is the **Tesla current,** commonly called the violet ray, used for both scalp and facial treatments.

The primary action of this current is thermal, or heat-producing. Because of its rapid oscillation, there are no muscular contractions. The physiological effects are either stimulating or soothing, depending on the method of application.

The electrodes for high-frequency current are made of glass or metal. Their shapes vary, the facial electrode being flat and the scalp electrode being rake shaped. As the current passes through the glass electrode, tiny violet sparks are emitted. All treatments given with high-frequency current should be started with a mild current and gradually increased to the required strength. The length of the treatment depends on the condition to be treated. About five minutes should be allowed for a general facial or scalp treatment.

For proper use, follow the instructions provided by the manufacturer of **Tesla** equipment.

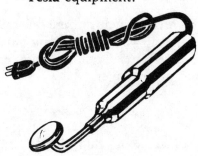

Facial electrode.

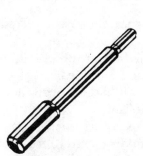

Metal electrode.

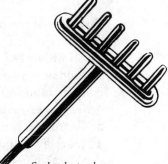

Scalp electrode.

There are three methods for using the Tesla current:

1. **Direct surface application.** The cosmetologist holds the electrode and applies it over the patron's skin. In facial treatments, the electrode is applied directly over facial cream which has been previously applied.

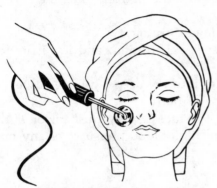

Applying high-frequency current to face using facial electrode.

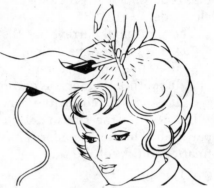

Applying high-frequency current to scalp using rake electrode.

2. **Indirect application.** The patron holds the metal or glass electrode, while the cosmetologist uses her fingers to massage the surface being treated. At no time is the electrode held by the cosmetologist. To prevent shock, the current is turned on after the patron has the electrode firmly in her hand; current is turned off before the electrode is removed from the patron's hand.

    Note: *Avoid contact by the patron with any metal, such as chair arms and stools. A burn may occur if such contact is made.*

3. **General electrification.** By holding a metal electrode in her hand, the patron's body is charged with electricity without being touched by the cosmetologist.

To obtain sedative, calming, or soothing effects with high-frequency current, the general electrification treatment is used, or the electrode is kept in close contact with the areas treated by the use of direct surface application.

To obtain a stimulating effect, lift the electrode slightly from the area to be treated and apply the current through the clothing or a towel.

Note: *When applying high-frequency current along with skin and scalp lotions containing an alcoholic content, you must apply the electricity first, and then the lotion.*

Benefits derived from the use of Tesla high-frequency current are as follows:

1. Stimulates circulation of the blood.
2. Increases glandular activity.
3. Aids in elimination and absorption.
4. Increases metabolism.
5. Germicidal action occurs during use.

The Tesla current may be used to treat falling hair, itchy scalp, tight scalp, and excessively oily or dry skin and scalp.

ELECTRICAL EQUIPMENT

The protection and safety of the patron are the primary concern of the cosmetologist. All electrical equipment should be regularly inspected to determine whether they are in safe working condition. Carelessness in making electrical connections and in applying various types of currents may result in a shock or a burn. Observing safety precautions will help to eliminate accidents and assure greater satisfaction to the patron.

The **vibrator** is an electric appliance used in massage to produce a mechanical succession of manipulations. It has a stimulating effect on the muscular tissues, increases the blood supply to the areas treated, is soothing to the nerves, increases glandular activities, and stimulates the functions of the skin and scalp.

The vibrator may be used by attaching it to the back of the hand. The vibrations are thus transmitted through the hand or fingers to the areas being treated.

The vibrator is used over heavy muscular tissue, such as the scalp, shoulders, and upper back. It is never used on a woman's face, but is used on a man's face.

Note: *The vibrator should never be used when there is a pronounced weakness of the heart, or in cases of fever, abscesses, or inflammation.*

The **steamer**, or **vaporizer**, is electrical equipment that is applied over the head or face to produce a moist, uniform heat.

The steamer may be used instead of hot towels to cleanse and steam the face. The steam warms the skin, inducing the flow of both oil and sweat. It thus helps to cleanse the skin, clean out the pores, and soften any scaliness on the surface of the skin.

The steamer also may be used for scalp and hair conditioning treatments. When fitted over the scalp, it produces controlled moist heat. Its action is to soften the scalp, increase perspiration, and promote the effectiveness of applied scalp cosmetics.

Another use for the steamer is to speed up the action of a lightener.

Electrically heated curling irons come in various types and sizes. They have built-in heating elements and operate from electrical outlets. One type has perforations. Oil is injected into the barrel of the curling irons where it is vaporized. The vapor leaves the irons through small perforations and conditions the hair as it curls.

Heating caps are electrical devices, applied over the head, which provide a uniform source of heat. Their main use is as part of corrective treatments for the hair and scalp. When used for this purpose, they recondition dry, brittle, and damaged hair, and also serve to activate a sluggish scalp.

The **processing machine**, or **accelerating machine**, has been designed as an aid to the professional hair colorist.

Its function is to reduce the processing time for lightening and tinting the hair. The processing time is reduced because the machine accelerates the molecular movement within the chemicals so that they work much faster.

SAFETY PRACTICES IN ELECTRICITY

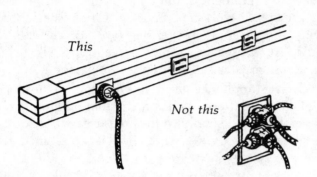

This

Not this

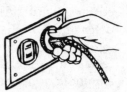

To disconnect current, *remove plug without pulling cord. Never pull on cord, as the wires may become loosened and cause a short circuit.*

Use only one plug to each outlet. *Overloading may cause fuse to blow out.*

WARNING

Keep a flashlight at top of steps, so you won't stumble down a dark stairway. Open fuse box and examine each fuse to locate "dead" one. When you replace a burned-out fuse, touch only its rim. Never put a coin in the fuse box instead of a fuse. Be sure to have some good fuses on hand. To test a fuse, use a flashlight battery, bulb (or bulb assembly), and a piece of wire—as shown at right. If fuse is good, bulb will light.

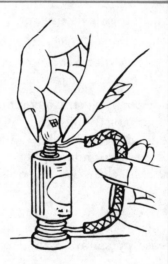

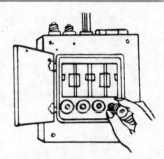

When replacing a blown-out fuse, *make sure you:*
1. *Use a new fuse with proper rating.*
2. *Stand on a dry surface.*
3. *Keep hands dry.*

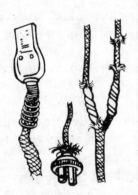

Examine cords regularly. *Repair or replace worn cords to prevent short circuit, shock, or fire.*

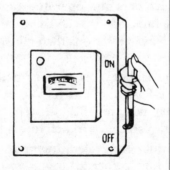

In an emergency, *turn off main switch, as illustrated, to shut off electricity for entire salon or building.*

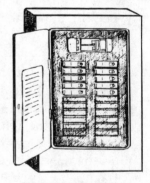

CIRCUIT BREAKER

The circuit breaker automatically disconnects any current with a defective appliance. It has the great advantage of restoring the current by a flick of the breaker switch to ON. This is very important in the beauty salon since it minimizes the possibility of long interruptions in the supply of electricity.

Accelerating machines may be used efficiently and successfully for various hair coloring treatments, such as hair lightening, tinting, frosting, tipping, streaking, and stripping. Accelerating machines must not be used over powdered lighteners.

The **electric chair hair dryer** delivers hot, medium, or cold air for the proper drying of the hair. It consists of an adjustable hood, or helmet, with deflectors that distribute the air evenly, and is capable of drying heavy hair in a comparatively short time. The **hand dryer** also delivers hot, medium, and cold air.

The **small electric oil heater** is used to heat oil and to keep the oil warm when giving an oil manicure.

SAFETY PRECAUTIONS

1. Study instructions before using any electrical equipment.
2. Disconnect appliances when you are finished using them.
3. Keep all wires, plugs, and equipment in a good condition.
4. Inspect all electrical equipment frequently.
5. Avoid wetting electric cords.
6. Sanitize all electrodes properly.
7. When using electrical equipment, protect the patron at all times.
8. Do not touch any metal while using an electrical apparatus.
9. Do not handle electric equipment with wet hands.
10. Do not allow patron to touch any metal surfaces when a treatment using electrical apparatus is being given.
11. Do not leave room when patron is attached to an electrical device.
12. Do not attempt to clean around an electric outlet when equipment is plugged in.
13. Do not touch two metallic objects at the same time while connected to an electric current.
14. Do not use any electrical equipment without first obtaining full instruction for its care and use.

LIGHT THERAPY

Light therapy (the'ra-pe) refers to treatment by means of light rays. Light or electrical waves travel at a tremendous speed—186,000 miles per second.

There are many kinds of light rays, but in salon work we are concerned with only three—those producing heat, known as **infra-red** (in'frah red) rays; those producing chemical and **germicidal** (jur-mi-si'dal) reaction, known as **ultra-violet** (ul'trah vi'o-let) rays; and visible lights, all of which are contained within the sun's rays.

If a ray of sunshine is passed through a glass **prism** (priz'm), it will appear in seven different colors, known as the **rainbow,** arrayed in the following manner: red, orange, yellow, green, blue, indigo, and violet. These colors, which are visible to the eye, constitute the **visible rays,** comprising about 12% of sunshine.

Scientists have discovered that at either end of the visible spectrum are rays of the sun that are **invisible** to us. The rays beyond the violet are the **ultra-violet rays,** also known as **actinic** (ak-tin'ik) **rays.** These rays are the shortest and least penetrating rays of the spectrum, comprising about 8% of sunshine. The action of these rays is both chemical and germicidal.

Beyond the red rays of the spectrum are the **infra-red rays.** These are pure heat rays, comprising about 80% of sunshine.

DISPERSION OF LIGHT RAYS BY A PRISM

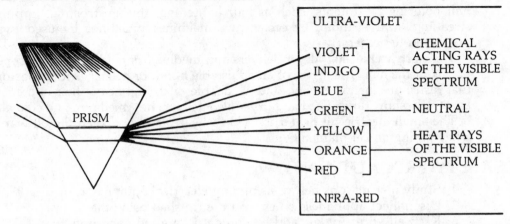

			ULTRA-VIOLET	
PRISM			VIOLET ⎤	CHEMICAL ACTING RAYS OF THE VISIBLE SPECTRUM
			INDIGO	
			BLUE ⎦	
			GREEN	NEUTRAL
			YELLOW ⎤	HEAT RAYS OF THE VISIBLE SPECTRUM
			ORANGE	
			RED ⎦	
			INFRA-RED	

Ultra-violet Rays			Solar Spectrum	Infra-red Rays
1847 AU to 3900 AU			3900 AU to 7700 AU	7700 AU to 14,000 AU
Far 1847-2200	Middle 2200-2900	Near 2900-3900	Violet Indigo Blue Green Yellow Orange Red	Penetrating
Germicidal	Therapeutic	Tonic		Analgesic
Cold Invisible Rays			Visible Rays	Invisible Heat Rays

PROPERTIES OF ULTRA-VIOLET RAYS:
1. Short wave length.
2. High frequency.
3. Weak penetrating power.

PROPERTIES OF INFRA-RED RAYS:
1. Long wave length.
2. Low frequency.
3. Deep penetrating power.

NATURAL SUNSHINE IS COMPOSED OF:
8% ultra-violet rays; 12% visible light rays; 80% infra-red rays.

HOW LIGHT RAYS ARE REPRODUCED

Glass bulb type.

A **therapeutic** (the-ra-pu'tik) **lamp** is an electrical apparatus capable of producing certain light rays. There are separate lamps for infra-red and for ultra-violet rays.

Ultra-violet lamps. There are three general types: the glass bulb, the hot **quartz** (kworts), and the cold quartz.

1. The **glass bulb lamp** is used mainly for cosmetic or tanning purposes.

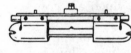

2. The **hot quartz lamp** is a general all-purpose lamp suitable for tanning, health, cosmetic, or germicidal purposes.
3. The **cold quartz lamp** produces mostly short ultra-violet rays. It is used primarily in hospitals.

Hot quartz type.

Infra-red rays give no light whatsoever. Special glass bulbs are used to produce infra-red rays.

The **visible rays,** or **dermal lights,** are reproduced by carbon or tungsten filament, in clear glass bulbs. They produce white light, or in colored bulbs, red or blue light.

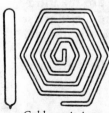

Cold quartz type.

Protecting the eyes. The patron's eyes always should be protected with cotton pads, saturated with a boric acid solution or witch hazel and placed on the eyelids during light ray treatments. The cosmetologist and patron always should wear safety eye goggles when using ultra-violet rays.

ULTRA-VIOLET RAYS

Ultra-violet rays are invisible rays. Their action is both chemical and germicidal. Plant and animal life need ultra-violet rays for healthy growth. In the human body, these rays produce changes in the chemistry of the blood and also stimulate the activity of body cells.

Ultra-violet rays increase resistance to disease by increasing the iron and vitamin D content and the number of red and white cells in the blood. They also increase elimination of waste products, restore nutrition where needed, stimulate the circulation, and improve the flow of blood and **lymph** (limf).

The slightest obstruction of any kind will keep ultra-violet rays from reaching the skin. Consequently, the skin must be entirely cleansed before being exposed to ultra-violet rays.

How applied. Ultra-violet rays are the shortest light rays of the spectrum. The farther they are from the visible light region, the shorter they become. The longer ultra-violet rays tend to increase the fixation of calcium in the blood. If the lamp is placed from 30-36" (76.2-91.4 cm) away, few of the shorter rays will reach the skin, so that the action is then limited to the effect of the longer rays.

The shorter rays are obtained when the lamp is within 12" (30.4 cm) from the skin. These rays are not only destructive to bacteria, but to tissue as well, if allowed to remain exposed for too long a period of time.

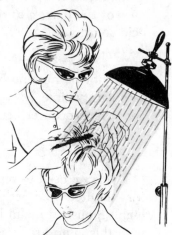

Applying ultra-violet rays to scalp.

Average exposure may produce redness of the skin, and overdoses may cause blistering. It is well to start with a short exposure of 2-3 minutes, and gradually increase the time to 7-8 minutes. **The cosmetologist and patron must wear eye goggles to protect their eyes.**

Skin tanning is the result of exposure to ultra-violet rays, which stimulate the production of pigment, or coloring matter, in the skin.

Sunburn may be produced by ultra-violet rays in various degrees; however, for cosmetic purposes, a first degree sunburn only is given. This is manifested by a slight reddening, appearing several hours after application, showing no signs of itching, burning, or peeling. Over-exposure produces third and fourth degree burns, which are destructive to the tissues.

Skin and scalp disorders. Ultra-violet rays are used for acne, tinea, seborrhea, and to combat dandruff. They also promote healing, and may stimulate the growth of hair.

INFRA-RED RAYS

Generally speaking, infra-red rays produce a soothing and beneficial type of heat, which penetrates into the tissues of the body.

Use and effects of infra-red rays on exposed areas:

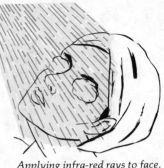

1. Heat and relax the skin without increasing temperature of the body as a whole.
2. Dilate blood vessels in the skin, thereby increasing blood flow.
3. Increase metabolism and chemical changes within skin tissues.
4. Increase the production of perspiration and oil on the skin.
5. Relieve pain.

Applying infra-red rays to face.

The lamp is operated at an average distance of 30" (76.2 cm). It is placed closer at the start, and to avoid the burning of the skin, is moved back gradually as the surface heat becomes more pronounced. **Always protect the eyes of the patron during exposure.** Place cotton pads saturated with boric acid solution or witch hazel over patron's eyelids.

CAUTION

Do not permit the light rays to remain on body tissue more than a few seconds at a time. Move the hand back and forth across the ray's path to break constant exposure. Length of exposure should be about five minutes.

VISIBLE LIGHTS

The **lamp** used to reproduce visible lights is usually a dome-shaped reflector mounted on a pedestal with a flexible neck. The dome is finished with a highly polished metal lining capable of reflecting heat rays. The bulbs used with this lamp are available in white, red, or blue.

Visible lights are used primarily in connection with facial and scalp treatments.

As with all other lamps, the patron's eyes must be protected from the glare and heat of the light. Cover the patron's eyes with cotton pads saturated with a boric acid solution or witch hazel.

Use and effect of white light: It relieves pain, especially in congested areas, and more particularly, around the nerve centers, such as in the back of the neck and across the shoulders.

Use and effects of blue light: It has a tonic effect on the bare skin and a soothing effect on the nerves. Blue light contains few heat rays. To obtain the desired result, always use it over the bare skin. Creams, oils, or powders must not be present on the skin.

Use and effects of red light: It has strong heat rays, providing a stimulating effect when used over the skin. Red light penetrates more deeply than the blue light. Its heat rays aid the penetration of cosmetic creams into the skin. It is recommended for dry, scaly, and shriveled skin, and is used over creams and ointments to soften and relax the tissues.

REVIEW QUESTIONS

ELECTRICITY

1. What is electricity?
2. What is a conductor?
3. What are electrodes?
4. What is a non-conductor or insulator? Give six examples.
5. What is a direct current (DC)?
6. What is an alternating current (AC)?
7. Which apparatus changes a direct current to an alternating current?
8. Which apparatus changes an alternating current to a direct current?
9. What is a volt?
10. What is an ampere?
11. What is an ohm?

GALVANIC, FARADIC, AND SINUSOIDAL CURRENTS

Galvanic Current

1. Describe galvanic current.
2. Give the chemical action of: a) the positive pole; b) the negative pole.
3. Name three effects of the positive pole on the body.
4. Name three effects of the negative pole on the body.
5. How is the galvanic current applied?

Faradic Current

1. What is faradic current? Its effects?
2. How is the faradic current applied?
3. In what cases should faradic current never be used?

Sinusoidal Current

1. What is sinusoidal current?
2. What is the difference between faradic and sinusoidal current?
3. How is the sinusoidal current applied?

HIGH-FREQUENCY CURRENT

1. What fact characterizes the high-frequency current?
2. Which type of high-frequency current is commonly used in the beauty salon?
3. What effects does the Tesla current produce on the body?
4. What type of glass electrode is used for the: a) face; b) scalp?
5. How much time should be allowed for a general facial or scalp treatment?
6. Name three methods of applying the Tesla current.
7. Briefly describe how to use direct surface application.
8. Briefly describe how to use indirect application.
9. Briefly describe how to use general electrification.
10. Which method of application produces soothing results?
11. How are stimulating effects produced?
12. What safety precaution should be observed when using skin and scalp lotions with an alcoholic content?
13. List five benefits obtained by using the Tesla current.
14. List five scalp conditions that may be treated with the Tesla current.

ELECTRICAL EQUIPMENT

1. What is a vibrator?
2. Over which areas of the body is the vibrator used?
3. Under what conditions should a vibrator never be used?
4. How is a steamer, or vaporizer, used?
5. What are the effects produced by the steamer when used over the face?
6. What are the effects produced by the steamer when used over the scalp?
7. What type of heating element do electrically heated curling irons have?
8. How does vapor from curling irons benefit the hair?
9. What are heating caps?
10. What is their main use?
11. How do heating caps aid in corrective scalp and hair treatments?
12. What is the function of a processing machine?
13. How does it reduce processing time?

LIGHT THERAPY

1. What is light therapy?
2. Which rays of the sun are invisible?
3. What is a therapeutic lamp?
4. Name three types of therapeutic lamps that produce ultra-violet rays.
5. Which ultra-violet lamps are desirable for cosmetic purposes?
6. Why do both plant and animal life need ultra-violet rays for healthy growth?
7. Which four blood constituents are increased by exposure to ultra-violet rays?
8. What effects do ultra-violet rays have on the body functions?
9. Why should the skin be clean before exposure to ultra-violet rays?
10. At what distance from the skin do the shorter ultra-violet rays become effective?
11. How long should the skin be exposed for the first time?
12. To how many minutes can exposure be gradually increased?
13. How should the eyes of both the patron and the cosmetologist be protected when using ultra-violet rays?
14. What causes the skin to tan?
15. What are the signs of first degree sunburn?
16. Why should prolonged exposure be avoided?
17. Which skin and scalp disorders are helped by ultra-violet rays?
18. What benefit does the hair receive from ultra-violet rays?
19. What are the five effects of infra-red rays on the body?
20. How far should the infra-red lamp be kept from the skin?
21. How should the patron's eyes be protected during exposure?
22. Why should infra-red light rays be broken with a hand movement?
23. Which type of lamp reproduces visible lights?
24. Why should the patron's eyes be protected during exposure?
25. What are the benefits of using a white light?
26. Which visible light lacks heat rays?
27. What are the benefits of using a blue light?
28. What are the three benefits of using a red light?

Chapter 31

CHEMISTRY

CHAPTER LEARNING OBJECTIVES

The student successfully mastering this chapter will know:
1. *The difference between organic and inorganic chemistry.*
2. *The nature and types of matter.*
3. *The composition of elements, compounds, and mixtures.*
4. *The properties of matter, elements, compounds, and mixtures.*
5. *The difference between acids and alkalies.*
6. *The chemistry of water.*
7. *The chemistry, types, and action of shampoos.*
8. *The chemistry of cosmetics.*
9. *The chemistry and use of rinses.*
10. *The chemistry of the various products used in grooming.*
11. *The composition of permanent wave solutions and how they act on the hair.*
12. *How chemical hair relaxers act on the hair.*
13. *The chemistry of hair coloring.*
14. *The action of hair lighteners.*

The professional cosmetologist must be more than a practicing technician. At various times, he or she must serve not only as a hairstylist, but also as a psychologist, a business executive, a chemist, an advisor, and an expert in every phase of good grooming.

In order to qualify for this unique position, it is now necessary that the cosmetologist possess a far greater knowledge and understanding of the many facets of the profession than ever before.

A basic knowledge of modern chemistry is an essential requirement for an intelligent understanding of the various products and cosmetics being used in the beauty salon. Through the advances in the science of chemistry, new and better products constantly are being developed for the benefit of both the cosmetologist and the patron. It is, therefore, important that the professional technician understand these products and learn how to use them for the maximum benefits to the patrons.

SCIENCE OF CHEMISTRY

Chemistry (kem'is-tre) is the science that deals with the composition, structure, and properties of matter, and how matter changes under different chemical conditions. The broad subject of chemistry is divided into two areas: 1) organic chemistry, and 2) inorganic chemistry.

Organic (or-gan'ik) **chemistry** is the branch of chemistry that deals with all substances in which carbon is present. Carbon can be found in all plants, animals, petroleum, soft coal, natural gas, and in many artificially pepared substances.

Most organic substances will burn. They are not soluble in water, but they are soluble in organic solvents, such as alcohol and benzene.

Examples of organic substances are grass, trees, gasoline, oil, soaps, detergents, plastics, and antibiotics.

Inorganic (in-or-gan'ik) **chemistry** is that branch of chemistry that deals with all substances that do not contain carbon. Inorganic substances will not burn and are usually soluble in water.

Examples are water, air, iron, lead, and iodine.

MATTER

Since chemistry is the science that deals with matter, it is essential that we develop an understanding of what matter really is. Matter may be defined as anything that occupies space. It exists in three physical forms: solids, liquids, and gases.

Solids. Look around the classroom and note what you see: hair, students, teachers, desks, chairs, walls. These are all matter in a solid state.

Liquids. In the clinic area of the school you see water, shampoos, lotions, hair tonics. These are matter in a liquid state.

Gases. Take a deep breath. The air you have just brought into your lungs also is matter. It is in a gaseous state.

It is not the purpose of this text to train scientists, but to help cosmetology students learn enough about matter to help them in their professional work. It is, therefore, advisable that we briefly examine the nature and the structure of matter.

ATOMS

An **atom** (at'um) is the smallest particle of an **element** (el'e-ment) that can exist and still retain the properties of the element. Therefore, an atom of hydrogen has the properties of hydrogen. Should this atom be shattered, it would no longer possess the properties of hydrogen, nor would it resemble a hydrogen atom.

MOLECULES

A **molecule** (mol'e-kul) is the smallest particle of an element or compound that possesses all the properties of the element or compound. If the molecule is of an element, the atoms are the same. If it is of a compound, the atoms are different. For example, a molecule of hydrogen contains two or more atoms of hydrogen, whereas a molecule of the compound of water is composed of two atoms of hydrogen and one atom of oxygen (H_2O).

CHEMICAL ACTIVITY

In general, when we talk about the chemical activity of an element, we refer to the tendency of its atoms to combine with other elements. For example, hydrogen is a very active element and readily combines with other elements, while neon is completely inactive and does not combine with other elements.

FORMS OF MATTER

Matter exists in an almost infinite variety. This variety is made possible because of the atomic structure of matter, which permits the joining of a number of elements in countless combinations.

Matter exists in the form of elements, compounds, and mixtures.

Elements. An element is the basic unit of all matter. It is a substance that **cannot** be made by the combination of simpler substances, and the element itself cannot be reduced to simpler substances. There are now more than 103 elements that are known, of which some of the more common are iron, sulfur, oxygen, zinc, and silver.

Each element is given a letter symbol. Iron is Fe; sulfur, S; oxygen, O; zinc, Zn; and silver, Ag. All symbols can be obtained by referring to a chart of elements.

Compounds. When two or more elements unite chemically, they form a compound. Each element loses its characteristic properties and the new compound develops its own individual properties. For example, iron oxide (rust) has different properties than the two elements of which it is comprised—iron and oxygen. The new substance, which is a compound, cannot be altered by mechanical means, but only by chemical methods.

ELEMENTS AND COMPOUNDS

MATTER	TYPES AND DEFINITION	SMALLEST PARTICLE	ELEMENTS FOUND IN HAIR
	ELEMENTS SIMPLEST FORM OF MATTER	ATOM *(Cannot be broken down by simple chemical reactions)* *About 103 different kinds*	CARBON NITROGEN OXYGEN SULFUR HYDROGEN PHOSPHORUS
FORMS GASES LIQUIDS SOLIDS	COMPOUNDS FORMED BY COMBINATION OF ELEMENTS	MOLECULE *(Consists of 2 or more atoms chemically combined)* *Unlimited kinds possible*	**COMPOUNDS USED ON HAIR** WATER HYDROGEN PEROXIDE AMMONIUM THIOGLYCOLATE ANILINE DERIVATIVE TINTS AMMONIA ALCOHOL ACIDS ALKALIES

Compounds can be divided into four classes:

1. **Oxides** are compounds of any element combined with oxygen. For example, one part carbon and two parts oxygen equal **carbon dioxide,** which might be recognized as dry ice. Or, one part carbon and one part oxygen equal **monoxide,** better known as the poisonous exhaust of an automobile.

2. **Acids** are compounds of hydrogen, a non-metal, such as nitrogen and, sometimes, oxygen. For example, hydrogen + sulfur + oxygen = **sulfuric acid** (H_2SO_4). Acids turn **blue** litmus paper **red,** providing a quick way to test a compound.

3. **Bases,** also known as **alkalies,** are compounds of hydrogen, a metal and oxygen. For example, sodium + oxygen + hydrogen = **sodium hydroxide** (NaOH), which is used in the manufacture of soap. Bases will turn **red** litmus paper **blue.**

4. **Salts** are compounds that are formed by the reaction of acids and bases, with water also produced by the reaction. Two common salts and their formulas are sodium chloride (table salt) (NaCl), which contains sodium and chloride, and magnesium sulphate (Epsom salts) ($MgSo_4.7H_2O$), which contains magnesium, sulfur, hydrogen, and oxygen.

Mixtures. A mixture is a substance that is made up of two elements combined **physically** rather than chemically.

The ingredients in a mixture do not change their properties as they do in a compound, but retain their individual characteristics. For example, concrete is composed of sand, gravel, and cement. While concrete is a mixture having its own functions, its ingredients never lose their characteristics. Sand remains sand, gravel is still gravel, and cement, cement.

CHANGES IN MATTER

Matter may be changed in two ways, either through physical or chemical means.

A **physical change** refers to an alteration of the properties without the formation of any new substance. For example, ice, a solid, melts at a certain temperature and becomes a liquid (water), and water, a liquid, freezes at a certain temperature and becomes a solid. There is no change in the inherent nature of the water, but merely a change in its form.

A **chemical change** is one in which a new substance or substances are formed, having properties different from the original substances. For example, soap is formed from the chemical reaction between an alkaline substance (potassium hydroxide) and an oil or fat. The soap resembles neither the alkaline substance nor the oil from which it is formed. Chemical reaction between the two forms a new substance, with its own characteristic properties.

PROPERTIES OF MATTER

Properties of matter refer to how we distinguish one form of matter from another.

Physical properties. These refer to properties such as density, specific gravity, odor, color, taste.

1. **Density** of a substance refers to its weight divided by its volume. For example, the volume of one cubic foot (0.03 m³) of water weighs 62.4 lbs. (28.08 kg). Therefore, its density is (weight) 62.4 lbs. (28.08 kg) ÷ (volume) 1 cubic foot (0.03 m³), or water has a density of 62.4 lbs. (28.08 kg) per cubic foot (0.03 m³).

2. **Specific gravity** of a substance also is referred to as its relative density. This means that substances are referred to as either more or less dense than water. For example, copper is 8.9 times as dense as water; therefore, the specific gravity (or relative density) of copper is 8.9.

3. **Odor** of a substance helps us to identify it in many instances. For example, the characteristic odor of ammonium thioglycolate, known as the thio odor, helps us identify this product.

4. **Color** helps us identify many substances. For example, we recognize the color of gold, silver, copper, brass, coal.

5. **Taste** has helped us identify many substances. For example, oil of wintergreen can be identified by its peppermint-like taste.

Chemical properties. The chemical properties of a substance refer to the ability of the substance to react, and the conditions under which it reacts. Two of the more widely known chemical properties a substance possesses are combustibility and the ability to **support combustion.** For example:

1. Phosphorus is a highly combustible substance. For that reason, it is used on the tips of matches. The heat produced by rubbing the match tip against a surface is enough to cause it to burst into flames.

2. One of the chemical properties of wood is its ability to support combustion. It is, therefore, used in the manufacture of matches. The phosphorous tip starts the fire and the wood supports the fire.

PROPERTIES OF COMMON ELEMENTS, COMPOUNDS, AND MIXTURES

Knowledge about the properties of the most common elements, compounds, and mixtures can be of great benefit to the student studying the reasons why certain chemical reactions take place.

Oxygen (O) (ok'si-jen) is the most abundant element, found both free and in compounds, and composes about half of the earth's crust, half of the rock, one-fifth of the air, and 90% of the water. It is a colorless, odorless, tasteless, gaseous substance, combining with most other elements to form an infinite variety of compounds called **oxides.** One of the chief characteristics of this element is that substances burn readily in oxygen.

Hydrogen (H) (hi'dro-jen) is a colorless, odorless, and tasteless gas. It is the lightest element known, being used as a unit of weight. It is inflammable and explosive when mixed with air. It is found in chemical combination with oxygen in water and with other elements in acids, bases, and organic substances, such as wood, meat, fish, sugar, and butter.

Air is the gaseous mixture that makes up the earth's atmosphere. It is odorless, colorless, and consists of about 1 part oxygen and 4 parts nitrogen.

These proportions vary somewhat according to conditions. It also contains a small amount of carbon dioxide, ammonia, nitrates, and organic matter, which are essential to plant and animal life.

Hydrogen peroxide (H_2O_2) (per-ok'side) is a compound of hydrogen and oxygen. It is a colorless liquid with a characteristic odor and a slightly acid taste. Organic matter, such as silk, hair, feathers and nails, are bleached by hydrogen peroxide because of its oxidizing power. The 20-40 volume hydrogen peroxide solution is used as a lightening agent for the hair. A 3-5% (6-10 volume) solution of hydrogen peroxide possesses antiseptic qualities.

Oxidizing (ok-si-diz'ing) **agents.** A substance that readily gives up its oxygen is known as an oxidizing agent. Hydrogen peroxide releases oxygen, which oxidizes the hair pigment to a colorless compound. The lightening agent is reduced and the pigment is oxidized. When oxygen is taken away from any substance, it is known as a **reduction.** The substance that attracts the oxygen is the **reducing agent.** Oxidation always is accompanied by reduction.

Nitrogen (N) (ni'tro-jen) is a colorless, gaseous element found free in the air. It constitutes part of the atmosphere, forming about four-fifths of the air. It is necessary to life because it dilutes the oxygen. It is found in nature chiefly in the form of ammonia and nitrates.

ACIDITY AND ALKALINITY

The **pH** of a liquid refers to its degree of acidity or alkalinity. Meters and indicators have been developed for the measurement of pH. Values are illustrated below.

The pH scale goes from 0-14. The neutral point is 7.

Cold wave solutions are alkaline up to 9.6.

Neutralizers are always acid.

Soaps up to 9.5 are satisfactory; higher, unsatisfactory.

Shampoos are 6-10. Depilatories, above 10.

AVERAGE pH VALUES

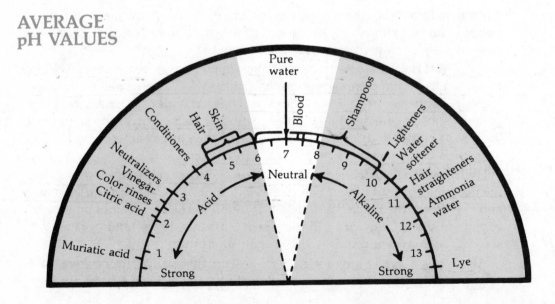

Acidity. Anything below 7 is acidic. The lower the pH, the greater is the degree of acidity.

Alkalinity. Anything from 7-14 is alkaline. The higher the pH, the greater is the degree of alkalinity.

Since cosmetics vary in their pH values, be guided in their use by your instructor.

Note: The cleansing action of soaps and shampoos depends on their alkalinity and contact time with the skin, scalp, or hair. Due to the short contact time, many alkaline products will achieve the desired results without damage to the skin, scalp, or hair.

CHEMISTRY OF WATER

Water (H_2O) is the most abundant of all substances, composing about 75% of the earth's surface and about 65% of the human body. It is the universal solvent. Demineralized or distilled water is used as a **non-conductor** of electricity. Water containing certain mineral substances is an excellent **conductor** of electricity.

Water serves many useful purposes in the beauty salon. Only water of known purity is fit for drinking purposes. Suspended or dissolved impurities render water unsatisfactory for cleaning objects and for use in salons.

Impurities can be removed from water by:

1. **Filtration**—passing water through a porous substance, such as filter paper or charcoal.
2. **Distillation**—heating water in a closed vessel arranged so that the resulting vapor passes off through a tube and is cooled and condensed to a liquid. This process purifies water used in the manufacture of cosmetics.

Boiling water at a temperature of 212° Fahrenheit (100° Celsius) will destroy most microbic life.

SOFT WATER

It is very important that soft water be used for shampooing, lightening, or tinting the hair. **Rain water** is the softest water. **Hard water** contains mineral substances, such as the salts of calcium and magnesium, which curdle or precipitate soap instead of permitting a permanent lather to form. Hard water may be softened by **distillation** or by use of **borax sodium carbonate** (washing soda) or **sodium phosphate**. Zeolite tanks are used to effectively soften hard water in beauty salons.

A good test for soft water uses a soap solution made by dissolving three-quarters of an ounce (22.5 ml) of pure powdered castile soap in a pint of distilled water. A pint (0.47 l) bottle is half filled with fresh water and one teaspoon (0.5 ml) of the soap solution is added. The bottle is then shaken vigorously. If a lather forms at once and persists, the water is very soft. If a lather does not appear at once, another teaspoon (0.5 ml) of soap solution is added and the shaking repeated. If an additional teaspoon (0.5 ml) of the soap solution is needed to produce a good lather, the water is hard and must be softened.

SHAMPOOING

All professional cosmetologists understand the importance of the shampoo and how the cleanliness of the hair affects other hair services. However, it is also important that they know how the shampoo cleanses the hair.

No discussion of the action of shampoos and how they function can be meaningful unless a study is made of the shampoo molecule.

SHAMPOO MOLECULES

Shampoo molecules are large molecules that have been specially treated. They are composed of a **head** and a **tail**, each with its own special function.

The **tail** of the shampoo molecule has an attraction for dirt, grease, debris, and oil, but has no attraction for or liking of water. The **head** of the shampoo molecule has a strong attraction for water, but does not like dirt.

Working as a team, both parts of the molecule do an effective job of cleansing the hair.

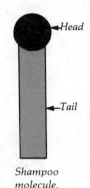

Shampoo molecule.

ACTION OF SHAMPOOS

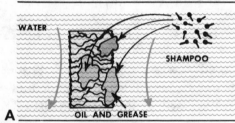

A

Sticky greasy surface attracts and holds dust and other particles of foreign matter to hair cuticle. Water alone is unable to clean hair because water molecules are unable to pull particles free from cuticle.

The tail of the shampoo molecule has a strong attraction for hair, grease and dirt, etc.

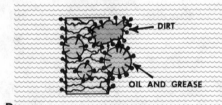

B

Proper massage of shampoo insures that shampoo molecules are brought in direct contact with these substances.

Each tail of a molecule is attracted to grease and dirt.

Action of shampoo causes grease and oils to roll up into small globules, reducing contact with hair cuticle.

EXCESS shampoo molecules are attracted to imbrications. Alkaline shampoos open imbrications, causing tangling and matting during massage movements as fibers rub together.

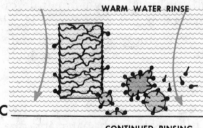

C

Currents of warm rinsing water remove dirt and grease because heads of shampoo molecules are attracted to passing water molecules. Tails of shampoo molecules, attached dirt and foreign matter are bound to heads of shampoo following the rinsing currents of water. Thus foreign matter is removed ONLY during rinsing stages of shampooing.

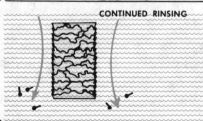

D

Excess shampoo molecules are less easily removed from hair shaft. Continued rinsing is essential to cleanse hair of shampoo. Time of rinsing is reduced by restricting amounts of shampoo. Excess swelling of imbrications is prevented by acid, soapless shampoos.

The shampoo is applied and thoroughly worked into the hair. The dirt, grease, debris, and oil in the hair are attracted to the tails of the shampoo molecules and become firmly attached to them.

Rinsing. During the rinsing step, as the stream of water is directed through the hair, the "water-loving" molecule heads attach themselves to the water molecules and are carried from the hair, taking with them the tails with the attached dirt.

CHEMISTRY OF SHAMPOOS

Shampoo soaps are formed by combining an alkali with an oil or fat. The oil used may be of vegetable origin, such as almond, peanut, coconut, olive, castor, and palm nut.

The fat used may be animal fat, lanolin, tallow, and synthetic compounds.

Most shampoos contain varying amounts of the same fatty acids. Therefore, the shampoo soap formed varies with the substances used.

Shampoos with a high pH factor, which are highly alkaline, are especially damaging to all types of hair.

TYPES OF SHAMPOOS

The main purpose of a shampoo is to cleanse the scalp and hair. This may be accomplished by a wet or dry shampoo. Wet shampoos are watery solutions of soap and various cleansing agents. Dry shampoos do not use water, but contain either powdery substances or cosmetic products in liquid form.

Wet shampoos, depending on their composition, are of three basic types:
1. Soap shampoos.
2. Soapless shampoos
   (foaming or foamless).
3. Cream or paste shampoos.

Soap shampoos are available in the form of cake, powder, gel, or liquid. The active cleansing agent is a soap made from olive oil, coconut oil, or other oils. Liquid soap shampoos contain more than 50% water. When used on the hair, a soap shampoo will produce an alkaline reaction. With soft water, soap shampoos lather readily. When used with hard water, soap shampoos will not lather, and tend to produce an insoluble soap residue on the hair.

Soapless shampoos come in the form of a powder, gel, cream, or liquid. They are effective cleansing agents. Their main ingredient is a sulfonated oil. Both the lathering and non-lathering types of soapless shampoos are available.

Soapless shampoos are just as effective in soft, hard, cold, or hot water. They should be used with discretion, since frequent applications not only dry the scalp and hair, but render the hair more absorptive than usual.

Cream or paste shampoos have a cleansing action due to soap, a synthetic detergent, or a combination of both. They also may contain a reconditioning agent for the hair. Cream shampoos, or pastes, without soap, are usually acid in reaction.

(For other types of shampoos, see chapter on **Shampooing And Rinsing.**)

CONDITIONERS

The professional treatment of hair requires the use of many chemicals. Certain chemicals remove excess amounts of natural oils and moisture from the hair, causing it to become dry and brittle (damaged). As a result, hair conditioners are required to help restore some of the natural oils and moisture and make the hair ready to accept other hair services. Patrons with naturally dry, brittle hair also will benefit from regular conditioning treatments.

Conditioners are primarily designed to coat and give body to damaged hair. They are available in cream and liquid forms. The formulation of the product varies with the manufacturer. It may contain lanolin, cholesterol, moisturizers, sulfonated oil, vegetable oils, proteins, or various combinations of these. For the best results, it is important that each product be applied exactly as indicated by manufacturer. Most conditioners are applied to hair that has been shampooed and towel dried.

There are four general groups of hair conditioners available. The selection of the type to be used depends on the texture and condition of the hair and the results to be achieved.

TIMED CONDITIONERS

These conditioners are applied to hair, allowed to stay on from 1-5 minutes, and then rinsed out. The hair is then set and styled, with setting lotion used as required. These conditioners usually have an acid pH; they do not penetrate into the hair shaft, but add natural oils and moisture to the hair.

CONDITIONERS COMBINED WITH STYLING LOTIONS

Protein or resin based conditioners are incorporated into the setting lotion and applied as part of the hair setting process. A little water, added during the hair setting procedure, helps to facilitate setting by keeping hair soft and manageable. This type of conditioner is designed to slightly increase hair diameter by coating action and to give it body. It is available in several strengths to accommodate the texture, condition, and quality of the hair.

PROTEIN PENETRATING CONDITIONERS

These conditioners utilize hydrolized protein (very small fragments) and are designed to pass through the cuticle, penetrate into the cortex, and replace the keratin that has been lost from the hair. They improve texture, equalize porosity, and increase elasticity. The excess conditioner must be rinsed from the hair before setting.

NEUTRALIZING CONDITIONERS

These conditioners neutralize an alkaline condition created by strongly alkaline hair products. They have an acid pH and are intended to prevent damage to the hair and alleviate scalp irritation. A neutralizing conditioner is allowed to remain on the hair from 1-5 minutes and is then rinsed out before the hair is set.

OTHER CONDITIONERS

In addition to the above, there are a number of other vegetable, protein, and synthetic polymer conditioners available. Each one of these conditioners is designed to deal with one or more of the hair and scalp problems facing the hairstylist.

Note: Regardless of the type of conditioner used, it is important that the cosmetologist follow manufacturer's directions at all times.)

PERMANENT WAVING

In order to understand the chemical actions of permanent waving, it is first necessary to understand the composition of hair and hair bonds.

COMPOSITION OF HAIR

Hair is made of a hard protein called **keratin**. It has three layers: **cuticle, cortex, medulla.** Since permanent hair waving takes place in the cortical layer, special attention is given to a study of the cortex.

The **cortex** is composed of numerous parallel fibers of hard keratin, referred to as **polypeptide chains.** These parallel fibers are twisted around one another in a manner resembling the twisting of the fiber strands in rope.

PEPTIDE BONDS

Each amino acid is joined to another by peptide bonds (end bonds), forming a chain as long as the hair. They are the strongest bonds in the cortex and most of the strength of hair is due to their properties.

Peptide bonds are chemical bonds, and if even a few are broken, the hair is weakened or damaged. If many of these bonds are broken, the hair will break off.

CROSS-BONDS

It is the presence of cross-bonds or links, however, that has given hair the ability to be permanently waved. There are two types of cross-bonds that are of major concern in hair work:

1. **Sulfur bonds** (chemical)—called **S-bonds.**
2. **Hydrogen bonds** (physical)—called **H-bonds.**

Hydrogen bonds are much more numerous than sulfur bonds, but they are much weaker and can be broken easily with water or chemicals.

Sulfur bonds are very strong and can only be broken by a strong chemical.

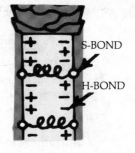

Cross-bonds

1. STRAIGHT HAIR (Both H- and S-Bonds in Straight Positions.)	2. HAIR WOUND ON RODS AND SOFTENED BY SHAMPOOING AND COLD WAVE SOLUTIONS. (H-Bonds and nearly all S-Bonds Broken.)	3. HAIR AFTER NEUTRALIZING. (Some H-Bonds and many S-Bonds Re-formed.)	4. HAIR ON ROLLERS AFTER PROPER DRYING. (Most H-Bonds and S-Bonds Re-formed.)	5. HAIR AFTER UNWINDING. (Original S-Bonds Stretched into Waved Positions.)

S-BOND
H-BOND

THIO SOLUTION IN PERMANENT WAVING

A thio (ammonium thioglycolate) solution with a pH of 9.4-9.6 causes the cuticle of the hair to swell and the imbrications to open, allowing the solution to penetrate into the cortex. The solution breaks down all the H-bonds and many of the S-bonds, permitting a slippage or alteration of the polypeptide chains. The chains assume the contour of the rods around which the hair is wound.

NEUTRALIZER

When sufficient processing has taken place, the thio is rinsed from the hair and neutralizer is applied. The neutralizer is an acid solution with a pH of 3 or 4. This solution stops the action of the thio and rehardens the hair by re-forming many of the S-bonds and some of the H-bonds. The rest of the H-bonds are re-formed during the drying of the hair. The S-bonds and H-bonds hold the polypeptide chains in their newly curled formation.

CAUTION

Caution must be exercised in the use of a thio solution. If it is permitted to remain in the hair too long, it could weaken and break the polypeptide chains by destroying the end bonds, thus causing hair breakage.

ACID AND NEUTRAL PERMANENT WAVING

In recent years, manufacturers have developed permanent wave solutions that are less damaging to the hair than thio. This type of permanent waving is developed from two solutions, one highly alkaline and the other very low in acidity, which must be mixed together immediately before use. When mixed, this combined solution has a pH factor that is slightly acid (4.5-6.5). The winding technique is the same as for the usual thio permanent wave.

Since this low pH causes no swelling of the hair, a new factor (heat) must be introduced to achieve penetration of the hair shaft. Heat is usually applied in one of two methods: 1) pre-heated clamps applied to each curl, or 2) a plastic cap fitted over the curls and the patron placed under a pre-heated hair dryer.

Advantages

1. No swelling of the hair shaft and less chance of over-processing.
2. Less hair damage.
3. Less chance of skin irritation.
4. No color removal from tinted hair.
5. Leaves hair feeling softer and more natural.

Disadvantages

1. Curls are not as tight.
2. Curls do not hold permanent as long as in the conventional thio permanent method.

PROTEIN FILLERS

Protein fillers are used to recondition over-porous or damaged hair before a permanent waving lotion is applied.

The filler is a jelly-like, colorless substance, made of a mixture of protein and keratin. Some fillers also contain lanolin and cholesterol, to protect the hair against the harshness of the permanent waving lotion.

The chemical properties of the filler are similar to those of the hair, so the filler is able to even out the hair's porosity along the entire hair shaft. This evening-out process takes place because the porous sections of the hair shaft absorb the filler more rapidly than do the less porous sections.

WET WAVING AND CURLING

A temporary hair set is produced by **physical changes** which occur within the hair cortex. Because of the nature of these physical changes, hair can be set as frequently as desired. This is the basis of finger waving, pin curling, roller curling, and all wet setting.

Water alone can be used because it has the ability to break down the hydrogen bonds in the cortex. These bonds, which occur between adjacent polypeptide chains, prevent them from moving. But, slippage of the chains must take place before a proper wave can be formed.

Stretching the part of each hair strand that is on the outside of the roller or curl must cause a temporary rearrangement of the chains. Water lubricates the chains so that they can move relative to one another. However, even though hydrogen bonds are broken, the total amount of movement is very small because the strong sulfur bonds are completely unaffected by the water and continue to restrict slippage of the polypeptide chains.

CHEMICAL HAIR RELAXING (STRAIGHTENING)

The procedure for chemical hair relaxing is very similar to the technique followed in permanent waving. However, since the objective to be attained is exactly the reverse of permanent waving, some of the techniques also must be reversed,

The cosmetologist starts with hair that is excessively curly, and her objective is to remove the curl permanently.

As in permanent waving, the process requires the breaking down of the S-bonds and the H-bonds in the cortex. The relaxing process, however, requires that the hair be held or directed in a straight position.

TWO TYPES OF CHEMICAL RELAXERS

The two types of chemical hair relaxers that are in general use by professional cosmetologists are thio (thioglycolate), pH 9.4-9.6, and sodium hydroxide, pH 10-14. The overall objective of both these products is exactly the same. Students must be cautioned, however, that sodium hydroxide is much stronger than thio, and, if not properly used, can cause great damage to the patron's hair. If left on the hair too long, it may change the color of the hair. If left on longer than 10 minutes, it may dissolve the hair.

Fixative. The neutralizer, or fixative, is used in an acid solution with a pH of 3-4.

Note: Before either of these products is used, it is extremely important to read the chapter on **Chemical Hair Relaxing and Chemical Blowout** for a detailed study of their application and the safety precautions required.

CHEMICAL HAIR STRAIGHTENING - SODIUM HYDROXIDE

1. CURLY HAIR	2. PROCESSING HAIR	3. HAIR BEING NEUTRALIZED	4. STRAIGHTENED HAIR . . .
Both H- and S-Bonds holding polypeptide chains in position.	All H-Bonds broken, most S-bonds broken. Hand and comb manipulations starting to relax wave. (Polypeptide chains shift.)	The neutralizer fixes polypeptide chains in a straight position after hair has been fully relaxed.	after rinsing and proper drying. LANTHIONINE cross links now exist between polypeptide chains, keeping the hair in a permanently straight form. Drying re-forms the physical bonds.

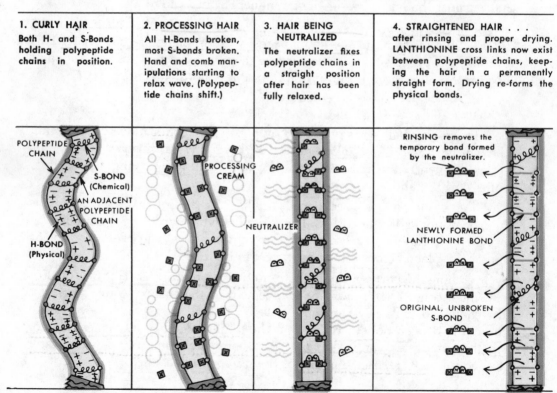

HAIR COLORING

This presentation is limited to a discussion of the chemical composition, actions, and reactions of the various types of hair colorings. (See chapter on **Hair Coloring** for information on techniques, application, and use of hair colorings.)

TEMPORARY HAIR TINTS

Temporary colorings for the hair come in various forms, such as color rinses, color sprays, and color shampoos. They come in a wide range of colors, and are easily applied. Temporary colors are washed out with the first shampoo. They are useful to a patron who is experimenting with new hair colors, or for a patron seeking a particular hair effect for a special occasion.

ACTION OF SIMPLE HAIR COLORINGS

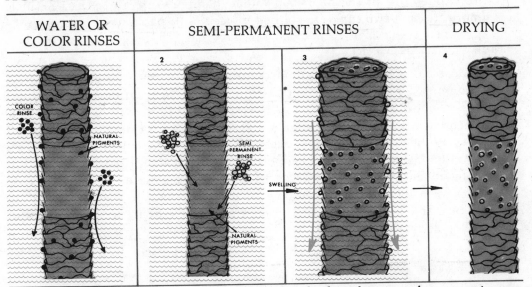

WATER OR COLOR RINSES	SEMI-PERMANENT RINSES		DRYING

Temporary colorings are harmless to the hair because they contain true stains, which are colors accepted by the government for use in foods, drugs, and cosmetics. They also are called **certified colors**. Temporary colorings are composed of large molecules that are acid in chemical composition and unable to penetrate into the cortical layer. They shrink the cuticle scales, closing the imbrications and preventing the entrance of the large color molecules into the cortex. The coloring substance can be trapped only behind the imbrications of the cuticle.

Temporary coloring is easily washed from the hair because the shampoo is alkaline and opens the imbrications. The rinsing action of the shampoo then easily washes out the coloring substance. Lightened hair is able to absorb more of the coloring substance because the lightener already has opened the cuticle, thus allowing more of the color to enter.

SEMI-PERMANENT TINTS

Semi-permanent colorings (tints) last from 4-6 weeks. They are aniline derivative tints, the same as permanent tints, but their molecules are larger than those of the permanent tints.

Semi-permanent tints offer patrons a number of benefits that are not found in other forms of hair coloring. Besides lasting from 4-6 shampoos, they have a very good range of colors. Semi-permanent tints are applied easily and do not require the use of hydrogen peroxide. They are effective in covering or blending partially grey hair without affecting the natural color. They also highlight and bring out the natural color of the hair.

Semi-permanent tints are alkaline in chemical composition and cause an alkaline reaction on the hair. The alkali swells the cuticle, opening the imbrications and permitting the color molecules to enter the cortex. However, since semi-permanent tints are only mildly alkaline, the swelling of the cuticle and the opening of the imbrications are limited, permitting only a small number of the large molecules to enter into the cortex.

A neutral or slightly acid rinse is used to close the imbrications and trap the colored molecules inside the cortex. Gradually, the semi-permanent tints are washed out of the hair by alkaline shampoos, which open the cuticle imbrications, permitting the colored molecules to pass out of the cortex.

PERMANENT HAIR TINTS

Most patrons prefer their hair coloring to last much longer than a few shampoos. Originally, hair tints were intended solely to hide greying hair. Today, patrons of all ages choose to color their hair simply to enhance their appearance. Permanent hair tints may be found in a number of different types: aniline derivative tints, vegetable tints, and metallic dyes.

Aniline derivative tints, or oxidizing tints, are the primary tints used in professional services. They offer a number of distinct advantages over all other forms of coloring. They give a permanent color to the hair, requiring no further coloring treatment, except for new growth. A wide range of aniline derivative colors has been developed to meet every patron's desires.

ACTION OF HAIR TINTS

TINT BASE PLUS DEVELOPER ON HAIR	1. TINT MIXTURE ENTERS INTO CORTEX	2. TINT PIGMENTS FORMED	3. SHRINKING OF CUTICLE SCALES TO TRAP PIGMENT

CONDITIONER

DRYING AND CONDITIONING

These tints are composed of very small, colorless molecules which experience no difficulty in passing through the cuticle imbrications and penetrating into the cortex. A developer, usually hydrogen peroxide, is added to the tint immediately before application. Once inside the cortex, the developer combines the small, colorless molecules into giant, colored molecules. These large molecules cannot be shampooed from the hair because they are too large to pass out through the imbrications. In addition, they form bonds with the keratin chains in the cortex, and thus become firmly affixed. These bonds are acid and, therefore, leave the H- and S-bonds free for other hair services.

VEGETABLE TINTS (HENNA)

Although vegetable henna has been used for hair coloring since the days of the early Egyptians, its use is very limited in the modern professional practice of hair coloring. The tint is formed by mixing henna powder with water and a mild acid to form a paste. This henna paste is applied to the hair, where it coats the shaft and some may penetrate into the cortex. It gives a reddish-orange color to hair which may vary in intensity with the quality of the powder used and the original color of the hair.

Although henna has very limited use as a hair coloring, it does have a number of important uses in the modern beauty salon. Several types of henna have been developed for a variety of uses.

1. **Brown henna**, made of old henna leaves, does not possess strong coloring properties and is used to provide a pale orange color. Its primary purpose is to give weak, warm highlights to light brown hair.

2. **Black henna** is used for its very good drabbing ability. This type of henna will turn light brown hair into a medium drab brown and medium brown brown hair into a dark ash brown. Black henna should never be used on light colored hair, blonde hair, and grey hair because it gives them a greenish color.

3. **Neutral henna** does not color the hair, but has wide popularity as a hair conditioner.

(See chapter on **Shampooing and Rinsing** for methods of application.)

METALLIC DYES

These dyes serve little purpose today. The metallic film on the hair cuticle, which gives the color, creates serious limitations. Some of the metallic salts enter the cortex and combine with the S-bonds. This interferes with permanent waving, hair relaxing, hair coloring, or hair lightening.

The metallic salts (lead, silver, copper) are very poisonous. They also cause a violent reaction with hydrogen peroxide on the hair.

Metallic dyes are not used professionally.

COMPOUND DYES

Compound dyes consist of a combination of vegetable dyes and metallic salts, to fix the color. These coloring agents are never used professionally, but are sometimes used at home. While they coat the hair shaft, some of the metallic salts may penetrate into the cuticle and combine with S-bonds. The action of compound dyes renders the hair unfit for permanent waving, tinting or lightening, and chemical hair straightening.

Color strippers are chemical agents that are designed to strip out color with the least risk of damage to the hair.

Tint (color) strippers are very strong oxidizing agents that reduce the giant color molecules in the cortex into small colorless particles. When these particles are small enough to pass through the imbrications of the cuticle, they may be easily rinsed from the hair.

Chemicals used in strippers may be inorganic sulfites or organic **reducing agents** with modifiers. Liquid 30 volume hydrogen peroxide, with excess ammonia to pH 10-12, also may be used as an effective color stripper.

HAIR LIGHTENING

Hair lightening is the process that decreases or removes the natural color pigments in the hair. Hair color pigments are: **melanin** (mel'a-nin)—black to brown shades; **oxymelanin**—red to yellow shades.

Hair lightening occurs in two ways: either through natural conditions or through artificial conditions.

Natural conditions—color may be removed from the hair by the sun's rays, chlorinated water, or other natural action.

Artificial conditions—this usually occurs through chemical means. Chemical hair lightening is a two-stage process: the first stage involves changing the melanin pigments into oxymelanin; the second stage, depending on the degree of lightening desired, involves the continued breaking down of the oxymelanin pigment until the desired effect is achieved.

REMOVING PIGMENTS

The chemical agent used for removing pigments from the hair shaft is a 6% (20 volume) solution of hydrogen peroxide.

The active ingredient of hydrogen peroxide is oxygen gas. To speed the liberation of oxygen gas, a small quantity of 28% ammonia water is added, which increases the pH to 10.

There are a number of commercial lighteners available to the cosmetologist. These products are:

1. **Oil lighteners**—mixtures of hydrogen peroxide and sulfonated oils.
2. **Cream lighteners**—containing conditioning agents, bluing, and thickener.
3. **Powder lighteners**—containing an oxygen releasing booster and inert substances.

The chemical action of all the commercial lighteners is basically the same as outlined above.

TONERS

Toners are permanent aniline derivative hair colorings. They consist primarily of pale, delicate colors requiring very careful application.

Since a toner is an aniline derivative tint, it must be handled exactly as other permanent aniline tints. The chemical actions are identical with those described for aniline derivative tints.

Toners are usually applied to lightened hair to add color and highlights.

COLOR FILLERS

Color fillers are used to equalize the porosity of abused or damaged hair. They also deposit a base color prior to a tinting service.

The color filler is a jelly-like substance, usually a mixture of protein, keratin, and certified color, which is applied directly to the cuticle.

Since the filler is composed of the same basic chemical properties as the hair itself, it evens out porosity along the entire hair shaft. Porosity is equalized because the porous sections of the hair shaft absorb the filler more rapidly than do the less porous areas.

The use of color fillers helps to make hair coloring services easier and more successful.

CHEMISTRY AS APPLIED TO COSMETICS

Cosmetic chemistry is both a science and an art. The **science** of chemistry consists of knowing what to do in the correct manner; **art** involves the proper methods of preparing and applying the cosmetic to the body.

Cosmetologists will be better equipped to serve the public if they have an understanding of the chemical composition, preparation, and use of cosmetics which are intended to cleanse and improve the hygiene of the external portions of the body.

Cosmetics may be classified according to their physical and chemical nature and the characteristics by which they are recognized. The object in classifyiing cosmetics is to assist in their study and identification.

PHYSICAL AND CHEMICAL CLASSIFICATIONS OF COSMETICS

1. Powders.　　　3. Suspensions.　　　5. Ointments.
2. Solutions.　　　4. Emulsions.　　　6. Soaps.

POWDERS

Powders are a uniform mixture of insoluble substances (inorganic, organic, and colloidal) that have been properly blended, perfumed, and/or tinted to produce a cosmetic that is free from coarse or gritty particles.

Mixing and sifting are used in the process of making powders.

SOLUTIONS

A **solution** (so-lu'shun) is a preparation made by dissolving a solid, liquid, or gaseous substance in another substance, usually liquid.

A **solute** (sol'ut) is a substance dissolved in a solution.

A **solvent** (sol'vent) is a liquid used to dissolve a substance.

Solutions are clear and permanent mixtures of solute and solvent which do not separate on standing. Since a good solution is clear and transparent, filtration is often necessary, particularly if the solution is cloudy.

Solutions are easily prepared by dissolving a powdered solute in a warm solvent and stirring at the same time. The solute may be separated from the solvent by applying heat and evaporating the solvent.

Water is a universal solvent. It is capable of dissolving more substances than any other solvent. Grain alcohol and glycerine are frequently used as solvents.

Water, glycerine, and alcohol readily mix with each other; therefore they are **miscible** (mis'i-b'l) (mixable). On the other hand, water and oil do not mix with each other; hence they are **immiscible** (unmixable).

The **solute** may be either a solid, liquid, or gas. For example: **boric acid solution** is a mixture of a solid in a liquid; **glycerine and rose water** is a mixture of two miscible liquids; **ammonia water** is a mixture of a gas in water.

Solutions containing **volatile** (vol'a-til) substances, such as ammonia and alcohol, should be stored in a cool place; otherwise the volatile substance will evaporate.

There are various kinds of solutions:

A **dilute** (di-lut') **solution** contains a small quantity of the solute in proportion to the quantity of solvent.

A **concentrated** (kon'sen-tra-ted) **solution** contains a large quantity of the solute in proportion to the quantity of solvent.

A **saturated** (sat'ur-a-ted) **solution** will not dissolve or take up more of the solute than it already holds at a given temperature.

SUSPENSIONS

Suspensions are temporary mixtures of insoluble powders in liquid. Since the particles have a tendency to separate on standing, a thorough shaking is required before using. A suspension should not be filtered. Some skin lotions are actually suspensions. (Example: calamine lotion.)

Suspensions are made by first mixing the powders, then adding a small amount of liquid to form a smooth paste, and finally adding the balance of the liquid.

EMULSIONS

Emulsions (e-mul'shunz) (creams) are permanent mixtures of two or more immiscible substances (oil and water) that are united with the aid of a binder (gum) or an emulsifier (soap). Emulsions are usually milky white in appearance. If a suitable emulsifier and the proper technique are used, the resultant emulsion will be stable. A stable emulsion can hold as much as 90% water. Depending on the amount of water and wax present, the cream may be either liquid or semi-solid in character. The amount of emulsifier used depends on its efficiency and the amount of water or oil to be emulsified.

Emulsions are prepared by hand or with the aid of a grinding and cutting machine, called a colloidal mill. In the process of preparing the emulsion, the emulsifier forms a protective film around the microscopic globules of either the oil or water. The smaller the globules, the thicker and more stable will be the emulsion.

Emulsions basically fall into two different classes: oil-in-water (O/W) and water-in-oil (W/O).

Oil-in-water (O/W) **emulsions** are made of oil droplets suspended in a water base. In addition to the emulsifier, which coats the oil droplets and holds them in suspension, there may be a number of additional ingredients present that are designed to cause certain reactions in the hair. (Examples: permanent wave solutions, lighteners (bleaches), neutralizers, and tints.)

Water-in-oil (W/O) **emulsions** are formed with drops of water suspended in an oil base. These are usually much thicker and oilier than the O/W emulsions. (Examples: hair grooming creams, cleansing creams, cold creams, and similar products.)

OINTMENTS

Ointments (oynt'ments) are semi-solid mixtures of organic substances (lard, petrolatum, wax) and a medicinal agent. No water is present. For the ointment to soften, its melting point should be below that of the body temperature (98.6° Fahrenheit [37° Celsius]).

Ointments are prepared by melting the organic substances and mixing the medicinal agent into the mixture.

Sticks are similar to ointments in that they are a mixture of organic substances (oils, waxes, petrolatum) that are poured into a mold to solidify. Sticks are a little harder than ointments. No water is present. Lipstick is an example of a cosmetic stick.

Pastes are soft, moist cosmetics, having a thick consistency. They are bound together with the aid of gum, starch, and water. If oils and fats are present, water is absent. The colloidal mill assists in the removal of grittiness from the paste.

Mucilages are thick liquids containing either natural gums (tragacanth or karaya) or synthetic gums, mixed with water. Since mucilages undergo decomposition, a preservative is required. Mucilages are used for hair setting lotions.

SOAPS

Soaps are compounds formed in a chemical reaction between alkaline substances (potassium or sodium hydroxide) and the fatty acids in oil or fat. Besides soap, glycerine also is formed. Potassium hydroxide produces a **soft soap**, whereas sodium hydroxide forms a **hard soap.** A mixture of the two alkalies will yield a soap of intermediate consistency.

A **good soap** does not contain an excess of free alkali and is made from pure oils and fats.

UNITED STATES PHARMACOPEIA (U.S.P.)

The cosmetologist should become familiar with the United States Pharmacopeia (U.S.P.), a book defining and standardizing drugs. The following are some of the terms of interest to cosmetologists:

Alcohol, also known as grain or ethyl alcohol, is a colorless liquid obtained by the fermentation of certain sugars. It is a powerful antiseptic and disinfectant; a 70% solution is used for sanitizing instruments, and a 60% solution can be applied to the skin. It is widely used in perfumes, lotions, and tonics.

Alum is an aluminum potassium or ammonium sulphate, supplied in the form of crystals or powder, which has a strong astringent taste and action.

It is used in skin tonics and lotions. It also is used in powder form as a styptic, which is applied to small cuts.

Ammonia water, as commercially used, is a colorless liquid with a pungent, penetrating odor. It is a by-product of the manufacture of coal gas. As it readily dissolves grease, it is used as a cleansing agent, and also is used with hydrogen peroxide in lightening hair. A 28% solution of ammonia gas dissolved in water is available commercially.

Bichloride of mercury is usually sold in tablet form of about 7½ grains each. It is shaped peculiarly for ready identification. It is a very strong poison and should be used very sparingly in beauty salons.

Boric acid, also called **boracic acid,** is a powder obtained from sodium borate, which is mined in the form of borax and crystallized with sulfuric acid. It is a mild healing and antiseptic agent. It is sometimes used as a dusting powder and, in solution, as a cleansing lotion or eyewash.

Formaldehyde is a gas, but in water solution containing from 37-40% of the gas by weight, it is known as **formalin.** Formaldehyde has a very disagreeable, pungent odor. It is very irritating to the eyes, nose, and mouth. Formalin may be used to sanitize instruments.

Glycerine is a sweet, colorless, odorless, syrupy liquid, formed by the decomposition of oils, fats, or molasses. It is an excellent skin softener, and is an ingredient of cuticle oil, facial creams, and lotions.

Phenol, or **carbolic acid,** is not actually an acid, but is a coal tar derivative, appearing as a crystalline substance having a slightly acid reaction. Glycerine is added to make it more readily soluble in water. A 5% solution of phenol is used to sanitize metallic instruments.

Potassium hydroxide (caustic potash) sticks are dissolved in distilled water to form an alkaline solution. When not in use, the sticks must be kept in sealed containers, as they tend to absorb moisture from the air and deteriorate. They are used in the making of soaps and cosmetic creams.

Quaternary ammonium compounds (quats) are a group of effective disinfectants used as sanitizing agents in beauty salons.

Sodium bicarbonate (baking soda) is a precipitate made by passing carbon dioxide gas through a solution of sodium carbonate. It is a white powder adapted for uses such as a neutralizing agent.

Sodium carbonate (washing soda) is prepared by heating sodium bicarbonate. It is used for water softening and in bath salts. Sodium carbonate also may be used with boiling water in the sterilization of metallic instruments. A small quantity is added to the water to keep the instruments bright.

Tincture of iodine is a 2% solution of iodine in alcohol. If the patron is not allergic to iodine, it can be used safely on the skin to treat minor cuts and bruises. Iodine stains are readily removed with alcohol. **Mercurochrome,** or a 3-5% peroxide solution, also may be used for cuts.

Witch hazel is a solution of alcohol and water containing an astringent agent extracted from witch hazel bark.

Zinc oxide is a heavy, white powder made by burning zinc carbonate with coal in a special furnace. It is used as a dusting powder and as an ointment for some skin conditions.

COSMETICS FOR BODY CLEANLINESS

The chemistry of cosmetics embraces the study of products designed to cleanse and beautify the skin, hair, and nails.

Cosmetics of this type are intended to cleanse the body by removing dirt, hair, or foreign odors from the skin. This classification includes soaps, bath accessories, deodorants, anti-perspirants, and depilatories.

KINDS OF SOAPS

Good toilet soaps should be made from purified fats that will not become rancid in the soap, and should not contain excessive free alkali. Soaps with a pH value above 9.5 tend to dry and roughen the skin. A pH value of about 8 is considered normal for the skin.

Kinds of Soaps

Soaps	Common Ingredients	Uses
Castile soap (pure)	Olive oil and soda.	Best for the skin — produces little lather.
Castile soap (other kinds)	Synthetic detergents, olive or other oils.	Used for normal skin.
Green soap	Made from potash and olive or linseed oil and glycerine.	A medicinal liquid soap, used for oily skin.
Tincture of green soap	Mixture of green soap in about 35% alcohol and a small amount of perfume.	Used for correcting oily skin and scalp. Very drying, if used on normal or dry skin over a period of time.
Medicated soap	Contains a small percent of cresol, phenol or other antiseptics.	Used for acne conditions.
Shaving soap	Contains alkalies, coconut oil, vegetable and animal fats and a small amount of gum.	Used for shaving. The alkalinity softens the hair. The thick lather keeps the hair erect.
Shaving soap in pressure can	Shaving soap and gas under pressure.	Used the same as shaving soap.
Carbolic soap	A disinfectant soap containing 10% phenol.	Used for oily skin and acne infection.
Transparent soap	Contains glycerine, alcohol and sugar which render it transparent.	Used for normal skin.
Super-fatted soap	Contains a fatty substance, such as lanolin or cocoa butter.	Recommended for dry or sensitive skin. Keeps the skin soft after washing. Not suitable for hard water.
Naphtha soap	Contains naphtha, obtained from petroleum.	Do not use on face or scalp. Use mainly for laundry purposes.
Hard water soap	Contains coconut oil, varying amounts of washing soda or borax, sodium silicate and a phosphate.	Use only on oily skin. The alkaline substances will dry the skin.

Bath accessories include soaps, bath salts, bath oils , bath powders, and body oils. Bath salts and oils are used during the bath, while bath powders and body oils are used after the bath.

Bath Accessories

Kind	Common Ingredients	Uses
Bath salts	Carbonates or phosphates of sodium, color and perfume.	Soften and perfume the bath water
Bath oils	Sulfonated oils (latherless) or sulfated fatty alcohols (produce lather), color and perfume.	Sulfonated oils are drying to the skin. If the body skin is dry, do not use them.
Bath dusting powders	Perfumed talc and other absorbent substances.	Impart a mild fragrance to the skin, and aid in drying body moisture.
Body oils	Vegetable and animal oils.	Replace natural oils removed by bathing.
Foam-bath salts	Sulfated compound related to coconut oil.	Drying to the skin.

DEODORANTS AND ANTI-PERSPIRANTS

Few preparations can be classified separately as deodorants or anti-perspirant products, since most combine the features of both. A deodorant is an agent that neutralizes or destroys disagreeable odors without suppressing the amount of perspiration. An anti-perspirant checks perspiration by its astringent action. The skin surrounding the pores swells, thereby temporarily closing the pores.

Deodorants and anti-perspirants are available in the form of creams, sticks, solutions, and powders.

Deodorants and Anti-Perspirants

Kind	Common Ingredients	Uses
Deodorant powders	Mixture of powder base, zinc compounds, boric acid, astringents, and antiseptics.	Destroy the odor of sweat without stopping perspiration.
Deodorant creams	Vanishing cream base, antiseptic and astringent.	Destroy the odor of sweat without stopping perspiration.
Deodorant solutions	Solution containing an antiseptic, an astringent, alcohol, glycerine and water.	Used to mask odor. The skin should be dry before ' wearing clothing. The acidity of the aluminum chloride will destroy clothing.
Deodorant sticks	Waxes and an astringent (zinc sulphocarbolate).	Easy to apply. Destroy odor without stopping perspiration.
Creams or liquids	Strong astringents, such as aluminum compounds.	Contract the sweat gland at the place of application. Prevent excessive sweating under the arms.

DEPILATORIES

Depilatories are preparations used for the temporary removal of superfluous hair in the armpits and on the legs. They consist of various alkali sulphides, calcium thioglycolate compounds, or resins and waxes. They are available in the form of a liquid, soft cream, paste, powder, or hard cake.

Chemical type. The chemical type of depilatory has the odor of spoiled eggs and is generally used over the legs and arms. It softens and dissolves the hair at the margin of the skin. To prevent irritation of the skin, use only as directed by manufacturer.

Wax type. The wax type of depilatory is odorless and is preferred for the face. After the melted wax hardens on the hairy surface, the patch is suddenly removed, and with it, the embedded hairs.

Before application, give a small patch test of the depilatory on the patron's skin. If skin redness or blisters do not develop, it is safe to use the depilatory over a larger skin surface.

(See chapter on **Removal of Superfluous Hair** for additional information.)

COSMETICS FOR SKIN AND FACE

Grouped under this heading are preparations designed to render the skin or face youthful and attractive in appearance. For this purpose, there are available creams, lotions, powders, makeup cosmetics, and miscellaneous products.

CREAMS

Of all cosmetics used for the skin or face, creams comprise the largest and most varied group. Basically, creams are either stable emulsions of oily and watery substances, or an ointment base without water. Creams do not actually feed the tissues, but they do lubricate the skin.

Creams

Kind	Common Ingredients	Uses
Cold cream	Beeswax, vegetable or mineral oil, borax (1%), water and perfume.	Suitable for cleansing dry or normal skin.
Liquefying cleansing cream	Mineral oil, petrolatum, mineral wax, perfume, small amount of water.	May be used on oily skin. Melts quickly, does not penetrate the skin. Long use will dry the skin.
Vanishing cream	75% water, stearic acid, combined with a small amount of an alkali. Cocoa butter, lanolin, glycerine and alcohol are also used.	Used before makeup is applied, and as a hand cream. Leaves a protective film on the skin. Skin may become very dry from its use.
Emollient cream (Also called tissue cream and lubricating cream)	Waxes, lanolin, vegetable fats and oils, fatty acids, alcohols and some mineral oil products.	Slightly penetrate and soften the skin. Used for the lubrication of the skin during massage.
Hormone cream	Emollient cream base containing sex hormones.	For women of middle age. Prevents dryness and age lines.
Moisturizing cream	Emollient cream base containing moisturizing agents.	For dryness in aging skin due to lack of moisture and natural oil.

Creams (continued)

Kind	Common Ingredients	Uses
Massage cream	Cold cream base, lanolin or casein (protein found in cheese).	For massage of normal or slightly dry skin.
Astringent cream	Mild ointment base containing zinc oxide and an astringent.	Recommended to correct excessive oiliness, and to close pores.
Acne cream	Boric acid, sulfur, zinc oxide, cade oil, camphor, benzoin and salicylic acids.	Helps clear the skin of simple acne and other minor lesions. Should be soft enough to spread easily without irritating the skin.
Foundation cream	Vanishing cream base is modified by increasing the glycerine content.	Applied to the face after cleansing, to provide a suitable base for makeup.
Eye cream and throat cream	Lanolin, vegetable oils, waxes and astringent substances.	Lubricate and soften fine lines. Make them less conspicuous.
Suntan cream	Contains a cream or ointment base and various color pigments.	Used to give the appearance of a darker skin color.

LOTIONS

Lotions are popular products used to a considerable extent in various kinds of hair and facial treatments. They are available as a clear solution or as a suspension, leaving an insoluble sediment at the bottom of the container.

Lotions

Kind	Common Ingredients	Uses
Aromatic water	Essential oil (oil of rose, geranium, lavender, etc.) dissolved in distilled water with the aid of talc.	Imparts a cooling and fragrant effect to skin tonics and lotions.
Cleansing lotions	Alcohol or a sulfonated compound.	For oily skin.
Astringent lotions	Zinc, alum, boric or salicylic acid, in solution of water, glycerine and alcohol.	For oily skin and large pores.
Skin freshener lotions	Witch hazel, camphor, boric acid, mild organic acids, perfume and coloring.	Slightly astringent solution for dry skin.
Acne lotions	Precipitated sulfur, glycerine, spirits of camphor and distilled water.	Used to sponge the skin where simple acne exists.
Witch hazel	A solution of alcohol and water containing the astringent from witch hazel bark.	Used as an astringent and cooling lotion.
Eye lotions	Boric acid, bicarbonate of soda, zinc sulfate and glycerine, witch hazel, or other herbs.	Used to soothe, cleanse, and brighten the eyes.

Lotions (continued)

Kind	Common Ingredients	Uses
Calamine lotion	Suspension of prepared calamine and zinc oxide in glycerine, bentonite and lime water.	Used as a soothing application to irritated surfaces of the skin and as a protective lotion.
✓ Hardy's lotion	Corrosive sublimate, alcohol, zinc sulfate, lead acetate and water.	Recommended by a physician to remove freckles. ✓
Medicated lotions	Antiseptics, sulfur compounds, or other medicinal agents.	Recommended by a physician for acne, or other skin eruptions.
Sunburn preventive lotion	Dilute solution of methyl salicylate in alcohol, glycerine and water.	Filters out most of the ultra-violet rays of the sun and produces a uniform tan.
✓ Sunburn remedial lotion	Dilute solution of astringent or cooling agent (camphor) in alcohol, glycerine and water.	Helps to heal a first degree burn. ✓

POWDERS

Powders are widely used, and constitute a profitable source of income. Since each kind of powder serves a particular purpose, the cosmetologist should be acquainted with the advantages of each powder used.

Face powder consists of a powder base, mixed with a coloring agent (pigment) and a suitable perfume. A good face powder for a normal skin should possess the following characteristics:

1. **Slip**—having a smooth feel to the skin. This quality is imparted by the talc or zinc stearate. The French or Italian talc, 200 mesh, is the best for face powders.
2. **Covering power**—having easy and even spread in order to cover skin shine, skin defects, and enlarged pores. Zinc oxide, kaolin, or titanium dioxide may be used.
3. **Adherency**—having the ability to remain on the skin. Zinc or magnesium stearate is used.
4. **Absorbency**—retaining the perfume, distributing the color, and absorbing perspiration and sebaceous secretions. Precipitated chalk and magnesium carbonate are used for this purpose.
5. **Bloom**—imparting a velvet-like appearance to the skin. Chalk is used for this purpose.
6. **Color and perfume**—having a fragrant odor and uniform shade.

Toilet powder is used after bathing and shaving to relieve irritated surfaces. Talcum is the most satisfactory base for a toilet powder, as it is not absorbent and is not affected by moisture.

Cream powder is composed of a vanishing cream base, to which is added a face powder. Cream powder combines both the face powder and the vanishing cream in one application.

Cake powder has 3% tragacanth mucilage mixed with a face powder. The tragacanth mucilage binds the substances together in a compact form.

Liquid powder may contain an oil, zinc oxide, stearates, talc, perfume, and coloring. It spreads quickly and uniformly over the skin, producing a non-drying, thin film, or foundation, over which facial cosmetics can be applied.

COSMETICS FOR MAKEUP

The selection and application of correct makeup are the primary requisites for improving the complexion and beautifying the facial features. The introduction of a personalized makeup service in beauty salons has increased the demand and sale of these cosmetics.

CHEEK COLOR (ROUGE)

Cheek color is available as a compact powder, paste, cream, and liquid.

Powder cheek color resembles the composition of a face powder, except that a suitable color is added and the entire mixture is moistened and molded with the aid of a binder. It is usually recommended for an oily skin.

Paste cheek color is composed of fats and waxes, having a red or brownish red color. It is recommended for a dry skin.

Liquid cheek color is composed of a dye dissolved in a solution of water, glycerine, alcohol, and wax.

Cream cheek color usually has a petrolatum base and contains lanolin, fats, and waxes. It is recommended for a dry skin.

The blood, as seen through the skin, reveals the natural coloring in the cheeks. The color of blood is bright red. Depending on the nature of the skin, it may acquire a bluish, purplish, or orange tone. The exact shade of cheek color should match the natural skin color tone.

LIP COLOR (LIPSTICK)

Lip color comes in stick, cream, and liquid form. Its three basic shades are blue-red, yellow-red, and true red.

Lip color contains high melting ingredients to which is added either an insoluble pigment (delible) or a soluble bromoacid dye (indelible).

The color of the inner mucous membrane of the lower lip is a guide to color selection.

EYE MAKEUP

Eyebrow pencil consists of a wax base with suitable coloring added. It comes in various shades and may be used to darken the brows and lashes.

Mascara is sometimes used to darken the brows and the lashes. It is available in the form of cake, cream, and liquid.

Cake mascara is a dehydrated cream into which color pigment is blended. A few drops of water is added to moisten the cake to a paste consistency when ready for use. The mascara is then applied with a brush.

Cream mascara contains a pigment in a vanishing cream base.

Liquid mascara usually consists of an alcoholic solution of resin colored with a dyestuff. It also is available as a suspension of pigment in a mucilage. A brush is used for direct application.

The following is a general guide to the selection of mascara:

Color of Eyes and Eyelashes	Shade of Mascara
Black eyelashes, with dark brown or black eyes	Black
Black eyelashes, with blue or grey eyes	Blue or black
Brown, golden, or reddish eyelashes, with brown eyes	Dark brown
Blonde, reddish, or light brown eyelashes, with green, grey, or hazel eyes	Brown or green

Indelible — that can't be blotted out; not erased by making of a mask or rubbing.

Eye shadow or eye color is usually a suspension of pigments in a fatty base. It is colored black, brown, blue, green, bronze, silver, or purple, and is carefully selected with regard to the color of the skin, hair, eyes, the time of day, and the occasion.

Eye shadow or eye color is used to emphasize the beauty of the eyes. It should be used sparingly and with good taste. The selected shade should blend with the tone of the natural shadow found between the inner corner of the eye and the root of the nose.

Color of Eyes	Eye Color or Eye Shadow
Dark brown or black	Green, violet, brown
Blue	Blue, grey, violet
Green	Green, grey, brown
Hazel	Green, grey, brown
Grey	Grey, green, blue
Tawny	Brown, green

MISCELLANEOUS COSMETICS

Grease paint is a mixture of fats, petrolatum and a coloring agent, and is used for theatrical purposes.

Cake or pancake makeup is available in a compressed or compact form. It contains a dehydrated cream into which a distinct color is blended. It is removed from the container with a moist applicator and then spread over the face. As the water evaporates, a thin film of cream and color adheres to the face.

Muscle oil is an oil in which either lecithin or cholesterol is dissolved. It is used around the eyes and over the throat. It lubricates and softens the outer layer of the epidermis.

Beauty clay is composed of substances (kaolin, bentonite, fuller's earth, or colloidal clay) to which is added honey, glycerine, zinc oxide, casein, oils, magnesium carbonate, starch, tragacanth gum powder, astringent, water, or milk, depending on the nature of the pack or mask.

A beauty clay, or pack, can exert a cleansing, softening, astringent, refreshing, or stimulating action on the skin.

SCALP LOTIONS AND OINTMENTS

Scalp lotions and ointments usually contain medicinal agents for the purpose of correcting a scalp condition and reconditioning the hair. The active ingredients of such preparations are irritants that stimulate the circulation of the scalp and hasten the shedding and renewal of epithelial tissue.

Scalp lotions contain such ingredients as lecithin, quinine, sulfur, salicylic acids, oils, resorcin, camphor, and capsicum. Resorcin and quinine, when used over a period of time, may discolor blonde hair.

Lotions for an oily scalp should contain a high percentage of alcohol and ingredients that possess astringent properties. On the other hand, lotions for a dry scalp should contain little or no alcohol or astringents. Instead, emulsified vegetable or animal oils should be the predominant ingredient.

Hair lotions or tonics are divided into groups according to the purpose for which they are used; some are used to regulate the activity of the oil glands of the scalp; others, to remove dandruff. They are found in liquid, oil, and cream form.

epithelial

For **dry scalp**, use olive oil, delicately perfumed.

For **oily scalp**, use sweet oil and alcohol.

Sulfur ointment contains precipitated sulfur in benzonated lard, and is used for skin and scalp disorders.

HAIR DRESSINGS

Hair dressings are used to impart a gloss or fragrance to the hair, and to keep unruly or curly hair in a fixed position.

Hair creams in both liquid and semi-solid form are used after a shampoo to give gloss to the hair. They may be applied to either wet or dry hair. Such creams consist of lanolin, oil emulsions, fatty acids, waxes, mild alkalies, and water. Hair creams generally are used on dry types of hair.

Other hair dressings that are used for oily types of hair and applied before the hair is set may contain resins, gums, starch, or other thickeners in water and alcohol. They hold the hair in place, leave a light film when dry, but give less gloss to the hair.

HAIR SPRAYS

Styling trends led to a demand for a quick-drying preparation that would impart sufficient rigidity to the hair to keep it in place, control loose ends, and not detract from hair's natural sheen.

A new type of hair spray was developed with the production of plastics, such as poly-vinyl-pyrrolidone (PVP). This hair spray gives a film with enough strength to control the hair, but with sufficient elasticity to allow combing without distorting the style. A product of this type can be used on wet hair as a setting lotion after the shampoo, thereby extending the duration of the style. The effect of this spray is better on weak, lightened, or over-processed hair.

REVIEW QUESTIONS

CHEMISTRY

1. Why is a basic knowledge of chemistry important to cosmetologists?
2. What is the chemical symbol of: a) water; b) hydrogen peroxide?
3. Name two methods for removing impurities from water.
4. What type of water is best for shampooing?
5. What two parts make up a shampoo molecule?
6. What is the purpose of: a) the tail of a shampoo molecule; b) the head?
7. What happens to the shampoo molecules during rinsing?
8. What part does the thio solution play in the permanent waving of hair?
9. What two types of chemical hair relaxers are in general use by professional cosmetologists?
10. What may happen to the hair if sodium hydroxide is left on the hair longer than 10 minutes?
11. Why do aniline derivative tints easily penetrate into the cortex?
12. What action takes place once the developer and tint are inside the cortex?
13. Why are aniline derivative tints permanent hair coloring?
14. What is: a) melanin; b) oxymelanin?
15. What is the difference between a solute and a solvent?

Chapter 32

SALON MANAGEMENT

CHAPTER LEARNING OBJECTIVES

The student successfully mastering this chapter will know:
1. *The many things to consider when opening a beauty salon.*
2. *Financial considerations involved in operating a beauty salon.*
3. *The importance of maintaining accurate business records.*
4. *The business laws to consider.*
5. *What constitutes good telephone usage and procedure.*
6. *Effective telephone techniques.*
7. *The principles and practices of good selling.*
8. *The basics of sales psychology.*
9. *The fundamental rules of first aid.*

Numerous management opportunities exist in the field of cosmetology. Many cosmetology school graduates want to advance themselves and become owners or managers of salons. However, only those who are adequately prepared to manage a business will be able to realize their ambitions.

The owner or manager of either a full service or special service salon must have the proper qualifications. In addition to formal training, working in different types of salons and dealing with a variety of patrons help to build valuable background and experience.

Going into your own business is a big responsibility and not a step to be taken without serious planning. A knowledge of business principles, bookkeeping, business laws, insurance, salesmanship, and psychology is crucial to the cosmetologist who aspires to be an owner and/or manager of a salon. In this chapter, you will learn about some of the advantages and disadvantages you will face in business management.

WHAT YOU SHOULD KNOW ABOUT OPENING A SALON

When planning to open a salon, give careful consideration to every aspect of running a business. The following topics will acquaint you with some of the things you must consider before going into business:

LOCATION

A good location has a population large enough to support the salon. When possible, the salon should be located near other active business places, such as restaurants, department stores, or supermarkets, which attract potential patrons. Unless you can afford to do a great deal of advertising, it is difficult to operate a successful salon in a low traffic area. Also, people are drawn to shopping areas where they can make one stop serve several purposes.

BE VISIBLE

The salon should be clearly visible and "eye catching" to attract the attention of people walking or driving by.

AVOID COMPETITION

Avoid too much competition in the immediate area. It is better to locate in an area where yours is the only salon.

STUDY THE AREA

Study the area for potential patrons. Find out about the size, income, and buying habits of the area's population. Talk to other business owners to see how well they think a salon would do in the area.

STUDY LEASE

Before signing a lease, be sure you understand all provisions that pertain to the landlord and to the tenant. The lease should provide for alterations that must be made by the landlord. Before signing a lease, have a lawyer help with your negotiations.

PARKING FACILITIES

When selecting a site for a new business, or when planning to take over an established business, you must consider parking facilities. People hesitate to patronize a business that is inconvenient to reach during bad weather. If possible, locate the salon near a bus line. This will attract patrons who do not drive. If your salon is open for evening service, the area should be well lighted.

WRITTEN AGREEMENTS

Written agreements for alterations will prevent disputes over who must pay for what.

PLANNING THE PHYSICAL LAYOUT

The layout of a salon takes a considerable amount of planning in order to achieve maximum efficiency and economy.

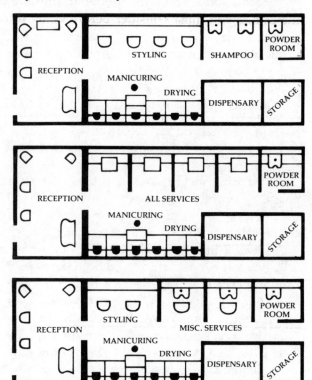

"OPEN" STYLE OF OPERATION
The plan opposite shows a 4-operator salon, with four styling stations. Shampooing, hair drying, and manicuring are done in separate sections.

"CLOSED" STYLE OF OPERATION
Four semi-private booths take care of all services, including hair coloring. Drying and manicuring are performed in a separate area.

"COMBINATION" (OPEN AND CLOSED) STYLE OF OPERATION
Two open stations are utilized for styling, while two closed booths may be used for other services. Drying and manicuring are performed in a separate area.

WHAT THE SALON SHOULD HAVE

1. Maximum efficiency of operation.
2. Adequate aisle space.
3. Flow of operational services toward the reception room.
4. Enough space for each piece of equipment.
5. Furniture, fixtures, and equipment chosen on the basis of cost, durability, utility, and appearance. The purchase of standard and guaranteed equipment is a worthwhile investment.
6. A color scheme that is restful and flattering.
7. A dispensary.
8. Adequate storage space.
9. A clean restroom containing toilet and basin.
10. Good plumbing and sufficient lighting for satisfactory services.
11. Good ventilation, air conditioning, and heating.

THE RECEPTION AREA

The reception area should not be overlooked when you plan the layout of your salon. This is the first contact a patron has with your establishment, and it sets the tone for the rest of the salon. An attractively decorated reception area can be one of your best promotional tools, since it immediately makes a patron comfortable. It gives the impression that this is a salon that cares about the comfort of its patrons. It also can attract the attention of people who pass by, and they may become patrons of your salon.

REGULATIONS, BUSINESS LAWS, AND INSURANCE

In conducting a business and employing help, it is necessary to comply with local, state, and federal regulations and laws.

Local regulations usually cover building renovations (local building code).

Federal law covers social security, unemployment compensation or insurance, and cosmetics and luxury tax payments.

State laws cover sales taxes, licenses, and workmen's compensation.

Income tax laws are covered by both the state and federal governments.

Insurance covers malpractice, premises liability, fire, burglary and theft, and business interruption.

ADVERTISING

Advertising includes all activities that attract attention to the salon and create a favorable impression on the public. The personality and ability of the manager and staff, the quality of work performed, and the attractiveness of the salon are all natural advertising assets.

A **pleased patron** is the best form of advertising.

Advertising must attract and hold the reader's, listener's, or viewer's attention and create a desire for the beauty service or merchandise.

1. Plan an advertising budget (about 3% of the gross income).
2. Use newspaper advertising as the first medium.
3. Use direct mail to create a more intimate contact with the reader.
4. Classified advertising in the yellow pages of your telephone book is comparatively inexpensive.
5. Radio advertising is more expensive, but is very effective.
6. TV is a dramatic, but expensive medium of advertising.
7. A window display acts as a salesman to every passerby.
8. Personal public appearances are excellent advertising, especially at women's and men's clubs, church functions, political gatherings, charitable affairs, and TV talk shows.

BUSINESS OPERATION AND PERSONNEL MANAGEMENT

Business problems are numerous, especially when you start a new salon. Contributing causes to salon failures are:

1. Inexperience in dealing with the public and with employees.
2. Not enough capital to carry the business through until established.
3. Poor location, and too high overhead expenses.
4. Lack of proper basic training in the field.
5. Business neglect and careless bookkeeping methods.

The owner or manager must have business sense, knowledge, ability, good judgment, and diplomacy. Smooth salon management depends on:

1. Sufficient investment capital.
2. Efficiency of management.
3. Cooperation between management and employees.
4. Good business procedures.
5. Trained and experienced personnel in the salon.

CREATE GOODWILL

Favorable impressions are made when the cosmetologist knows her work and merchandise, and is able to talk in clear and vivid language. The keynote to patron goodwill is satisfactory service. Efficient service will create goodwill, confidence, and satisfaction. Favorable impressions start with the courteous reception of the patron, and continue for as long as the patron obtains the desired results from repeated services.

BE A LEADER OF BEAUTY FASHION

There is no surer way of introducing your services than by using them yourself. You can be your own best advertisement of the services you perform. In addition, by looking attractive, you can motivate your patrons to do the same.

ALLOCATION OF MONEY

As part of your business operation, you must always know where your money is being spent. It is a good idea to apportion your money so that maximum benefit is derived from it.

Note: The following figures may vary in different localities. In large towns and cities items such as rent may run higher, while in small towns rent may be lower and utilities and telephone higher. The figures are suggested merely as a general guide.

AVERAGE EXPENSES FOR SALONS IN THE UNITED STATES
(Based on total gross income)

	Percent
Salaries and commissions (including payroll taxes)	53.5
Rent	13
Supplies	5
Advertising	3
Depreciation	3
Laundry	1
Cleaning	1
Light and power	1
Repairs	1.5
Insurance	.75
Telephone	.75
Miscellaneous	1.5
Total expenses	85
Net profit	15
	100%

You will note that the largest items of expense are salaries, rent, supplies, and advertising. The first three merit your closest attention. The advertising item can be adjusted at your discretion.

When opening a salon, it is important to have enough working capital. It often takes time for a new business to build a clientele, so money must be available to take care of necessary expenses. As overhead is met and profits become greater, the budget may be increased to cover more advertising and to expand in other areas.

BOOKING APPOINTMENTS

Booking appointments must be done with care, because the efficient scheduling of appointments can make the difference between success and failure. Services are sold in terms of time on the appointment page. Depending on how it is used, time may spell either a gain or a loss.

The size of the salon determines who books the appointments. This may be done by a full time receptionist, the owner or manager, or any of the cosmetologists working in the salon.

A receptionist with a pleasing voice and personality is a valuable asset to the beauty salon. In addition, she must have:

1. An attractive appearance.
2. Knowledge of the various beauty services and how much time they require.
3. Unlimited patience with both patrons and salon personnel.

GOOD BUSINESS ADMINISTRATION

Good business administration requires the keeping of a simple and efficient record system. Records are of value only if they are correct, concise, and complete. Bookkeeping means keeping an accurate record of all income and expenses. Income is usually classified as receipts from services and retail sales. Expenses include rent, utilities, insurance, salaries, advertising, equipment, and repairs. The assistance of an accountant is recommended to help keep records accurate. Retain check stubs, cancelled checks, receipts, and invoices.

Proper business records are necessary to meet the requirements of local, state, and federal laws regarding taxes and employees.

All business transactions must be recorded in order to maintain proper records. These are required by the owner, or manager, for the following reasons:

1. For efficient operation of the salon.
2. For determining income, expenses, profit or loss.
3. For proving the value of the salon to prospective buyers.
4. For arranging a bank loan.
5. For such reports as income tax, social security, unemployment and disability insurance, wage and hour law, accident, compensation, and labor tax.

DAILY RECORDS IMPORTANT

Keeping daily records enables the owner, or manager, to know just how the business is progressing. A weekly or monthly summary helps to:

1. Make comparisons with other years.
2. Detect any changes in demands for different services.
3. Order necessary supplies.
4. Check on the use of materials according to the type of service rendered.
5. Control expenses and waste.

Each expense item affects the total gross income. Accurate records show the cost of operation in relation to income.

Keep daily sales slips, appointment book, and a petty cash book for at least six months. Payroll book, cancelled checks, monthly and yearly records are usually held for at least seven years. Service and inventory records also are important to keep. Sales records help to maintain a perpetual inventory which can be used to:

1. Prevent overstocking.
2. Prevent running short of supplies needed for services.
3. Help in establishing the net worth of the business at the end of the year.

KEEP SERVICE RECORDS

A service record should be kept of treatments given and merchandise sold to each patron. Such information is the basis for suggested services that result in increased sales. For this purpose, use a card file system or memorandum book.

All service records should contain the name and address of the patron, date, amount charged, product used, and results obtained. Also, note the patron's preferences and taste.

Keep a running inventory of all supplies. Classify them as to their use and retail value. Those to be used in the business are **consumption** supplies. Those to be sold are **retail** supplies.

Inventory records indicate which merchandise is most popular, and prevent running short of any item. When reordering, buy enough merchandise that can be used or sold within a reasonable period of time. It is better to have a slight excess rather than a deficiency of supplies.

APPOINTMENT RECORD

The use of a private appointment record helps the cosmetologist arrange working time to suit the patron's convenience. The appointment book accurately reflects what is taking place in the salon at a given time. The cosmetologist who makes advance preparation can render prompt and efficient service when the patron arrives. Besides, waste in time and money is prevented.

BUSINESS LAW FOR THE SALON

A salon may be owned and operated by an **individual,** a **partnership,** or a **corporation.** Before deciding which type of ownership is most desirable, you should be acquainted with the relative merits of each.

INDIVIDUAL OWNERSHIP

1. The proprietor is owner and manager.
2. The proprietor determines policies and makes decisions.
3. The proprietor receives all profits and bears all losses.

PARTNERSHIP

1. More capital is available for investment.
2. The combined ability and experience of each partner make it easier to share work and responsibilities, and to make decisions.
3. Profits are equally shared.
4. Each partner assumes each other's unlimited liability for debts.

CORPORATION

1. A charter is obtained from the state.
2. A corporation is subject to taxation and regulation by the state.
3. The management is in the hands of a board of directors who determine policies and makes decisions in accordance with the corporation's charter.
4. The dividing of profits is proportionate to the number of shares owned by each stockholder.
5. The stockholder is not personally responsible for losses.

BEFORE BUYING OR SELLING AN ESTABLISHED SALON

1. A written purchase and sale agreement should be formulated in order to avoid any misunderstandings between the contracting parties.
2. The buyer and seller should make and sign a complete statement of inventory (goods, fixtures, etc.) indicating the value of each article.
3. If there is a transfer of chattel mortgage, notes, lease, and bill of sale, an investigation should be made to determine if there is any default in the payment of debts.
4. Consult your lawyer for additional guidance.

AGREEMENT TO BUY SALON

An agreement to buy an established salon should include the following:
1. Correct identity of owner.
2. True representations concerning the value of the salon and inducements offered to buy.
3. Use of salon's name and reputation for a definite period of time.
4. An understanding that the seller will not compete with the prospective owner within a reasonable distance from present location.

PROTECTION IN MAKING A LEASE

1. Secure exemption of fixtures or appliances that may be attached to the store or loft, so that they can be removed without violating the lease.
2. Insert into the lease an agreement relative to necessary renovations and repairs, such as painting, plumbing, fixtures, and electrical installation.
3. Secure an option from the landlord to assign the lease to another person; in this way, the obligations for the payment of rent are kept separate from the responsibilities of operating the business.

PROTECTION AGAINST FIRE, THEFT, AND LAWSUITS

1. Employ honest and able employees, and keep premises securely locked.
2. Follow safety precautions to prevent fire, injury, and lawsuits. Liability, fire, malpractice, and burglary insurance should be obtained.
3. Do not violate the medical practice law of your state by attempting to diagnose, treat, or cure a disease.
4. Become thoroughly familiar with all laws governing cosmetology and with the sanitary codes of your city and state.
5. Keep accurate records of number of workers, salaries, lengths of employment, and social security numbers, required by various state and federal laws that affect the social welfare of employees.

Note: Ignorance of the law is no excuse for its violation.

SUMMARY

Important things to consider when going into business:

CAPITAL: Amount available, amount required.

ORGANIZATION: Individual, partnership, corporation.

BANKING: Opening a bank account, deposits, drawing checks, monthly statements, notes and drafts.

SELECTING LOCATION: Population, transportation facilities, transients, trade possibilities, space required, zoning ordinances, parking.

DECORATING AND FLOOR PLAN: Selection of furniture, floor covering, installing telephone, electric signs, exterior decorating, window displays, interior decorating.

EQUIPMENT AND SUPPLIES: Selecting equipment, comparative values, installation, labor-saving steps.

ADVERTISING: Planning, direct mail, local house organs, newspaper, radio, television, classified yellow pages.

LEGAL: Lease, contracts, claims, lawsuits.

BOOKKEEPING SYSTEM: Installation, record of appointments, receipts, disbursements, petty cash, profit and loss, inventory.

COST OF OPERATION: Supplies, depreciation, rent, light, salaries, telephone, linen service, sundries, taxes.

MANAGEMENT: Methods of building goodwill, analysis of materials and labor in relation to service charges, greeting patrons, adjusting complaints, handling employees, selling merchandise, telephone techniques.

OFFICE ADMINISTRATION: Stationery, office supplies, inventory.

INSURANCE: Public liability and malpractice, compensation, unemployment, social security, fire, theft and burglary, business interruption.

METHODS OF PAYMENT: In advance, C.O.D., open account, time payments.

COMPLIANCE WITH LABOR LAWS: Minimum wage law, hours of employment, minors.

ETHICS: Courtesy, observation of professional trade practices.

COMPLIANCE WITH STATE COSMETOLOGY LAW governing salon physical layout and equipment.

LICENSING of salons, salon managers, and cosmetologists.

CAUTION:

Do not have business transactions with a total stranger, and never give cash to a stranger. Never make out a check to an individual who is working for a firm; make check payable to the firm.

THE USE OF THE TELEPHONE IN THE SALON

An important part of the salon business is handled over the telephone. Good telephone habits and techniques make it possible for the salon owner and cosmetologist to increase business and win friends. With each call, you have a chance to build up the salon's reputation by rendering high caliber service.

The telephone serves many useful purposes in the salon, such as, to:
1. Make or change appointments.
2. Go after new business, or strayed or infrequent patrons.
3. Remind patrons of needed services.
4. Answer questions and render friendly service.
5. Adjust complaints and satisfy patrons.
6. Receive messages.
7. Order equipment and supplies.

Your success in using the phone depends to a large extent on your observation of certain fundamental principles. To the extent that these requirements are fulfilled, the telephone can be a very helpful aid to the success of the salon.

Business in the salon can be promoted effectively over the phone, provided there is:
1. Good planning.
2. Good telephone usage.

GOOD PLANNING

Good planning consists mainly of assigning the right person and giving him/her the necessary information with which to do a good telephone job.

An understanding and capable person should be put in charge of telephone calls. He/she should be thoroughly familiar with the prices charged for the various beauty services, and be able to recommend appropriate services to fit the needs of the patron. A reliable substitute should be trained to handle the salon's calls when the regular person is absent.

Next in importance is locating the phone in a convenient and quiet place. A comfortable seat should be provided. Near the phone there should be readily accessible an appointment book, patron's record cards, pencil or ball-point pen, and paper pad. To save time, there should be available an up-to-date list of telephone numbers commonly used and a recent telephone directory.

Good business practice requires that the salon's telephone number be freely and prominently displayed on stationery, advertising circulars, newspaper ads, and appointment cards. Business cards should be readily available on the receptionist's desk and in the reception area. They save patrons the trouble of looking up the salon's phone number, making it easier for them to call your salon.

GOOD TELEPHONE USAGE

Good telephone usage can best be described as the golden rule of dealing with others as you would have them deal with you. The motto should be "Phone as you would like to be phoned to." When put into daily practice, it really means saying or doing the right thing at the right time, and in the right manner. Good telephone usage requires the application of a few basic principles which add up to common sense and common courtesy.

YOUR GREETINGS

The first thing the caller wants to know is the name of the speaker and the salon he/she represents. The proper way to answer the telephone is to say, "Good morning (afternoon or evening), (your name) speaking. This is (name of your salon)." Following this brief introduction, you may say, "May I help you?"

The first few words you say over the phone immediately register your personality and give prestige to the salon. That is why it is so important to greet every caller with a cordial welcome. It shows that you are pleased to receive the call and want to be of service.

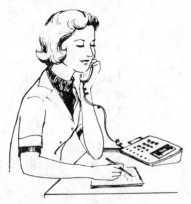

Example: "Good morning. This is Mary Dore from the East Park Beauty Salon. May I help you?"

BASIC RULES

The person answering the salon telephone should follow these four basic rules for good telephone usage:

1. Display an interested, helpful attitude, as revealed by the tone of your voice and what you have to say.
2. Be prompt. Answer all calls as quickly as possible. Nothing irritates the caller more than waiting for you to answer.
3. Practice giving all necessary information to the caller. This means identifying yourself and your salon when making or receiving a call. If the requested information is not readily available, be courteous enough to say, "Will you please hold the line while I get the information for you?" Then put the caller on "hold."
4. Be tactful. Avoid saying or doing anything that may offend or irritate the caller. The tactful telephone user is careful to:
   a) Inquire who is calling by saying, "May I tell Mr. Smith who is calling, please?" or "May I have your name, please?" Refrain from using such blunt questions as "Who's calling?"
   b) Address people by their last names. Make use of such expressions as "Thank you," "I'm sorry," or "Excuse me."
   c) Avoid making side remarks during a call.
   d) Let the caller end the conversation. Do not bang down the receiver at the end of a call.

YOUR VOICE AND SPEECH

Every time you telephone someone, you make a definite impression— good, bad, or indifferent. Your voice, what you say, and how you say it are what reveal you to others. If you want a good telephone personality, then be sure to acquire the habit of:

1. Clear speech.　　2. Correct speech.　　3. Pleasing tone of voice.

In this way, the other person hearing your voice will readily understand what you are saying.

As a general rule, the most effective speech is that which is correct and at the same time natural. A cheerful, alert, and enthusiastic voice most often comes from a person who has these desirable qualities as part of his/her personality.

To make a good impression over the phone, relax and draw a deep breath before answering the phone. Open your mouth, pronounce the words distinctly, use a low-pitched natural voice, and speak at a moderate pace. Clear voices carry better than loud voices over the phone.

If your listeners sometimes break in with such remarks as "What was that?" or "I'm sorry, I didn't get that," it may mean that your voice is not doing its job well. In that event, you should try to find out what is wrong and correct it. The more common causes of this condition may be:

1. You are speaking too loudly or too softly.
2. Your lips are too close or too far away from the mouthpiece. They should be about the width of two fingers from the mouthpiece.
3. The pitch of your voice is too low or too high.
4. Your pronunciation is not precise.

PLANNING YOUR TELEPHONE CONVERSATION

Whether it be a friendly chat or a business conversation, list the main points on your pad so you will know what to say. In this way, you will project an image of someone who knows how to handle all types of situations in an efficient manner. The salon will benefit from this image as patrons will obtain a favorable impression of the people who are employed there.

If you are having a lengthy conversation with the patron, take notes of the main points of the conversation. When you answer, you will be able to address yourself to the points in which the patron expressed interest.

EFFECTIVE TELEPHONE TECHNIQUES

Regular observance of the simple requirements of good telephone practice will help you make friends, bring in more business, and create goodwill for the salon.

To acquire skill in handling different situations and patrons, you should study and practice the following effective telephone techniques:

1. Booking appointments by phone.
2. Adjusting complaints over the phone.
3. Answering price objections over the phone.

BOOKING APPOINTMENTS BY PHONE

Whoever is assigned to handle salon appointments has an important responsibility. For this task, special qualifications and experience are required, such as:

1. Being familiar with all types of services and products available in the salon, and the prices to be charged.
2. Being familiar with the quality of work done by each cosmetologist.

3. Using judgment in giving assignments and being fair.
4. Being accurate in recording name, service, and time when making appointments.
5. Spacing appointments uniformly to permit the efficient functioning of the salon.

HOW TO HANDLE A PROSPECTIVE PATRON

The proper way to handle a prospective patron is illustrated in the following telephone conversation:

Receptionist (R): "Good afternoon. Miss Jones of the Milady Beauty Salon speaking. May I help you?"

Patron (P): "I am Mrs. Brown and would like to have a permanent."

R: "At what time, please?"

P: "Two o'clock on Wednesday."

R: "I am sorry, Mrs. Brown. That time is already taken. We have a 4 o'clock opening. Would that time meet with your convenience?"

P: "Yes, that's fine. But, I want that blond young girl."

R: "Do you mean Miss Paul? She has no openings for Wednesday. But we have Miss Dell, a very capable hairstylist, who can take care of you at 4 o'clock."

P: "I would really prefer Miss Paul."

R: "I am sorry that we cannot accommodate you this time. Could you take another time instead? Perhaps, at your next appointment, if made early enough, we can arrange to have Miss Paul serve you."

P: "All right, then. I will be in at 4 o'clock on Wednesday."

R: "Very well, Mrs. Brown. Thank you. Good-bye."

HOW TO HANDLE A REGULAR PATRON

How to arrange a convenient appointment for the patron is illustrated by the following telephone conversation:

Patron (P): "This is Mrs. West. Can Stella give me a shampoo and set any time on Friday? I'd rather come in the afternoon."

Receptionist (R): "Just a moment, Mrs. West, I'll check. Stella is booked both Friday and Saturday. How about tomorrow?"

P: "Tomorrow is rather inconvenient for me."

R: "Then I would suggest an appointment with Mary on Friday afternoon. Mary is new with us, but she does very good work, and I'm sure you will be satisfied. Stella could take care of you tomorrow at one, or Mary on Friday, at three."

P: "I do like to have Stella do my hair, but I simply can't come in then. I don't know what to do."

R: "If any appointments are cancelled, I'll be glad to call you, Mrs. West. I have your number—536-4327. But in case there isn't a cancellation, should I give you the appointment on Friday at three with Mary? Stella could show Mary how to style your hair."

P: "All right, I'll try Mary."

R: "Friday at three, then, unless I call. Thank you, Mrs. West. Good-bye."

Some beauty salons resent complaints; they take it as a personal affront. Such an attitude only makes matters worse and frequently results in a loss of business. Instead, the patron's complaint should be given **careful consideration**. It affords an opportunity to improve service and retain the patron's goodwill.

Adjusting complaints, particularly over the phone, is a difficult task. Since the complainant is probably upset and short-tempered, try to use **self-control, tact,** and **courtesy**, no matter how trying the circumstances may be. Only in this way will the complainant be made to feel that she has been fairly treated.

Remember that the tone of your voice must be sympathetic and reassuring. Your manner of speaking and the words you use should make the caller believe that you are really concerned about the complaint. Get the patron to tell you the whole story. **Avoid interrupting.**

After hearing the complaint in full, your next move is to adjust it quickly and effectively. Any of the following techniques will accomplish good results:

1. Tell the unhappy patron that you are sorry for what happened and explain the reason for the difficulty. Inform her that it will not happen again.

2. Sympathize with the patron by telling her you understand how she feels and regret the inconvenience suffered. Express thanks for calling this matter to your attention.

3. Ask the caller how the beauty salon can remedy the complaint. If the request is fair and reasonable, agree and comply with it.

4. If the patron is dissatisfied with the results of the beauty service, try to correct the complaint to her satisfaction. Pacify the patron by arranging for a corrective service free of charge.

How to adjust a complaint over the phone is illustrated by the following conversation:

R: "Good morning, Miss Jones of the Milady Beauty Salon speaking."

P: "May I speak to Mr. Charles?"

R: "I'm sorry, but he can't come to the phone now. May I help you?"

P: "Well . . . This is Mrs. Bell and I wanted to talk to Mr. Charles because I'm not satisfied with my permanent."

R: "I'm sorry to hear that, Mrs. Bell. I'm sure Mr. Charles would want to talk with you himself. Would it be convenient for you to come to the salon so that he can see your hair? If you could do that sometime within the next few days, I'll be glad to make an appointment for a consultation."

P: "I'm going to be near the shop tomorrow morning. Would 11 o'clock be all right?"

R: Yes, or it would be even better if you could see him a few minutes before 11:00. Shall I tell him to expect you then?

P: "Yes, thank you."

R: "Thank you, Mrs. Bell. I'm so glad you called."

ANSWERING PRICE OBJECTIONS

A patron may phone in to ask for the price of a permanent wave. After being told what the cost is, the patron says, "I can get the same permanent wave around the corner for less." How will you answer this objection?

The best way to overcome such an objection is to build up more value in the patron's mind. You can appeal to her better judgment by presenting logical reasons. Try to show her how she will profit from the greater value and better service offered by your beauty salon.

In the telephone conversation, first get the patron to agree with you. You might say in a calm, assuring voice, "I quite agree, Mrs. Brown, but you can also get a pair of shoes for less. Yet, you prefer to pay more and get only the best for your feet. Why, Mrs. Brown? Because you know that although shoes may look the same, there may be a vast difference in the quality of the leather, the skill of the shoemaker, and the fit of the shoes. In the long run, the higher-priced shoe will give you better wear, and, therefore, cost less.

"By the same token, our permanent wave costs more because we use only the highest quality materials for your hair, and take great care to produce a natural-looking permanent. You can rest assured that the reason we charge more is to enable us to provide you with better service and a higher quality permanent."

REMINDERS FOR PROPER TELEPHONE USAGE

1. Be prompt. When the telephone rings, answer it immediately, after the first ring, if possible.

2. Be prepared. Know in advance what you intend to say. Be able to provide accurate information to any inquirer. Always keep a pencil, ball point pen and pad handy for messages.

3. Identify both yourself and your salon for every incoming and outgoing call.

4. Speak clearly into the phone. Don't mumble or shout. Use good English and avoid slang.

5. Be tactful and courteous when speaking over the phone. Refer to the caller by last name. Try to leave a good impression on your listener.

6. Be interested in and helpful to the people who call the beauty salon.

7. Avoid arguments and interruptions while on the phone.

SELLING IN THE BEAUTY SALON

Selling is becoming an increasingly important responsibility of the cosmetologist as salons add wig and boutique departments to their beauty culture operations. The cosmetologist who is equally proficient as both a hairstylist and a salesperson is most likely to be the one to succeed in business.

No attempt is made here to cover all aspects of selling, but if students use this material as a basis upon which to build, they will find that effective selling techniques will become part of their repertoire of skills.

Successful salesmanship requires ambition and determination. Effective salesmanship is a necessity in any business.

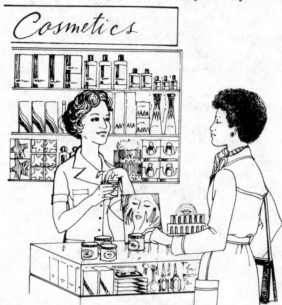

The first step in selling is to "Sell Yourself." Patrons must like and trust the cosmetologist in order for them to buy beauty services, cosmetics, wigs, or other merchandise.

Every patron who enters a salon is a prospective purchaser of additional services or merchandise. The manner in which you greet her lays the foundation for suggestive selling. Greet her with a smile and say, "May I help you?" Be ready and eager to serve her. Recognizing the needs and preferences of patrons makes the intelligent use of suggestive selling possible.

SELLING PRINCIPLES

The cosmetologist who is to become a proficient salesperson must understand, and be able to apply, the following principles of selling:

1. Be familiar with the merits and benefits of each service and product.
2. Adapt the approach and selling method to the needs and psychology of each patron.
3. Be self-confident. It is essential to make selling agreeable and productive.
4. Stimulate attention, interest, and desire, which are the steps leading up to a sale.
5. Never misrepresent your service or product.
6. Use tact in handling a patron. Avoid being rude or offensive.
7. Understand human nature so that you can apply appropriate sales technique.
8. Don't be negative.
9. To sell a product or service, deliver a sales talk in a relaxed, friendly manner and, if possible, demonstrate its use.
10. Recognize the right psychological moment to close any sale.

TYPES OF PATRONS AND WAYS OF HANDLING THEM

The cosmetologist who is most likely to be successful in selling additional services or merchandise to patrons is the one who can recognize the many different types of people and knows how to handle each type.

The following material describes seven of the most common types you are likely to deal with, and suggests ways on how each should be treated.

1. **Shy, timid.** Make her feel at ease. Lead the conversation. Don't force her to talk. Cheer her up.
2. **Talkative type.** Be a good, patient listener. Tactfully switch the conversation to her beauty needs.
3. **Nervous, irritable type.** Does not want much conversation. Wants simple, practical hairdo and fast worker. Get her started and finished as fast as possible.
4. **Inquisitive, over-cautious type.** Explain everything in detail. Show her facts—sealed bottles, brand names. Ask her opinion.
5. **Conceited "Know-It-All" type.** Agree with her. Cater to her vanity. Suggest things in question form. Don't argue with her. Compliment her.
6. **Teenager.** Don't oversell her. Leave her hair longer. Give her special advice on hair care and proper makeup.
7. **Old-timer** (60 and over). Be extra courteous and solicitous of her comfort. Suggest a permanent and hairstyle more becoming to a mature woman.

PERSONALITY IN SELLING

Greeting the patron. Your selling power will increase progressively as you make patrons aware of your personal interest in their welfare. Treat patrons with friendliness and extend such little courtesies as a warm greeting and a pleasant smile. Hang up patron's coat in designated area, and do not let her wait too long for her services. Attention to these little details is greatly appreciated by patrons. The beauty service may be obtained elsewhere, but the personality and friendliness behind the service are what bring the patron back again to you.

Personal magnetism is a valuable asset in selling. Each person creates an atmosphere that may either attract or repel patrons. Since an attractive personality is conducive to making friends and increasing sales, the cosmetologist should develop the qualities that make for an outstanding personality.

The following are positive qualities necessary for a successful selling career:

Optimism—the expectation that things will come out all right.

Acquisitiveness—the desire to acquire wealth and improve one's position in life.

Self-assertiveness—the ability to face and overcome problems and obstacles.

Initiative—the ability to do what is necessary without being told what or how to do it.

Cheerfulness—a congenial spirit that makes the work of selling agreeable both to the cosmetologist and the patron.

Tact—saying or doing the right thing, at the right time, in the right place, without offense.

Sincerity—making your suggestions because you really believe the sale will be a good one for the patron.

Ability to smile—a smiling face tells the patron that you are pleased to be of service to her.

SALES PSYCHOLOGY

No matter how good a beauty service or product may be, you will find it difficult to make a sale if there is no need for it. Before attempting to sell anything, first determine whether the patron has a need for it. Every person who enters a salon is an individual with specific wants and needs. Determine how the patron can use a particular item before attempting to sell it to her.

Motives for buying. What are the motives that prompt women to buy beauty services and merchandise? Women want to make the most of their natural endowments or substitute for what is lacking. A modern hairstyle, a youthful complexion, sparkling eyes, a tender skin, stylish clothes, and correct makeup are among the most cherished desires of women. Personal influence and social prestige can be enhanced by a youthful appearance. Vanity, personal satisfaction, and aesthetic gratification are other reasons why patrons desire beauty services. The buying motive that predominates and is the strongest is the one to which the cosmetologist should make her most successful appeal.

Help patron make decision. If a patron is doubtful or undecided, help her make a decision by giving honest and sincere advice. For instance, if a patron wants a permanent wave and you see that her hair is very dry, it is your responsibility to recommend the use of a conditioner and to fully explain how it will help her hair.

In the beauty profession, you should instill ideas in conjunction with selling services and merchandise. Show the patron not only what the beauty service is, but also what it can mean to her in terms of results and benefits. Sell her the idea that a beauty treatment or product will improve her feminine attractiveness and personality. The selling of ideas along with beauty services gives greater value to the patron and more sales to the cosmetologist.

SALES TECHNIQUES

The best interests of the patron should be your first consideration. Under no circumstances should you approach a patron with the thought of the amount of money you can get from her. Sincerity and honesty are the foundation of good salesmanship.

Careful consideration on your part will acquaint you with the patron's needs, and those needs can be fulfilled to the complete satisfaction of the patron and to your financial advantage. Tact and diplomacy must be used, as well as courtesy.

USE ATTRACTIVE DISPLAYS

To acquaint new and old patrons with the quality and cost of beauty services and merchandise, use attractive displays in the window, at the reception desk, cosmetic counter, service booth, and boutique area. Dress the windows so that they carry a definite message and appeal to the people passing the salon. Frequent rearrangement of case displays and changes in the featured service or merchandise will draw attention to new items. Price signs should accompany the placards. If the price is within reach of the patron, there will be no hesitation or embarrassment in obtaining more particulars about the advertisement.

An effective display can create interest in a particular service or product and help in its sale. Beauty products should appeal to the eye through color, and to the imagination through suggestion of feminine loveliness. Manufacturers and wholesale dealers will cooperate in arranging for well-lighted and attractive displays of their products.

DESCRIBE BENEFITS OF BEAUTY SERVICE

Each beauty service requires a suitable sales technique, employing simple and suggestive language that will make the patron feel like buying. In creating interest and desire, use picture words and descriptive adjectives charged with feeling. Present to the patron a verbal picture of herself as a relaxed, refreshed, and more charming individual after using the recommended beauty service.

Facial. Say to Mrs. Smith, "Our beauty facial invigorates the skin, making it radiant and lovely. A smooth and velvety skin will prompt others to remark 'what beautiful skin you have'." An emotional appeal is often more effective than the use of cold, reasoned facts.

For salesmanship to be successful, the language should be positive rather than negative. Refrain from using the word "don't" in selling language.

Hair shaping. A patron makes an appointment for a shampoo and set. Her hair needs shaping. (Use the term "shaping" instead of "cutting" because it sounds softer and is easier to sell.) The conversation might be as follows:

Cosmetologist: "Mrs. Jones, your hair is a little too long and not right for the style I'd like to give you. I would like to shape it a little so that it will conform to your head, and also frame your face. The set will last longer, your hair will be more manageable, and it will dry in less time."

Mrs. Jones: "I didn't realize my hair was that long. Go ahead and shape it for I want my hairstyle to look as good as possible. Don't take off too much, please."

Cosmetologist: "Don't be concerned. I will take off only what is really necessary."

DON'T UNDERESTIMATE PATRON

At no time should you underestimate either the patron's intelligence or ability to pay for what she actually wants or needs. A simple dress and lack of pretentiousness on the part of the patron are no indications that she is not able to afford anything she wants. Regardless of financial status, each patron is entitled to courteous treatment and sincere consideration, whether her purchase is for a large or small amount. When making a sale, you should refrain from mentioning price until the patron's interest is sufficiently aroused. Then it should be given in a casual manner, without attaching too much importance to it.

SELLING BEAUTY SERVICES AND ACCESSORIES

Learn to identify patrons not only by appearance, but also by name. Address the patron as "Miss Jones" or "Mrs. Smith" and not by "dearie" or "honey." Keep a reminder file of the patron's type of skin, hair, and scalp; also include the type and price of service rendered and merchandise sold. When the patron calls again, you can refresh your memory as to previous work. Reminder forms help not only to sell more beauty services and products, but also assure the patron that you have a personal interest in her problems.

Another source of income is keeping up with the latest hairstyles. The progressive cosmetologist can create new coiffures whenever the occasion arises.

Every patron is a potential source of new patrons and additional beauty services. A fashionable hairstyle will boost the reputation of the cosmetologist and, as a result, bring in new patrons. For complete grooming, beauty services should supplement one another. For example, reconditioning and corrective scalp treatments can be recommended between permanents. Explain to the patron that a much more satisfactory permanent wave will be achieved and the coiffure will be kept looking smarter and more vibrant if dry and brittle hair is treated first. Encourage the patron to take a series of corrective treatments at a special price. For complete personal grooming, other services may be required, such as a facial, eyebrow shaping, and manicure.

In selling beauty services and merchandise, stress quality and other advantages over cheaper substitutes. The cosmetologist should have a ready answer for a price objection. She can say, "Although you are paying a higher price, you will be getting greater value and superior results from the money expended." The cosmetologist also can explain that the higher price is occasioned by the use of standard top quality materials and highly skilled cosmetologists.

SELLING SUPPLIES

Before the cosmetologist tries to sell accessory supplies, such as cosmetics, compacts, perfumes, atomizers, hair nets, wigs, jewelry, combs, and brushes, she should have correct information concerning the following:

1. Location of the product.
2. Name and brand of product.
3. Contents and price of product.
4. Comparative merits of similar products that differ in price.

There should be a complete assortment of beauty accessories to meet the demand and to fit the pocketbook of all patrons. The range in shade and color of cosmetics should be large enough to suit all types of skin tones. The sale of one item leads to the sale of other items, if they are in stock. Reorder regularly, to assure a fresh and complete stock at all times.

Most women are anxious to know whether the color of the powder, cheek color, and lip color they are using is correct. A question of this nature may open the door to cosmetic sales. A complimentary skin analysis and makeup should be given to show the patron the cosmetics that are most suitable for her. Once the patron begins to buy her cosmetics through the beauty salon, she will establish the buying habit that will continue as long as high quality merchandise is sold.

The most effective way to convince women of the value of professional beauty services and accessories is to show them an actual treatment or application. Depend more on demonstration than on spoken claims or promises.

FIRST AID

Emergencies arise in every line of business, and a knowledge of first aid measures is invaluable to the salon manager and staff.

A physician (or emergency ambulance) should be called as soon as possible after any accident has occurred, both as a courtesy to the patron and as a protection to the salon. There are certain first aid treatments, however, that the layman can give while awaiting medical assistance. Have a well equipped first aid kit where it is within easy access. When possible the salon owner, manager, and employees should take a course in first aid.

For more information about emergency care, consult the latest edition of the First Aid Manual published by the American Red Cross.

Abrasions. When the skin is cut or broken by accident, an antiseptic, such as tincture of iodine, hydrogen peroxide, or mercurochrome, should be applied.

Burns. Burns may be caused by electricity or flames, while scalds usually are due to exposure to hot liquids or live steam. Burns are classified as first degree, characterized by redness; second degree, having watery blisters; and third degree, involving deeper structures of the flesh with possible charring of tissues. In case of accidental burns, see that the patron gets immediate medical attention by a physician.

A quick, safe, and temporarily effective method of treating burns is to immediately apply ice or cold water to the affected area.

Electric shock. The clothing should be loosened and the patron removed to a cool place. The head should be raised and the tongue drawn forward to prevent strangulation. Apply artificial respiration. Stimulants should not be given.

Heat exhaustion. Heat exhaustion is a general functional depression due to heat. It is characterized by a cool, moist skin and collapse. Clothing should be loosened and the patron removed to a cool, dark, quiet place. The patron should be kept lying down for several hours, as rest and quiet will hasten recovery.

Nose bleed. Nose bleed is a hemorrhage from the nose, and is treated by loosening the collar and applying pads saturated with cool water to the face and back of the neck.

Foreign body in the eye. If this is under the lower lid, pull the lid down gently while the patron looks up. If the hair or speck of dust can be seen, it should be removed with the corner of a clean, moistened handkerchief or with a twist of clean cotton.

If it is under the upper lid, pull the lid down over the eye and the speck should then be apparent when the patron opens her eye again. Remove in same way as above.

Fainting. Fainting is caused by a lack of blood flow to the brain, bad air, indigestion, nervous condition, unpleasant odors, etc., and is characterized by pallor and loss of muscular control. There is a temporary suspension of respiration and circulation. If there is a sign of fainting, and before it actually occurs, have the patron hold his/her head between the knees, as this action may check the faintness by causing the blood to flow quickly to the head. **Treatment for fainting** consists of loosening all tight clothing, being sure there is fresh air in the room, and placing the patron in a reclining position with the head slightly lower than the body. If the patron is conscious, hold aromatic spirits of ammonia near his/her nose or offer stimulants, such as hot coffee, tea, or milk. If the patron is unconscious, apply cold applications to the face, chest, and over the heart. Do not dash cold water in the patron's face.

Epileptic fit. An epileptic fit is a nerve disorder characterized by unconsciousness, convulsions, contortions of the face, foaming at the mouth, and rolling of the eyes. In such a case, call for immediate medical attention.

Emergency treatment consists of lying patron on the side and fixing a wad of cotton between the teeth to prevent biting of the tongue. Mild stimulants may be administered in moderation after recovery. If the patron falls into a deep sleep after the attack, he/she should not be disturbed, but allowed to awaken naturally.

In case of emergency. Every salon should have information that may be needed in case of an emergency, posted or placed (in clear view) near the telephone. The owner of the salon or manager should have the names, addresses, and telephone numbers of employees on file in case of an emergency. The file that is kept for regular patrons also should have information that might be needed in case of an emergency. Addresses and telephone numbers for the following services should be placed near the salon telephone: fire station; police (local and state); emergency ambulance; nearest hospital emergency room; doctors; taxi service; telephone company and telephone numbers of persons and organizations that provide service.

Utility service companies, such as electricity, water, heat, air-conditioning, etc. also should be posted. Additional information to be included are the names and telephone numbers of the owner and/or manager, custodian, and others who might need to be called if something goes wrong in the salon.

Each employee should know where exits are located and how to evacuate a building quickly in case of fire or other emergencies. Fire extinguishers should be placed where they can be reached easily, and employees should know how to use them. A well-stocked first aid kit should be kept within easy reach.

ARTIFICIAL RESPIRATION

To deal with occurrences such as severe electric shock, protracted fainting, poisoning, and gas suffocation, the most currently acceptable methods are mouth-to-mouth breathing or mouth-to-nose breathing.

Procedure

1. Place patron on a flat surface.
2. Place one hand on back of patron's neck, one hand on forehead, and tilt the head backward until the chin is pointed upward.
3. Lift patron's lower jaw forward to move the tongue away from the throat.
4. Pinch patron's nose closed.

5. Seal your mouth on patron's mouth and give four quick breaths.
6. Listen for patron's breathing and check pulse. (Pulse can be checked by placing fingers on carotid artery.)
7. If there is no pulse, continue giving at least one breath every five seconds until you see patron's chest rising and falling.
8. For mouth-to-nose breathing, follow the same procedure as for mouth-to-mouth breathing, except that you close the patron's mouth with your hand and blow into the nose.

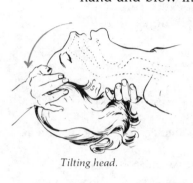
Tilting head.

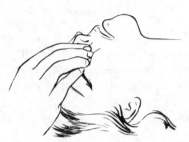
Holding nose.

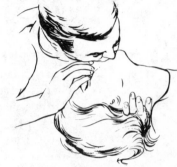
Giving four quick breaths.

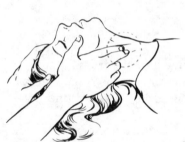
Checking pulse.

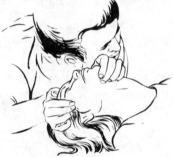
Checking breathing.

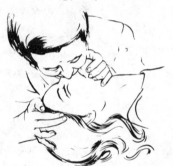
Mouth-to-nose breathing.

BREATHING OBSTRUCTION (ABDOMINAL THRUST)

If patron's breathing becomes obstructed due to choking, immediate help must be given.

Procedure

1. Standing behind patron, hit patron rapidly between the shoulder blades.
2. Wrap your arms around patron's waist. Make a fist and place the thumb just below the breastbone.
3. Hold your fist with your other hand and press it into patron's abdomen, using four quick upward thrusts.
4. Repeat the procedure if necessary.

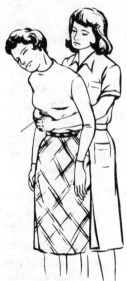

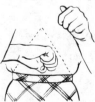
Positioning hand.

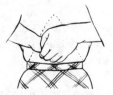
Positioning hand.

Thrusting upward.

REVIEW QUESTIONS

SALON MANAGEMENT

Opening A Beauty Salon

1. What constitutes a good location for a beauty salon?
2. Why must parking and transportation facilities be considered?
3. Why is the reception area of a beauty salon important?
4. What should advertising accomplish for a beauty salon?
5. What are five contributing causes of beauty salon failure?

Good Business Administration

1. How should records be kept in order to be effective?
2. What purpose do accurate records serve?
3. How long should sales slips, appointment book, and petty cash book be kept?
4. How long should payroll book, cancelled checks, monthly and yearly records be kept?
5. What two types of supplies make up a beauty salon's inventory?
6. Under what three types of ownership may a beauty salon be operated?

Using The Telephone In The Salon

1. Name seven uses a telephone has in a beauty salon.
2. Describe good telephone usage.
3. What are four basic rules to follow when using the telephone?
4. What three speech characteristics contribute to good telephone personality?
5. What should a cosmetologist do before undertaking a telephone conversation?
6. How will the use of good telephone techniques help a salon?
7. How should a patron's complaint be handled?
8. How should a price objection be handled?

Selling In The Beauty Salon

1. What are the ten principles of selling?
2. Name seven of the most common types of salon patrons.
3. Before attempting to sell a service or a product, what must a cosmetologist determine?
4. What is the foundation of good salesmanship?
5. What type of language is most effective for selling?
6. How should beauty products make their appeal?
7. What potential does every patron have?
8. What is one of the most effective selling tools?
9. What factors should be stressed in selling beauty services or mechandise?
10. In what four areas must the cosmetologist have the correct information before trying to sell beauty accessories?

First Aid

1. When an accident occurs, when should a physician be called?
2. What should be done when the skin is accidentally cut?
3. What causes heat exhaustion?
4. How is a nose bleed treated?
5. Give the procedure for the abdominal thrust.

METRIC SYSTEM

Wherever possible, metric equivalents are indicated in the text alongside the measurement system commonly used in the United States. Conversions have been made strictly in accordance with conversion tables and information supplied by the U.S. Department of Commerce.

EVERYDAY METRIC-AID

Spoonfuls

¼ tsp.	1.25 milliliters
½ tsp.	2.5 milliliters
¾ tsp.	3.75 milliliters
1 tsp.	5 milliliters
¼ tbls.	3.75 milliliters
½ tbls.	7.5 milliliters
¾ tbls.	11.25 milliliters
1 tbls.	15 milliliters

Fluid Ounces

¼ oz.	7.5 milliliters
½ oz.	15 milliliters
¾ oz.	22.5 milliliters
1 oz.	30 milliliters

Cups

¼ cup	59 milliliters
⅓ cup	78 milliliters
½ cup	118 milliliters
⅔ cup	157 milliliters
¾ cup	177 milliliters
1 cup	236 milliliters

Pints-Quarts-Gallons

½ pint	236 milliliters
1 pint	473 milliliters
1 quart	946.3 milliliters
1 gallon	3785 milliliters

Weight in Ounces

¼ oz.	7.1 grams
½ oz.	14.17 grams
¾ oz.	21.27 grams
1 oz.	28.35 grams

Pounds

¼ lb.	.113 kilograms
½ lb.	.227 kilograms
¾ lb.	.340 kilograms
1 lb.	.454 kilograms
2.205 lbs.	1 kilogram

Length

1 inch	2.544 centimeters
1 foot	30.48 centimeters
1 yard	91.44 centimeters
100 ft.	30.48 meters
1 mile	1.609 kilometers
50 mph	80.45 kilometers/hr.

Temperature

32° F.	0° Celsius
68° F.	20° Celsius
212° F.	100° Celsius

Square Measure

1 sq. in.	6.452 sq. cm.
1 sq. ft.	929 sq. cm.
1 sq. yd.	.8361 sq. meters
1 acre	4047 sq. meters

Volume

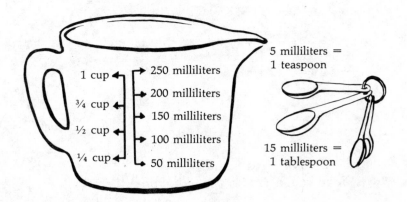

1 cup → 250 milliliters
→ 200 milliliters
¾ cup → 150 milliliters
½ cup → 100 milliliters
¼ cup → 50 milliliters

5 milliliters = 1 teaspoon

15 milliliters = 1 tablespoon

METRIC CONVERSION FACTORS

Approximate Conversions to Metric Measures

Symbol	When You Know	Multiply by	To Find	Symbol
LENGTH (speed)				
in	inches	2.5	centimeters	cm
ft	feet	30	centimeters	cm
yd	yards	0.9	meters	m
mi	miles	1.6	kilometers	km
AREA				
in²	square inches	6.5	square centimeters	cm²
ft²	square feet	0.09	square meters	m²
yd²	square yards	0.8	square meters	m²
mi²	square miles	2.6	square kilometers	km²
a	acres	0.4	hectares	ha
MASS (weight)				
oz	ounces	28	grams	g
lb	pounds	0.45	kilograms	kg
	short tons (2000 lb)	0.9	tonnes	t
VOLUME				
tsp	teaspoon	5	milliliters	ml
tbsp	tablespoon	15	milliliters	ml
fl oz	fluid ounces	30	milliliters	ml
c	cups	0.24	liters	l
pt	pints	0.47	liters	l
qt	quarts	0.95	liters	l
gal	gallons	3.8	liters	l
ft³	cubic feet	0.03	cubic meters	m³
yd³	cubic yards	0.76	cubic meters	m³
TEMPERATURE (exact)				
°F	Fahrenheit temperature	5/9 after subtract-ing 32)	Celsius tempera-ture	°C

GLOSSARY

Compiled of words used in connection with beauty culture, defined in the sense of anatomical, medical, electrical and beauty culture relationship only. Key to pronunciation is as follows:

fāte, senᶏte, câre, ăm, finâl,

ärm, ȧsk, sofȧ; ēve, ȇvent, ĕnd,

recênt, evẽr; īce, ĭll; ōld, ȯbey,

ôrb, ŏdd, cônnect, sŏft, fo͞od,

fo͝ot; ūse, ᴜ̇nite, ûrn, ŭp, circᴜ̂s; thóse

abdomen (ăb-dō'měn): the belly; the cavity in the body between the thorax and the pelvis.

abducent nerve (ăb-dū'sênt): the sixth cranial nerve; a small motor nerve supplying the external rectus muscle of the eye.

abductor (ăb-dŭk'tēr): a muscle that draws a part away from the median line (opp., adductor). i.e.: spreads the fingers.

abrasion (ă-brā'zhûn): scraping of the skin; excoriation.

abscess (ăb'sĕs): a circumscribed cavity containing pus.

absorption (ăb-sôrp'shûn): assimilation of one body by another; act of absorbing.

accessory nerve (ăk-sĕs'ô-rē nûrv): spinal accessory nerve; eleventh cranial nerve; affects the sterno-cleido-mastoid and trapezius muscles of the neck.

acetic (ă-sĕt'ĭk): pertaining to vinegar; sour.

acetone (ăs'ĕ-tōn): a colorless, inflammable liquid, miscible with water, alcohol, and ether, and having a sweetish, ethereal odor and a burning taste.

acid: a sour substance; any chemical compound having a sour taste.

acid rinse: a solution of water and lemon juice or vinegar.

acne (ăk'nē): inflammation of the sebaceous glands from retained secretion.

acoustic (ă-kōos'tĭk): auditory; eighth cranial nerve; controlling the sense of hearing.

activator (ăk'tĭ-vā-tēr): a substance employed to start the action of hair coloring products.

acute (ă-kūt'): attended with severe symptoms; having a short and relatively short course; not chronic; said of a disease.

additive: a substance which is to be added to another product.

adductor (ă-dŭk'tēr): a muscle that draws a part toward the median line. i.e.: draws fingers together.

adipose tissue (ăd'ĭ-pōs): fatty tissue; areolar connective tissue containing fat cells; subcutaneous tissue.

adrenal (ăd-rē'nâl): an endocrine gland situated on the top of the kidneys.

adulterate (ă-dŭl'tēr-āt): to falsify; to alter, make impure by combining other substances.

aeration (ā-ēr-ā'shûn): airing; saturating a fluid with air, carbon dioxide or other gas; the change of venous into arterial blood in the lungs.

aerosol (â'rô-sōl): colloidal suspension of liquid or solid particles in a gas; aerosol container filled with liquified gas and dissolved or suspended ingredients which can be dispersed as a spray or aerosol.

afferent nerves (ăf'ēr-ênt): convey stimulus from the external organs to the brain.

agnail (ăg'nāl): hangnail.

affinity (ă-fĭn'ĭ-tē): 1) inherent likeness or relationship; 2) chemical attraction; the force that unites atoms into molecules.

albinism (ăl'bĭ-nĭz'm): congenital leucoderma or absence of pigment in the skin and its appendages; it may be partial or complete.

albino (ăl-bī'nō): a subject of albinism; a person with very little or no pigment in the skin, hair or iris.

albumin (ăl-bū'mĭn): a simple, naturally-occurring protein soluble in water, coagulated by heat; found, in egg white (ovalbumin), in blood (serum albumin), in milk (lactalbumin).

alcohol (ăl'kô-hŏl): a readily evaporating colorless liquid with a pungent odor and burning taste; powerful stimulant and antiseptic.

alkali (ăl'kă-lī): an electropositive substance; capable of making soaps from fats; used to neutralize acids.

alkaline (ăl'kâ-līn): having the qualities of, or pertaining to, an alkali.

alkalinity (ăl-kâ-lĭn'ĭ-tē): the quality or state of being alkaline.

allergy (ăl'ēr-jē): a disorder due to extreme sensitivity to certain foods or chemicals.

alopecia (ăl-ô-pē'shē-â): deficiency of hair; baldness.

alopecia adnata (ăl-ô-pē'shē-â ăd-nă'tâ): baldness at birth.

alopecia areata (ăl-ô-pē'shē-â ā-rê-ă'tâ): baldness in spots or patches.

alopecia prematura (ăl-ô-pē'shē-â): prē-mă-tū'râ): baldness beginning before middle age.

alopecia senilis (ăl-ô-pē'shē-â sĕ-nĭl'ĭs): baldness occurring in old age.

alum, alumen (ăl'ŭm, ă-lū'mên): sulphate of potassium and aluminum; an astringent; used as a styptic.

amino-acid (ăm'ĭ-nō): an important constituent of proteins.

amitosis (ăm-ĭ-tō'sĭs): cell multiplication by direct division of the nucleus in the cell.

ammonia (ă-mō'nē-â): a colorless gas with a pungent odor; very soluble in water.

ammonium sulphide (ă-mō'nē-ŭm sŭl'fīd): a combination of ammonia and sulphur.

ammonium thioglycolate (ă-mō'nē-ŭm thī-ō-glī'kô-lāt) (thio; thio relaxer): a chemical relaxer, similar in acid content to chemicals used in permanent waving and hair relaxing.

ampere (ăm-pâr): the unit of measurement of strength of an electric current.

anabolism (ăn-ăb'ō-lĭz'm): constructive metabolism; the process of assimilation of nutritive matter and its conversion into living substance.

analysis, hair: an examination to determine the condition of the hair prior to a hair treatment.

anatomy (â-năt'ō-mē): the study of the gross structure of the body which can be seen with the naked eye.

angiology (ăn-jē-ŏl'ô-jē): the science of the blood vessels and lymphatics.

angular artery (ăng'û-lăr): supplies the lacrimal sac and the eye muscle.

anidrosis, anhidrosis (ăn-ĭ-drō'sĭs): a deficiency in perspiration.

aniline (ăn'ĭ-lĭn, -lēn): a product of coal tar used in the manufacture of artificial dyes.

antibody (ăn'tĭ-bŏd-ē): a substance in the blood which builds resistance to disease.

antidote (ăn'tĭ-dōt): an agent preventing or counteracting the action of a poison.

anti-perspirant (ăn-tĭ-pēr-spī'rânt): a strong astringent liquid or cream used to stop the flow of perspiration in the region of the armpits, hands or feet.

antiseptic (ăn-tĭ-sĕp'tĭk): a chemical agent that prevents the growth of bacteria.

antitoxin (ăn-tĭ-tŏk'sĭn): a substance in serum which binds and neutralizes toxin (poison).

aorta (ā-ôr'tă): the main arterial trunk leaving the heart, and carrying blood to the various arteries throughout the body.

aponeurosis (ăp-ô-nū-rō'sĭs): a broad, flat tendon; attachment of muscles.

appendage (â-pĕn′dêj): that which is attached to an organ, and is a part of it.

aqueous (ā′kwē-ûs): watery; pertaining to water.

aromatic (ăr-ô-măt′ĭk): pertaining to or containing aroma; fragrant.

arrector pili (ă-rĕk′tôr pī′lĭ): plural of arrectores pilorum.

arrectores pilorum (â-rĕk-tō′rēz pĭ-lôr′ûm): the minute involuntary muscle fibers in the skin inserted into the bases of the hair follicles.

artery: a vessel that conveys blood from the heart.

articulation (ăr-tĭk-û-lā′shŭn): joint; a connection between two or more bones, whether or not allowing any movement between them.

asepsis (ă-sĕp′sĭs): a condition in which pathogenic bacteria are absent.

aseptic (ă-sĕp′tĭk): free from pathogenic bacteria.

asteatosis (ăs-tē-ă-tō′sĭs): a deficiency or absence of the sebaceous secretions.

astringent (ăs-trĭn′jênt): a substance or medicine that causes contraction of the issues, and checks secretions.

athlete's foot: a fungus foot infection; epidermophytosis.

atom: the smallest quantity of an element that can exist and still retain the chemical properties of the element.

atrium (ăt′rē-ûm); pl., **atria** (-ă): the auricle of the heart.

atrophy (ăt′rô-fē): a wasting away of the tissues of a part of or of the entire body from lack of nutrition.

auditory (ô′dĭ-tô-rē): eighth cranial nerve; controlling the sense of hearing.

auricle (ô′rĭ-k'l): the external ear; one of the upper cavities of the heart.

auriculo-temporal (ô-rĭk′û-lô tĕm′pôr-âl): sensory nerve affecting the temple and pinna.

auricular (ô-rĭk′û-lâr): pertaining to the ear or cardiac auricle.

auricularis (ô-rĭk′û-lâr′ĭs): a muscle of the ear.

autonomic nervous system (ô-tô-nŏm′ĭk): the sympathetic nervous system; controls the involuntary muscles.

axon (ăk′sŏn): a long nerve fiber extending from the nerve cell.

B

bacillus (bă-sĭl′ûs); pl., **bacilli** (-ī): rod-like shaped bacterium.

back-combing: combing the short hair toward the scalp while the hair strand is held in a vertical position; also called teasing.

bacteria (băk-tē′rē-ă): microbes, or germs.

bactericide (băk-tē′rĭ-sīd): an agent that destroys bacteria.

bacteriology (băk-tē-rē-ŏl′ô-jē): the science which deals with bacteria.

bacterium (băk-tē′rē-ûm); pl., **bacteria** (-ă): unicellular vegetable micro-organism.

baldness: a deficiency of hair; hair loss.

bandeau hairpiece (băn-dō′): hairpiece sewn to a headband covering the hairline.

band wig (bănd): see bandeau hairpiece.

bang: the front hair cut so as to fall over the forehead; often used in the plural, as to wear bangs.

basal layer (bās′âl): the layer of cells at base of epidermis closest to the dermis.

base: the lower part or bottom; chief substance of a compound; an electropositive element that unites with an acid to form a salt.

base, protective (prō-tĕk′tĭv): the material to which the hair is attached in order to form a wig.

benign (bê-nīn′): mild in character.

benzine (bĕn′zēn): an inflammable liquid derived from petroleum and used as a cleansing fluid.

benzoin (bĕn′zō-ĭn, -zoin): a balsamic resin used as a stimulant, and also as a perfume.

bicarbonate of soda (bī-kär′bôn-āt): baking soda; relieves burns, itching, urticarial lesions and insect bites; is often used in bath powders as an aid to cleansing oily skin.

biceps (bī′sĕps): having two heads; a muscle producing the contour of the front and inner side of the upper arm.

bichloride (bī-klō′rīd): a compound having two parts or equivalents of chlorine to one of the other element.

biology (bī-ŏl′ô-jē): the science of life and living things.

blackhead: a comedone; a plug of sebaceous matter.

bleach: see hair lightening.

bleb (blĕb): a blister of the skin filled with watery fluid.

blending (blĕnd′ĭng): the physical act of fusing the color of hair during tinting and lightening applications.

block: a head-shaped form upon which a wig is placed for a specific purpose.

blocking: the act of dividing the hair into practical working parts.

blonde; blond: a person of fair complexion, with light hair and eyes.

blood: the nutritive fluid circulating through the arteries and veins.

blood vascular system (văs′kû-lăr sĭs′tĕm): comprised of structures (the heart, arteries, veins and capillaries) which distribute blood throughout the body.

blood vessel: an artery, vein or capillary.

blue light: a therapeutic lamp used to soothe the nerves.

bluing rinse: a solution used to neutralize the unbecoming yellowish tinge on gray or white hair.

blunt cutting: cutting the hair straight off without thinning or slithering.

boil: a furuncle; a subcutaneous abscess. It is caused by bacteria which enter through the hair follicles.

boiling point: 212° F. or 100° C. The temperature at which a liquid begins to boil.

bond: 1) the linkage between different atoms or radicals of a chemical compound, usually effected by the transfer of one or more electrons from one atom to another; 2) it can be found represented by a dot or a line between atoms shown in various formulas.

booster (bōōs′tĕr): oxidizer added to hydrogen peroxide to increase its chemical action; such chemicals as ammonium persulfate or percarbonate are used.

borax (bō′răks): sodium tetraborate; a white powder used as an antiseptic and cleansing agent.

boric acid (bō′rĭk): acidum boricum; used as an antiseptic dusting powder; in liquid form, as an eye wash.

bouffant (bōō′fänt): the degree of height and fullness in a finished hairstyle.

brachial artery (brā′kĭ-âl): the main artery of the upper arm.

braid: to weave, interlace, or entwine together.

brain: that part of the central nervous sysem contained in the cranial cavity, and consisting of the cerebrum, the cerebellum, the pons, and the medulla oblongata.

brilliantine (brĭl-yân-tēn′): an oily composition that imparts luster to the hair.

bristle: the short, stiff hair of a brush; short, stiff hairs of an animal, used in brushes.

brittle: easily broken or shattered.

bromidrosis (brō-mĭ-drō′sĭs): perspiration which smells foul.

buccal nerve (bŭk′âl): a motor nerve affecting the buccinator and the orbicularis oris muscle.

buccinator (bŭk′sĭ-nā-tẽr): a thin, flat muscle of the cheek, shaped like a trumpet.

bulbous (bŭl′bûs): pertaining to, or being like a bulb in shape or structure.

bulla (bōōl′ă): a large bleb or blister.

C

calamine lotion (kăl′ă-mĭn; -mĭn): zinc carbonate in alcohol used for the treatment of dermatitis in its various forms.

calcium (kăl′sē-ŭm): a brilliant silvery-white metal; enters into the composition of bone.

callous, callus (kăl′ŭs): skin which has become hardened; thick-skinned.

camphor (kăm′fẽr): a mild cutaneous stimulant; it produces redness and warmth, and has a slightly anaesthetic and cooling effect.

cancellous (kăn′sē-lûs): having a porous or spongy structure.

caninus (kă-nīn′ûs): the muscle which lifts the angle of the mouth.

canities (kă-nĭsh′ĭ-ēz): grayness or whiteness of the hair.

cap: the netting and binding of a wig which together form the base to which the hair is attached.

capillary (kăp′ĭ-lâ-rē): any one of the minute blood vessels which connect the arteries and veins; hair-like.

capitate (kăp′ĭ-tāt): the large bone of the wrist.

caput (kă′pût); poss., **capitis** (kăp′ĭ-tĭs): pertaining to the head.

carbohydrate (kär-bō-hī′drāt): a chemical containing carbon, hydrogen, and oxygen.

carbolic acid (kär-bŏl′ĭk): phenol made from coal tar; a caustic and corrosive poison; used in dilute solution as an antiseptic.

carbon: coal; an elementary substance in nature which predominates in all organic compounds and occurs in three distinct forms: black lead, charcoal, and lampblack.

carbon-arc lamp: an instrument which produces ultra-violet rays.

carbon dioxide (dī-ŏk′sīd): carbonic acid gas; product of the cumbustion of carbon with a free supply of air.

carbonic acid (kär-bŏn′ĭk): a weak, colorless acid, formed by the solution of carbon dioxide in water, and existing only in solution.

carbuncle (kär′bŭn-k'l): a large circumscribed inflammation of the subcutaneous tissue that is similar to a furuncle, but much more extensive.

cardiac (kär′dē-ăk): pertaining to the heart.

carotid (kă-rŏt′ĭd): the principal artery of the neck.

carpus (kär′pûs): the wrist; the eight bones of the wrist.

cartilage (kär′tĭ-lâj): gristle; a non-vascular connective tissue softer than bone.

catabolism (kă-tăb′ŏ-lĭz′m): chemical changes which involve the breaking down process within the cells.

catalyst (kăt′â-lĭst): a substance having the power to increase the velocity of a chemical reaction.

caustic (kôs′tĭk): an agent that burns and chars tissue.

caustic soda: sodium hydroxide.

cell: a minute mass of protoplasm forming the structural unit of every organized body.

cell division: the reproduction of cells by the process of each cell dividing in half and forming two cells.

cellular (sĕl′û-lăr): consisting of, or pertaining to cells.

centrosome (sĕn′trô-sōm): a cellular body which controls the division of the cell.

cerebellum (sĕr-ê-bĕl′ûm): the posterior and lower part of the brain.

cerebral (sĕr′ê-brâl): pertaining to the cerebrum.

cerebrospinal system (sĕr-ê-brô-spī′nâl sĭs′tĕm): consists of the brain, spinal cord, spinal nerves and the cranial nerves.

cerebrum (sĕr′ê-brûm): the superior and larger part of the brain.

certified color (sûr′tĭ-fīd): a commercial coloring product which temporarily coats the hair shaft.

chemical change: alteration in the chemical composition of a substance.

chemical dye remover: a dye remover containing a chemical solvent.

chemical hair relaxer (rē-lăks′ẽr): a chemical agent which is employed to straighten over-curly hair.

chemistry (kĕm′is-trē): the science dealing with the composition of substances; the elements and their mutual reactions, and the phenomena resulting from the formation and decomposition of compounds.

chignon (shēn′yŏn): a knot or coil of hair worn at the crown or nape, created from natural hair or from a hairpiece.

chloasma (klō-ăz′mă): irregular large brown patches on the skin, such as liver spots.

chlorine (klō′rĭn, -rēn): greenish yellow gas, with a disagreeable suffocating odor; used in combined form as a disinfectant and a bleaching agent.

cholesterin; cholesterol (kô-lĕs′tẽr-ĭn; -ōl): a waxy alcohol found in animal tissues and their secretions; it is present in lanolin, and used as an emulsifier.

chronic (krŏn′ĭk): long-continued; the reverse of acute.

cicatrix (sĭ-kā′trĭks, sĭk′ă-trĭks); pl., **cicatrices** (sĭk ă-trī′sēz): the skin or film which forms over a wound, later contracting to form a scar.

cilia (sĭl′ĭ-ă): the eyelashes; microscopic hair-like extensions which assist bacteria in locomotion.

circuit: the path of an electric current.

circulation: the passage of blood throughout the body.

citric acid (sĭt′rĭk): acid found in the lemon, orange, grapefruit; used for making a rinse.

clavicle (klăv′ĭ-k'l): collarbone, joining the sternum and scapula.

clipping (klĭp′ĭng): the act of cutting split hair ends with the shears or the scissors.

clockwise: the movement of hair, in shapings or curls, in the same direction as the hands of a clock.

coagulate (kô-ăg′û-lāt): to clot; to convert a fluid into a soft, jelly-like solid.

coccus (kŏk′ûs); pl., **cocci** (kŏk′sī): spherical cell bacterium.

coiffure (kwä-fūr′): an arrangement or dressing of the hair.

cold waving: a system of permanent waving involving the use of chemicals rather than heat.

collodion (kô-lō′dē-ôn): a thick liquid used to form an adhesive covering.

color blender: a preparation which cleanses, highlights and blends in gray hair.

color filler: a preparation used to recondition lightened, tinted or damaged hair.

color remover: a prepared commercial product which removes tint from the hair.

color rinse: a rinse which gives a temporary tint to the hair.

color shampoo: a preparation which colors the hair permanently without requiring presoftening treatment.

color test: a method of determining the action of a selected tint on a small strand of hair.

comedone (kŏm′ê-dōne): blackhead; a worm-like mass in an obstructed sebaceous duct.

comedone extractor (ĕks′trăk′tĕr): an instrument used for the removal of blackheads.

compact tissue (kŏm′păkt): a dense, hard type of bony tissue.

compound henna (kŏm′pound hĕn′ă): Egyptian henna to which has been added one or more metallic preparations.

compounds (kŏm′poundz): 1) made of two or more parts or ingredients; 2) in chemistry, a substance which consists of two or more chemical elements in union.

concentrated (kŏn′sên-trāt-ĕd): condensed; increasing the strength by diminishing the bulk.

conditioning (kŏn-dĭ′shŭn-ĭng): the application of special chemical agents to the hair, to help restore its strength, and give it body in order to protect it against possible breakage.

conducting cords (kŏn-dŭckt′ĭng): insulated copper wires which convey the current from the wall plate to the patron and operator.

conductor: any substance which will attract or allow a current to flow through it easily.

configuration (kŏn-fĭg′û-rā′shŭn): the arrangement and spacing of the atoms of a molecule.

congeal (kŏn-jēl′): to change from a fluid to a solid state.

congenital (kŏn-jĕn′ĭ-tâl): existing at birth; born with.

congestion (kŏn-jĕs′chŭn): overfullness of the capillary and other blood vessels in any locality or organ; local hyperemia.

connecting cords: the insulated strands of copper wires which join together the apparatus and the commercial electric current.

constitutional (kŏn-stĭ-tū′shŭn-âl): belonging to or affecting the physical or vital powers of an individual.

contagion (kŏn-tā′jŭn): transmission of specific diseases by contact.

contraction (kŏn-trăk′shŭn): the act of shrinking, drawing together.

converter (kŏn-vŭr′tĕr): an apparatus used to convert the direct current to alternating current.

corium (kō′rē-ŭm): the derma or true skin.

cornification (kŏr-nĭ-fĭ-kā′shŭn): the process of becoming a horny substance or tissue; a callosity.

corpuscles, red (kôr′pŭs′lz): cells in blood, whose function is to carry oxygen to the cells.

corpuscles, white: cells in the blood whose function is to destroy disease germs.

corrosive (kŏ-rō′sĭv): something causing corrosion.

corrugations (kŏr-û-gā′shŭns): alternate ridges and furrows; wrinkles.

corrugator supercilli (kŏr′û-gā-tĕr sū-pĕr-sĭl′ē-ī): draws eyebrows inward and downward, thus causing vertical wrinkles at the root of the nose.

cortex (kôr′tĕks): the second layer of the hair.

cortical (kôr′tĭ-kâl): pertaining to the cortex.

cosmetic dermatology (kŏz-mĕt′ĭk dŭr-mă-tŏl′ŏ-jē): a branch of dermatology devoted to improving the health and beauty of the skin and its appendages.

cosmetology (kŏz-mĕ-tŏl′ŏ-jē): the science of beautifying and improving the complexion, skin, hair and nails.

counterclockwise: the movement of hair, in shapings or curls, in the opposite direction to the hands of a clock.

cowlick: a tuft of hair standing up.

cranium (krā′nē′ûm): the bones of the head excluding bones of the face; bony case for the brain.

crayon: a temporary hair coloring, massaged or brushed on with a lipstick-like applicator.

cream: a semi-solid cosmetic.

crepe wool (krăp wŏŏl): a sheep wool substance used as tissue strips, headbands, fillers or for confining hair ends in winding.

cresol (krē′sōl): a colorless, oily liquid or solid derived from coal tar and wood tar and used as a disinfectant.

crest: a ridge, line or thin mark made by folding or doubling, as a crest between two waves.

croquignole (krō′kĭ-nōl): winding of the hair under from ends to the scalp.

cross bonds: the bonds holding together the long chains of amino-acids, which compose hair; the bonds holding together the parallel chains of amino-acids to form hair.

crown: the top part of the head.

crust (krŭst): a scab.

curd (kûrd): soap residue found on the hair after an unsatisfactory shampoo.

curl: a circle, or circles, within a circle.

curl, base: the stationary or immovable foundation of the curl, which is attached to the scalp.

curl, cascade (kăs′kād): a "stand-up" curl which is wound from the hair ends to the scalp.

curl direction: see direction, curl.

curl, Maypole (Mā′pōl): see curl, overlapping.

curl, overlapping: a strand of wet hair wound around the finger with the hair ends on the outside.

curl, pin: a strand of hair which is combed smooth and ribbon-like and wound into a circle with the ends on the inside; sometimes called a flat curl —sculpture curl.

curl, ridge: a curl placed behind and close to the ridge of a finger wave, and pinned across its stem.

curl, roller: a curl formed over a specially made roller.

curl, sculpture (skŭlp′tyûr): same as pin curl.

curl, stand-up: see curl, cascade.

curl stem: that part of the pin curl between the base and the first arc of the circle.

curl, thermal (thûr′mâl): a curl formed with thermal irons.

current, alternating; A.C. (kŭr′ênt, ôl′tĕr-nāt-ĭng): a rapid and interrupted current, flowing first in one direction and then in the opposite direction.

current, direct; D.C. (dĭ′rĕkt): a constant and even flowing current, travelling in one direction.

current, high-frequency (hī-frē′kwĕn-sē): an electric current characterized by a high rate of vibration.

cutaneous (kû-tā′nē-ûs): pertaining to the skin.

cuticle (kū′tĭ-k'l): the outer layer of the skin or hair.

cutis (kū′tĭs): the deeper layer of the skin (dermis).

cyst (sĭst): a closed, abnormally developed sac containing fluid, semi-fluid or morbid matter.

cysteine (sĭs′tĭ-ēn): an amino-acid produced by digestion; it is easily **oxidized** to cystine; obtained by reduction of cystine.

cystine (sĭs'tĭn): a sulphur containing amino-acid found in hair and nails.

cytoplasm (sī'tō-plăz'm): the protoplasm of the cell body, exclusive of the nucleus.

D

dandricide (dăn'drĭ-sīd): a chemical substance; counteracts the effects of dandruff.

dandruff (dăn'drŭf): pityriasis; scurf or scales formed in excess upon the scalp.

decolorize: see hair lightening.

deltoid (dĕl'toid): a muscle of the shoulder.

demarcation (dē-mär-kā'shŭn): a line setting bounds or limits.

dendrite (dĕn'drīt): a tree-like branching of nerve fibers extending from a nerve cell.

deodorant (dē-ō'dĕr-ănt): a substance that removes or conceals offensive odors.

depilatory (dĕ-pĭl'ă-tō-rē): a substance, usually a caustic alkali, used to destroy the hair; having the power to remove hair.

depressor (dē-prĕs'ĕr): that which presses or draws down; a muscle that depresses.

dermatitis (dûr-mă-tī'tĭs): inflammation of the skin.

dermatitis, contact: an inflammation of the skin caused by coming in contact with chemicals, dyes, etc., to which the individual may be allergic.

dermatitis, cosmetic: an inflammation of the skin caused by coming in contact with some cosmetic product to which the individual may be allergic.

dermatitis, occupational (ŏk-û-pā'shŭn-ăl): an inflammation of the skin caused by the kind of employment in which the individual is engaged.

dermatology (dûr-mă-tŏl'ō-jē): the science which treats of the skin and its diseases.

dermis, derma (dûr'mĭs, dûr'mă): the layer below the epidermis; the corium or true skin.

detergent (dē-tûr'jĕnt): an agent that cleanses.

developer: an oxidizing agent, such as 20-volume hydrogen peroxide solution; when mixed with an aniline derivative tint it supplies the necessary oxygen gas.

diagnosis (dī-ăg-nō'sĭs): the recognition of a disease from its symptoms.

dialysis (dī-ăl'ĭ-sĭs): the process of separating different substances in solution by diffusion through a moist membrane or septum; separation.

diathermy (dī'ă-thûr-mē): a method of raising the temperature in the deep tissues, using high-frequency current.

diffusion (dĭ-fū'zhŭn): a spreading out; dialysis.

digits (dĭj'ĭts): fingers or toes.

dilator (dī-lā'tĕr; dĭ-): that which expands or enlarges.

dilute (dĭ-lūt'; dī-): to make thinner by mixing, especially with water.

diplococcus (dī-plō-kŏk'ŭs): bacteria exhibiting pairs.

direction, curl: the movement of hair in order to form a particular pattern or style. Forward: toward the face. Backward (reverse): away from the face.

direction, stem: the direction in which the stem moves from the base to the first arc.

disease: a pathologic condition of any part or organ of the body, or of the mind.

disease carrier: a healthy person capable of transmitting disease germs to another person.

disinfectant (dĭs-ĭn-fĕk'tănt): an agent used for destroying germs.

dispensary (dĭs-pĕn'sà-rē): a place where medicines or other supplies are prepared and dispensed.

dispersion (dĭs-pûr'shŏn): 1) the act of scattering o separating; 2) the incorporation of the particles c one substance into the body of another, comprising solutions, suspensions and colloid solutions.

distill (dĭs-tĭl'): to extract the essence or active principle of a substance.

disulfide (dī-sŭl'fīd): (sulphur): a chemical compound in which two sulphur atoms are united with a single atom of an element; i.e., carbon.

dormant (dôr'mănt): inactive; asleep.

double application tints: products requiring two separate applications; also called two process tint or two step tints.

duct: a passage or canal for fluids.

dye remover: see color remover.

E

eczema (ĕk'zĕ-mă): an inflammatory itching disease of the skin.

efferent (ĕf'ĕr-ĕnt): motor nerves conveying impulses away from the central nervous system.

effilate (ĕf'ĭ-lāt): to cut the hair strand by a sliding movement of the scissors.

effleurage (ĕ-flū-razh'): a stroking movement in massage.

Egyptian henna (ē-jĭp'shân hĕn'ă): a pure vegetable hair dye.

elasticity (ē-lăs'tĭs'ĭ-tē): the property that allows a thing to be stretched, and to return to its former shape.

electricity: a form of energy, which, when in motion exhibits magnetic, chemical or thermal effects.

electrode (ē-lĕk'trōd): a pole of an electric cell; an applicator for directing the use of electricity on a patron.

electrolysis (ē-lĕk-trŏl'ĭ-sĭs): decomposition of a chemical compound or body tissues by means of electricity.

electron (ē-lĕk'trŏn): an extremely minute corpuscle or charge of negative electricity, the smallest known to exist.

electropositive (ē-lĕk'trō-pŏz'ĭ-tĭv): relating to or charged with positive electricity.

electro-static (ē-lĕk'trō-stăt'ĭk): pertaining to static electricity.

element (ĕl'ê-mĕnt): 1) a simple substance which cannot be decomposed by chemical means, and which is made up of atoms which are alike in their peripheral electronic configurations and in their chemical properties; 2) any one of the 103 ultimate chemical entities of which matter is believed to be composed.

emollient (ē-mŏl'yĕnt): an agent that softens or soothes the surface of the skin.

emulsifier (ē-mŭl'sĭ-fī-ēr): a substance, as gelatin gum, etc., for emulsifying a fixed oil.

emulsion (ē-mŭl'shŭn): a product consisting of minute globules of one liquid dispersed throughout the body of a second liquid.

end bonds (peptide bonds) (pĕp'tīd): the chemical bonds which join together the amino-acids to form the long chains which are characteristic of all proteins.

endocrine (ĕn'dō-krĭn): any internal secretion or hormone.

enzyme (ĕn'zīm): a substance which induces a chemical change in other substances, without undergoing any change itself.

epicranius (ĕp-ĭ-krā'nē-ûs): the occipito-frontalis; the scalp muscle.

epidemic (ĕp-ĭ-dĕm'ĭk): common to many people; a prevailing disease.

epidermis (ĕp-ĭ-dûr'mĭs): the outer layer of the skin.

epilation (ĕp-ĭ-lā'shŭn): the removal of hair by the roots.

epithelium (ĕp-ĭ-thē'lē-ûm): a cellular tissue or membrane, with little intercellular substance, covering a free surface or lining a cavity.

eponychium (ĕp-ō-nĭk'ē-ûm): the extension of cuticle at base of nail-body.

erythrocyte (ĕ-rĭth'rō-sīt): a red blood cell; red corpuscle.

esophagus; oesophagus (ē-sŏf'ă-gûs): the canal leading from the pharynx to the stomach.

ester (ĕs'tĕr): an organic compound formed by the reaction of an acid and an alcohol.

esthetic (ĕs-thĕt'ĭk): sensitive to art and beauty; showing good taste; artistic.

ethics: principles of good character and proper conduct.

ethmoid (ĕth'moid): resembling a sieve; a bone forming part of the walls of the nasal cavity.

etiology (ē-tē-ŏl'ō-jē): the science of the causes of disease.

evaporation: change from liquid to vapor form.

excoriation (ĕks-kō-rē-ā'shŭn): act of stripping or wearing off the skin; an abrasion.

excrete (ĕks-krēt'): to separate (waste matter) from the blood or tissue and eliminate from the body as through the kidneys or sweat glands.

excretion (ĕks-krē'shŭn): that which is thrown off or eliminated from the body.

exhalation (ĕks-hà-lā'shŭn): the act of breathing outward.

extensibility (ĕks-tĕn-sĭ-bil'ĭ-tē): capable of being extended or stretched.

extensor (ĕks-tĕn'sôr): a muscle which serves to extend or straighten out a limb or part.

extremity (ĕks-trĕm'ĭ-tē): the distant end or part of any organ; a hand or foot.

exudation (ĕks-û-dā'shŭn): act of discharging from the body through pores as sweat, moisture or other liquid.

eye-shadow: a cosmetic applied on the eyelids to accentuate their brilliance.

F

facial (fā'shăl): pertaining to the face; the seventh cranial nerve.

Fahrenheit (fä'rĕn-hīt): pertaining to the Fahrenheit thermometer or scale; water freezes at 32° F. and boils at 212° F.

fall: an artificial section of hair running across the back of the head.

fascia (făsh'ē-ă): a sheet of connective tissue covering, supporting, or binding together internal parts of the body.

felon (fĕl'ûn): paronychia of the nail.

fermentation (fûr-mĕn-tā'shŭn): a chemical decomposition of organic compounds into more simple compounds, brought about by the action of an enzyme.

fetid (fĕt'ĭd): having a foul smell; stinking.

fever blister: an acute skin disease characterized by the presence of vesicles over an inflammatory base; herpes simplex.

fiber: a slender, threadlike structure that combines with others to form animal or vegetable tissue.

fibrin (fī'brĭn): the active agent in coagulation of the blood.

filler: a commercial product used to provide fill for porous spots in the hair during tinting, lightening and permanent waving.

finger test: a test given to determine the degree of porosity in the hair.

fission (fĭsh'ŭn): reproduction of bacteria by cellular division; any splitting or cleaving; atomic f.: the splitting of the neutrons of an atom in two main fragments.

fissure (fĭsh'ûr): a narrow opening made by separation of parts; a furrow; a slit.

fixative (fĭk'să-tĭv): a chemical agent capable of stopping the processing of the permanent wave solution or the chemical hair relaxer and hardening the hair in its new form; neutralizer; stabilizer.

flagella (flă-jĕl'ă): slender whip-like processes which permit locomotion in certain bacteria.

flexor (flĕk'sôr): a muscle that bends or flexes a part or a joint.

fluorescent (floo'ôr-ĕs'n't): an ability to emit light after exposure to light, the wave length of the emitted light being longer than that of the light absorbed.

"fly away": an excessive electrostatic condition of hair which causes individual hair strands to repel one another and stand away from the head.

foamer (fō'mĕr): a substance which creates an excessive amount of foam.

follicle (fŏl'ĭ-k'l): the depression in the skin containing the hair root.

formaldehyde (fôr-măl'dĕ-hīd): a pungent gas possessing powerful disinfectant properties.

Formalin (fôr'mă-lĭn): a 37% to 40% solution of formaldehyde.

formula (fôr'mû-lă): a prescribed method or rule; a recipe or prescription.

fragilitas crinium (fră-jĭl'ĭ-tăs krĭ'nē-ûm): brittleness of the hair.

freckle: a yellow or brown spot on the skin; lentigo.

free edge: part of the nail body extending over the fingertip.

French lacing: see teasing.

frequency (frē'kwĕn-sē): the number of complete cycles per second of current produced by an alternating current generator. Standard frequencies are 25 and 60 cycles per second.

friction: the resistance encountered in rubbing one body on another.

frizz: hair having too much of a curl.

frontal: in front; relating to the forehead; the bone of the forehead.

frontalis (frŏn-tā'lĭs): anterior portion of the muscle of the scalp.

frosting (frŏst'ĭng): to lighten or darken small selected strands of hair over the entire head to blend with the rest of the hair.

fulling (fool'ĭng): a massage movement in which the limb is rolled back and forth between the hands.

fumigate (fū'mĭ-gāt): disinfect by the action of fumes.

fungus (fŭn'gŭs): a vegetable parasite; a spongy growth of diseased tissue on the body.

furuncle (fū-rŭn'k'l): a small skin abscess (boil).

fuse: to liquefy by heat; a special device which prevents excessive current from passing through a circuit.

fusion (fū'zhŭn): the act of uniting or cohering.

G

ganglion (găn′glē-ôn); pl., **ganglia** (-ă): bundles of nerve cells in the brain, in organs of special sense, or forming units of the sympathetic nervous system.

gastric juice (găs′trĭk): the digestive fluid secreted by the glands of the stomach.

gauze: a thin, open-meshed cloth used for dressings.

gel: comprised of a solid and a liquid which exist as a solid or semi-solid mass.

gelatine: the tasteless, odorless, brittle substance extracted by boiling bones, hoofs and animal tissues used in various foods, medicines, etc.

gene: the ultimate unit in the transmission of hereditary characteristics.

genetic (jĕ-nĕt′ĭk): the genesis or origin of something.

gentian violet jelly: (jĕn′shän): an antiseptic used in the first aid treatment of a scalp burn.

germ: a bacillus; a microbe; an embryo in its early stages.

germicide (jûr′mĭ-sīd): any chemical, especially a solution that will destroy germs.

germinative layer (jûr-mĭ-nā′tĭv): stratum germinativum; the deepest layer of the epidermis resting on the corium.

gland: a secretory organ of the body.

globule (glŏb′ūl): a small, spherical droplet of fluid or semi-fluid material.

glossopharyngeal (glŏs-ô-fâ-rĭn′jĕ-āl): pertaining to the tongue and pharynx; the ninth cranial nerve.

glycerin; glycerine (glĭs′ĕr-ĭn): sweet, oily fluid, used as an application for roughened and chapped skin; also used as a solvent.

granules (grăn′ūlz): small grains; small pills.

granulosum (grăn-û-lōs′ûm): granular layer of the epidermis.

great auricular (grāt ô-rĭk′û-lär): a nerve affecting the face, ear, neck and parotid gland.

greater occipital (ŏk-sĭp′ĭ-tâl): sensory and motor nerve affecting the back part of the scalp.

gristle (grĭs″l): cartilage.

grooming (grōōm′ĭng): to make neat or tidy.

ground wire (ground wĭr): a wire which connects an electric current to a ground (waterpipe or radiator).

H

hacking (hăk′ĭng): a chopping stroke made with the edge of the hand in massage.

hair: pilus; a slender threadlike outgrowth on the body.

hair bulb: the lower extremity of the hair.

hair clipping: removing the hair by the use of hair clippers; removing split hair ends of the hair with the scissors.

hair coloring: artificially changing the color of the hair.

haircutting: shortening and thinning of the hair, and molding the hair into a becoming style; hair shaping.

hair density: the number of hairs per square inch on the scalp.

hair dressing: the art of arranging the hair into various becoming shapes or styles.

hair follicle (fŏl′ĭ-k′l): the depression of the skin containing the root of the hair.

hair lightener: a chemical substance used to remove the natural color pigment from the hair.

hair lightening: the removal of natural pigment c artificial color from the hair.

hair papilla (hâr pă-pĭl′ă): a small, cone-shape elevation at the bottom of the hair follicle.

hairpiece: an artificial section of woven hair use in place of or in conjunction with the natura hair.

hair pressing: a method of straightening curly c kinky hair by means of heated irons or a press ing comb.

hair pressing oil: an oily or waxy mixture used i hair pressing.

hair relaxing, chemical: a permanent method c straightening over-curly hair.

hair restorer: a preparation containing a metall dye (not used professionally).

hair root: that part of the hair contained withi the follicle.

hair shaft: the portion of the hair which projec beyond the skin.

hair shaping: the art of haircutting.

hair straightener: a physical or chemical agent use in straightening kinky or over-curly hair.

hair stream: the natural direction in which the ha grows after leaving the follicle.

hair, superfluous (sŭ-pûr′flōō-ûs): unwanted or ex cess hair, usually found on the faces of wome See: hirsuties.

hair test: a sampling of how the hair will react a particular treatment.

hair texture (tĕks′tŭr): the general quality of hai as to coarse, medium or fine; the feel of the hair

hair tinting: the physical act of adding color pigme to either virgin or tinted hair.

halitosis (hăl-ĭ-tō′sĭs): offensive odor from th mouth; foul breath.

hangnail (hăng′nāl): a tearing up of a strip epidermis at the side of the nail; agnail.

H-bond: see hydrogen bond.

heating cap: an electrical device, applied over th head, to provide a uniform source of heat.

heating coil: an electric coil which heats the a in a hair dryer.

helix (hē′lĭks; hĕl′ĭks): the fleshy tip of the ea (ear lobe).

hematocyte (hĕ′mă-tô-sīt): a blood corpuscle.

hemoglobin; haemoglobin (hē-mô-glō′bĭn): the co oring matter of the blood.

hemorrhage (hĕm′ô-râj): bleeding; a flow of bloo especially when profuse.

henna (hĕn′ă): the leaves of an Asiatic thorny tr or shrub used as a dye, imparting a reddish tir it is also used as a cosmetic.

henna, compound (kŏm′pound): Egyptian henna which has been added one or more metall preparations.

heredity (hĕ-rĕd′ĭ-tē): the inborn capacity of th organism to develop ancestral characteristics.

herpes (hûr′pēz): an inflammatory disease of th skin having small vesicles in clusters.

herpes simplex (sĭm′plĕks): fever blister; cold sor

hexachlorophenol (hĕks-ă-klō-rō-fē′nōl): white, fr flowing powder, essentially odorless; used as bactericidal agent in antiseptic soaps, deodora products, including soaps and various cosmetics.

high-frequency (hī-frē′kwĕn-sē): violet ray; electric current of medium voltage and mediu amperage.

highlighting shampoo tint: a preparation used wi shampoo when a very slight change in hair sha is desired.

hirsute (hûr′sūt, hĕr-sūt′): hairy; having coars long hair; shaggy.

hirsuties (hûr-sū'shǐ-ēz): hypertrichosis; growth of an unusual amount of hair in unusual locations, as on the faces of women or the backs of men; hairy; superfluous hair.

histology (hǐs-tŏl'ô-jē): the science of the minute structure of organic tissues; microscopic anatomy.

hives: urticaria; a skin eruption.

homogeneous (hō-môj'ê-nūs): having the same nature or quality; a uniform character in all parts.

homogenizer (hō-mŏj'ê-nīz-ẽr): serving to produce a uniform suspension of emulsions from two or more normally immiscible substances.

hormone (hôr'mōn): a chemical substance formed in one organ or part of the body and carried in the blood to another organ or part which it stimulates to functional activity or secretion.

humerus (hū'mẽr-ûs): the bone of the upper part of the arm.

humidity: moisture; dampness.

hydro (hī'drô): a prefix denoting water; hydrogen.

hydro carbon: any compound composed only of hydrogen and carbon.

hydrogen: the lightest element; it is an odorless, tasteless, colorless gas found in water and all organic compounds. **h. acceptor:** a substance which, on reduction, accepts hydrogen atoms from another substance called a hydrogen donor.

hydrogen bond (physical bond): that bond formed between two molecules when the nucleus of a hydrogen atom, originally attached to a florine, nitrogen or oxygen atom of a molecule, is attracted to the florine, nitrogen or oxygen atom of a second molecule of the same or different substance.

hydrogen peroxide: a powerful oxidizing agent; in liquid form it is used as an antiseptic and for the activation of lighteners and hair tints.

hydrophilic (hī-drô-fīl'ĭk): capable of combining with or attracting water.

hygiene: the science of preserving health.

hygroscopic (hī-grŏ'skŏp'ĭk): readily absorbing and retaining moisture.

hyoid (hī'oid): the "u" shaped bone at the base of the tongue.

hyperhidrosis, hyperidrosis (h-'pẽr-ǐ-drŏ'sǐs): excessive sweating.

hypertrophy (hī'pẽr-trŏ'fē): abnormal increase in the size of a part or an organ; overgrowth.

hypoglossal (h:'pô-glŏ'sâl): the twelfth cranial nerve; motor nerve to base of tongue.

hyponychium (hī-pô-nǐk'ē-ûm): the portion of the epidermis upon which the nail-body rests under the free edge.

I

imbrications (ǐm-brǐ-kā'shŭnz): cells arranged in layers overlapping one another; found in cuticle layer of hair.

immerse (ǐ-mûrs'): to plunge into; dip; submerge in a liquid.

immersion (ǐ-mûr'chŭn): plunging or dipping into a liquid, especially so as to cover completely.

immunity (ǐ-mūn'ǐ-tē): freedom from, or resistant to disease.

incubation (ǐn-kû-bā'shûn): the period of a disease between the implanting of the contagion and the development of the symptoms.

index: the forefinger; the pointing finger.

infection (ǐn-fĕk'shûn): the invasion of the body tissues by disease germs.

infection, general: the result of the disease germs gaining entrance into the blood stream and thereby circulating throughout the entire body.

infection, local: confined to only certain portions of the body, such as an abscess.

infectious (ǐn-fĕk'shûs): capable of spreading infection.

inflammation (ǐn-flâ-mā'shûn): the reaction of the body to irritation with accompanying redness, pain, heat, and swelling.

infra-orbital (ǐn-frǎ ôr'bǐ-tâl): below the orbit; a sensory and motor nerve affecting the cheek muscles, nose, and upper lip.

infra-red: rays pertaining to that part of the spectrum lying outside of the visible spectrum and below the red rays.

infra-trochlear (trŏk'lē-âr): sensory nerve affecting the skin of the nose and the inner muscle of the eye.

ingredient: any one of the things of which a mixture is made up.

ingrown hair: a wild hair that has grown underneath the skin, which may cause an infection.

ingrown nail: the growth of the nail into the flesh instead of toward the tip of the finger or toe, which may cause an infection.

inhalation (ǐn-hǎ-lā'shûn): the inbreathing of air or other vapors.

inoculation (ǐn-ŏk-û-lā'shûn): the process by which protective agents are introduced into the body.

inorganic (ǐn-ôr-gǎn'ǐk): composed of matter not relating to living organisms.

insanitary; unsanitary: not sanitary or healthful; injurious to health; unclean.

insoluble (ǐn-sŏl'û-b'l): incapable of being dissolved or very difficult to dissolve.

insulator (ǐn'sû-lā-tẽr): a non-conducting material or substance; materials used to cover electric wires.

intensity (ǐn-tĕn'sǐ-tē): the amount of force or energy of heat, light, sound, electric current, etc., per unit area; the quality of being intense.

intercellular (ǐn-tẽr-sĕl'û-lär): between or among cells.

intestine (ǐn-tĕs'tǐn): the digestive tube from the stomach to the anus.

involuntary muscles (ǐn-vŏl'ûn-tâ-rē): function without the action of the will.

iodine: a non-metallic element used as an antiseptic for cuts, bruises, etc.

ion: an atom or group of atoms carrying an electric charge.

ionization (ī-ŏn-ǐ-zā'shûn): the separating of a substance into ions.

iris: the colored, muscular, disk-like diaphragm of the eye which regulates the pupil or opening in the center.

irradiation (ī-rā'dē-ā'shûn): the process of exposing an object to the natural or artificial sunlight.

irreversible (ǐr-ê-vẽr'sǐ-b'l): not capable of being reversed.

irritability (ǐr-ǐ-tà-bǐl'ǐ-tē): readily excited or stimulated.

J

joint: a connection between two or more bones.

jowl: the hanging part of a double chin.

jugular (jōō'gû-lâr): pertaining to the neck or throat; the large vein in the neck.

K

keratin (kĕr′ă-tĭn): a fiber protein characteristic of horny tissues: hair, nails, feathers, etc.; it is insoluble in protein solvents and has a high sulfur content.

keratinization (kĕr′ă-tĭn-ĭ-zā′shŭn): the process of being keratinized.

keratoma (kĕr-ă-tō′mă): a callosity; a horny tumor; an acquired thickened patch of the epidermis.

kidney: a glandular organ which excretes urine.

kilowatt (kĭl′ō-wŏt): one thousand watts of electricity.

knead (nēd): to work and press with the hands as in massage.

L

labii (lā′bē-ī): of or pertaining to the lip.

labium (lā′bē-ûm); pl., **labia** (-ă): lip.

laceration (lăs′ĕr-ā′shŭn): a tear of the skin or tissues.

lachrymal; lacrimal (lăk′rĭ-mâl): pertaining to tears or weeping; bone at the front of the orbits.

lacquer, nail (lăk′ĕr): a thick liquid which forms a glossy film on the nail.

lanolin (lăn′ō-lĭn): purified wool fat.

lanugo (lă-nū′gō): the fine hair which covers most of the body.

larynx (lăr′ĭnks): the upper part of the trachea or wind pipe; the organ of voice production.

lather: froth made by mixing soap and water.

latissimus dorsi (lă-tĭs′ĭ-mŭs dôr′sī): a broad, flat superficial muscle of the back.

lecithin (lĕs′ĭ-thĭn): a colorless crystalline compound, soluble in alcohol; it is found in animal tissues, especially nerve tissue, and the yolk of egg.

lemon rinse: a product containing lemon juice or citric acid; used to eliminate soap curds.

lentigo (lĕn-tī′gō); pl., **lentigines** (lĕn-tĭ-jī′nēz): a freckle; circumscribed spot or pigmentation in the skin.

lesion (lē′zhŭn): a structural tissue change caused by injury or disease.

lesser occipital (lĕs′ĕr ŏk-sĭp′ĭ-tâl): the nerve supplying muscles at the back of the ear.

leucocyte (lū′kŏ-sīt): a white corpuscle; white blood cell.

leucoderma (lū-kŏ-dûr′mă): abnormal white patches on the skin; absence of pigment in the skin.

leuconychia (lū-kŏ-nĭk′ē-ă): a whitish discoloration of nails; white spots.

ligament (lĭg′ă-mênt): a tough band of fibrous tissue, serving to connect bones, or to hold an organ in place.

lightener (bleach): the chemical employed to remove color from hair.

lightening (bleaching): see: hair lightening.

light therapy: the application of light rays for treatment of disorders.

lipophilic (lĭp-ō-fĭl′ĭk): having an affinity or attraction to fat and oil.

liquefy (lĭk′wĕ-fī): to reduce to the liquid state; said of both solids and gases.

liquor cresolis compound (lĭk′ĕr krē-sōl′ĭs kŏm′pound): a powerful germicide.

litmus paper (lĭt′mûs): a blue coloring matter that is reddened by acids and turned blue again by alkalies.

liver spots: the discolorations of chloasma.

lobe: a branch extending from a body; ear lobe.

lock-jaw: tetanus; specifically trismus; a firm closing of the jaw due to tonic spasm of the muscles of mastication.

lotion: a liquid solution used for bathing the sk

louse; pl., **lice**: pediculus; an animal parasite infe ing the hairs of the head.

lubricant: anything that makes things smooth a slippery, such as oil.

lucidum (lū′sĭ-dŭm): the clear layer of t epidermis.

lung: one of the two organs of respiration.

lunula (lū′nū-lă): the half-moon shaped area at t base of the nail.

lymph (lĭmf): a clear yellowish or light stra colored fluid, which circulates in the lym spaces, or lymphatics of the body.

lymphatic system (lĭm-făt′ĭk): consists of lym flowing through the lymph spaces, lymph vesse lacteals, and lymph nodes or glands.

Lysol (lī′sōl): a trade name; a disinfectant a antiseptic; a mixture of soaps and phenols.

M

macroscopic (măk-rō-skŏp′ĭk): visible to the u aided eye.

macula (măk′ū-lă); pl., **maculae** (-lē): a spot discoloration level with skin; a freckle; macule.

magnetism (măg′nĕ-tĭz'm): the power possessed a magnet to attract or repel other masses.

malar (mā′lăr): of or pertaining to the cheek; t cheek bone.

malformation (măl-fôr-mā′shûn): an abnormal shap or structure; badly formed.

malignant (mă-lĭg′nânt): resistant to treatmen growing worse; occurring in severe form; a tum recurring after removal.

malpighian (măl-pĭg′ē-ân): stratum mucosum; t deeper portion of the epidermis.

mandible (măn′dĭ-b'l): the lower jaw bone.

mandibular nerve (măn-dĭb′û-lăr): the fifth crani nerve which supplies the muscles and skin of th lower part of the face.

manganese (măn′gă-nēs): a grayish-white, metall chemical element which rusts like iron, but is n magnetic.

manicure: the artful care of the hands and nails.

manipulation (mă-nĭp-û-lā′shûn): act or process treating, working or operating with the hands by mechanical means, especially with skill.

marcel: a series of even waves or tiers put in th hair with the aid of a heated iron.

marrow: a soft, fatty substance filling the caviti of bone.

mascara (măs-kă′ră): a preparation used to darke the eyelashes.

mask: a special cosmetic formula used to beautif the face.

massage (mă-säzh′): manipulation of the body b rubbing, pinching, kneading, tapping, etc., increase metabolism, promote absorption, reliev pain, etc.

matting (măt′ĭng): tangling together into a thic mass.

matrix (mā′trĭks): the formative portion of a nai

maxilla (măk-sĭl′ă): upper jaw bone.

medulla (mĕ-dŭl′ă): the marrow in the various bon cavities; the pith of the hair.

melanin (mĕl′ă-nĭn): the dark or black pigment i the epidermis and hair, and in the choroid coat of the eye.

melanophore (mĕl-ân′ō-fôr): a pigment cell contain ing melanin.

membrane (mĕm′brăn): a thin sheet or layer o pliable tissue, serving as a covering.

mental nerve: a nerve which supplies the skin of the lower lip and chin.

mentalis (měn-tā'lǐs): the muscle that elevates the lower lip, and raises and wrinkles the skin of the chin.

metabolism (mě-tăb'ō-lǐz'm): the constructive and destructive life process of the cell.

metacarpus (mět-ă-kär'pûs): the bones of the palm of the hand.

metatarsus (mět-ă-tär'sǔs): the bones which comprise the instep of the foot.

metallic salts: a compound of a base and an acid.

meta-toluene-diamine (mět'ă-tŏl'ū-ēn-dī-ăm'ĭn): the name given to an oxidation dye used to provide lighter shades of red and blonde; it is an aniline derivative type.

meter: an instrument used for measuring.

microbe: a micro-organism; a minute one-celled animal or vegetable bacterium.

micrococcus (mī-krō-kŏk'ŭs): a minute bacterial cell having a spherical shape.

micro-organism (mī'krō-ôr'gân-ĭz'm): microscopic plant or animal cell; a bacterium.

microscope (mī'krō-skōp): an instrument for making enlarged views of minute objects.

miliaria rubra (mĭl-ē-ā'rē-ă rōōb'ră): prickly heat; burning and itching usually caused by exposure to excessive heat.

milium (mĭl'ē-ûm); pl., **milia** (-ă): a small whitish pearl-like mass due to a retention of sebum beneath the epidermis; a whitehead.

mineral salts: salts derived from an inorganic chemical compound.

miscible (mĭs'ĭ-b'l): the property of certain liquids to mix with each other in equal proportions.

mixture: a preparation made by incorporating an insoluble ingredient in a liquid vehicle; sometimes used to identify an aqueous solution containing two or more solutes.

modifier (mŏd'ĭ-fī-ēr): anything that will change the form or characteristics of an object or substance.

mole: a small brownish spot on the skin.

molecule (mŏl'ê-kūl): the smallest unit of any substance having all the properties of the substance.

monilethrix (mô-nĭl'ê-thrĭks): beaded hair; a condition in which the hairs show a series of constrictions, giving the appearance of a string of fusiform beads.

mordant (môr'dânt): a substance, such as alum, phenol, aniline oil, which fixes the dye used in coloring.

motor nerves: carry impulses from nerve centers to muscles for certain motions.

mould: to form or to shape into a definite pattern.

mucous membrane (mū'kûs měm'brăn): a membrane secreting mucus which lines passages and cavities communicating with the exterior.

muscle: the contractile tissue of the body by which movement is accomplished.

muscle tone: the normal degree of tension in a healthy muscle.

myology (mī-ŏl'ō-jē): the science of the function, structure, and diseases of muscles.

N

naevus; nevus (nē'vûs); pl., **naevi; nevi** (-vī): a birthmark; a congenital skin blemish.

nail: unguis; the horny protective plate located at the end of the finger or toe.

nail-bed: that portion of the skin on which the body of the nail rests.

nail-body: the horny nail blade resting upon the nail-bed.

nail-grooves: the furrows on the sides of the nail upon which the nail moves as it grows.

nail lacquer: a thick liquid which forms a glossy film on the nail.

mantle: the fold of the skin into which the nail root is lodged.

nail matrix (mā'trĭks): the portion of the nail-bed extending beneath the nail-root.

nail-root: located at the base of the nail, imbedded underneath the skin.

nail-wall: folds of skin overlapping sides and base of the nail-body.

nape: the back of the neck.

naris (nā'rĭs); pl., **nares** (-rēz): a nostril

nasalis (nâ-zā'lĭs): a muscle of the nose.

neck line: in haircutting, where the hair growth of the head ends and the neck begins; hairline.

nerve: a whitish cord, made up of bundles of nerve fibers, through which impulses are transmitted.

neuritis (nū-rī'tĭs): inflammation of nerves, marked by neuralgia.

neurology (nū-rŏl'ō-jē): the science of the structure, function and pathology of the nervous system.

neuron (nū'rŏn): the unit of the nervous system, consisting of the nerve cell and its various processes.

neutral: exhibiting no positive properties; indifferent; in chemistry, neither acid nor alkaline.

neutralization (nū-trăl-ĭ-zā'shûn): a chemical reaction between an acid and a base; rehardening the hair in cold waving or in chemical hair relaxing.

neutralizer (nū'trâl-ĭz-ēr): an agent capable of neutralizing another substance. (See fixative.)

nit: the egg of a louse, usually attached to a hair.

nitrate (nī'trāte): an oxidizing agent.

nitrite (nī'trīte): a reducing agent; sodium nitrite is used as a sanitizing agent and acts as an anti-rusting agent.

nitric acid (nī'trĭk): concentrated acid employed as a caustic.

nitro-cellulose (nī-trō-sěl'û-lōs): used in nail polishes.

nitrogen (nī'trō-jěn): a colorless, gaseous element, tasteless and odorless, found in air and living tissue.

nodule (nŏd'yūle): a small, circumscribed, solid elevation that usually extends into the deeper layers of the skin.

non-conductor (kôn-dŭk'těr): any substance that resists the passage of electricity, light or heat towards or through it.

non-pathogenic (păth-ô-jěn'ĭk): non-disease producing; growth promoting.

non-striated (strī'ăt-ěd): involuntary, smooth muscle which functions without the action of the will.

nucleus (nū'klê-ûs); pl., **nuclei** (-ī): the active center of cells.

nutrition (nū-trĭsh'ûn): the process of nourishment.

O

oblique (ôb-lēk'; lĭk'); **obliquus** (-ûs): slanting, or inclined.

obsolete (ŏb-sô-lēt'): old; gone out of date.

occipital (ŏk-sĭp'ĭ-tâl): the bone which forms the back and lower part of the head.

occipito-frontalis (ŏk-sĭp'ĭ-tō-frŏn-tā'lĭs): epicranius; the scalp muscle.

occupational disease (ŏk-û-pā'shûn-âl): due to certain kinds of employment, in which contact with chemicals, dyes is involved.

oculist (ŏk'û-lĭst): a specialist in diseases of the eyes.

oculomotor (ŏk'û-lō-mō'tēr): third cranial nerve; controlling the motion of the eye.

oculus (ŏk'û-lŭs); pl., **oculi** (-lī): the eye.

ohm (ōm): a unit of measurement used to denote the amount of resistance in an electrical system or device.

Ohm's law (ōmz lô): the simple statement that the current in an electric circuit is equal to the pressure divided by the resistance.

ointment: a fatty, medicated mixture used externally.

oleic acid (ō-lē'ĭk): an oily acid used in making soap and ointments.

olfactory (ŏl-făk'tô-rē): relating to the sense of smell; first cranial nerve, the special nerve of smell.

onychatrophia (ŏn-ĭ-kă-trō'fē-ă): atrophy of the nails.

onychauxis (ŏn-ĭ-kôk'sĭs): enlargement of the nails.

onychia (ô-nĭk'ē-ă): inflammation of the matrix of the nail with pus formation and shedding of the nail.

onychoclasis (ŏn-ĭ-kô-klā'sĭs): breaking of the nail.

onychocryptosis (ŏn-ĭ-kô-krĭp-tō'sĭs): ingrowing nail.

onychogryposis (ŏn-ĭ-kô-grī-pō'sĭs): denotes enlargement with increased curvature of the nail.

onycholysis (ŏn-ĭ-kŏl'ĭ-sĭs): loosening of the nail without shedding.

onychomycosis (ŏn-ĭ-kô-mī-kō'sĭs): refers to any parasitic disease of the nails.

onychophagy (ŏn-ĭ-kŏf'ă-jē): the morbid habit of eating or biting the nails.

onychophosis (ŏn-ĭ-kŏf-ō'sĭs): growth of horny epithelium in the nail-bed.

onychophyma (ŏn-ĭ-kŏf-ī'mă): a morbid degeneration of the nail.

onychoptosis (ŏn-ĭ-kŏp-tō'sĭs): falling off of the nails.

onychorrhexis (ŏn-ĭ-kô-rĕk'sĭs): abnormal brittleness of the nails with splitting of free edge.

onychosis; onychonosus (ŏn-ĭ-kō'sĭs; ŏn-ĭ-kô-nō'sûs): any disease of the nails.

onyx (ō'nĭks): a nail of the fingers or toes.

opaque (ō-pāk'): impervious to light rays; neither transparent nor translucent.

optic (ŏp'tĭk): second cranial nerve; the nerve of sight; pertaining to the eye, or to vision.

orangewood stick: a stick made of orangewood used in manicuring the nails.

orbicularis oculi (ôr-bĭk-û-lā'rĭs ŏk'û-lī): orbicularis palpebrarum; the ring muscle of the eye.

orbicularis oris (ō'rĭs): orbicular muscle; muscle of the mouth.

orbit: the bony cavity of the eyeball; the eye-socket.

organic (ôr-găn'ĭk): relating to an organ; pertaining to substances derived from living organisms.

organism (ôr'găn-ĭz'm): any living being, either animal or vegetable.

origin: the beginning; the starting point of a nerve; the place of attachment of a muscle to a bone.

oris (ō'rĭs): peraining to the mouth; an opening.

os (ŏs): a bone.

oscillation (ŏs-ĭ-lā'shûn): movement like a pendulum; a swinging or vibration.

osmidrosis (ŏs-mĭ-drō'sĭs; ŏz-): bromidrosis; foul smelling perspiration.

osmosis (ŏs-mō'sĭs; ŏz-): the passage of fluids a solutions through a membrane or other poro substance.

osseous; osseus (ŏs'ê-ûs): bony.

osteology (ŏs-tê-ŏl'ô-jē): science of the anatom structure, and function of bones.

ovary (ō'vă-rē): one of the two reproductive glan in the female, containing the ova or germ cells

oxidation (ŏk-sĭ-dā'shûn): the act of combin oxygen with another substance.

oxygen: a gaseous element, essential to animal a plant life.

oxygenation (ŏk'sĭ-jê-nā'shûn): saturation w oxygen, noting especially the aeration of the blo in the lungs.

oxymelanin (ŏk'sĭ-mĕl'ă-nĭn): a compound form by a combination of an oxidizing agent with t dark melanin (color) pigments in the hair; (ge erally found in the red to yellow shades).

P

pack: a special cosmetic formula used to beauti the face.

palatine bones (păl'ă-tĭn): situated at the back pa of the nasal depression.

palmar (păl'măr): referring to the palm of the han

papilla, hair (pă-pĭl'ă): a small cone-shaped eleva tion at the bottom of the hair follicle in t dermis.

papillary layer (păp'ĭ-lă-rē): the outer layer of t dermis.

papule (păp'ūl): a pimple; a small, circumscribe elevation on the skin containing no fluid.

para (păr'ă): see para-phenylene-diamine.

para-phenylene-diamine (păr-ă-fēn'ĭ-lēn-dĭ-ăm'ĭ dĭ'ă-mēn): an aniline derivative used in ha tinting.

parasite (păr'ă-sīt): a vegetable or animal organis which lives on or in another organism, and draw its nourishment therefrom.

parasiticide (păr-ă-sĭt'ĭ-sīd): a substance th destroys parasites.

para tint: a tint made from an aniline derivative.

para toluene diamine (păr'ă tŏl'ū-ēn dī-ăm'ĭn): variety of aniline derivative dyes commonly use in preparations compounded to provide red an blonde tones. (meta: prefix meaning higher, c change relating to the position of the amine fre arm on the toluene ring.)

parietal (pă-rī'ê-tâl): pertaining to the wall of cavity; a bone at the side of the head.

paronychia (păr-ô-nĭk'ē-ă): felon; an inflammatio of the tissues surrounding the nail.

parotid (pă-rŏt'ĭd): near the ear; a gland near th ear.

patch test: see predisposition test.

pathogenic (păth-ô-jĕn'ĭk): causing disease; diseas producing.

pathology (păth-ŏl'ô-jē): the science of the natur of disease.

pectoralis (pĕk-tô-rā'lĭs): a muscle of the breast.

pediculosis capitis (pê-dĭk'û-lō'sĭs kăp'ĭ-tĭs): lousi ness of the hair of the head.

pedicure (pĕd'ĭ-kūr): care of feet and toe nails.

penetration (pĕn-ē-trā'shûn): act or power of pene trating.

peptide (pĕp'tīd): a compound of two or more amino acids containing one or more peptide groups continuous filaments in the case of fiber protei or keratin.

peptide bonds: see end bonds.

percarbonate (pĕr-kär′bô-nāt): quantity of salts or esters of carbonic acid.

percussion (pĕr-kŭsh′ûn): a form of massage consisting of repeated light blows or taps of varying force.

pericardium (pĕr-ĭ-kär′dē-ûm): the membranous sac around the heart.

peripheral nervous system (pê-rĭf′ĕr-âl): consists of the nerve endings in the skin and sense organs.

permanent wave, cold: a system of permanent waving employing chemicals rather than heat.

permanent wave, heat: accomplished by changing the hair structure from an ordinary and natural straightness to one of permanent curliness or waviness.

permeable (pûr′mê-ă-b′l): permitting the passage of liquids.

peroxide of hydrogen: a powerful oxidizing agent; in liquid solution it is used as an antiseptic; used in tinting and lightening treatments.

perspiration (pûr′spĭ-rā′shûn): sweat; the fluid excreted from the sweat glands of the skin.

persulfate (pĕr-sŭl′fât): a sulfate which contains more sulfuric acid than the ordinary sulfide.

petrissage (pĕt-rĭ-säj): the kneading movement in massage.

petrolatum (pĕt-rô-lā′tûm): petroleum jelly; Vaseline; a purified, yellow mixture of semi-solid hydrocarbons obtained from petroleum.

petroleum (pê-trô′lê-ûm): an oily liquid coming from the earth and consisting of a mixture of hydrocarbons.

pH: symbol for potential hydrogen concentration; the relative degree of acidity or alkalinity.

pH number: a measure of the degree of acidity or alkalinity of a solution.

phalanx (fā′lănks); pl., **phalanges** (fă-lăn′jēz): the long bone of the finger or toe.

pharynx (făr′ĭnks): the upper portion of the digestive tube, behind the nose and mouth.

phenol (fē′nŏl): carbolic acid; caustic poison; in dilute solution is used as an antiseptic and disinfectant.

phyma (fī′mă); pl., **phymata** (fī′mă-tă): a circumscribed swelling on the skin, larger than a tubercle.

physics (fīz′ĭks): the branch of science that deals with matter, motion, light, heat, electricity, sound and mechanics.

physiology (fīz-ē-ŏl′ô-jē): the science of the functions of living things.

pigment (pĭg′mênt): any organic coloring matter, as that of the red blood cells, the hair, skin, iris, etc.

pigmentation (pĭg′mên-tā′shûn): the deposition of pigment in the skin or tissues.

pilus (pī′lûs); pl., **pili** (-lī): hair.

pimple: any small, pointed elevation of the skin; a papule or small pustule.

pituitary (pĭ-tū′ĭ-târ-ē): a ductless gland located at the base of the brain.

pityriasis (pĭt-ĭ-rī′ă-sĭs): dandruff; an inflammation of the skin characterized by the formation and flaking of fine branny scales.

pityriasis capitis simplex (kăp′ĭ-tĭs sĭm′plĕks): a scalp inflammation marked by dry dandruff or branny scales.

pivot, hair shaping: the exact point from which the hair is directed in forming a curvature or shaping.

plasma (plăz′mă): the fluid part of the blood and lymph.

platelets (plāt′lĕts): blood cells which aid in the forming of clots.

platysma (plă-tĭz′mă): a broad, thin muscle of the neck.

pledget (plĕj′ĕt): a compress or small, flat mass of lint, absorbent cotton, or the like.

plexus (plĕk′sûs): a network of nerves or veins.

pliability (plī-ă-bĭl′ĭ-tē): flexibility.

pneumogastric nerve (nū-mô-găs′trĭk nûrv): vagus nerve; tenth cranial nerve.

polypeptide (pŏl-ē-pĕp′tĭd): strings of amino-acids joined together by peptide bonds, the prefix "poly" meaning many.

pollex (pŏl′ĕks): the thumb.

pomade (pô-mād′): a medicated ointment for the hair.

pore: a small opening of the sweat glands of the skin.

porosity (pô-rŏs′ĭ-tē): ability of the hair to absorb moisture.

porous: full of pores.

positive: affirmative; not negative; the presence of abnormal condition; having a relatively high potential in electricity.

posterior (pōs-tē′rē-ēr): situated behind; coming after or behind.

posterior auricular (ô-rĭk′û-lăr): a nerve which supplies muscles in the posterior surface of the ear.

postiche (pôs-tēsh′): artificial hairpiece; curls, braids, or other extra hairpiece used in creating coiffures.

potassium hydroxide (pô-tăs′ē-ûm hī-drŏk′sīd): a powerful alkali, used in the manufacture of soft soaps.

potassium permanganate (pĕr-măn′gâ-nāt): a salt of permanganate acid; used as an antiseptic and deodorant.

precipitate (prê-sĭp′ĭ-tāt): to cause a substance in solution to settle down in solid particles; to decrease solubility.

predisposition (prē-dĭs-pô-zĭsh′ûn): a condition of special susceptibility to disease; allergy.

predisposition test: a skin test designed to determine an individual's over-sensitivity to certain chemicals (patch test, allergy test, skin test).

pressing: a method of straightening over-curly or kinky hair with a heated comb or iron.

primary colors: pigments or colors that are, or thought to be, fundamental; red, yellow and blue are the primary colors in pigments.

primary hair: the baby fine hair that is present over almost the entire smooth skin of the body.

prism (prĭz′m): a transparent solid with triangular ends and two converging sides; it breaks up white light into its component colors.

procerus (prô-sē′rûs): muscle that covers bridge of the nose.

processing (prŏs′ĕs-ĭng): the action of a chemical in softening and reforming the structure of the hair. (In permanent waving and hair relaxing.)

processing machine: an apparatus employed to hasten the action of the chemical in hair tinting or lightening.

prognosis (prŏg-nō′sĭs): the foretelling of the probable course of a disease.

progressive tints (prô-grĕs′ĭv): hair restorers requiring time to oxidize; color develops gradually.

prong: the round rod of the thermal (marcel) iron.

properties (prŏp′ĕr-tēz): the identifying characteristics of a substance which are observable; a peculiar quality of anything; i.e., color, taste, smell, etc.

prophylaxis (prô-fĭ-lăk′sĭs): prevention of disease.

protective base (prô-tĕk′tĭv): a petroleum base, applied to the entire scalp in order to protect it from the active agents contained in the chemical hair relaxer.

protein: a complex organic substance present in all living tissues, such as skin, hair and nails; necessary in the daily diet; also present in skin and hair conditioners.

protoplasm (prō'tô-plăz'm): the material basis of life; a substance found in all living things.

protozoa (prō-tô-zō'å): subkingdom of animals, including all the unicellular animal organisms.

psoriasis (sô-rī'å-sĭs): a skin disease with circumscribed red patches, covered with adherent white silver scales.

puberty (pū'bĕr-tē): the period of life in which the organs of reproduction are developed.

pull burn: scalp irritation resulting from uneven winding of the hair during permanent waving.

pull test: a test to determine the degree of elasticity of the hair.

pulmonary (pŭl'mô-nâ-rē): relating to the lungs.

pumice (pŭm'ĭs): hardened volcanic substance, white or gray in color, used for buffing in manicuring; also called pumice stone.

purification (pū-rĭ-fĭ-kā'shŭn): the act of cleaning or removing foreign matter.

pus: a fluid product of inflammation, consisting of a liquid containing leucocytes and the debris of dead cells and tissue elements.

pusher: a steel instrument used to loosen the cuticle from the nail.

pustule (pŭs'tūl): an inflamed pimple containing pus.

Q

quadratus labii superioris (kwŏd-rā'tŭs lā'bē-ī sû-pē'rē-ôr'ĭs): a muscle of the upper lip.

quarantine (kwŏr'ân-tēn): the isolation of a person to prevent spread of a contagious disease.

quinine (kwī'nĭn): enters into the composition of many hair lotions in small quantities; its effect is slightly antiseptic.

R

radial nerve (rā'dê-ăl): a nerve which affects the arm and hand.

radiation (rā-dê-ā'shŭn): the process of giving off light or heat rays.

radius (rā'dê-ûs): the outer and smaller bone of the forearm.

rash: a skin eruption having little or no elevation.

ratting: see teasing.

reconditioning (rē-kŏn-dĭ'shŭn-ĭng): the application of a special substance to the hair in order to improve its condition.

rectifier (rĕk'tĭ-fĭ-ēr): an apparatus to change an alternating current of electricity into a direct current.

rectus (rĕk'tûs): in a straight line; the name of small muscles of the eye.

reddish cast: a tinge of red.

reducing agent: a substance capable of adding hydrogen; in cosmetology, a cold wave solution would be a reducing agent.

reflex: an involuntary nerve reaction.

relaxer (rē-lăk'sēr): a chemical applied to the hair to remove the natural curl.

relaxer testing: checking the action of the relaxer in order to determine the speed at which the natural curl is being removed.

reproductive (rē-prô-dŭk'tĭv): pertaining to reproduction or the process by which plants and animals give rise to offspring.

resilient (rê-zĭl'ĭ-ĕnt): elastic.

resistance (rē-zĭst'âns): the difficulty of moisture or chemical solutions to penetrate the hair shaft.

respiration (rĕs-pĭ-rā'shŭn): the act of breathing; the process of inhaling air into the lungs and expelling it.

respiratory system (rê-spīr'å-tô-rē): consists of the nose, pharynx, larynx, trachea, bronchi and lungs which assist in breathing.

rete (rē'tê): any interlacing of either blood vessels or nerves.

reticular layer (rê-tĭk'û-lâr): the inner layer of the corium.

retina (rĕt'ĭ-nă): the sensitive membrane of the eye which receives the image formed by the lens.

retouch: application of hair color, lightener or chemical hair relaxer to new growth of hair.

reversible (rē-vērs'ĭ-b'l): capable of going through a series of changes in either direction, forward or backward, as a reversible chemical reaction.

rhagades (răg'å-dēz): cracks, fissures or chaps on the skin.

rickettsia (rĭk-ĕt'sê-ä): a type of pathogenic microorganism, capable of producing disease.

ringed hair: a variety of canities in which the hair appears white or colored in rings.

ringworm: a vegetable parasitic disease of the skin and its appendages which appears in circular lesions and is contagious.

rinse: to cleanse with a second or repeated application of water after washing; a prepared rinse water.

risorius (rĭ-zôr'ē-ûs): muscle at the side of the mouth.

rolling: a massage movement in which the tissues are pressed and twisted.

root: in anatomy, the base; the foundation or beginning of any part.

rotary (rō'tå-rē): circular motion of the fingers as in massage.

ruffing (rŭf'ĭng): back combing; teasing of the hair.

S

saccular (săk'û-lâr): consisting of little sacs, such as oil glands.

sachet (så-shā'): a perfumed bag or pad.

saline (sā'līn): salty; containing salt.

saliva (så-lī'vå): the secretion of the salivary glands; spittle.

salt: in chemistry, the union of a base with an acid.

sanitary (săn'ĭ-tâ-rē): pertaining to cleanliness in relation to health; tending to promote health.

sanitation (săn-ĭ-tā'shŭn): the use of methods to bring about favorable conditions of health.

sanitize: to make sanitary.

saprophyte (săp'rô-fĭt): a micro-organism which grows normally on dead matter, as distinguished from a parasite.

S-bonds: see: sulphur bonds.

scab: a crust formed on the surface of a sore.

scabies (skā'bĭ-ēz): a skin disease caused by an animal parasite, attended with intense itching; the itch.

scale: any thin plate of horny epidermis; regular markings used as a standard in measuring and weighing.

scalp: the skin covering of the cranium.

scapula (skăp'û-lå): the shoulder blade; a large, flat, triangular bone of the shoulder.

scar: a mark remaining after a wound has healed.

scarf skin: epidermis.

science: knowledge duly arranged and systematized

scurf (skûrf): thin, dry scales or scabs on the body, especially on the scalp; dandruff.

sebaceous cyst (sē-bā'shŭs sĭst): a distended, oily or fatty follicle or sac.

sebaceous glands: oil glands of the skin.

seborrhea (sĕb-ō-rē'ā): an oily condition caused by the over-action of the sebaceous glands.

seborrhea capitis (kăp'ĭ-tĭs): seborrhea of the scalp, commonly called dandruff; pityriasis.

seborrhea oleosa (ō-lē-ō'sā): excessive oiliness of the skin, particularly of the forehead and nose.

seborrhea sicca (sĭk'ā): an accumulation on the scalp, of greasy scales or crusts, due to over-action of the sebaceous glands; dandruff or pityriasis.

seborrheic (sĕb-ō-rē'ĭk): seborrheal; pertaining to the over-action of the sebaceous glands.

sebum (sē'bŭm): the fatty or oily secretions of the sebaceous glands.

secondary hair: the stiff, short, coarse hair found on the eyelashes, eyebrows and within the openings or passages of the nose and ears.

secretion (sē-krē'shŭn): a product manufactured by a gland for a special purpose.

sectioning (sĕk'shŭn-ĭng): dividing the hair into separate parts.

senility (sē-nĭl'ĭ-tē): quality or state of being old.

sensation (sĕn-sā'shŭn): a feeling or impression arising as the result of the stimulation of an afferent nerve.

sensitivity (sĕn-sĭ-tĭv'ĭ-tē): the state of being easily affected by certain chemicals or external conditions.

sensory nerve: afferent nerve; a nerve carrying sensations.

sepsis (sĕp'sĭs): the presence of various pus-forming and other pathogenic organisms, or their toxins, in the blood or tissues; septicemia.

septic (sĕp'tĭk): relating to or caused by sepsis.

septum (sĕp'tŭm): a dividing wall; a partition.

serratus anterior (sē-rā'tŭs ăn-tē'rē-ôr): a muscle of the chest assisting in breathing and in raising the arm.

shaft: slender, stem-like structure; the long, slender part of the hair above the scalp.

shampoo: to subject the scalp and hair to washing and massaging with some cleansing agent, such as soap and water.

shaping, haircutting: the process of shortening and thinning the hair to a particular style or to the contour of the head.

shaping, hairstyling: the formation of uniform arcs or curves in wet hair, thus providing a base for finger waves, pin curls or various patterns in hairstyling.

sheath: a covering enclosing or surrounding some organ.

shingling: cutting the hair close to the nape of the neck and gradually longer toward the crown.

shortwave: a form of high-frequency current used in permanent hair removal.

singeing: process of lightly burning hair ends with a lighted wax taper.

single application tints: products which lighten and add color to the hair in a single application; also called one process or one step tints.

sinus (sī'nŭs): a cavity or depression; a hollow in bone or other tissue.

skeletal muscles (skĕl'ē-tâl): muscles connected to the skeleton.

skeleton: the bony framework of the body.

skin: the external covering of the body.

skin texture: the general feel and appearance of the skin.

skull: the bony case or the framework of the head.

slicing: carefully removing a section of hair from a shaping in preparation for making a pin curl.

slip: a smooth and slippery feeling imparted by talc to face powder.

slippage: the shifting and changing of position of the sulphur bonds.

slithering (slĭth'ĕr-ĭng): tapering the hair to graduated lengths with scissors.

smaller occipital (ŏk-sĭp'ĭ-tâl): sensory nerve affecting skin behind the ear.

soap cap: a solution of equal parts of shampoo, hydrogen peroxide and tint; employed when a slight change in color is desired.

soapless shampoo: a shampoo made with sulfonated oil, alcohol, mineral oil and water; this type of shampoo does not foam, and is usually alkaline in reaction.

sodium (sō'dē-ŭm): a metallic element of the alkaline group.

sodium bicarbonate (bī-kär'bôn-āt): baking soda; it relieves burns, bites; is often used in bath powders as an aid to cleansing oily skin.

sodium carbonate (kär'bôn-āt): washing soda; used to prevent corrosion of metallic instruments when added to boiling water.

sodium hydroxide (hī-drŏk'sīd): a powerful alkaline product used in some chemical hair relaxers; caustic soda.

sodium lauryl sulfite (lô'rĕl sŭl'fīt): a metallic element of the alkaline group, in white or light yellow crystals; used in detergents.

sodium perborate (pēr'bō-rāt): a compound, formed by treating sodium peroxide with boric acid; on dissolving the substance in water, peroxide of hydrogen is generated; used as an antiseptic.

sodium sulphite (sŭl'fīt): a soft, white metallic salt of sulphurous acid.

softening: the application of a chemical product to hair in order to make it more receptive to hair coloring or permanent waving.

solar (sō'lâr): pertaining to the sun.

solarium (sō-lă'rē-ŭm): a sun parlor.

solubility (sŏl-û-bĭl'ĭ-tē): the extent to which a substance (solute) dissolves in a liquid (solvent) to produce a homogeneous system (solution).

solute (sŏl'ūt): the dissolved substance in a solution.

solution: the act or process by which a substance is absorbed into a liquid.

solvent (sŏl'vĕnt): an agent capable of dissolving substances.

spatula (spăt'û-lă): a flexible, knife-like implement for handling creams and pomades, etc.

spectrum (spĕk'trŭm): the band of rainbow colors produced by decomposing light by means of a prism.

sphenoid (sfē'noid): wedge-shaped; a bone in the cranium.

spinal accessory (spī'nâl ăk-sĕs'ō-rē): eleventh cranial nerve.

spinal column: the backbone or vertebral column.

spinal cord: the portion of the central nervous system contained within the spinal, or vertebral canal.

spinal nerves: the nerves arising from the spinal cord.

spine: a short process of bone; the backbone.

spiral: coil; winding around a center, like a watch spring.

spirillum (spī-rĭl'ûm); pl., **spirilla** (-ă): curved bacterium.

splash neutralizer: a chemical agent capable of stopping the action of the cold waving solution and setting or hardening the hair in its new form.

spore (spôr): a tiny bacterial body having a protective wall to withstand unfavorable conditions.

spray gum: a sticky juice applied as a liquid going through the air in small drops.

squama (skwā'mă): an epidermic scale made up of thin, flat cells.

stabilized: made stable or firm, preventing changes.

stabilizer: see fixative.

stable: in a balanced condition; not readily destroyed or decomposed; resisting molecular change.

stain: an abnormal skin discoloration.

staphylococcus (stăf-ĭ-lō-kŏk'ŭs): cocci which are grouped in clusters like a bunch of grapes; found in pustules and boils.

static electricity: a form of electricity generated by friction.

steamer, facial: an apparatus, used in place of hot towels, for steaming the scalp or face.

stearic acid (stē-ăr'ĭk): a white, fatty acid, occuring in solid animal fats and in some of the vegetable fats.

steatoma (stē-ă-tō'mă): a sebaceous cyst; a fatty tumor.

steatosis (stē-ă-tō'sĭs): fatty degeneration; adiposis.

stem direction: the direction in which the stem moves from the base to the first arc.

stem, pin curl: that part of the pin curl between the base and the first arc of the circle.

sterilization: the process of making sterile; the destruction of germs.

sterno-cleido-mastoideus (stûr'nō-klī'dō-măs-toid'ê-ŭs): a muscle of the neck which depresses and rotates the head.

stimulation (stĭm-û-lā'shŭn) the act arousing increased functional activity.

stomach: the dilated portion of the alimentary canal, in which the first process of digestion takes place.

strand test: a preliminary test given before a tint or lightening application to determine the required development time; a test to determine the degree of porosity and elasticity of the hair, as well as the ability of the hair to withstand the effects of chemicals.

stratum (strā'tŭm); pl., **strata** (-ă): layer of tissue.

stratum corneum (kôr'nê-ŭm): horny layer of the skin.

stratum germinativum (jûr-mĭ-nā'tĭv-ŭm): the deepest layer of the epidermis resting on the corneum.

stratum granulosum (grăn-û-lō'sŭm): granular layer of the skin.

stratum lucidum (lū'sĭ-dŭm): clear layer of the skin.

stratum mucosum (mū-kō'sŭm): mucous or malpighian layer of the skin.

streaking (strēk'ĭng): lightening broad sections of hair attractively placed around the face.

streptococcus (strĕp-tō-kŏk'ŭs): pus-forming bacteria that arrange in curved lines resembling a string of beads; found in erysipelas and blood poisoning.

striated (strī'ăt-ĕd): marked with parallel lines or bands; striped; voluntary muscle.

stripping: the removal of color from the hair shaft; lightening. Strong shampoos or soap removing some of the color from the hair is also known as stripping.

stroking: a gliding movement over a surface; to pass the fingers or any instrument gently over a surface; effleurage.

strontium sulphide (strŏn'shê-ŭm sŭl'fīd): a light gray powder capable of liberating hydrogen sulphide in the presence of water; used as a depilatory.

styptic (stĭp'tĭk): an agent causing contraction living tissue; used to stop bleeding; an astring

subcutaneous (sŭb-kū-tă'nē-ŭs): under the skir

subcutis (sŭb-kū'tĭs): subdermis; subcutane tissue; under or beneath the corium or derr the true skin.

subdermis (sŭb-dûr'mĭs): subcutis or subcutane tissue of the skin.

submental artery (sŭb-mĕn'tâl är'tĕr-ē): suppl blood to the chin and lower lip.

sudamen (sû-dā'mĕn); pl., **sudamina** (sû-dăm'ĭ-n a disorder of the sweat glands with obstruct of their ducts.

sudoriferous glands (sū-dôr-ĭf'ĕr-ûs glăndz): sw glands of the skin.

sulfite (sŭl'fīt): any salt or sulfurous acid.

sulfonated oil (sŭl'fôn-āt-êd): an organic substa prepared by reacting oils with sulphuric acid; an alkaline reaction and is miscible with wat used as a base in soapless shampoos.

sulphide (sŭl'fīd): a compound of sulphur w another element or base.

sulphur (sŭl'fûr): a chemical element whose co pounds are used in lightening, in hair preparatic and in medicine.

sulphur bonds: sulphur cross bonds in the ha which hold the chains of amino-acids together order to form a hair strand.

supercilium (sū-pĕr-sĭl'ē-ûm); pl., **supercilia** (- the eyebrow.

suppuration (sŭp-û-rā'shûn): the formation of p

supraorbital (sū-pră-ôr'bĭ-tâl): above the orbit eye.

supra-trochlear (sū-pră-trŏk'lē-âr): above t trochlea or pulley of the superior oblique musc

surface tension: the tension or resistance to ruptu possessed by the surface film of a liquid.

susceptible (sû-sĕp'tĭ-b'l): capable of being inf enced or easily acted on.

suspension (sû-spĕn'shûn): a mixture of a liqu and insoluble particles which have a tenden to settle on standing.

swirl: formation of a wave in a diagonal directi from back to side of head.

switch: long wefts of hair, tail-like in formatic mounted with a loop at the end.

sympathetic nervous system (sĭm-pă-thĕt'ĭk): co trols the involuntary muscles which affe respiration, circulation and digestion.

symptom, objective (sĭmp'tôm, ŏb-jĕk'tĭv): th which can be seen, as in pimples, pustules, etc.

symptom, subjective (sŭb-jĕk'tĭv): can be felt, in itching.

system: a group of organs which especially co tribute toward one of the more important vit functions.

systematic: proceeding according to system regular method.

systemic (sĭs-tĕm'ĭk): pertaining to a system or the body as a whole.

T

tactile corpuscle (tăk'tĭl kôr'pŭs-'l): touch nerv endings found within the skin.

tannic acid (tăn'ĭk): a plant extract used as astringent.

tapotement (tà-pôt-män'): a massage moveme using a short, quick slapping or tapping mov ment.

tapping: a massage movement; striking lightly wit partly flexed fingers.

tartaric acid (tär′tâ-rĭk): a colorless crystalline acid compound.

teasing: combing small sections of hair from the ends toward the scalp, causing the shorter hair to mat at the scalp, forming a cushion or base. Also known as ratting, French lacing or ruffing.

temple: the flattened space on the side of the forehead.

temporal bone (tĕm′pô-râl): the bone at the side and base of the skull.

temporalis (tĕm-pô-rā′lĭs): the temporal muscle.

tendon: fibrous cord or band connecting muscle with bone.

tensile (tĕn′sĭl): capable of being stretched.

tension: stress caused by stretching or pulling.

terminology (tĕr-mĭ-nŏl′ô-jē): the special words or terms used in science, art or business.

tertiary (terminal) hair (tĕr′shĕ-â-rē hâr): the long, soft hair found on the scalp.

test curls: a method to determine how the patron's hair will react to permanent waving solution and neutralizer.

test, hair tint: a test made upon the scalp, behind the ear, or in the bend of the arm, for predisposition to the agent used; a test to determine the reaction of the color upon the sample strand, regarding both color and breakage.

tetanus (tĕt′â-nŭs): a disease with spasmodic and continuous contraction of the muscles; lockjaw.

textometer (tĕks-tŏm′e-tĕr): a device used to measure the elasticity and reaction of the hair to alkaline solutions.

texture of hair: the general quality as to coarse, medium or fine; feel of the hair.

texture of skin: the general feel and appearance of the skin.

thallium (thă′lĭ-ŭm): a bluish-white metallic element, the salts of which have been used for epilation; thallium is highly toxic to humans.

therapeutic lamp (thĕr-â-pū′tĭk): an electrical apparatus producing any of the various rays of the spectrum; used for skin and scalp treatments.

therapy (thĕr′â-pē): the science and art of healing.

thermal (thûr′mâl): relating to heat.

thermal curling: the process of forming curls with thermal irons.

thermal hair straightening: straightening over-curly hair with heated thermal irons.

thermal irons: an implement used to curl, wave or straighten hair by the application of heat.

thermal waving: forming waves in the hair with heated thermal iron.

thermostat (thûr′mô-stăt): an automatic device for regulating temperature.

thinning, hair: decreasing the thickness of the hair where it is too heavy.

thio (thī′ō): see ammonium thioglycolate.

thioglycolic acid (thī-ô-glĭ′kô-lĭk): a colorless liquid or white crystals with a strong unpleasant odor, miscible with water, alcohol or ether; (used in permanent wave solutions, hair relaxers and depilatories.)

thorax (thō′răks): the part of the body between the neck and the abdomen; the chest.

thrombocyte (thrŏm′bô-sīt): a blood platelet which aids in clotting.

thyroid gland (thī′roid): a large, ductless gland situated in the neck.

tincture (tĭnk′tûr): an alcoholic solution of a medicinal substance.

tinea (tĭn′ē-â): a skin disease, especially ringworm.

tint: to give a coloring to; as used in cosmetology, pertaining to hair tinting; to color the hair by means of a hair tint or color rinse.

tinting: the process of adding artificial color to hair.

tipping: similar to frosting, but the darkening or lightening is confined to small strands of hair at the front of the head.

tissue: a collection of similar cells which perform a particular function.

tissue, connective (kŏ-nĕk′tĭv): binding and supporting tissue.

toluene diamine (tŏl′ū-ēn dī-ăm′ĭn): a colorless liquid, obtained from a coal tar product, used as a solvent and also in a drug designed to increase the amount of bile secreted.

tone: healthy functioning of the body or its parts.

toner: an aniline derivative tint applied to highly lightened hair to achieve a pale, delicate color.

tonic: increasing the strength or tone of the system.

toupee (tōō-pē′): a small wig used to cover the top or crown of a man's head.

toxemia (tŏk-sē′mē-â): form of blood poisoning.

toxin; toxine (tŏk′sĭn; -sēn): a poisonous substance of undetermined chemical nature, elaborated during the growth of pathogenic micro-organisms.

tracheo (trā′kĕ-â; tră-kē′â): wind pipe.

translucent (trăns-lū′sênt): somewhat transparent.

transformation (trăns-fôr-mā′shŭn): an artificial band of hair worn over a person's own hair.

transformer (trăns-fôr′mĕr): used for the purpose of increasing or decreasing the voltage of the current used; it can only be used on an alternating current.

transverse facial (trăns-vûrs′): an artery supplying the skin, the parotid gland and the masseter muscle.

trapezius (tră-pē′zē-ûs): muscle that draws the head backward and sideways.

triangularis (trī-ăn-gû-lā′rĭs): a muscle that pulls down the corner of the mouth.

triceps (trī′sĕps): three-headed.

trichology (trĭ-kŏl′ô-jē): the science of the care of the hair.

trichonosus (trĭk-ô-nō′sûs): any disease of the hair.

trichophytosis (trĭ-kŏf-ĭ-tō′sĭs): ringworm of the skin and scalp, due to growth of a fungus parasite.

trichoptilosis (trĭ-kŏp-tĭ-lō′sĭs): a splitting of the hair ends, giving them a feathery appearance.

trichorrhexis (trĭk-ô-rĕk′sĭs): brittleness of the hair.

trichosis (trĭ-kō-sĭs): abnormal growth of hair.

trifacial: the fifth cranial nerve; also known as the triceminal nerve.

trigeminal (trī-jĕm′ĭ-nâl): relating to the fifth cranial or trigeminus nerve.

true skin: the corium.

trypsin (trĭp′sĭn): an enzyme in the digestive juice secreted by the pancreas; trypsin changes proteins into peptones.

tubercle (tū′bĕr-k′l): a rounded, solid elevation on the skin or membrane.

tumor: a swelling; an abnormal enlargement.

turbinal; turbinate (tûr′bĭ-nâl; -năt): a bone in the nose; turbinated body.

tweezers: a pair of small forceps to remove or extract hair.

tyrosine (tī-rō′sĭn): an amino-acid widely distributed in proteins, particularly in casein.

U

ulcer (ŭl′sĕr): an open sore not caused by a wound.

ulna (ŭl′nă): the inner and larger bone of the forearm.

ultra-violet: invisible rays of the spectrum which are beyond the violet rays.

unadulterated (ŭn-â-dŭl′tĕr-āt-ĕd): pure.

undulation (ŭn-dû-lā′shûn): a wave-like movement or shape.

unguentum (ŭn-gwĕn′tûm); pl., **unguenta** (-ă): a salve or ointment.

unguis (ŭn′gwĭs)); pl., **ungues** (-gwēz): the nail of a finger or toe.

unguium, tinea (ŭn′gwē-ŭm, tĭn′ê-ă): ringworm of the nails.

unit: a single thing or value.

United States Pharmacopeia (U.S.P.) (fär-mà-kô-pē′yà): an official book of drug and medicinal standards.

unstable: liable to fade.

urea (ū-rē′à): a diuretic; also employed externally in treating infected wounds; occurs as colorless to white crystals or powder; soluble in water.

urea peroxide: a combination of urea and peroxide in the form of a cream developer or activator; employed in hair tinting.

V

vaccination (văk-sĭ-nā′shûn): inoculation with the virus of cowpox, or vaccina, as a means of producing immunity against small pox.

vaccine (văk′sĭn; -sēn): any substance used for preventive inoculation.

vacuum (văk′ū-ûm): a space from which most of the air has been exhausted.

vagus (vā′gûs): pneumogastric nerve; tenth cranial nerve.

vapor: the gaseous state of a liquid or solid.

varicose veins (văr′ĭ-kōs): swollen or knotted veins.

vascular (văs′kû-lăr): supplied with small blood vessels; pertaining to a vessel for the conveyance of a fluid as blood or lymph.

Vaseline (văs′ê-lĭn; ēn): a tradename; petrolatum; a semi-solid greasy or oily mixture of hydrocarbons obtained from petroleum.

vein; vena (vē′nà): a blood vessel carrying blood toward the heart.

vena cava (kā′và): one of the large veins which carries the blood to the right auricle of the heart.

ventilate: to renew the air in a place.

ventricle (vĕn′trĭ-k′l): a small cavity; particularly in the heart.

vermin (vûr′mĭn): parasitic insects, as lice and bedbugs.

verruca (vĕ-rōō′kà): a wart; a growth of the papillae and epidermis.

vertebra (vûr′tĕ-brà); pl., **vertebrae** (-brē): a bony segment of the spinal column.

vesicle (vĕs′ĭ-k′l): a small blister or sac; a small elevation on the skin.

vibrator (vī′brà-tēr): an electrically driven massage apparatus causing a swinging, shaking sensation on the body, producing stimulation.

violet-ray: high-frequency; Tesla; an electric current of medium voltage and medium amperage.

virgin hair: normal hair which has had no previous lightening or tinting treatments.

virus (vī′rûs): poison; the specific poison of an infectious disease.

viscid (vĭs′ĭd): sticky or adhesive.

viscosity (vĭs-kŏs′ĭ-tē): 1) resistance to change of form; 2) a resistance to flow that a liquid exhibits; 3) the degree of density, thickness, stickiness and adhesiveness of a substance.

viscous (vĭs′kûs): sticky or gummy.

visible rays: light rays which can be seen; are visible to the eye.

vitiligo (vĭt-ĭ-lī′gō): milky-white spots of the skin.

volatile (vŏl′à-tĭl): easily evaporating; diffusing freely; not permanent.

volt: the fractional unit of electromotive force.

voltage: electrical potential difference expressed in volts.

voluntary: under the control of the will.

vomer (vō′mēr): the thin plate of bone between the nostrils.

W

wart (wôrt): verruca.

water, hard: water containing certain minerals; does not lather with soap.

water, soft: water which readily lathers with soap; relatively free of minerals.

water softener: certain chemicals, such as the carbonate or phosphate of sodium, used to soften hard water to permit the lathering of soap.

wattage (wŏt′åj): amount of electric power expressed in watts.

wave, cold: a method of permanent waving requiring the use of certain chemicals rather than heat.

wave, finger: arranging waves into the hair, which has been wet with fingers and comb.

wave, marcel: thermal wave produced by means of heated thermal irons.

wave, permanent: a wave given to the hair which is of permanent duration.

wave, pin curl: alternating the direction of rows of pin curls in order to form a wave pattern.

wave, shadow: a wave with low ridges and shallow waves.

wave, skip: a pattern formed by a combination of alternating ridges and curls.

weft (wĕft): an artificial section of woven hair used for practice work or as a substitute for natural hair.

wen (wĕn): a sebaceous cyst, usually on the scalp.

wetting agent: a substance that causes a liquid to spread more readily on a solid surface, chiefly through a reduction of surface tension.

wheal (whēl): a raised ridge on the skin, usually caused by a blow, a bite of an insect, urticaria, or sting of a nettle.

whitehead (whĭt′hĕd): milium.

whorl (whûrl; whôrl): a spiral turn, in general; a hair whorl or cowlick; a spiral turn causing a tuft of hair which goes contrary to the usual growth of the hair.

wig: an artificial covering for the head consisting of a network of interwoven hair.

wiglet: a hairpiece with a flat base which is used in special areas of the head.

winding, croquignole (krō′kwĭ-nōl): winding under the hair, from the hair ends towards the scalp.

winding, spiral (spī′râl): winding the hair from the scalp to the ends.

wind pipe: trachea.

wrapping: winding hair on rollers or rods in order to form curls.

wrinkle: a small ridge or a furrow.

Z

zinc sulphate (sŭl′fāt): a salt often employed as an astringent, both in lotions and creams.

zinc sulphocarbonate (zĭnk sŭl-fô-kär′bôn-āt): a fine white powder having the odor of carbolic acid; used as an antiseptic and astringent in deodorant preparations.

zygomatic (zī-gô-măt′ĭk): pertaining to the malar or cheek bone.

zygomaticus (zī-gô-măt′ĭ-kûs): a muscle that draws the upper lip upward and outward.

CROSS INDEX

BIBLIOGRAPHY

In the revision of this textbook, the following basic references and authorities were consulted. The books herein listed can be purchased directly from the Milady Publishing Corp., 3839 White Plains Road, Bronx, New York 10467.

BASIC REFERENCES:

Air Jet Hairstyling—Michael D. Morro
A Man's Guide to Business and Social Success—Ruth Tolman
Beautician's Guide to Beauty, Charm and Poise—Ruth Tolman
Chemistry in Your Beauty Shop—Arnold Lowman, Ph.D.
Common Skin Diseases—H. Goodman, M.D.
Curling Iron Techniques with Directional Design—Mary Lou Augustine
Electricity and Light—Noble M. Eberhart, M.D.
Electrolysis, Thermolysis and the Blend—Arthur R. Hinkel
Gray's Anatomy—Warren H. Lewis
Hair Structure and Chemistry Simplified—A. H. Powitt
Harry's Cosmetology—Ralph G. Harry
Human Anatomy and Physiology—Dr. King and Dr. Showers
New Gould's Medical Dictionary—G. M. Gould, A.M., M.D.
Salesmanship in the Beauty Salon—Margaret B. Fleck
Standard Textbook for Professional Estheticians—Joel Gerson
Stedman's Practical Medical Dictionary—Norman B. Taylor, M.D.
Synopsis of Diseases of the Skin—Sutton and Sutton
The Complete Guide to Wigs and Hairpieces—Rebecca Hyman
The Make-Up Artist in the Beauty Salon—Vincent J-R Kehoe
The Scalp in Health and Disease—Howard T. Behrman, A.B., M.D.
Van Dean Manual—Dean Barrett
Your Skin and Its Care—Dr. Behrman and Dr. Levin

TRADE PERIODICALS:

National Beauty School Journal
Modern Salon
American Hairdresser/Salon Owner

The publisher expresses sincere thanks to those manufacturers and cosmetology educators who so willingly cooperated in the revision of this text.

ANSWERS TO REVIEW QUESTIONS

Chapter 1
HYGIENE AND GOOD GROOMING
(Answers to Questions on Page 4)

1. a) The science of healthful living. b) The care given by the individual to preserve his/her health. c) Sanitary measures taken by the government to promote public health. d) Keeping teeth and gums in good condition by brushing at least twice a day and using a mouth wash to sweeten the breath.
2. Cleanliness, oral hygiene, good posture, sufficient exercise, relaxation, adequate sleep, balanced diet, and wholesome thoughts.
3. Providing pure air, pure food, pure water, adequate sewerage, control of disease, and adequate medical facilities.
4. Cheerfulness, courage, and hope.
5. Worry and fear.
6. Clean.
7. Deodorant.
8. Mouth wash.

Chapter 2
VISUAL POISE
(Answers to Questions on Page 10)

1. Prevents fatigue, improves personal appearance, permits moving with ease and grace.
2. Regular exercise keeps the muscles of the body in good condition.
3. 45.
4. Up; floor; up; flat.
5. Together.
6. Floor.
7. Chair.
8. It will help to avoid fatigue and back strain.
9. Sit towards the back of the chair.
10. They give the body support and balance which help maintain good posture.
11. Low-heeled.
12. Daily foot care helps to maintain good posture.

Chapter 3
PERSONALITY DEVELOPMENT
(Answers to Questions on Page 16)

1. Personality is the outward reflection of your inner feelings, habits, attitudes, and values.
2. By developing the ability to handle both the good and bad experiences of life.
3. A pleasing personality is vital to a successful career in cosmetology.
4. A smile of greeting and a word of welcome.
5. Thoughtfulness of others.
6. Success.
7. Sincerity, intelligence, friendliness, vitality, flexibility, and expressiveness.
8. Because patrons will enjoy being with you and, therefore, they will seek your services.
9. Liveliness.
10. The use of voice, words, intelligence, charm, and personality.
11. Grammar.
12. Fashions, personal grooming, education, and literature.
13. Manners.

Chapter 4
PROFESSIONAL ETHICS
(Answers to Questions on Page 20)

1. Ethics deal with proper conduct and business dealings in relation to employers, patrons, and co-workers.
2. Courtesy, honesty, obeying the cosmetology law, and keeping your word.
3. Repeating gossip will cause loss of confidence.
4. Slovenliness in dress or hygiene is offensive.
5. Harsh, rough treatment chases patrons away.
6. Lowers the dignity of cosmetology as a profession.
7. State board members are acting in line of duty and contribute to the higher standards of cosmetology.
8. By complying with the cosmetology laws, the cosmetologist is contributing to the health, welfare, and safety of the community.

Chapter 5
BACTERIOLOGY
(Answers to Questions on Page 26)

1. Bacteriology is the science or study of microorganisms, called bacteria.
2. A knowledge of the relationship between bacteria and disease will help students to understand the need for salon cleanliness and sanitation.
3. Bacteria are minute, one-celled, vegetable microorganisms found nearly everywhere.
4. Germs and microbes.
5. They are very small; 1500 rod-shaped bacteria barely reach across a pinhead.
6. a) Non-pathogenic bacteria—non-disease producing, beneficial or harmless type. b) Pathogenic bacteria—disease producing and harmful type.
7. a) Parasites are bacteria that live on living matter. b) Saprophytes are bacteria that live on dead organic matter.
8. Cocci—round shape; bacilli—rod shape; and spirilla—corkscrew shape.
9. a) Staphylococci. b) Streptococci.
10. Each bacteria divides in the middle, forming two cells that grow to full size and then produce again.
11. Staphylococci and streptococci.
12. a) Certain bacteria form spherical spores with tough outer coverings during their inactive stage in order to withstand adverse conditions. b) Anthrax and tetanus.
13. An infection occurs when pathogenic bacteria and other harmful toxins enter the body and the body is unable to cope with them.
14. A local infection is indicated by a boil or pimple that contains pus. A general infection, such as blood poisoning, results when bacteria or their poisons enter the bloodstream and are carried to all parts of the body.
15. One that may be spread from one person to another by contact.
16. Tuberculosis, common cold, ringworm, scabies, head lice, and virus infections.
17. Through the mouth, nose, eyes or ears, and a break in the skin.

18. Unbroken skin; body secretions, such as perspiration; white blood cells; and antitoxins.
19. By the practice of personal hygiene and public sanitation at all times.
20. Immunity is the ability of the body to resist infection by destroying bacteria once they have gained entrance.
21. Natural immunity means natural resistance to disease. Acquired immunity is achieved after the body has overcome certain diseases by itself or has received inoculations against these diseases.
22. A human disease carrier is a person who, although immune to the disease himself, can infect other persons with the germs of the disease. Two examples are diphtheria and typhoid fever.
23. Disinfectants, intense heat such as boiling, steaming or burning, and ultra-violet rays.

Chapter 6
STERILIZATION AND SANITATION
(Answers to Questions on Page 35)
Sterilization and Sanitation
1. Sterilization is the process of making an object germfree by the destruction of all kinds of bacteria, whether beneficial or harmful.
2. Sanitize.
3. Those germs responsible for infections and communicable diseases.
4. Infections and communicable diseases.
5. Asepsis—freedom from disease germs; sterile—free from all germs; and sepsis—poisoning due to pathogenic bacteria.
6. A chemical agent that may kill or retard the growth of bacteria.
7. No. All have the power to destroy bacteria, both harmful and harmless.
8. A chemical agent that destroys bacteria.
9. A vapor used to keep clean objects sanitary.
10. Chemical.
11. Ultra-violet rays and vapors keep objects clean after they have been sanitized.
12. Convenient to prepare, quick acting, practically odorless, non-corrosive, economical, and non-irritating to skin.
13. Quats.
14. A receptacle containing a disinfectant solution in which objects to be sanitized can be completely immersed.
15. Remove all hair. Wash them thoroughly with hot water and soap. Rinse them thoroughly.
16. To prevent contamination of the solution.
17. They are removed from the disinfectant solution, rinsed in clear water, wiped dry with a clean towel, and stored in a dry cabinet sanitizer until needed.
18. An airtight cabinet containing an active fumigant.
19. Place one tablespoon of borax and one tablespoon of formalin on a small tray on the bottom of a cabinet sanitizer.
20. Short disinfection time, odorless, non-toxic, and stable.
21. 1:1000 solution.
22. a) 1-5 minutes. b) 10 minutes. c) 20 minutes.
23. Formalin.
24. Formalin is a 37-40% solution of formaldehyde gas in water.
25. 25%.
26. Rub the surface with a cotton pad dampened with 70% alcohol.

27. Gently rub exposed surface of electrodes with a cotton pad dampened with 70% alcohol.
28. Any six of the following: a) Purchase in small quantities. b) Carefully weigh and measure chemicals. c) Keep all containers labeled, covered, and under lock and key. d) Do not smell chemicals or solutions. e) Avoid spilling when diluting chemicals. f) Prevent burns by using forceps to insert and remove objects from source of heat.

Public Sanitation
1. Public sanitation is the application of measures to promote public health and prevent spread of infectious diseases.
2. To insure protection of the patron's health.
3. To prevent disease.
4. A patron with an infectious disease is a source of contagion to others.
5. State board of cosmetology and board of health.
6. Keep in closed container and remove it regularly.
7. Before and after serving a patron and after leaving the rest room.
8. In a sanitized, closed cabinet.
9. Headrest coverings must be changed for each patron.
10. Remove creams with a clean spatula.
11. Face powder must be kept in closed containers and applied to the face with sterile cotton pledgets.
12. The responsibility for sanitation rests with each student.
13. It should be sanitized before being used on a patron.

Chapter 7
DRAPING
(Answers to Questions on Page 42)
1. Protection of the patron.
2. a) To provide for patron's comfort. b) To protect patron's clothing from damage. c) To protect patron from injury. d) To provide competent, professional services.
3. Proper draping of the patron.
4. a) Seat patron comfortably. b) Select and arrange required materials and supplies. c) Wash and sanitize hands. d) Ask patron to remove all neck and hair jewelry, earrings, and glasses and place in her purse for safekeeping. e) Turn dress or blouse collar to the inside. f) Place neck strip or towel around patron's neck. g) Adjust cape over neck strip or towel. h) Fold neck strip or towel over cape neck band. i) Remove all hairpins and combs from hair.
5. It prevents the cape from coming into direct contact with the patron's skin.
6. The cape is used on many patrons, and it could be a carrier of disease or infection.
7. By draping a sanitized towel around the neck and over the cape to form a protective shield.
8. In draping for dry services, less emphasis is placed on the use of towels, with neck strips more commonly used.
9. The neck strip is used for sanitary as well as protective purposes.
10. The cape used for a comb-out is usually shorter and is fastened in the front to avoid interference with the back and nape comb-out. Comb-out capes do not have to be waterproof.

Chapter 8
SHAMPOOING AND RINSING
(Answers to Questions on Page 54)

Shampooing

1. Because a patron who is pleased with the way her hair has been shampooed will look favorably upon a recommendation for additional services.
2. It must remove all dirt, oils, cosmetics, and debris from the scalp and hair shaft without affecting the scalp or hair.
3. A shampoo with a high alkaline content.
4. To prevent oils and perspiration from mixing with scales and dirt and forming a breeding place for disease-producing bacteria.
5. Hair should be shampooed as often as necessary, depending on how quickly the hair and scalp become soiled.
6. Hard water or soft water.
7. The minerals it contains and its ability to lather freely.
8. Selecting and arranging required materials; draping patron properly; examining hair and scalp; and brushing hair.
9. Natural bristles have tiny imbrications which clean and add luster to the hair. Nylon bristles are shiny and smooth and are used primarily for hairstyling.
10. Brushing stimulates the blood circulation to the scalp, helps remove dust and dirt from the hair, and gives hair added sheen.
11. a) Prior to a lightener; b) prior to a tint or toner; c) prior to a permanent wave; d) prior to a chemical hair relaxer; e) if scalp is irritated.
12. Wet the hair thoroughly with warm water. Work liquid shampoo into the hair to form a thick lather. Massage entire scalp. Rinse hair thoroughly. Repeat shampoo and rinse. Dry hair.
13. They are placed in their proper places.
14. Before and after the shampoo.
15. Plain shampoos, soapless oil shampoos, liquid cream shampoos, liquid dry shampoos, cream or paste shampoos, acid-balanced shampoos, anti-dandruff shampoos, and henna shampoos.
16. When the hair has been tinted or toned.
17. When the patron is prevented by illness from having a wet shampoo.

Rinses

1. Hair rinses consist of water alone or a mixture of water with a mild acid, coloring agent, or special ingredients.
2. Acid rinses.
3. Citric acid, tartaric acid, acetic acid, and lactic acid.
4. Acid rinses dissolve soap curds, separate the hair, and make the hair soft, pliable, and bright.
5. After a tint, lightener, or cold wave application.
6. It softens the hair, adds luster, and makes tangled hair easier to comb.
7. An acid-balanced rinse.
8. They usually last from one shampoo to the next.
9. It is used as a final rinse to give an auburn tinge to the hair.
10. Blonde, grey, or white hair.

Chapter 9
SCALP AND HAIR CARE
(Answers to Questions on Page 62)

1. To preserve the health and beauty of the hair and scalp.
2. Scalp manipulations stimulate the blood circulation to the scalp, relax and soothe nerves, stimulate the muscles and activity of the glands, render a tight scalp more flexible, and help maintain the growth and health of the hair.
3. Because the scalp and hair are vitally related. A healthy scalp contributes to the growth of healthy hair.
4. The cosmetologist treats only common and minor conditions.
5. If there are scalp abrasions or a scalp disorder present, or immediately prior to the application of a lightener, tint, toner, permanent wave, or a chemical hair relaxing treatment.
6. Hairbrushing removes dust and dirt, gives the hair added luster, and stimulates the blood circulation to the scalp.
7. Scalp massage should be given as a series of treatments, once a week for normal scalp and more frequently for scalp disorders.
8. Scalp treatments for normal hair and scalp keep the scalp and hair in a clean, healthy condition, and prevent baldness.
9. Dandruff may be caused by poor blood circulation to the scalp, improper diet, uncleanliness, and infection.
10. Over-activity of the sebaceous glands.
11. Hair tonics or lotions with alcoholic content may be applied only after the application of high-frequency current.
12. Dry hair can be softened quickly with a conditioning preparation containing cholesterol and related compounds applied directly on the hair shaft.
13. Alopecia is a condition of premature baldness or excessive hair loss.
14. Alopecia areata is a disorder causing baldness in spots.

Chapter 10
HAIR SHAPING
(Answers to Questions on Page 78)

1. A good hair shaping serves as the foundation for beautiful coiffures.
2. Hair shaping scissors, thinning shears, straight razor (with or without guards), combs, hair clippers.
3. Thinning the hair removes excess bulk without shortening the length of the hair.
4. If coarse hair is thinned too close to the scalp, the short, stubby ends could protrude through the top layer of hair.
5. Fine hair—½-1″ from scalp; medium hair—1-1½″ from scalp; coarse hair—1½-2″ from scalp.
6. At the nape of the neck (ear to ear); at the side of the head (above ears); around facial hairline; and in the hair part.
7. The cut ends would be seen in the finished hairstyle.
8. Thinning too much hair could prevent the development of the desired style.
9. Cutting the hair close to the nape and gradually longer toward the crown, without showing a definite line.
10. To clean the neckline.
11. In order to avoid pulling the hair and to prevent dulling the razor.
12. The bridge of the nose.
13. Combing the short hairs of a strand towards the scalp.
14. Thinning and tapering the hair at the same time with scissors.
15. Shortening the hair in a graduated effect.

Chapter 11
FINGER WAVING
(Answers to Questions on Page 84)

1. Finger waving is the art of shaping and directing the hair into waves and designs using the fingers, comb, waving lotion, and hairpins or clippies.
2. Because it teaches them the techniques of moving and directing hair. It also helps to develop dexterity, coordination, and finger strength.
3. Training in creating hairstyles and in molding hair to the curved surface of the head.
4. By proper draping with a clean towel and shampoo cape.
5. Naturally wavy hair and permanently waved hair.
6. It makes the hair pliable and keeps it in place during finger waving procedure.
7. By placing a net over the hair.
8. To protect the patron's forehead and ears from the intense heat of the hair dryer.

Chapter 12
HAIRSTYLING
(Answers to Questions on Page 129)

1. A cosmetologist must have a knowledge of basic hairstyling in order to keep up with the ever-changing fashions.
2. A cosmetologist must understand hair structure and the overall importance of hair shaping, permanent waving, hair straightening, thermal waving and curling, hair coloring, hair chemistry, and the action of hair conditioners.
3. The hair should be in good condition.
4. Removing tangles in a systematic manner prevents hair damage.
5. Sculpture curls.
6. The hair should be properly tapered and pin curls wound smoothly.
7. Naturally or permanently waved hair.
8. Base, stem, and circle.
9. The base is the stationary, or immovable, foundation of the curl, which is attached to the scalp.
10. The stem of a pin curl is located between the base and the first arc of the circle.
11. It gives the circle its direction, action, and mobility.
12. The pin curl circle governs the width and strength of the wave.
13. The stem.
14. No-stem, half-stem, and full-stem.
15. A no-stem curl is used when a strong, long-lasting curl is desired.
16. It gives the base of the curl a firm, immovable position, permitting only the curl to move.
17. The half-stem curl is used when the hairstyle requires some freedom of movement.
18. Movement occurs because the half-stem allows the circle to move away from its base.
19. The full-stem curl is used when the hairstyle requires a great deal of movement.
20. By using a full-stem curl.
21. The size of the curl.
22. To obtain an even, smooth wave and a uniform end curl.
23. For fine hair, when a fluffy comb-out is desired.
24. Forward curl—toward the face. Reverse curl—away from the face.
25. A shaping is a section of hair that has been molded into a design to serve as a base for a curl or wave pattern.
26. Forward and reverse.
27. The hair is directed in a circular motion, following the side hair part, downward and towards the face.
28. Square, triangular, rectangular, and arc (half moon or "C" shape).
29. The shape of the base has no effect upon the resulting curl.
30. To prevent splits or breaks in the finished hairstyle.
31. For even construction suitable for combing and brushing into curls or waves.
32. In the direction in which they are intended to be combed.
33. Ridge curls are pin curls placed behind the ridge of a shaping or finger wave when a loose wave is desired.
34. The skip wave is a combination finger wave and pin curl pattern, the pin curls being placed in alternate finger wave formations.
35. When wide, smooth-flowing vertical waves are desired.
36. The hair should be 3-5" in length.
37. Stand-up curl.
38. The cascade curl may be used to create a lift to the hairstyle.
39. Roller curls are used to create volume and/or indentation wherever needed in a hairstyle.
40. Stand-up curls are formed one at a time, while rollers can accommodate the equivalent of 2-4 stand-up curls at one time.
41. By making the base ¼" shorter than the roller.
42. End papers may be used for easier winding.
43. A barrel curl is used when there is insufficient room to place a roller.
44. Volume means lift in a hairstyle.
45. Indentation means valleys and hollowness in a hairstyle.
46. Volume is created by directing the hair up from the head, rolling the ends under, and then rolling the hair down to the scalp on its base.
47. Indentation is achieved by keeping hair close to the head level and rolling the hair over on the rollers.
48. The texture of the hair.
49. The shape of her head, her facial type, and the desired hairstyle.
50. They form a cushion or base for the top or covering hair.
51. Teasing, ratting, matting, and French lacing.
52. Ruffing.
53. Brush out curls. Place general wave. Accentuate and develop lines and style. Finish.
54. To hold the hair in place.
55. Shape of the entire head; characteristics of features; and body structure, posture, and poise.
56. The oval facial type.
57. To create the illusion of length.
58. Style the hair to create the illusion of width in the forehead and to minimize the width at the jawline.
59. Style the hair to create the illusion of width at the jawline and to minimize the width at the forehead.
60. The hair should be styled with a smooth, head-hugging napeline.
61. Cover the neck with soft waves or curls.

Chapter 13
THE CARE AND STYLING OF WIGS
(Answers to Questions on Page 148)

1. How wigs and hairpieces improve the patron's appearance; how wigs are made and fitted; how to select and style wigs; and how to clean and service wigs.

2. Fashion, necessity, and practicality.
3. Wigs can be made from human hair, synthetic or animal hair, and a blend of both.
4. By a simple match test. Human hair burns slowly and gives off a strong odor. Synthetic hair burns quickly and gives off little or no odor.
5. The quality of hair it contains; the way it is constructed; and how it is fitted to the patron's measurements.
6. Wigs may be constructed by hand or by machine.
7. Brush the hair down smoothly and pin it as flat and tight as possible.
8. To keep the wig in shape so that it will not stretch.
9. A canvas block.
10. Styrofoam block.
11. For better block control.
12. The wig may shrink when the cap is wetted (if the cap is made of cotton).
13. The wig is stretched by turning wig inside out, wetting foundation with hot water, and pinning wig carefully to a larger block.
14. Tucks are used.
15. So that the hair will stand away from the wig in the comb-out.
16. A wig should be dry-cleaned every 2-4 weeks, depending on how often it is worn and when it is ready for restyling.
17. Cover block with plastic cover to protect canvas.
18. Switches are long wefts of hair mounted with a loop at the end.
19. Wiglets are hairpieces with flat bases which are used in special areas of the head.
20. Bandeau type is a hairpiece that is sewn to a headband.

Chapter 14
PERMANENT WAVING
(Answers to Questions on Page 179)

1. Relatively inexpensive, much faster, and more comfortable for patron.
2. Physical and chemical.
3. The two types of permanent waving solution are processing solution and neutralizer (fixative).
4. It breaks the chemical cross-bonds and thus softens the hair.
5. The neutralizer.
6. It stops the action of the waving lotion and re-forms the physical and chemical cross-bonds in the cortical layer.
7. A correct analysis of the patron's scalp and hair condition.
8. Scalp condition, hair porosity, hair texture, hair elasticity, hair density, and hair length.
9. The texture and porosity of the hair.
10. Elasticity is the ability of the hair to stretch and contract. Without elasticity there will be no curl in the hair.
11. Thick hair requires smaller blockings and larger rods, while thin hair requires smaller blockings and smaller rods.
12. Shampoo is given with an acid-balanced or mild shampoo.
13. In rinsing the hair, make sure that all the shampoo has been removed. A residue of shampoo could destroy the effectiveness of the waving lotion.
14. Proper rinsing helps to equalize the porosity of the hair.

15. The condition of the patron's hair.
16. A conditioner is used to replace the natural oils removed by the permanent wave lotion.
17. An extra mild waving lotion.
18. The size of the blockings is determined by the diameter of the rods.
19. Elasticity and texture.
20. The size of the rods and blockings.
21. Hair wrapped smoothly and without tension permits better penetration of the waving lotion, which causes the hair to expand and form uniform waves with strong ridges.
22. Tight wrapping or stretching interferes with the expansion of the hair, prevents penetration of solutions, and could cause hair breakage.
23. Test curls help to determine in advance how the patron's hair will react to the cold waving process.
24. Immediately after the last rod is secured, following the re-wet application of lotion, and frequently thereafter, every 30 seconds.
25. To protect the patron's skin and scalp against chemical injury.
26. Absorb the waving lotion with cotton pledgets saturated with cold water or neutralizer.
27. Apply the lotion on top of a section and comb through from underneath with an upward motion.
28. When the wave forms a well defined letter "S."
29. Weak or fine hair.
30. It is very curly when wet, completely frizzy when dry, and refuses to be combed into a suitable wave pattern.
31. a) Acid-Balanced—4.5 to 6.5. b) Neutral—7.0 to 7.9.
32. The permanent waving techniques are substantially the same. The only difference is in the styling patterns. Men do not want end curls.
33. Men may want a permanent wave to maintain proper hair control.
34. It relieves the salon owner to some extent from responsibility for accidents or damage.
35. It contains all essential information and eliminates guesswork.
36. To relax an over-curly permanent, carefully comb cold waving lotion through the hair to widen and loosen the wave. When sufficiently relaxed, the hair is rinsed, towel blotted and neutralized.

Chapter 15
HAIR COLORING
(Answers to Questions on Page 219)
Hair Coloring

1. Hair tinting is both the science and the art of changing the color of hair.
2. a) To restore grey hair to its natural color; b) to change the natural shade of hair to a more attractive color; c) to restore hair to its natural color; d) to create decorative effects.
3. a) The general structure of the hair and scalp; b) the proper selection and application of hair tints and lighteners; c) chemical reactions to tints and lighteners.
4. Temporary, semi-permanent, and permanent.
5. Color rinses contain certified colors and remain on the hair until the next shampoo.
6. Semi-permanent hair coloring is a tint that is formulated to last 4-6 weeks.
7. Aniline derivative tints.

8. Pure vegetable tints (henna); metallic or mineral dyes; and compound dyes.
9. Metallic dyes and compound dyes.
10. Aniline derivative tints.
11. The coloring penetrates through the cuticle into the cortex of the hair and cannot be washed out.
12. To determine whether the patron is allergic to the tint; because it is required by the U.S. Federal Food, Drug and Cosmetic Act.
13. Behind the ear or on the inner fold of the elbow.
14. The patron's skin tone and the color that suits the patron's age group.
15. A strand test determines whether the proper color was selected, the condition of the patron's hair, and the correct processing time.
16. a) Positive results of patch test; b) scalp irritations or eruptions; c) contagious scalp or hair disorders; and d) presence of metallic or compound dyes.
17. Soft water.
18. One-step tints.
19. One-process and single-application tints.
20. Hair that has neither been lightened nor tinted.
21. New growth only.
22. To cleanse the hair and highlight its natural color in a single application.
23. If the patron's hair is resistant.

Hair Lightening

1. Hair lightening is the partial or total removal of the natural pigment or artificial color from the hair.
2. If the patron wishes a drastic color change and when a toner is to be used.
3. Two-process and double-application tints.
4. The application of a toner or tint.
5. The hair becomes more porous during the lightening treatment.
6. Oil lighteners, cream lighteners, and powder (paste) lighteners.
7. They are easy to apply and will not run, drip, or dry out.
8. To speed the liberation of the oxygen gas.
9. 6% solution (20 volume strength).
10. The hydrogen peroxide solution softens the cuticle of the hair shaft and lightens the shade of the coloring pigment in the cortical layer.
11. It makes the hair porous and lighter in color.
12. Hydrogen peroxide softens the cuticle and makes it more receptive to the pentrating action of the aniline derivative tint.
13. Hydrogen peroxide acts as a developer by liberating oxygen gas, which changes para-phenylene-diamine into a dark-colored compound capable of tinting the hair.
14. Toners are aniline derivative tints which consist of pale or delicate colors.
15. They are aniline derivative tints and are a permanent, penetrating type of hair coloring.
16. To make the hair porous enough to receive the toner.
17. To new growth only.
18. Frosting—strand of hair lightened in various parts of head; tipping—wisps of hair lightened in various areas; and streaking—lightened strand, usually at front hairline.
19. Any seven of the following: over-porous; dry and brittle; breaks easily; no elasticity; rough and harsh to the touch; over-lightened; rejects color; and absorbs too much color.

20. Fillers are used to revitalize, recondition and correct abused, lightened, tinted, or damaged hair.
21. Conditioner fillers and color fillers.
22. To recondition lightened, tinted, or damaged hair before beauty salon services.
23. If the hair is in a damaged condition; and if there is any doubt that the finished color will be an even shade.
24. To match the same basic shade as the toner or tint to be used.
25. To correct a previous tinting, or to apply a new shade.
26. As an individual problem.
27. A dye that deposits a coating of the color substance over the hair shaft. It does not penetrate into the hair shaft.
28. Check natural shade of hair next to scalp. Select an appropriate shade of filler. Take two or more strand tests.
29. An aniline derivative tint.

Chapter 16
CHEMICAL HAIR RELAXING AND CHEMICAL BLOWOUT
(Answers to Questions on Page 235)

1. Chemical hair relaxing is the process of permanently rearranging the basic structure of over-curly hair into a straight form.
2. Sodium hydroxide and ammonium thioglycolate.
3. Ammonium thioglycolate requires pre-shampooing. Sodium hydroxide does not require pre-shampooing.
4. It has a softening· and swelling action on the hair fibers.
5. 8 minutes. After 8 minutes the hair may turn a reddish color or it may become brittle and break. After 10 minutes the hair may dissolve.
6. The neutralizer.
7. Stabilizer or fixative.
8. The protective base is designed to protect the patron's skin and scalp during a sodium hydroxide chemical straightening process.
9. Hair that has had a recent tinting, lightening, thermal comb or thermal irons treatment, and also hair that has been treated with a metallic dye.
10. It is important that the cosmetologist know the quality of the hair.
11. Texture, porosity, elasticity, and the extent, if any, of damage to the hair.
12. The patron's record card is important to assure consistent satisfactory results.
13. The signed release card is designed to protect the cosmetologist to some extent from responsibility for accidents or damages.
14. Because a chemical hair relaxing treatment should not be given if scalp eruptions, scratches, or abrasions are present.
15. Strand test.
16. A strand test determines the results to be expected.
17. A strand test should be given on either the crown area or any other area where the hair is wiry and resistant.
18. The hair must be rapidly and thoroughly rinsed to remove all the relaxer, because if it is left in the hair it continues to process.
19. The stream of water should be directed from the scalp to the hair ends.

20. A non-alkaline or cream shampoo.
21. Because the hair is very fragile at this point and tangled ends can easily be broken.
22. It helps to keep the hair in a relaxed state.
23. After the hair has been saturated with neutralizer.
24. To avoid hair breakage.
25. To offset the harshness of the sodium hydroxide in the relaxer, and to help restore some of the natural oils to the scalp and hair.
26. Because of the fragile condition of the hair.
27. The same as for a regular chemical hair relaxing treatment, except that the relaxer is applied only to the new growth.
28. By a three-step rinsing process. 1) 50% of the re- laxer is rinsed out with warm water. 2) Comb hair smooth and straight for five minutes. 3) Rinse re- maining relaxer from head.
29. The chemical blowout is a combination of chemical hair straightening and hairstyling.
30. In a chemical blowout only a small amount of the curl is removed from the hair, leaving it manageable for styling. In a regular hair straightening service, all the curl is removed.
31. Not to over-relax the hair to the point where the blowout process becomes impossible to perform.
32. The hair is shampooed before the application of the thio.

Chapter 17
THERMAL HAIR STRAIGHTENING
(HAIR PRESSING)
(Answers to Questions on Page 244)

1. Over-curly hair is temporarily straightened.
2. A soft press is accomplished with a thermal pressing comb.
3. A hard press is accomplished with thermal irons over the comb press. It also may be accomplished by a double comb press.
4. Cuticle, cortex, and medulla.
5. Wiry, curly hair.
6. Hair that has been abused by lightening and tinting services.
7. If the patron has a scalp abrasion, a contagious scalp condition, or a scalp injury.
8. a) Form of hair; b) texture of hair; c) elasticity of hair; d) condition of hair; e) length of hair; f) feel of hair; g) shade of hair; h) and condition of scalp.
9. Conditioning treatments require the application of special cosmetic preparations to the hair and scalp; thorough brushing; and scalp massage.
10. Soft pressing requires pressing comb, heating ap- pliance, pressing oil, hair brush and comb, brillian- tine or pomade, shampoo, towels and cape, spatula, neck strips, and thermal irons.
11. Apply pressing oil to hair. Divide into four main sections. Subdivide hair into small sections. Test temperature of heated comb. Press hair with press- ing comb.
12. Apply brilliantine or pomade to the hair near the scalp, and brush it through the hair. Comb and style the patron's hair. Place supplies in their proper places.
13. Burning of the hair, skin or scalp; and hair breakage.
14. Immediately apply 1% gentian violet jelly to the burn.

Chapter 18
THERMAL WAVING, CURLING
AND BLOW-DRY STYLING
(Answers to Questions on Page 265)

Thermal Waving and Curling
1. Thermal waving and curling is the art of waving and curling straight or pressed hair with thermal irons by using special manipulative techniques.
2. a) Conventional (regular) stove heated; b) electric self-heated; and c) electric self-heated (vaporizing).
3. Because the moisture from the irons could cause the hair to revert to its natural over-curly form.
4. The rod and the shell.
5. Lukewarm.
6. The temperature of the irons is tested on a piece of tissue paper.
7. In a position that is comfortable and permits com- plete control.
8. Combs made of hard rubber or another non-flam- mable substance and should have fine teeth.
9. Spiral curls are hanging curls.
10. They are used to give a finished appearance to hair ends.
11. They are used to create volume or lift in a finished hairstyle.
12. Metal combs become hot and burn the scalp.
13. The comb is placed between the scalp and thermal irons to protect scalp from burn.
14. Fish hooks occur when hair ends protrude over the heated irons.

Blow-Dry Styling
1. Blow-dry styling is basically the technique of drying and styling damp hair in one operation.
2. Blow-dry curling with a brush and blow-dry waving with a comb.
3. A blow dryer is an electrical device especially de- signed for drying and styling the hair in a single operation.
4. Both hard rubber combs and those made of metal.
5. Styling lotions, hair conditioners, and hair sprays.
6. The carefully planned hair shaping.
7. Tapered.
8. To avoid scalp burns.
9. It will not hold.

Chapter 19
MANICURING
(Answers to Questions on Page 290)

Manicuring
1. Manicuring is the care of the hands and nails.
2. Equipment and implements.
3. Cosmetics and materials.
4. Any five of the following: orangewood stick, nail file, cuticle pusher, cuticle nippers, nail brush, emery board, nail buffer, fine camel's hair brush, tweezers.
5. Nail polish remover, cuticle solvent, cuticle oil, cuti- cle cream, base coat, nail polish, and top coat.
6. With its application, the nail polish adheres readily to the nail surface.
7. It protects the polish and minimizes its chipping or cracking.
8. So that it will be ready for the next patron.
9. After seating patron and prior to giving the manicure.
10. To stop bleeding from a small cut.

11. Remove old polish. Shape nails. Soften cuticles. Dry fingertips. Apply cuticle remover. Loosen cuticles. Clean under free edges. Trim cuticles. Bleach under free edges. Apply cuticle oil or cream. Cleanse nails. Dry hands and nails thoroughly. Apply base coat. Apply liquid polish. Remove excess polish. Apply top coat. Apply hand lotion.
12. Filing with the growth of the nails avoids splitting.
13. Soap bath softens the cuticle.
14. It softens cuticle and helps to remove dead cuticle.
15. They should be sanitized and placed in a cabinet sanitizer.
16. To help prevent accidents and injury to the patron or manicurist.
17. Apply styptic powder or alum solution to stop the bleeding.
18. Oval, slender tapering (pointed), square or rectangular, and clubbed (round).
19. Oval.
20. The nail should be tapered somewhat longer than usual.
21. It should extend only slightly passed the tip of the finger with the nail tip rounded off.
22. It should be slightly tapered and extend just a bit past the tip of the finger.
23. It keeps the hands flexible, well-groomed, and smooth.
24. A manicure given with the aid of a portable device operated by a small motor.
25. It is beneficial for ridged and brittle nails and for dry cuticles.
26. A manicure given in a booth and not at the manicure table.
27. Capping of fragile tips; repairing of partially broken or split nails; and re-attaching tips that are broken off completely.
28. Nail wrapping is used to strengthen soft and fragile nails.
29. For women who cannot grow natural nails of the desired strength and length.
30. Not more than 48 hours.

Pedicuring
1. Pedicuring is the care of the feet, toes, and toenails.
2. Corns, callouses, ingrown nails, foot infections, and ringworm of the foot (athlete's foot).
3. It is an infectious condition which can be spread from one person to another.
4. Watery blisters, and thick, white skin between the toes.
5. To avoid ingrown nails, do not file into corners of nails.

Chapter 20
THE NAIL AND DISORDERS OF THE NAIL
(Answers to Questions on Page 297)
The Nail
1. A healthy nail is firm and flexible and appears to be slightly pink in color. Its surface is smooth, curved, and unspotted, without any hollows or wavy ridges.
2. Nails are horny, translucent plates.
3. To protect the tips of the fingers and toes.
4. Onyx.
5. A nail is composed mainly of keratin, a protein substance.
6. The nail plate seems to be one piece, but actually it is constructed in layers.
7. a) The nail root is located at the base of the nail, embedded underneath the skin. b) The nail body is the visible portion of the nail that rests upon, and is attached to, the nail bed. c) The free edge is the end portion of the nail plate that reaches over the fingertip. d) The nail bed is the portion of the skin upon which the nail body rests.
8. The matrix.
9. Poor health, if a nail disorder or disease is present, or if there is an injury to the nail matrix.
10. In the matrix.
11. From the matrix, which contains nerves, lymph, and blood vessels.
12. At the base of the nail.
13. The light color of the lunula may be due to the reflection of light where the matrix and the connective tissue of the nail bed join.
14. Eponychium is the extension of the cuticle at the base of the nail body that partly overlaps the lunula.
15. a) Cuticle is the overlapping epidermis around the nail. b) Mantle is the deep fold of skin in which the nail root is embedded. c) Nail grooves are slits or tracks on the sides of the nail upon which the nail moves as it grows.
16. Hyponychium is that portion of the epidermis under the free edge of the nail.
17. Perionychium is that portion of the cuticle surrounding the entire nail border.
18. Nutrition and health.
19. The nail grows forward, starting at the matrix and extending over the tip of the finger.
20. 1/8″ per month.
21. It will be replaced only as long as the matrix remains in good condition.

Nail Disorders
1. No. The patron should be referred to a doctor.
2. Uneven growth of the nails, usually the result of illness or injury.
3. a) 4, b) 5, c) 3, d) 2, e) 1.
4. Corrugations, furrows, white spots, hypertrophy, atrophy, pterygium, bitten nails, brittle nails, hangnails, eggshell nails, blue nails, bruised nails.
5. Onychorrhexis.
6. Oil manicures.
7. Hangnail is a condition in which the cuticle splits around the nail. Dryness of the cuticle, cutting off too much cuticle, or carelessness in removing the cuticle may cause hangnails.
8. With proper nail care, such as hot oil manicures.
9. An antiseptic is applied immediately.
10. Onychosis is the technical term for any nail disease.
11. A vegetable parasite.
12. A vegetable parasite.
13. Deep, itchy, colorless vesicles appear.
14. A bacterial infection.
15. Onychia is an inflammation of the nail matrix, accompanied by pus formation.
16. Paronychia is identified by an inflammatory condition of the tissues surrounding the toenails.
17. Onychia.
18. Onychocryptosis.
19. a) 3. b) 1. c) 2.

Chapter 21
THEORY OF MASSAGE
(Answers to Questions on Page 304)
1. Massage is used to exercise facial muscles, maintain muscle tones, and stimulate circulation.

2. Massage is the application of external manipulations to the head and body.
3. Therapeutic lamps, high-frequency current, facial steamers, scalp steamers, heating caps, and vibrators.
4. Heart condition; high blood pressure; inflamed and swollen joints; or glandular swelling.
5. Strong, flexible hands; a quiet temperament; and self-control.
6. a) Effleurage—stroking movement; b) petrissage—kneading movement; c) friction—deep rubbing movement; d) percussion or tapotement—tapping, slapping and hacking movements; e) vibration—shaking movement.
7. The fixed attachment of one end of the muscle to a bone or tissue.
8. The attachment of the opposite end of the muscle (opposite to the origin) to another muscle or to a movable bone or joint.
9. Massaging always should be from the insertion toward the origin of a muscle.
10. Massaging the muscle in the wrong direction may result in the loss of resiliency and the sagging of the skin and muscles.
11. Effleurage movements, which are soft, light, slow, and in rhythmic manner.
12. a) Chucking—grasping the flesh firmly in one hand and moving the hand up and down along the bone. The other hand keeps the arm or leg steady. b) Rolling—compressing the tissues firmly against the bone and twisting around the arm or leg. Both hands twist the flesh in the same direction. c) Wringing—the hands are placed on the sides of the arm or leg a little distance apart. While both hands are working downward, the flesh is twisted against the bone in opposite directions.
13. a) The skin and all its structures are nourished. b) Muscle fibers are stimulated and strengthened. c) Fat cells are reduced. d) Blood circulation is increased. e) Nerves are soothed and rested. f) Pain is sometimes relieved.
14. Weekly.

Chapter 22
FACIALS
(Answers to Questions on Page 318)

1. Improvement in the patron's skin tone, texture, and appearance.
2. Skin diseases.
3. Preservative and corrective.
4. By using correct cleansing methods, increasing circulation, relaxing the nerves, and activating the skin glands and metabolism through massage.
5. Dryness, oiliness, blackheads, aging lines, and minor conditions of acne.
6. Any six of the following: a) Cleanse the skin. b) Increase circulation. c) Activate glandular activity. d) Relax the nerves. e) Maintain muscle tone. f) Strengthen weak muscle tissue. g) Correct certain skin disorders. h) Help prevent formation of wrinkles and aging lines. i) Soften and improve skin texture and complexion. Give a youthful feeling to skin.
7. Once a week.
8. To protect the patron's hair.
9. a) To determine if the skin is dry; b) if the skin is oily; c) if comedones or acne are present; d) if broken capillaries are visible; e) if the skin texture is soft or

harsh and rough; and f) the skin's color and fine lines.
10. a) Choice of cream to use; b) amount of pressure to use; c) areas that need extra attention; d) if special lubricating oil is needed around the eyes and/or throat; e) type of astringent to use; and f) color of makeup to apply.
11. A spatula.
12. With an even tempo or rhythm.
13. Origin of the muscle.
14. Insufficient flow of sebum (oil) from the sebaceous glands.
15. Lotions with a large percentage of alcohol.
16. Hardened masses of sebum formed in the ducts of the sebaceous glands.
17. By applying an astringent lotion.
18. a) Reducing the oiliness of the skin by local applications; b) removing blackheads with a sanitized comedone extractor; c) cleansing the skin; d) using special medicated pre-preparations; and e) suggesting a regulated diet.
19. Packs are recommended for normal and oily skin.
20. Masks are recommended for dry skin.
21. a) Bleach pack—to reduce visibility of freckles. b) Clay pack—for normal or oily skin. c) Lemon pack—for normal or oily skin. d) Egg pack—to cleanse pores and tighten skin.
22. For dry skin and for skin inclined to wrinkle.

Chapter 23
FACIAL MAKEUP
(Answers to Questions on Page 339)
Facial Makeup

1. Makeup is applied to the face for the purpose of improving its appearance. The main objective is to emphasize good facial features and minimize defects.
2. Proper application of foundation creates a pleasing facial contour. Evens out skin color. Provides a base for color harmony. Conceals minor imperfections. Protects the skin against soil, wind, and weather.
3. It makes the face look pale and artificial.
4. Cream, liquid (lotion), and cake.
5. a) Cake foundation. b) Cream foundation.
6. Stick foundation and blemish masking cream.
7. a) Conceal skin blemishes. b) Tone down excessive coloring, gloss, or shine. c) Enhance the natural skin coloring. d) Makes skin soft and velvety to the touch.
8. To give a soft glow of color to the face.
9. Liquid, cream, dry (compact), and brush-on (powdered).
10. a) Liquid cheek color blends well and is suitable for all skin types. b) Cream cheek color is preferred for dry and normal skin. c) Dry (compact) cheek color blends harmoniously with the facial makeup. d) Brush-on (powdered) cheek color is easy to use.
11. It adds color to the lips and helps correct the shape of the mouth.
12. Blue-red, yellow-red, orange, and true red.
13. To the eyelids, close to the lashes.
14. a) Eye shadow is applied to upper lids. b) Mascara is applied to eyelashes and eyebrows. c) Eyebrow pencil is applied to eyebrows.
15. a) Eye shadow complements the eyes by making them look brighter and more expressive. b) Mascara makes the eyelashes appear fuller and longer. c) Eyebrow pencil darkens and fills in the eyebrows and corrects misshapen brows.

Eyebrow Arching

1. Correctly shaped eyebrows have a marked effect on the beauty and contour of the face.
2. Stretch the skin taut with the index finger and thumb of left hand. Grasp each hair individually with tweezers and pull with a quick motion in the direction in which the hair grows.
3. To avoid infection.
4. To contract the skin.
5. About once a week.
6. With hair-like strokes of an eyebrow pencil.

Chapter 24
FALSE EYELASHES
(Answers to Questions on Page 348)

1. Strip eyelashes and semi-permanent individual eyelashes.
2. They are made with a permanent curl and do not react to changes in weather conditions.
3. Eye tabbing.
4. About 6-8 weeks.
5. Wearers can participate in all normal activities with the same freedom as with natural eyelashes.
6. Because some women may be allergic to the adhesive being used.
7. They are used on the lower lashes or in combination with others to achieve special effects.
8. Oily eyelashes present a problem because the oil dissolves the adhesive and the lashes fall off.
9. Apply more adhesive over entire length of natural eyelash. Hold false eyelash in place several additional seconds to permit the adhesive to dry.
10. By a special procedure. The false lash is applied to both top and bottom of the natural lash. The false lashes are angled inward slightly to fill in all the gaps. A second set of eyelashes is cemented on top of the first set, also angled inward slightly to completely fill in the gaps.
11. Since the false lash is firmly cemented to the natural lash, by pulling out the false lash you also will pull out the natural lash.

Chapter 25
SUPERFLUOUS HAIR REMOVAL
(Answers to Questions on Page 356)

1. Permanent and temporary.
2. Electrolysis is the process of removing hair permanently by means of electricity.
3. Thermolysis, diathermy, and high-frequency.
4. By the rapid shut off of current.
5. All areas of the body may be treated by electrolysis, except the eyelids, insides of ears, nostrils, and moles.
6. Heredity, more common in certain races, and glandular disturbances.
7. The galvanic method and the shortwave method.
8. The galvanic method destroys the hair by decomposing the papilla. The shortwave method destroys the hair by coagulating the papilla through the use of heat.
9. The shortwave method.
10. The coarseness of the hair.
11. 15-90°.
12. Shaving, tweezing, and depilatories.
13. For shaping the eyebrows and for removing superfluous hairs from around the mouth and chin.
14. Physical (wax) and chemical.
15. Cheeks, chin, upper lip, nape area, arms, legs.

16. a) To prevent burns, test temperature of wax. b) Keep wax from running into the patron's eyes or other unwanted areas. c) Do not use wax under the arms, over warts, on moles, abrasions, and irritated or inflamed skin.
17. For those patrons who cannot tolerate heated wax.
18. Cream, paste, and powder.
19. Because some people may be sensitive to the action of the depilatory being used.

Chapter 26
CELLS
(Answers to Questions on Page 360)

1. Cells are the basic units of all living things.
2. Cells differ as to size, shape, structure, and function.
3. Protoplasm.
4. Nucleus and cytoplasm.
5. a) Nucleus—important to reproduction of the cell. b) Cytoplasm—contains food materials necessary for growth, reproduction, and self-repair.
6. The human cell reproduces by indirect division.
7. Metabolism is the chemical process whereby body cells are nourished and supplied with energy.
8. Anabolism and catabolism.
9. During anabolism, the cells absorb water, food, and oxygen for growth, reproduction, and repair.
10. During catabolism, the cells consume what they have absorbed in order to perform their special functions, such as muscular effort, secretions, or digestion.
11. Tissues are composed of groups of cells of the same kind.
12. Connective, muscular, nerve, epithelial, and liquid tissues.
13. An organ is a structure containing two or more tissues that are combined to accomplish a specific function.
14. The heart.
15. The lungs.
16. Systems are groups of organs that cooperate for a common purpose.
17. Skeletal, muscular, nervous, circulatory, endocrine, excretory, respiratory, digestive, and reproductive systems.
18. The skeletal system.
19. The muscular system.
20. The nervous system.
21. The circulatory system.

Chapter 27
THE SKIN AND DISORDERS OF THE SKIN
(Answers to Questions on Page 373)
The Skin

1. A healthy skin is slightly moist; soft and flexible; possesses a slightly acid reaction; and is free from any disorder or disease.
2. A good complexion is an indication of the fine texture and healthy color of the skin.
3. Epidermis and dermis.
4. The epidermis is the outermost layer of the skin. Its main function is to form a protective covering of the body.
5. Stratum corneum (horny layer); stratum lucidum (clear layer); stratum granulosum (granular layer); and stratum germinativum.
6. Stratum corneum.
7. Stratum lucidum.
8. Stratum granulosum.
9. Stratum germinativum.

10. It is a highly sensitive and vascular layer of connective tissue.
11. Papillary and reticular.
12. Papillae and tactile corpuscles.
13. Fat cells; blood vessels; lymph vessels; oil glands; sweat glands; hair follicles; and arrector pili muscles.
14. It gives smoothness and contour to the body; contains fat for use as energy; and acts as a protective cushion to the outer skin.
15. Through a network of arteries and lymphatics.
16. Motor, sensory, and secretory nerve fibers.
17. To arrector pili muscles.
18. The sensory nerves of the skin react to heat, cold, touch, pressure, and pain.
19. Secretory nerve fibers.
20. The fingertips.
21. The elasticity of the skin. The ability of the skin to stretch and immediately regain its former shape when released.
22. Aging skin loses its elasticity.
23. The color of the skin depends on the blood supply to the skin and primarily on the melanin, the coloring matter.
24. In the stratum germinativum and in the papillary layer of the dermis.
25. This is an hereditary trait and varies among races and nationalities.
26. Sudoriferous (sweat) glands and sebaceous (oil) glands.
27. The sweat glands consist of a coiled base and a tube-like duct that terminates at the skin surface to form a sweat pore.
28. Sweat glands are found all over the body, but are more numerous on the palms, soles, forehead, and in the armpits.
29. The sweat glands regulate body temperature and help to eliminate waste products from the body.
30. Their activity is increased by heat, exercise, emotions, and certain drugs.
31. The sweat glands.
32. Oil glands consist of little sacs whose ducts open into the hair follicles.
33. Sebum, an oily substance.
34. Oil glands lubricate the skin and preserve the softness of the hair.
35. Oil glands are found in all parts of the body, with the exception of the palms and soles.
36. Protection, sensation, heat regulation, excretion, secretion, and absorption.
37. 98.6° Fahrenheit.
38. Female hormones, when an ingredient of a face cream may enter the body through the skin.
39. Hair, nails, sweat glands, and oil glands.

Disorders of the Skin

1. There are only few disorders of the skin or scalp that logically come within the province of the cosmetologist.
2. Refer the patron to a physician.
3. To safeguard her own health as well as the health of the public.
4. Dermatology is the study of the skin, its nature, structure, functions, diseases, and treatment.
5. A dermatologist is a skin specialist.
6. A lesion is a structural change in the tissues caused by injury or disease.
7. An objective lesion is one that can be seen, such as pimples, pustules, and inflammations. A subjective lesion is one that can be felt, such as itching, burning, and pain.
8. Macule, papule, wheal, tubercle, tumor, vesicle, bulla, and pustule.
9. Scale, crust, excoriation, fissure, ulcer, scar, and stain.
10. Disease is any departure from a normal state of health.
11. a) Comedones—blackheads; b) milia—whiteheads.
12. When the hair follicle fills up with an excess of oil from the sebaceous gland, a blackhead forms and creates a blockage at the mouth of the follicle.
13. Acne is a chronic inflammatory disorder of the sebaceous (oil) glands.
14. Milia, acne, comedones, and seborrhea.
15. a) Bromidrosis—foul smelling perspiration; b) anidrosis—lack of perspiration; c) hyperidrosis—excessive perspiration; and d) miliaria rubra—an acute inflammatory disorder of the sweat glands.
16. Dermatitis is an inflammatory condition of the skin.
17. Eczema is an inflammation of the skin of acute or chronic nature.
18. Lesions that are round, dry patches covered with coarse, silvery scales.
19. On the scalp, elbows, knees, chest, and lower back.
20. Herpes simplex is a virus infection of unknown origin, commonly called fever blisters.
21. Lips, nostrils, or other parts of the face.
22. Dermatitis venanata is an eruptive skin infection caused by cold waving lotion or hair tinting (aniline derivatives).
23. Freckles (lentigines) are small yellow to brown colored spots caused by exposure to the sun.
24. Moth patches or liver spots.
25. Naevus is commonly known as a birthmark.
26. a) Leucoderma are abnormal white patches in the skin due to congenital defective pigmentation. b) Vitiligo is an acquired condition of leucoderma affecting the skin or hair.
27. Albinism is a congenital absence of melanin pigment in the body, including the skin, hair, and eyes.
28. Keratoma.
29. A mole is a small brownish spot or blemish on the skin.
30. Verruca.

Chapter 28
THE HAIR AND DISORDERS
OF THE HAIR AND SCALP
(Answers to Questions on Page 389)
Hair

1. Hair is a slender, thread-like outgrowth of the skin and scalp of the human body.
2. The study of hair is of paramount importance to cosmetologists because hair is what they primarily deal with.
3. The main purposes of hair are adornment and protection of the head from heat, cold, and injury.
4. Abuse of the hair by harmful cosmetic applications or faulty hair services can cause the hair structure to become weakened or damaged.
5. Keratin.
6. Hair root and hair shaft.
7. The hair root is that portion of the hair located beneath the skin surface.
8. The hair shaft is that portion of the hair structure extending above the skin surface.

9. Hair follicle is a tube-like depression, or pocket, in the skin that encases the hair root.
10. The direction of the natural flow of hair on the scalp.
11. Germs and dirt.
12. Hair bulb is a thickened, club-shaped structure forming the lower part of the hair root.
13. Hair papilla is a small cone-shaped elevation at the bottom of the hair follicle that fits into the hair bulb.
14. The papilla has a supply of rich blood and nerves. These contribute to the growth and regeneration of the hair. Through the papilla nourishment reaches the hair bulb. The papilla has the ability to produce hair cells.
15. Through the papilla.
16. Arrector pili muscle and sebaceous (oil) glands.
17. Fear or cold contracts the arrector pili muscle causing the hair to stand up straight.
18. The oil glands secrete an oily substance (sebum) which gives luster and pliability to the hair.
19. Diet; blood circulation; emotional disturbances; stimulation of endocrine glands; and drugs.
20. The shape, size, and direction of the hair follicle.
21. Straight, wavy, and curly or kinky.
22. Cuticle, cortex, and medulla.
23. The cuticle.
24. The cortex.
25. The medulla.
26. Palms, soles, lips, and eyelids.
27. Lanugo hair is the fine, soft, downy hair of the cheeks, forehead, and nearly all other areas of the body.
28. It helps in the efficient evaporation of perspiration.
29. Hair cycle is the growth, fall, and replacement of the hair.
30. About ½" per month.
31. a) Moisture in the air will deepen the natural wave. b) Cold air will cause hair to contract. c) Heat will cause hair to swell or expand and absorb moisture.
32. 50-80 hairs.
33. The bulb loosens and separates from the papilla. The bulb moves upward in the follicle. The hair moves slowly to the surface, where it is shed. The new hair is formed by cell division at the root of the hair around the papilla.
34. 2-4 years.
35. a) Blonde hair—140,000. b) Brown hair—110,000. c) Black hair—108,000. d) Red hair—90,000.
36. Melanin is the coloring matter or pigment in the hair.
37. Grey hair is caused by the absence of hair pigment in the corticle layer. In most cases, the hair greying is caused by age. It also can result from a serious illness or nervous shock.
38. An albino is a person born with white hair, the result of an absence of coloring matter in the hair shaft, accompanied by no marked pigment coloring in the skin or irises of the eyes.
39. a) A cowlick is a tuft of hair standing up. b) A whorl is hair that forms in a swirl effect.
40. Sight, touch, hearing, and smell.
41. Texture, porosity, elasticity, and condition of the hair.
42. Degree of coarseness or fineness of the hair.
43. Ability of hair to absorb moisture.
44. Ability of hair to stretch and return to its original form without breaking.
45. a) Dry hair can be stretched about one-fifth its length. b) Wet hair can be stretched from 40-50% of its length.

Disorders of the Scalp and Hair

1. Dandruff is recognized by small, white scales that usually appear on the scalp and hair.
2. The excessive shedding of the epithelial cells.
3. Poor circulation; infection; injury; lack of nerve stimulation; improper diet; uncleanliness.
4. a) Pityriasis. b) Pityriasis capitis simplex. c) Pityriasis steatoides.
5. Alopecia is the technical term for any abnormal form of hair loss.
6. No. When hair has grown to its full length, it comes out by itself and is replaced by a new hair.
7. In the spring and fall.
8. Alopecia senilis is a form of baldness occurring in old age.
9. Alopecia prematura is a form of baldness beginning any time before middle age with a slow thinning process.
10. Alopecia areata is the sudden falling out of hair in round patches or baldness in spots.
11. Ringworm.
12. It is caused by vegetable parasites.
13. It is commonly carried by scales or hairs containing fungi. Shower baths, swimming pools, and unsanitized articles also are sources of transmission.
14. Head louse. No.
15. A boil.
16. Canities.
17. Worry, anxiety, nervous strain, prolonged illness, various wasting diseases, and heredity.
18. Alternate bands of grey and dark hair.
19. a) Trichoptilosis is the technical name for split hair ends. b) Hypertrichoses means superfluous hair—an abnormal development of hair on areas of the body normally bearing only downy hair.
20. Hirsuties.
21. a) Trichorrhexis nodosa. b) Monilethrix.
22. Term used for hair that is split at any part of the hair length.

Chapter 29
ANATOMY
(Answers to Questions on Page 413)

1. Knowledge of the structure and functions of the human body forms the scientific basis for the proper application of cosmetic services.
2. Anatomy is the study of the organs and systems of the body.
3. The head, face, neck, arms, and hands.
4. Histology is the study of the minute structure of the various parts of the body.
5. The skin and its appendages.
6. Hair, nails, sweat glands, and oil glands.
7. Physiology is the study of the functions or activities performed by the various parts of the body.

THE SKELETAL SYSTEM
Bones of the Skull

1. Bone is the hardest structure of the body.
2. a) Give shape and strength to the body. b) Protect organs from injury. c) Serve as attachments for muscles. d) Act as levers for all bodily movements.
3. The skull is the skeleton of the head.
4. The skull is divided into two parts: the cranium and the skeleton of the face.
5. 8 bones.
6. Occipital; 2 parietal; frontal; and 2 temporal.
7. Forms the lower back part of the cranium.

8. The sides and top of head.
9. Frontal bone.
10. Temporal bones.
11. Sphenoid bone.
12. 14 bones.
13. 2 nasal; 2 zygomatic; 2 maxillae; and mandible.
14. The upper jaw.
15. The lower jaw.
16. Zygomatic bones.
17. Hyoid bone is located in the front part of the throat.
18. Cervical vertebrae form the top part of the spinal column and are located in the neck region.
19. Thorax.

Bones of the Shoulder, Arm, and Hand

1. Clavicle and scapula.
2. a) Upper arm—humerus. b) Forearm—ulna and radius.
3. a) Wrist—8. b) Palm—5. c) Fingers—14.
4. Carpus.
5. Metacarpus.
6. Digits.
7. Phalanges are the 3 bones in each finger and the 2 in each thumb.

THE MUSCULAR SYSTEM

1. Muscle is a contractile fibrous tissue on which the various movements of the body depend for their variety and action.
2. Muscles cover, shape, and support the skeleton and produce all body movements.
3. a) Voluntary, or striated. b) Involuntary, or non-striated. c) Cardiac, or heart.
4. Voluntary muscles, such as those of the face, arms, and legs, are controlled by the will. Involuntary muscles, such as those of the stomach and intestines, are not controlled by the will.
5. The skeletal and nervous systems.
6. a) Origin of the muscle refers to the more fixed attachment. b) Insertion of a muscle refers to the more movable attachment.
7. Chemicals; massage; electric current; light rays; heat rays; moist heat; and nerve impulses.

Muscles of the Head, Face, and Neck

1. The epicranius covers the top of the skull. The occipitalis is the back portion, and the frontalis is the front portion.
2. Frontalis raises the eyebrows, draws the scalp forward, and causes wrinkles across the forehead.
3. Orbicularis oculi.
4. Corrugator.
5. Procerus.
6. Orbicularis oris.
7. Platysma.
8. Trapezius.

Muscles of the Shoulder, Arm, and Hand

1. Deltoid, biceps, and triceps.
2. Pronators, supinators, flexors, and extensors.
3. The pronators turn the palm downward. The supinators turn the palm upward.
4. The flexor muscles bend the wrist, draw the hand up, and close the fingers toward the forearm. The extensor muscles straighten the wrist, hand, and fingers.

THE NERVOUS SYSTEM

1. a) To understand how to administer scalp and facial treatments for the patron's benefit. b) To understand what effects these treatments have on the nerves in the skin and scalp and on the body as a whole.
2. The brain, spinal cord, and their nerves.
3. The cerebro-spinal, the peripheral, and the sympathetic nervous systems.
4. Controls consciousness and all mental activities; controls the voluntary functions of the five senses; and controls the voluntary muscle actions.
5. The peripheral system is made up of sensory and motor nerve fibers that carry messages to and from the cerebro-spinal nervous system.
6. The main functions of the sympathetic nervous system are independent of the will. It controls internal body functions, such as breathing, circulation, digestion and glandular activity.
7. A neuron is the structural unit of the nervous system.
8. It is composed of a cell body and long and short fibers called cell processes.
9. Nerves are long white cords made up of fibers which carry messages to and from various parts of the body.
10. Sensory and motor nerves.
11. a) Sensory nerves—afferent nerves. b) Motor nerves—efferent neves.
12. Sensory nerves carry impulses or messages from sense organs to the brain regarding sensations of touch, heat, cold, sight, hearing, smell, taste, and pain.
13. Motor nerves carry impulses from the brain to the muscles which produce movement.
14. The quick removal of the hand away from a hot object.
15. There are 12 pairs of cranial nerves and 31 pairs of spinal nerves.
16. Worry; excessive mental work; and excessive muscular activity.
17. Chemicals; massage; electrical currents; light rays; heat rays; and moist heat.
18. The fifth, or trigeminal nerve; the seventh, or facial nerve; and the eleventh, or accessory nerve.

Nerves of the Head, Face, and Neck

1. The fifth cranial nerve.
2. It is the chief sensory nerve of the face and the motor nerve of the muscles of mastication.
3. The seventh cranial nerve.
4. a) Supra-orbital. b) Nasal. c) Infra-orbital. d) Mental. e) Auriculo-temporal. f) Zygomatic.
5. The scalp, as far up as the top of the head.
6. The spinal portion of the eleventh cranial nerve.
7. a) Temporal. b) Mandibular. c) Cervical. d) Posterior auricular. e) Buccal. f) Zygomatic.

Nerves of the Arm and Hand

1. The ulnar nerve supplies the little finger side of the arm and palm of the hand. The radial nerve supplies the thumb side of the arm and back of the hand. The median nerve with its branches supplies the arm and hand.
2. The digital nerve.

THE CIRCULATORY SYSTEM

1. Because the circulatory system is vitally related to the maintenance of good health.
2. It keeps the blood moving within the circulatory system.
3. Arteries, veins, and capillaries.
4. The arteries.
5. The smaller arteries and the veins.

6. They carry impure blood from the various capillaries back to the heart.
7. a) Pulmonary circulation. b) General circulation.
8. 98.6° Fahrenheit.
9. The blood is composed of two-thirds plasma, and one third red and white corpuscles, and blood platelets.
10. Blood plasma is composed of about 9/10ths water, and carries food and secretions to the cells and carbon dioxide from the cells.
11. Red blood cells carry oxygen to the cells.
12. White blood cells destroy disease-causing germs.
13. Lymph is a colorless, watery fluid circulating through the lymphatic system.
14. Lymph is derived from the blood plasma.
15. It carries nourishment from the blood to the cells and removes waste material from the cells.

Blood Vessels of the Head, Face, and Neck
1. Common carotid arteries.
2. Internal common carotid artery and external common carotid artery.
3. Internal branches of the common carotid arteries.
4. External branches of the common carotid arteries.
5. Facial artery.
6. Submental artery.
7. Frontal artery.
8. a) Superior labial artery. b) Inferior labial artery.
9. Parietal artery—the crown and side of the head. Frontal artery—forehead.
10. Frontal; parietal; transverse; middle temporal and anterior auricular.
11. The back of the head, up to the crown.
12. Posterior auricular artery.
13. Infra-orbital artery.
14. Internal jugular and external jugular.

Blood Circulation of Arm and Hand
1. Ulnar and radial arteries.
2. Ulnar artery.
3. Radial artery.

GLANDS AND OTHER SYSTEMS
1. Duct glands and ductless glands.
2. The kidneys; liver; skin; large intestine; and lungs.
3. With each cycle an exchange of gases takes place. During inhalation, oxygen is absorbed into the blood, while carbon dioxide is expelled during exhalation.
4. Mouth; pharynx; esophagus; stomach; and small intestine.

Chapter 30
ELECTRICITY AND LIGHT THERAPY
(Answers to Questions on Page 429)
Electricity
1. Electricity is a form of energy that produces magnetic, chemical, and heat effects when in motion.
2. A conductor is a substance that readily transmits an electric current.
3. Electrodes, composed of good conductors, serve as points of contact when applying electricity to the body.
4. A non-conductor, or insulator, is a substance that resists the passage of an electric current. Rubber, silk, dry wood, glass, cement, and asbestos.
5. Direct current (DC) is a constant and even-flowing current traveling in one direction.

6. Alternating current (AC) is a rapid and interrupted current flowing first in one direction and then in the opposite direction.
7. A converter.
8. A rectifier.
9. A volt is the unit of pressure that forces the current forward.
10. An ampere is the unit of current flow (strength).
11. An ohm is the unit of resistance to flow of current.

Galvanic Current
1. Galvanic current is a constant and direct current, whose action is chemical, having a positive and negative pole.
2. a) Acidic reaction. b) Alkaline reaction.
3. Soothes nerves; decreases blood supply; and hardens tissues.
4. Stimulates nerves; increases blood supply; and softens tissues.
5. The active electrode, applied by the cosmetologist, is connected to the particular pole whose action is desired. The inactive electrode, connected to the other pole, is held by the patron.

Faradic Current
1. a) Faradic current is an alternating and interrupted current whose action is mechanical. b) Muscular contractions.
2. The cosmetologist wears a wrist electrode with a moistened pad, while the patron holds a carbon electrode wrapped in damp absorbent cotton.
3. It should never be used if a) it causes pain or discomfort; b) if the face is very florid; c) if the patron has many gold filled teeth; d) if there are broken capillaries in the skin; e) if patron has high blood pressure; or f) if any pustular conditions of the skin exist.

Sinusoidal Current
1. Sinusoidal current is an alternating current that produces mechanical contractions in muscles.
2. Sinusoidal current supplies greater stimulation, deeper penetration, and less irritation than faradic current.
3. The cosmetologist wears a wrist electrode with a moistened pad, while the patron holds a carbon electrode wrapped in damp absorbent cotton.

High-Frequency Current
1. High-frequency current is characterized by a high rate of oscillation.
2. The Tesla current.
3. Tesla current is heat producing and may be either stimulating or soothing.
4. a) face—flat electrode; b) scalp—rake electrode.
5. About five minutes.
6. Direct surface application; indirect application; and general electrification.
7. The cosmetologist holds the electrode and applies it over the patron's skin.
8. The patron holds the metal or glass electrode while the cosmetologist uses her fingers to massage the surface being treated.
9. By holding a metal electrode in her hand, the patron's body is charged with electricity without being touched by the cosmetologist.
10. General electrification.
11. By lifting the electrode slightly from the area to be treated and applying the current through the clothing or a towel.

12. The high-frequency current must be applied first, and then the lotion.
13. a) Stimulates circulation of the blood. b) Increases glandular activity. c) Aids in elimination and absorption. d) Increases metabolism. e) Germicidal action occurs during use.
14. Falling hair; itchy scalp; tight scalp; excessively oily scalp; and excessively dry scalp.

Electrical Equipment

1. A vibrator is an electric appliance used in massage to produce a mechanical succession of manipulations.
2. It is used over heavy muscular tissue, such as the scalp, shoulders, and upper back. It may be used on a man's face.
3. The vibrator should not be used when there is a pronounced weakness of the heart, or in cases of fever, abscesses, or inflammation.
4. The steamer, or vaporizer, may be used instead of hot towels to cleanse and steam the face. The steamer also may be used for scalp and hair conditioning treatments.
5. It is used on the face to produce a moist, uniform heat. The steam warms the face, inducing the flow of both oil and sweat. It helps cleanse the skin, clean out the pores, and soften any scaliness on the surface of the skin.
6. It produces controlled moist heat; softens the scalp; increases perspiration; and promotes the effectiveness of applied scalp cosmetics.
7. Built-in heating elements that operate from electrical outlets.
8. Vapor conditions the hair as it curls.
9. The main use of heating caps are electrical devices which are applied over the head and provide a uniform source of heat.
10. Their main use is as part of corrective treatments for the hair and scalp.
11. They recondition dry, brittle, and damaged hair, and also serve to activate a sluggish scalp.
12. A processing machine reduces the processing time for lightening and tinting the hair.
13. The machine accelerates the molecular movement within the chemicals used so that they work much faster.

Light Therapy

1. Light therapy refers to treatment by means of light rays.
2. Ultra-violet rays and infra-red rays.
3. A therapeutic lamp is an electrical apparatus capable of producing certain light rays.
4. Glass bulb lamp, hot quartz lamp, and cold quartz lamp.
5. Glass bulb lamp and hot quartz lamp.
6. They produce changes in the chemistry of the blood and stimulate the activity of body cells.
7. Iron, vitamin D, and red and white blood cells.
8. They improve the blood and lymph flow; restore nutrition where needed; increase the elimination of waste products; and stimulate circulation.
9. The skin must be entirely clean because the slightest obstruction will keep the ultra-violet rays from reaching the skin.
10. About 12".
11. About 2-3 minutes.
12. About 7-8 minutes.
13. Both should wear eye goggles.

14. Skin tanning is the result of exposure to ultra-violet rays, which stimulate the production of pigment, a coloring matter in the skin.
15. Slight reddening of the skin, appearing several hours after application, without any signs of itching, peeling, or burning.
16. Over-exposure produces third and fourth degree burns which are destructive to the tissues.
17. Acne, tinea, seborrhea, and dandruff.
18. Ultra-violet rays stimulate growth of hair.
19. a) Heat and relax the skin without increasing body temperature. b) Dilate blood vessels in the skin, thereby increasing blood flow. c) Increase metabolism and chemical changes within skin tissues. d) Increase the production of perspiration and oil on the skin. e) Relieve pain.
20. About 30".
21. Place cotton pads saturated with boric acid solution or witch hazel over patron's eyelids.
22. To break constant exposure on body tissues.
23. Dome-shaped reflector mounted on a pedestal with a flexible neck.
24. To protect the eyes from the heat and glare of the light.
25. It relieves pain, especially in congested areas and nerve centers.
26. Blue light.
27. It has a tonic effect on the bare skin and a soothing effect on the nerves.
28. a) Stimulating effect when used over the skin. b) Its heat rays aid the penetration of cosmetic creams into the skin. c) It softens and relaxes the tissues.

Chapter 31
CHEMISTRY
(Answers to Questions on Page 460)

1. For an intelligent understanding of the various products and cosmetics being used in the beauty salon.
2. a) Water—H_2O. b) Hydrogen peroxide—H_2O_2.
3. Filtration and distillation.
4. Soft water.
5. Head and tail.
6. a) The tail attracts dirt, grease, debris, oil, etc. (it collects the dirt). b) The head loves water (it washes it out).
7. During rinsing the shampoo molecules are carried from the hair by the stream of water, taking with them the tails with the attached dirt.
8. It causes the cuticle of the hair to swell and the imbrications to open, allowing the solution to penetrate into the cortex.
9. Thio (thioglycolate), with a pH of 9.4-9.6, and sodium hydroxide, with a pH of 10-14.
10. The hair may dissolve.
11. They are composed of very small, colorless molecules.
12. The developer combines the small, colorless molecules into giant, colored molecules.
13. The large colored molecules cannot be shampooed from the hair because they are too large to pass through the imbrications.
14. a) Hair color pigments of the black to brown shades. b) Hair color pigments of the red to yellow shades.
15. A solute is a substance dissolved in a solution. A solvent is a liquid used to dissolve a substance.

Opening a Beauty Salon

1. A good location has a population large enough to support the salon. It should be located near other active business places that attract potential patrons.
2. People hesitate to patronize a salon that is inconvenient to reach, especially in bad weather. Bus facilities should be available for patrons who do not drive.
3. It is the first contact the patron has with the salon and sets the tone for the rest of the salon. It also can attract the attention of potential patrons passing the salon.
4. Advertising must attract and hold the reader's, listener's, or viewer's attention and create a desire for the services or merchandise offered by the salon.
5. a) Inexperience in dealing with employees and public. b) Not enough capital. c) Poor location and too high an overhead. d) Lack of proper basic training. e) Business neglect and careless bookkeeping methods.

Good Business Administration

1. The records system should be simple and efficient. It must be correct, concise, and complete.
2. a) Contribute to the efficient operation of the beauty salon. b) Determine income, expense, profit and loss. c) Prove the value of the salon to a prospective buyer. d) To arrange a bank loan. e) For government reports.
3. At least 6 months.
4. At least 7 years.
5. Consumption and retail supplies.
6. Individual, partnership, and corporation.

Using the Telephone in the Salon

1. Make or change appointments; go after new business; remind patrons of needed services; answer questions; adjust complaints; receive messages; and order equipment and supplies.
2. Phone as you would like to be phoned to.
3. a) Display an interested, helpful attitude. b) Be prompt in answering the phone. c) Give all necessary information to the caller. d) Be tactful.
4. Clear speech; correct speech; and pleasing tone of voice.
5. Plan her telephone conversation and list the main points on a pad so that she will know what to say.
6. They help make new friends; bring in more business; and create good-will for the salon.
7. The patron's complaint should be given careful consideration. Use self-control, tact, courtesy, and a sympathetic and reassuring tone of voice.
8. Build up more value in the patron's mind by pointing out benefits of receiving the better service offered by your salon.

Selling in the Beauty Salon

1. a) Be familiar with merits and benefits of service or product. b) Adapt approach and selling method to the needs and psychology of each patron. c) Be self-confident, but agreeable and productive. d) Stimulate attention, interest, and desire. e) Never misrepresent service or product. f) Use tact; avoid being rude or offensive. g) Apply appropriate sales technique. h) Don't be negative. i) Deliver sales talk in a relaxed, friendly manner. j) Recognize the right psychological moment to close the sale.

2. a) Shy; b) timid; c) talkative; d) nervous, e) irritable; f) inquisitive, g) over-cautious; h) conceited, "know it all;" i) teenager; j) old-timer.
3. Whether the patron has a need for the service or product.
4. Sincerity and honesty.
5. Simple and suggestive language that will make the patron feel like buying. The language should be positive, not negative. Use picture words and descriptive adjectives charged with feelings.
6. Beauty products should appeal to the eye through color and to the imagination through suggestion of feminine loveliness.
7. Every patron is a potential source of new patrons and additional beauty services.
8. Showing an actual treatment or application to patrons.
9. Stress quality and other advantages over cheaper substitutes.
10. a) Location of the product. b) Name and brand of product. c) Contents and price of product. d) Comparative merits of similar products that differ in price.

First Aid

1. As soon as possible after any accident has occurred.
2. An antiseptic, such as tincture of iodine, hydrogen peroxide, or mercurochrome, should be applied.
3. A general functional depression due to heat.
4. By loosening the collar and applying pads saturated with cool water to the face and back of the neck.
5. a) Standing behind patron, hit patron rapidly between the shoulder blades. b) Wrap your arms around patron's waist. Make a fist and place the thumb just below the breastbone. c) Hold your fist with your other hand and press it into patron's abdomen, using four quick upward thrusts. d) Repeat the procedure if necessary.